OFFICE OF MULTICULTURAL AFFAIRS
SCHOOL OF MEDICINE
UNIVERSITY OF WASHINGTON
BOX 357430
SEATTLE, WA 98195

MULTICULTURAL MEDICINE AND HEALTH DISPARITIES

► NOTICE

Medicine is an ever-changing science. As new research and clinical experience broaden our knowledge, changes in treatment and drug therapy are required. The authors and the publisher of this work have checked with sources believed to be reliable in their efforts to provide information that is complete and generally in accord with the standards accepted at the time of publication. However, in view of the possibility of human error changes in medical sciences, neither the editors nor the publisher nor any other party who has been involved in the preparation or publication of this work warrants that the information contained herein is in every respect accurate or complete, and they disclaim all responsibility for any errors or omissions or for the results obtained from use of the information contained in this work. Readers are encouraged to confirm the information contained herein with other sources. For example and in particular, readers are advised to check the product information sheet included in the package of each drug they plan to administer to be certain that the information contained in this work is accurate and that changes have not been made in the recommended dose or in the contraindications for administration. This recommendation is of particular importance in connection with new or infrequently used drugs.

MULTICULTURAL MEDICINE
AND
HEALTH DISPARITIES

DAVID SATCHER, MD, PhD

Director
National Center for Primary Care
Morehouse School of Medicine
Atlanta, Georgia

RUBENS J. PAMIES, MD, FACP

Vice Chancellor for Academic Affairs
Dean for Graduate Studies
Professor of Internal Medicine
University of Nebraska Medical Center
Omaha, Nebraska

CONTRIBUTING EDITOR

NANCY N. WOELFL, PhD

Professor and Director
McGoogan Library of Medicine
University of Nebraska Medical Center
Omaha, Nebraska

McGraw-Hill

MEDICAL PUBLISHING DIVISION

New York   Chicago   San Francisco   Lisbon
London   Madrid   Mexico City   Milan   New Delhi
San Juan   Seoul   Singapore   Sydney   Toronto

Multicultural Medicine and Health Disparities

1234567890   DOC DOC   098765

ISBN: 0-07-143680-4

This book was set in Garamond Light by TechBooks.
The editors were Jim Shanahan, Karen G. Edmonson, and Karen Davis
The production supervisor was Catherine H. Sagesse.
The copyeditor was Donna M. Frassetto.
The cover illustrator was Phoebe Beasley. "Slow Sojourn" (1987).
The cover designer was Aimeé Nordin.
The indexer was Andover Publishing Services.
RR Donnelley was printer and binder.

This book is printed on acid-free paper.

Library of Congress Cataloging-in-Publication Data
Multicultural medicine and health disparities / [edited by] David Satcher, Rubens J. Pamies.
    p.   cm.
Includes bibliographical references and index.
ISBN 0-07-143680-4
1. Transcultural medical care.   2. Ethnic groups—Health and hygiene.   3. Minorities—Health and hygiene.
4. Medicine—Cross-cultural studies.   5. Social medicine—Cross-cultural studies.   6. Health services accessibility—Cross-cultural studies.   I. Satcher, David, 1941–   II. Pamies, Rubens J.
    RA418.5.T73M855   2005
    362.1—dc22   2005052218

Contents

SECTION II

The Disparate Burden of Disease / 165

SECTION III

Issues in Health-Care Policy and Delivery   /   369

Contributors

TANYA R. ANDERSON, MD

Medical Director, Comprehensive Assessment and
  Treatment Unit for Adolescents
Assistant Professor of Psychiatry,
  Department of Psychiatry
University of Illinois at Chicago
Chicago, Illinois

CAROLYNE W. ARNOLD, ScD

Associate Professor of Health and Social Research
University of Massachusetts, Boston
Brookline, Massachusetts

HANI K. ATRASH, MD, MPH

Associate Director for Program Development
National Center on Birth Defects and
  Developmental Disabilities
Centers for Disease Control and Prevention
Atlanta, Georgia

SAMIR K. BALLAS, MD

Professor of Medicine and Pediatrics
Director, Blood Bank/Sickle Cell Center
Thomas Jefferson University
Cardeza Foundation for Hematologic Research
Philadelphia, Pennsylvania

CARL C. BELL, MD

President and CEO, Community Mental
  Health Council, Inc.
Professor of Psychiatry and Public Health
  Department of Psychiatry
University of Illinois at Chicago
Chicago, Illinois

WILLIAM J. BLOT, PhD

Professor of Medicine
Vanderbilt University
Nashville, Tennessee

CHRISTINE M. BRANCHE, PhD

Director, Division of Unintentional Injury
  Prevention
National Center for Injury Prevention and Control
Centers for Disease Control and Prevention
Atlanta, Georgia

OTIS W. BRAWLEY, MD

Professor of Hematology, Oncology, Medicine,
  and Epidemiology
Associate Director for Cancer Control,
  Winship Cancer Institute
Emory University
Atlanta, Georgia

NATHANIEL C. BRIGGS, MD, MSc

Assistant Professor, Preventive Medicine
Meharry Medical College
Nashville, Tennessee

LAWRENCE S. BROWN, JR, MD, MPH, FASAM

Senior Vice President, Division of Medical Services,
  Evaluation, and Research
Addiction Research and Treatment Corporation and
  Department of Public Health
Weill Medical College, Cornell University
Brooklyn, New York

JADA BUSSEY-JONES, MD

Assistant Professor of Medicine
Emory University School of Medicine
Atlanta, Georgia

CLIVE O. CALLENDER, MD

LaSalle D. Leffall, Professor and Chairman,
  Department of Surgery
Howard University Hospital
National Minority Organ Tissue Transplant Education
  Program (MOTTEP)
Washington, DC

JOHN CAPITMAN, PhD

Central Valley Health Policy Institute
California State University at Fresno
Fresno, California

ALICE HM CHEN, MD, MPH

Assistant Clinical Professor of Medicine
Division of General Internal Medicine
University of California at San Francisco
Medical Director, General Medicine Clinic
San Francisco General Hospital
San Francisco, California

JORDAN J. COHEN, MD

President
Association of American Medical Colleges
Washington, DC

LOIS COLBURN

Executive Director, Center for Continuing Education
University of Nebraska Medical Center
Omaha, Nebraska

COLLEEN CONWAY-WELCH, PhD, RN, FAAN

Dean, Nancy and Hilliard Travis Professor of Nursing
Vanderbilt University School of Nursing
Nashville, Tennessee

ALEX E. CROSBY, MD, MPH

Medical Epidemiologist, Division of Violence
  Prevention
National Center for Injury Prevention and Control
Centers for Disease Control and Prevention
Atlanta, Georgia

SAMUEL DAGOGO-JACK, MD, FRCP

Professor of Medicine
Department of Medicine and General Clinical
  Research
University of Tennessee Health Sciences Center
Memphis, Tennessee

EZRA C. DAVIDSON, JR, MD

Associate Dean, Primary Care
Professor, Obstetrics and Gynecology
Charles R. Drew University of Medicine and Science
David Geffen School of Medicine at UCLA
Los Angeles, California

JAMEHL L. DEMONS, MD

Assistant Professor
Section on Gerontology and Geriatric Medicine
Sticht Center on Aging and Rehabilitation
Wake Forest University School of Medicine
Winston-Salem, North Carolina

ROBERT S. DITTUS, MD, MPH

Albert and Bernard Wethan Professor of Medicine
Division of General Internal Medicine,
  Department of Medicine
GRECC, VA Tennessee Valley Health Care System
Vanderbilt University Medical Center
Nashville, Tennessee

HENRY W. DOVE, MD

Associate Professor of Clinical Psychiatry
Acting Head, Department of Psychiatry
Director, Residency Education
Associate Professor of Clinical Psychiatry
Department of Psychiatry
University of Illinois at Chicago
Chicago, Illinois

MARILYN DUBREE, MSN, RN

Associate Hospital Director, Patient Care Services
Chief Nursing Officer, Vanderbilt University Medical Center
Nashville, Tennessee

FRANCES J. DUNSTON, MD, MPH

Professor and Chairperson
Department of Pediatrics
Morehouse School of Medicine
Atlanta, Georgia

GEORGIA M. DUNSTON, PhD

Professor and Chair, Department of Microbiology
Founding Director, National Human Genome Center
Director, Molecular Genetics, NHGC
Howard University
Washington, DC

KATHI A. EARLES, MD, MPH

Assistant Clinical Professor
Department of Pediatrics
Morehouse School of Medicine
Atlanta, Georgia

MICHAEL D. FLOYD, MD, MSCI

Assistant Professor of Medicine
Meharry Medical College
Nashville, Tennessee

DANIEL J. FRANCE, PhD, MPH

Research Assistant Professor
Departments of Medicine and Anesthesiology
Vanderbilt University
Nashville, Tennessee

RANDOLPH FRASCH, PhD, RN

Professor of Nursing
Vanderbilt University School of Nursing
Nashville, Tennessee

JOHN S. FRIEDMAN, PhD

Addiction Research and Treatment
Brooklyn, New York

VANESSA NORTHINGTON GAMBLE, MD, PhD

Director, Tuskegee University National Center
  for Bioethics in Research and Health Care
106 Drew Hall
Tuskegee, AL 36088

JAMES R. GAVIN III, MD, PhD

President and Professor of Medicine
Morehouse School of Medicine
Atlanta, Georgia

ERIC P. GOOSBY, MD

Chief Executive Officer and Chief Medical Officer
Pangaea Global AIDS Foundation
San Francisco, California

MARK GRABER, MD

Associate Professor
Departments of Family Medicine and Emergency Medicine
Roy J and Lucille A Carver College of Medicine
University of Iowa
Iowa City, Iowa

DAVID GRANDISON, MD, PHD

Director, Clinical Research Center
Interim Chair, Department of Internal Medicine
Associate Professor of Medicine
Meharry Medical College
Nashville, Tennessee

CARMEN RENEE' GREEN, MD

Associate Professor, Department of Anesthesiology
University of Michigan Medical School
Ann Arbor, Michigan

KIMBERLY D. GREGORY, MD, MPH

Director, Division Maternal–Fetal Medicine
Director, Women's Health Services Research
Cedars Sinai Medical Center
Associate Professor in Residence
David Geffen School of Medicine at UCLA and
    UCLA School of Public Health
Los Angeles, California

MARGARET K. HARGREAVES, PHD

Associate Professor of Internal Medicine
Meharry Medical College
Nashville, Tennessee

CHARLES H. HENNEKENS, MD, DRPH

Visiting Professor of Medicine and Epidemiology
    and Public Health
University of Miami School of Medicine
Miami, Florida

GEORGE C. HILL, PHD

Professor, Department of Microbiology and Immunology
Vanderbilt University School of Medicine
Nashville, Tennessee

STEVEN H. HINRICHS, MD

Stokes-Shackleford Professor of Pathology
Director, University of Nebraska Center for Biosecurity
Director, Nebraska Public Health Laboratory
University of Nebraska Medical Center
Omaha, Nebraska

CAROL R. HOROWITZ, MD, MPH

Assistant Professor, Health Policy and Medicine
Mount Sinai School of Medicine
New York, New York

HANS HOUSE, MD

Assistant Professor and Residency Director
The Iowa Emergency Medicine Program
Roy J and Lucille A Carver College of Medicine
University of Iowa
Iowa City, Iowa

MELISSA D. HUNTER, MPH

Fellow, National Center on Birth Defects and
    Developmental Disabilities
Centers for Disease Control and Prevention
Atlanta, Georgia

BAQAR A. HUSAINI

Professor and Director, Center for Health Research
Tennessee State University
Nashville, Tennessee

SONJA S. HUTCHINS, MD, MPH, DRPH

National Immunization Program
Centers for Disease Control and Prevention
Atlanta, Georgia

SHARON JONES, MSN, RN

Instructor, Clinical Nursing
Vanderbilt University School of Nursing
Nashville, Tennessee

CHARLOTTE JONES-BURTON, MD

Fellow, Nephrology
Internal Medicine Division of Nephrology
University of Maryland School of Medicine
Baltimore, Maryland

ADAM M. KINGSTON, BA

Coordinator
University of Nebraska Center for Biosecurity
University of Nebraska Medical Center
Omaha, Nebraska

OLADIPO KUKOYL, MD

Departments of Family Medicine and Psychiatry
Roy J and Lucille A Carver College of Medicine
University of Iowa
Iowa City, Iowa

ROBERT S. LEVINE, MD

Professor, Preventive Medicine
Meharry Medical College
Nashville, Tennessee

GWENDOLYN D. MADDOX, MSN

Executive Director, National MOTTEP
Washington, DC

MARY J. MCNAMEE, PHD, RN

Assistant Vice Chancellor for Student Equity
    and Multicultural Affairs
University of Nebraska Medical Center
Omaha, Nebraska

ALAN MEYERS, MD, MPH

Assistant Professor, Pediatrics Department
Boston University School of Medicine
Boston Medical Center
Boston, Massachusetts

PATRICE MILES

Director, Corporate and Community Relations,
National MOTTEP
Washington, DC

SUSAN G. MOORE, MD, MPH

Fellow, Department of Hematology and Oncology
Winship Cancer Institute
Emory University
Atlanta, Georgia

MARSHA MORIEN, MSBA, FACHE

Assistant Director
University of Nebraska Center for Biosecurity
Administrator, Center for Biosecurity
Computer Assisted Medicine and Surgery
Omaha, Nebraska

HARVEY J. MURFF, MD, MPH

Assistant Professor
Division of General Internal Medicine,
Department of Medicine
GRECC, VA Tennessee Valley Healthcare System
Nashville, Tennessee

ANA NÚÑEZ, MD

Associate Professor of Medicine
Director, Women's Health Education Program
Institute for Women's Health and Leadership
Drexel University College of Medicine
Philadelphia, Pennsylvania

WALTER A. ORENSTEIN, MD

Assistant Professor of Medicine
Emory University School of Medicine
Emory Vaccine Center
Atlanta, Georgia

RUBENS J. PAMIES, MD, FACP

Vice Chancellor for Academic Affairs
Dean for Graduate Studies
Professor of Internal Medicine
University of Nebraska Medical Center
Omaha, Nebraska

MAGDA G. PECK, ScD

Professor of Pediatrics and Public Health
CEO, CityMatCH
University of Nebraska Medical Center
Omaha, Nebraska

ANNELLE B. PRIMM, MD, MPH

Director of Minority and National Affairs, American
Psychiatric Association
Johns Hopkins University School of Medicine
Baltimore, Maryland

BENY J. PRIMM, MD

Executive Director
Addiction Research and Treatment Corporation
Brooklyn, New York

NICOLE PRUDENT, MD, MPH

Assistant Professor of Pediatrics
Boston University School of Medicine
Director of Project HEALTHY CHOICE
Co-Founder and Director of Haitian Health Institute
Boston Medical Center
Boston, Massachusetts

RANDOLPH F. R. RASCH, PhD, RN

Professor of Nursing
Vanderbilt University School of Nursing
Nashville, Tennessee

JOHN W. REINHARDT, DDS, MS, MPH

Professor and Dean, College of Dentistry
University of Nebraska Medical Center
Lincoln, Nebraska

CANDACE ROBERTSON, MPH

Research Manager, Women's Health Education Program
Institute for Women's Health and Leadership
Drexel University College of Medicine
Philadelphia, Pennsylvania

LANCE RODEWALD, MD

National Immunization Program
Centers for Disease Control and Prevention
Atlanta, Georgia

MATHILDA B. RUWE, MD, MPH

Schneider Institute for Health Policy
Heller School for Social Policy and Management
Brandeis University
Waltham, Massachusetts

DAVID SATCHER, MD, PhD

Director, National Center for Primary Care
Morehouse School of Medicine
Atlanta, Georgia

ELIJAH SAUNDERS, MD, FACC, FACP

Professor of Medicine (Cardiology)
University of Maryland School of Medicine
Baltimore, Maryland

G. BRADLEY SCHAEFER, MD, FAAP, FACMG

Omaha Scottish Rite, Masonic Professor of Child Health
Associate Director, Munroe-Meyer Institute for Genetics
and Rehabilitation
Associate Chairman for Faculty Development, Department
of Pediatrics
University of Nebraska Medical Center
Omaha, Nebraska

JEANNE CRAIG SINKFORD, DDS, MS, PhD

Associate Executive Director, American Dental
Education Association
Professor and Dean Emeritus
Howard University College of Dentistry
Washington, DC

WALLY R. SMITH, MD

Associate Professor of Medicine
Chairman, Division of Quality Health Care
Medical Director, Center on Health Disparities
Virginia Commonwealth University
Richmond, Virginia

GREGORY STRAYHORN, MD, MPH, PhD

Morehouse School of Medicine
Atlanta, Georgia

RAMON VELEZ, MD, MPH, MS

Professor of Medicine
Department of Internal Medicine
Wake Forest University School of Medicine
Winston-Salem, North Carolina

LEVI WATKINS, JR, MD

Professor of Surgery, Department of
    Cardiac Surgery
Associated Dean, School of Medicine
Johns Hopkins University
Baltimore, Maryland

MICHELLE WHITEHURST-COOK, MD

Associate Professor of Medicine
Department of Family Practice
Virginia Commonwealth University
Richmond, Virginia

JASON WILBUR, MD

Assistant Professor (Clinical)
Department of Family Medicine
Roy J and Lucille A Carver College of Medicine
University of Iowa
Iowa City, Iowa

WALTER W. WILLIAMS, MD, MPH

Office of the Director
Centers for Disease Control and Prevention
Atlanta, Georgia

KRISTI F. WOODS, MD, MPH

Professor of Medicine
Director, Maya Angelou Research Center on
    Minority Health
Wake Forest University School of Medicine
Winston-Salem, North Carolina

Foreword I

Before the formation of the United States from the 13 English colonies in 1776, diversity was already a reality in the populations in our lands—primarily the result of immigration of whites from Europe, the importation of black slaves from Africa, and the preexisting Native American populations. Although the founding fathers employed noble words to describe the goals of the new nation, nearly 230 years later the United States still struggles to fulfill their inspiring vision of equality among all citizens. We are making progress, but that progress is far too slow.

One of the important, long-standing priorities for our nation and its people is good health. Good health (or the lack thereof) influences virtually everything that an individual, a population, or a society does or aspires to do. It influences our nation's social, economic, and political discourse. This text, *Multicultural Medicine and Health Disparities,* edited by Drs. David Satcher, and Rubens J. Pamies, includes a comprehensive and impressive range of scholarship and policy discussions on health disparities. Health disparities in children and among senior citizens, as well as the adverse impact of specific diseases and conditions on the nation's minority populations and the poor are presented and analyzed, and remedies are proposed.

The past two to three decades have seen a remarkable increase in the diversity of our population, and the rate of change in the national diversity is accelerating. Today, there are more people in the United States from Latin America, Eastern Europe, Southeast Asia, and Africa than ever before. They have brought with them their languages, cultures, customs, and beliefs. If the United States is to continue to be a cohesive society, and to benefit from this rich diversity as in the past, we must redouble our efforts to welcome these recently arrived brothers and sisters with understanding, sensitivity, and respect. All of these factors influence their health status and their access to health care.

Today in our nation there is a growing understanding of the importance of recognizing, studying, treating, and ultimately preventing or eliminating disparities in health status and in access to health care. This book is an important contribution that will be of value to those in the health professions, government, business, education, sociology, and many other arenas.

I salute the many contributors to this book and express my gratitude to Drs. Satcher and Pamies for shepherding its assembly and its publication.

Louis W. Sullivan, MD
President Emeritus, Morehouse School of
    Medicine
US Secretary of Health and Human Services,
    1989–1993

Foreword II

Racial and ethnic disparities have been identified as an enduring characteristic of the US health-care system. Over the past several years, many studies have defined the presence and severity of disparities in both health status and the related but separate area of health care. The US health system seems replete with these disparities. With respect to health status one need not look far, for it seems that all stages of life and all diseases and clinical conditions are affected—as if there is a disparity "beneath every rock and behind every tree." Just as troubling are the disparities in health care, as summarized by the Institute of Medicine's report, *Unequal Treatment*. Minorities receive less care than others for the same conditions, and when they receive care, it is often of lower quality.

At Aetna, a large national provider of primarily employer-based health insurance benefits, we turned to the issue of disparities as part of our overall efforts to provide our members with access to high-quality care. We were concerned that emerging research findings showed that, although importantly influenced by socioeconomic conditions, disparities persisted in the presence of health insurance. Equally disturbing was the lack of data collection by commercial insurers relating to race, ethnic background, and language preference of those they insured. We viewed collection of these data as essential if we were to truly understand the needs of our customers and identify those individuals or groups at special risk. As we began systematically to collect this information about our membership, we were heartened by the collaboration of the employers who purchase our products as well as the strong support we received from the US Department of Health and Human Services. We are very encouraged that other health plans are beginning to collect this information and that the Agency for Healthcare Research and Quality is coordinating efforts to standardize and increase such efforts.

As our program has advanced, in addition to collecting data on our membership and analyzing it for the presence of disparities, we have introduced mandatory cultural competency training for all clinical personnel in our company, provided our members with access to information on the languages spoken in the offices of our network physicians, and launched initiatives in health literacy and health benefits literacy. These efforts have strengthened our capacity to work effectively with employers to provide their employees and family members with high-quality care.

Health plans can and should play an important role in a comprehensive, coordinated effort to reduce or eliminate health and health-care disparities in the United States.

This comprehensive volume, edited by Drs. Satcher and Pamies, marks a significant milestone in our progress against disparities. By bringing together expert analyses from many points of view, it provides a truly interdisciplinary body of work that can inform the development of an effective strategy going forward.

John W. Rowe, MD
Chairman and CEO, Aetna, Inc
Hartford, Connecticut

Foreword III

"Disease and disasters come and go like rain, but health is like the sun that illuminates the entire village." —African proverb

The preceding proverb is an apt way to think about the purpose and power of *Multicultural Medicine and Health Disparities,* edited by Drs. Satcher and Pamies. Having the sun illuminate all parts and the people within our village is what we seek, but that is not possible without understanding the "rain"—those diseases and disasters that have long plagued our communities. Now, at the beginning of the 21st century, the health status and health care available to Americans is, for some, the best ever. Yet for many populations—African Americans, Hispanics, Native Americans, and many Asian groups, among others—health status is embarrassingly wanting and the health-care system fails them continually. The reasons for the disparities in health status and health care that haunt people of color are complex. However, it is possible to dissect them and extract answers to the questions long posed by students of racial and ethnic disparities in health care and health status. The reader will find the questions and the best available answers in this book.

▶ DISEASES AND DISASTERS

The metaphorical diseases and disasters that rob so many people and populations of color of their health are too numerous to describe exhaustively here, but a few questions illuminate the scope of the problem.

- Why are African Americans and Hispanics overrepresented among the 45 million uninsured people in the United States?
- Why is the infant mortality rate for black infants nearly two-and-a-half times higher than the rate for white infants?
- Why are diabetes rates more than 30% higher in Native Americans than in Hispanics and whites?
- Why are mortality rates for cancer, diabetes, and stroke significantly higher in African Americans than in whites?
- Why is the highest prevalence of childhood obesity among Mexican American boys and African American girls?
- Why do people of color continue to be underrepresented in medicine, dentistry, nursing, and public health?
- Why is life expectancy for black men and women in the United States nearly 10 years less than that of their white counterparts?

▶ SEEKING THE SUN

To find the answers to these questions, Satcher and Pamies have called on the scholarship of a diverse group of experts who collectively examine health policy, the social determinants of health, the implications of recent discoveries in biology, and the role of the environment. Answering these and other questions is a crucial step in developing a strategy and road map to eliminate disparities in health status and health care. In the end, however, we must heed Goethe's admonition that "Knowing is not enough; we must apply. Willing is not enough; we must do." My hope is that everyone who reads this important text will gain the knowledge and inspiration to take action against disparities.

Risa Lavizzo-Mourey, MD, MBA
President and CEO
The Robert Wood Johnson Foundation
Princeton, New Jersey

Preface

With the publication of the IOM report *Unequal Treatment* in 2003, health disparities finally emerged as a topic of national importance and worthy of much attention and discussion. As a result of the IOM work, Congress charged the Agency for Healthcare Research and Quality with compiling an annual report on the status of disparities. Increasingly more research funding from the government and foundation community is being directed toward the study of health disparities and more sophisticated analyses of health disparities are being published in some of this country's leading health journals.

The concept of health disparities, however, did not suddenly emerge with publication of the IOM report. Two other important events preceded the IOM report on health disparities. In January, 2000, the *Healthy People 2010* report targeted the elimination of disparities in health as two of its primary goals. In addition, the US Congress passed legislation creating the National Center for Minority Health and Health Disparities (NCMHD) at NIH later the same year. It was following these actions that the IOM report was commissioned. As early as 1985, the US Department of Health and Human Services' landmark *Report of the Secretary's Task Force on Black & Minority Health* noted "...there was a continuing disparity in the burden of death and illness experienced by black Americans and other minority Americans as compared with our nation's population as a whole." Those of us who are health professionals have always been aware that some populations—our patients, our friends, even our own families—do not share the same health outcomes as those of white Americans despite their level of education, insurance status, or socioeconomic resources.

The two editors of this book have a deep and abiding passion for these issues and have spent much of their careers trying to energize the nation's health care professionals and others to get involved in finding a solution to this silent epidemic. To address our nation's health care practitioners, policy makers, students, and community advocates, we conceived a textbook that brought together leading practitioners and scholars to discuss a broad range of health and policy issues related to health disparities and multicultural medicine. Our chapter authors bring highly informed perspectives on the broad sociopolitical parameters of health disparities as well as knowledge of diseases as they specifically present among racial and ethnic minorities.

This book is organized into three broad sections. The first addresses health disparities from a developmental perspective, across the lifespan. The second focuses on health disparities as they present in the clinical setting. The final section addresses key concepts, skills, and case examples in multicultural medicine, as well as larger policy issues that may be helpful in mitigating healthcare disparities.

Data presented in many of these chapters are sobering and speak for themselves. It is our sincerest hope that by documenting the nature and extent of health disparities, we will provide a platform for discussion and strengthen resolve among people of all racial and ethnic backgrounds to address, reduce, and eventually eliminate them. It is our hope that the issues we raise in this book will increase awareness of health disparities among students, health practitioners, educators, policy makers, and the American people and lead them to ask, as we do, "What can be done?"

David Satcher, MD, PhD
Rubens J. Pamies, MD, FACP

Acknowledgments

► FROM DS

I want to first acknowledge my co-editor, Dr Pamies, for the energy and passion he brought to this important project. He and his staff at the University of Nebraska kept us headed toward our goal even when my own schedule greatly limited my day-to-day involvement. In addition, I want to acknowledge all of those who made the commitment to deliver a quality chapter and followed through—keeping their word. Their commitment to excellence and to the elimination of disparities in health is greatly appreciated.

Moreover, my own staff at the National Center for Primary Care at the Morehouse School of Medicine is also to be commended for managing, not only my complex schedule as former Surgeon General, but my involvement as co-editor and the writer of two chapters—one with Dr Kathi Earles. Cynthia Bennett, who served as my speechwriter while I was in the Office of the Surgeon General, also assisted with this very important project as she did with the development of *Healthy People 2010,* which set the national goal of eliminating disparities in health.

Finally, my strongest supporter and most valued ally continues to be my wife, Nola, who is always there to support me and encourage me in any endeavor. I owe her more than I can ever repay.

David Satcher, MD, PhD
Director, National Center for Primary Care
Sixteenth US Surgeon General

► FROM RJS

First and foremost, I want to acknowledge my co-editor, Dr David Satcher and to commend him for his life-long commitment to addressing health disparities. His wisdom, guidance, hard work, and dedication to this project have made this a uniquely enjoyable experience for me, for which I thank him.

Special thanks are offered to the following people: the staff at the Morehouse Center for Primary Care at the Morehouse School of Medicine, for their hard work, patience, and professionalism throughout this project; the contributing authors, for their outstanding work in preparing the manuscripts; and the editors at McGraw-Hill, especially Jim Shanahan, Executive Editor, for their willingness to support this project.

I also wish to acknowledge my colleagues at the University of Nebraska Medical Center, in particular Dr Harold M. Maurer, Chancellor; Dr David A. Crouse, Associate Vice Chancellor; and members of my office staff, Ms Marcia L. Beer and Mrs Margaret T. Robinson, for their assistance and support.

A special thank-you is in order to Dr Nancy Woelfl, Director of the McGoogan Library of Medicine at the University of Nebraska Medical Center. Without her dedication, hard work, and many services in assisting the authors, this project could not have been completed.

Additionally, I want to acknowledge and thank all of the wonderful students, residents, and colleagues with whom I have been privileged to work over the years. They have inspired me to work harder and motivate me to always strive for excellence in everything I do.

To my family, especially my children and the Boucard family; to my very close friends and mentors, Drs. Nathan Berger, David Harmond, L. Kent Smith, and Robert Haynie; to the Mesa and Hatcher families—my sincerest thanks for your unwavering encouragement and support throughout my career.

Finally, I want to dedicate this book in memory of my mother and father, Lilliane and Georges Pamies, for the unconditional love and support they gave me, and for teaching me that with faith, a dream, and hard work, anything is possible.

Rubens J. Pamies, MD, FACP
Vice Chancellor for Academic Affairs
Dean for Graduate Studies
Professor of Internal Medicine

SECTION I

---

*Health-Care Disparities
Across the Life Span*

CHAPTER 1

Health Disparities in the United States: A Continuing Challenge

HANI K. ATRASH, MD, MPH

MELISSA D. HUNTER, MPH

▶ INTRODUCTION

The 20th century brought significant improvements in the health and longevity of the American public. However, some segments of the American public have not benefited fully from this progress. The disproportionate burden of poor health status and premature mortality in the United States, often referred to as health disparity, has been well documented for over two centuries. Health disparity was defined by the National Institutes of Health as "the differences in the incidence, prevalence, mortality, and burden of disease and other adverse health conditions that exist among specific population groups in the United States."[1] Many studies have documented widespread racial and ethnic disparities in health status and the many factors that contribute to these disparities: inequalities in income and education, environmental and economic conditions, specific health behaviors and life style patterns, access to care, and even quality of services. Health disparities have also been observed in other segments of the population characterized by geographic location, age, gender, disability status, and sexual orientation.

For example, Casey et al reported that people living in rural areas are less likely to use preventive services such as mammograms, Pap smears, proctosigmoidoscopy, and influenza and pneumococcal vaccinations.[2]

Health disparities are evident in almost all measures of well-being in the United States. For example, the average American life expectancy at birth in 2001 was 77.2 years; for blacks or African Americans, life expectancy was 72.2 years, whereas for whites, it was 77.7 years.[3] Furthermore, in 1990, blacks or African Americans experienced 56 years of healthy life compared with 64.7 years of healthy life for Hispanics and 65 years of healthy life for white Americans.[4] The mortality rate due to heart disease among blacks or African Americans in 2000 was 324.8 deaths per 100,000 population compared with 255.5 deaths per 100,000 population among non-Hispanic whites.[5] In 2000, the death rate due to cancer was 200.6 per 100,000 among non-Hispanic whites compared with 248.5 per 100,000 among blacks or African Americans.[5] The incidence of serious morbidity is also higher among minority populations; for example, in 2001 the incidence of human immunodeficiency virus (HIV) infection or acquired immunodeficiency syndrome (AIDS) was 60.45 per 100,000 among blacks or African Americans compared with 6.67 among whites.[6] Disparities also exist in access to services and quality of health care; for example, in 1999, a much higher proportion of blacks or African Americans (56%) and Hispanics (44%) who needed HIV combination drug therapy were unable to receive it compared with whites (32%).[7]

► CHALLENGES TO UNDERSTANDING HEALTH DISPARITIES

Several issues face program managers and policy makers who seek to understand health disparities and develop and implement effective strategies to reduce or eliminate disparities. These issues start with a limited ability to accurately assess the magnitude and types of problems, because of issues related to the reliability of data and information, and are further complicated by the increasing diversity of the American public in both racial and ethnic composition. There is also wide diversity within each racial and ethnic group by health status and the various factors that contribute to good or poor health status, such as socioeconomic, environmental, educational, cultural, and other factors.

Although many of the observed differences are large, average differences between racial and ethnic groups may mask important differences within the society. For example, there is evidence that blacks or African Americans who live in very poor urban areas suffer extreme health disadvantages relative not only to non-Hispanic whites but also to blacks or African Americans who live in poor rural areas or middle-class urban neighborhoods.[8] In addition, health differences by national origin, socioeconomic status, and age, particularly within the Hispanic and Asian populations, are not apparent when statistics are reported at this level of aggregation. There is evidence, for example, that the health status of younger cohorts of Hispanics may be declining; and, among Asian

and Pacific Islanders, those with low incomes and those with origins in South and Southeast Asia are disadvantaged relative to other Asian groups and non-Hispanic whites.[9,10] Hispanics from Cuba have much better health indicators than Hispanics from Central and South American countries, whereas Hispanics from Mexico tend to have the worst indicators.[5] In 2001, for example, 91.8% of Cuban American mothers had early prenatal care compared with 79.1% of Puerto Ricans, 74.6% of Mexican Americans, and 77.4% of other Hispanics.[5] The infant mortality rate was 4.3 per 1000 live births among Cuban Americans compared with 8.1 among Puerto Ricans, 5.5 among Mexican Americans, and 4.9 among other Hispanics.[5] Finally, in 2001, 19.2% of Cuban Americans younger than 65 years of age had no health insurance coverage compared with 16.0% of Puerto Ricans, 39% of Mexican Americans, and 33.1% of other Hispanics.[5]

Increasing Diversity of the American Public

During the past 20 years, the diversity of the US population has increased. The proportion of white Americans decreased from 83.2% in 1970 to 69.1% in 2000; the proportion of blacks or African Americans increased from 11.1% in 1970 to 12.1% in 2000; and the proportion of Hispanics living in the United States increased from 4.7% in 1970 to 12.5% in 2000[11,12] (see Appendix A, Fig. A–1).* The Census Bureau further projects that by 2050, nearly one in every two Americans will be a member of a racial or ethnic minority[13] (see Fig. A–2). Concurrent with this increased population diversity, there has been an increase in the numbers of interracial marriages, resulting in an increase in the number of children of mixed race or ethnicity. For example, in the 1970 census, there were about 321,000 interracial unions. By 1980, the number had increased to about 1 million; and by 1990 there were about 1.5 million interracial couples.

---

* Figures illustrating statistical information presented in this chapter are included in Appendix A at the end of the book.

Census data indicate that the number of children in interracial families grew from less than 500,000 in 1970 to about 2 million in 1990.[14,15]

Minority populations are also unevenly distributed around the country. In 2000, blacks or African Americans constituted 0.5% of the population of Montana compared with 61.3% of the population of the District of Columbia and 32.9% of the population of Louisiana,[16] Hispanics constituted 32.4% of the population of California compared with 0.7% of the population of West Virginia, and American Indians lived mostly in western and northeastern states.[17] With the steady increase in the minority population, the persistent barriers to care, and continuing inequity in the quality of health care, the issue of health disparity will only become more challenging.

Data Collection

The collection of information about race and ethnicity is essential for the development and implementation of targeted strategies for the elimination of racial and ethnic health disparities. Currently, information on race and ethnicity to calculate health status indicators and health-care utilization measures is obtained from numerous sources collected by multiple agencies at the local, state, and federal levels. Categories and types of information collected include natality, mortality, morbidity, health behavior and attitude, health service utilization, health-care financing, population size and migration, and socioeconomic data.[18,19] Although data are collected by different agencies and from different sources, these data often need to be combined to estimate health-related indicators, such as using vital statistics and census data to estimate birth and death rates. Because these sources use different methods to determine the race and ethnicity of individuals, substantial inconsistencies may result in the categorization of race and ethnicity in data collecting and reporting. For example, information regarding race and ethnicity in the census depends on self-identification,

which may differ from race and ethnic categorizations assigned by an interviewer or reported by a health-care provider.

Collection of vital statistics data in the United States dates to 1632, when the Grand Assembly of Virginia passed a law requiring a minister or warden from every parish to appear annually at court on the first of June to present a register of christenings, marriages, and burials for the year.[20] Since then, various colonies and states have initiated and implemented their own requirements for vital registration and data compilation and reporting.[20] In 1842, Massachusetts adopted the first State Registration Law in America, which required central state filing; provided for standard forms, fees, and penalties; specified types of information, including causes of death; and lodged responsibility for each kind of record in designated officials. The Seventh Federal Census of 1850 was the first attempt in 150 years of census data collection to collect information on births, deaths, and marriages.[20]

Census enumeration of vital events continued to serve as the source of national vital statistics data, while encouraging states to intensify their efforts to register vital events, and included mortality information from these registration systems in the census data for areas having records in satisfactory detail. This approach was not entirely abandoned until the census of 1910, when the developing vital registration area was large enough to provide national statistics. In 1900, the census office recommended a death certificate and requested each area to adopt it by January 1, 1900. In 1902, the census office, which had previously been disbanded between censuses, was made a permanent, full-time agency of the federal government and was given its present name, the Bureau of the Census.

For more than 30 years, the fundamental task of the Bureau of the Census in the field of vital statistics was to extend the registration area for births and deaths. This primary responsibility was accomplished with the admission of Texas into the birth and death registration areas in 1933. Alaska was added in 1950, Hawaii in

1917, Puerto Rico in 1932, and the Virgin Islands in 1924. By the early 1930s, responsibility for vital records had been largely transferred from civil offices to health departments. In 1946, the National Office of Vital Statistics was established in the Public Health Service. Before 1900, mortality rates by race were reported based on data obtained through the census. Starting in 1900, mortality was reported annually by race through the Annual Mortality Statistics Reports.[20–22]

Race and Ethnicity Classification

The terminology used to classify the US public by race and ethnicity has changed over the years to be more consistent with current language and as a result of emerging changes in the composition of the population. The first census of the United States in 1790 enumerated three racial groups: "Whites," "Blacks," and "Civilized Indians" (ie, those who paid taxes).[23] During the 1800 and early 1900s, census and vital statistics reports classified the US public as "White," "Black," and "Other Colored" (which included Indians, with a few Chinese and Japanese).[21–28] New racial categories were added in the late 19th century and beyond (Chinese in 1870, Japanese in 1890) as the need arose to track new immigrant groups.[23] Starting in 1930, a new category, "Other," was added to the "Colored" group. The new category was added to include Mexicans, who were given a separate classification in the population census of 1930, "as the number of Mexicans in the population had increased very rapidly."[29] From 1930 through the 1970s, categorization by race always included a "White" category, the rest of the population was categorized as "Other," "All Other," "Non-White," and occasionally broken down further into "Black" and "Other."[21–28] The growth of the Hispanic population in the United States starting in the early 1970s stimulated interest in obtaining vital statistics information pertaining to that group. However, the ability to obtain reliable and accurate health-indicator rates for racial and ethnic groups in the United States has been seriously limited by the lack of clear guidance for classification and categorization and by the use of different systems by the various agencies collecting data.

In June 1976, a joint resolution of Congress (Public Law 94-311) required federal agencies to begin collecting and publishing data on Americans of Spanish origin or descent. During the 1980s, the number of states including a Hispanic identifier on their birth and death certificates steadily increased. In 1978, the Office of Management and Budget issued Directive 15, titled "Race and Ethnic Standards for Federal Statistics and Administrative Reporting."[14] The standards provided a minimum set of categories for data on race and ethnicity and called for four categories on race ("American Indian or Alaska Native," "Asian or Pacific Islander," "Black," and "White") and two categories for data on ethnicity ("Hispanic Origin," and "Not Of Hispanic Origin"). The directive further stated that "Self identification is the preferred means of obtaining information about individual's race and ethnicity, except in instances where observer identification is more practical (eg, completing a death certificate)." The directive was to apply immediately to all new and revised record-keeping systems; all existing record-keeping or reporting requirements were required to comply with the new directive at the time of extension or no later than January 1, 1980.[14]

In 1993, because of continuing concerns related to the accuracy and reliability of race- and ethnicity-specific information, the Office of Management and Budget (OMB) undertook a 4-year comprehensive review of the race and ethnicity categories under Directive 15 in collaboration with representatives from more than 30 agencies representing diverse federal needs for data on race and ethnicity. In October 1997, OMB issued its decision to introduce two modifications to Directive 15, as follows: (1) the Asian or Pacific Islander category will be separated into two categories—"Asian" and "Native Hawaiian or Other Pacific Islander," and (2) the term "Hispanic" will be changed to "Hispanic or Latino."[15] The revised standards will have five minimum categories for data on race: "American Indian or Alaska Native," "Asian," "Black or African American," "Native Hawaiian or Other Pacific Islander," and "White." There will be two categories for data on ethnicity: "Hispanic or Latino" and "Not Hispanic or Latino." OMB provided definitions to each of these categories as follows:

- **American Indian or Alaska Native.** A person having origins in any of the original peoples of North and South America (including Central America), and who maintains tribal affiliation or community attachment.
- **Asian.** A person having origins in any of the original peoples of the Far East, Southeast Asia, or the Indian subcontinent, including Cambodia, China, India, Japan, Korea, Malaysia, Pakistan, the Philippine Islands, Thailand, and Vietnam.
- **Black or African American.** A person having origins in any of the black racial groups of Africa. Terms such as "Haitian" or "Negro" can be used in addition to "Black or African American."
- **Hispanic or Latino.** A person of Cuban, Mexican, Puerto Rican, South or Central American, or other Spanish culture or origin, regardless of race. The term, "Spanish Origin," can be used in addition to "Hispanic or Latino."
- **Native Hawaiian or Other Pacific Islander.** A person having origins in any of the original peoples of Hawaii, Guam, Samoa, or other Pacific Islands.
- **White.** A person having origins in any of the original peoples of Europe, the Middle East, or North Africa.

The revised directive also requires that respondents be offered the option of selecting one or more racial designations. OMB further recommended that two formats be used for data on race and ethnicity. Self-reporting or self-identification using two separate questions is the preferred method for collecting data on race and ethnicity. In situations where self-reporting is not practicable or feasible, the combined format may be used. OMB directed that the new standards be used by the Bureau of the Census in the 2000 decennial census. Other federal programs were to adopt the standards as soon as possible, but not later than January 1, 2003, for use in household surveys, administrative forms and records, and other data collections.[15]

Data Accuracy and Reliability

Studies have repeatedly demonstrated that a nontrivial proportion of non–black or African American minorities are misclassified as white on the death certificate. This numerator problem leads to an underestimate of the death rates for American Indians, Asian and Pacific Islanders, and Hispanics.[30–32] Additional bias in the reliability of health indicators for minority populations is related to the considerable heterogeneity within each of the major racial and ethnic populations with significant variation in health status within each group. Moreover, a relatively high proportion of Hispanics and other minorities, especially Asian Americans, is foreign-born, and their health profile reflects in part the impact of immigration. Immigrants tend to enjoy better health status than the native-born population, even when those immigrants are lower in socioeconomic status.[30,33] However, with increasing length of stay in the United States and adaptation to mainstream behavior, the health status of immigrants deteriorates.

Misclassification

The current methods used for assigning race and ethnicity to population, deaths, and births are not consistent and therefore may cause a bias in estimating the race- and ethnicity-specific birth and death rates.

Births

Racial classification of births is based on information provided by the family or based on observation. By law, the registration of births is the direct responsibility of the professional attendant at birth, generally a physician or midwife. In their absence, the parents of the child are responsible for the report. Each birth must be reported promptly; the reporting requirements vary from state to state, ranging from 24 hours after the birth to as much as 10 days. Certificates must be filed with the local registrar of the district in which the birth occurs.

The birth certificate does not provide for reporting of race of the newborn. Prior to 1989, for statistical purposes, classification of the child's race or national origin was based on the race or national origin of the parents. When both parents were not of the same race or national origin, rules had been established for coding various combinations. If only one parent was white, the child was assigned the race of the other parent. If neither parent was white, the child was assigned the race of the father, with one exception: if either parent was Hawaiian or part Hawaiian, the child race was assigned to Hawaiian. Beginning with the 1989 data, natality tabulations were modified to show race of the mother rather than race of the child.[20]

Deaths

Race classification for deaths is recorded by the funeral director based on information provided by an informant or based on observation. The registration of deaths is the direct responsibility of the funeral director, or person acting as such. The funeral director obtains the data required other than the cause of death. The person who supplies the information to the funeral director is usually required to sign the certificate as informant to attest to the truth of the facts entered. The physician in attendance at the death is required to indicate the cause of death. If no physician was in attendance, the coroner, or person acting as such, is required to enter the cause of death. Where death is from other than natural causes, the coroner may be required to examine the body and report the cause of death, even though a physician was in attendance.[20]

Population

Information on population in the census by race or ethnicity is based on information reported through self-reports of people who respond for themselves or others in their household.[18]

Potential Bias

The multiple sources of data, together with the multiple means for classifying persons by race and ethnicity, have resulted in biases when data sources are combined to estimate health indicators for the various racial and ethnic groups. In general, studies have demonstrated good agreement between race reported on death certificates and other sources for white and black or African American decedents, but poorer consistency between the two sources for other racial groups.[18] An early study by Hambright compared race reported on death certificates with race reported for the same individuals on the 1960 census.[34] The study showed greater than 98% agreement between the two sources for white and black or African American decedents but poorer agreement for other groups (American Indians, 79.2%; Japanese, 97%; Chinese, 90.3%; and Filipino, 72.6%). Rosenberg et al compared race reported on death certificates for 1979 to 1989 with response to race questions on the Current Population Survey, a monthly survey comprising about 60,000 US households. The survey, which is carried out by the Census Bureau, asks questions about labor force participation and is the source of national unemployment figures. During certain months of the year, the survey asks supplemental questions on various social, demographic, and economic topics. Again, as in the earlier study, the level of agreement for the two major race groups was greater than 98%. In contrast, for American Indians, the level of agreement was 57%; for Asian or Pacific Islanders, 82.5%; for

Hispanics, 89.7% (Mexican, 84.9%; Puerto Rican, 85.9%; Cuban, 80%; other Hispanic, 47.6%); and for non-Hispanic, 99.8%.[18]

Thus, the quality, reliability, and accuracy of death rates by race and Hispanic origin vary among population groups. Generally, death rates are reliable for the white and black or African American populations, and the overall effect of black or African American and white undercounts does not seriously distort analysis or interpretation of the resulting mortality data.[35] However, for the other minority population groups, levels of mortality are seriously biased from misreporting in the numerator and undercoverage in the denominator of the death rates.

► DATA AND STATISTICS

Health Monitoring

The number of measures of health status, health outcomes, behaviors, access, and quality of care is potentially unlimited. A simple way to obtain a general understanding of racial and ethnic disparities in health is to examine health indicators developed by the US Department of Health and Human Services (DHHS) to monitor the health of the nation: the Healthy People 2000 Health Status Indicators and the Healthy People 2010 Leading Health Indicators.

Starting in the late 1970s, the DHHS initiated a process for developing and setting national health targets based on scientific knowledge and for use in decision making and action. This process is used to identify the most significant preventable threats to health and to focus public and private sector efforts to address them. The first set of national health targets, the 1990 Health Objectives, was published in 1979 as part of "Healthy People: The Surgeon General's Report on Health Promotion and Disease Prevention."[36] The second set of targets, "Healthy People 2000: National Health Promotion and Disease Prevention Objectives,"

was released in 1990, and is a comprehensive agenda organized into 22 priority areas with 319 supporting objectives and three overarching goals: increase years of healthy life, reduce disparities in health among different population groups, and achieve access to preventive health services.[37] *Healthy People 2010* builds on both the 1979 Surgeon General's Report and Healthy People 2000 to set national objectives for 2010.[38] *Healthy People 2010* was designed to achieve two overarching goals: increase quality and years of healthy life, and eliminate health disparities.

Healthy People 2000 Objective 22.1 called for the development of a set of Health Status Indicators (HSIs) to facilitate the comparison of health status measures at the national, state, and local levels.[39,40] A group of public health professionals, known as Committee 22.1, developed and published a list of 18 HSIs in 1991[40,41] (Table 1–1). The process involved intensive consultation and review with over 200 public health professionals representing state and local health departments, professional organizations, and the academic community.[40]

The Leading Health Indicators were developed in conjunction with *Healthy People 2010,* with 10 areas of emphasis: physical activity, overweight and obesity, tobacco use, substance abuse, responsible sexual behavior, mental health, injury and violence, environmental quality, immunization, and access to health care.[38,42] The Leading Health Indicators serve as a link to the 467 objectives in *Healthy People 2010* and as the basic building blocks for community health initiatives. For each of the Leading Health Indicators, specific objectives derived from *Healthy People 2010* will be used to track progress[42] (Table 1–2). Like its predecessors, *Healthy People 2010* was developed through a broad consultation process, built on the best scientific knowledge and designed to measure progress over time. Healthy People 2000 Health Status Indicators measure health status outcomes and factors that put individuals at increased risk of disease or premature

▶ **TABLE 1–1.** Healthy People 2000 Health Status Indicators

1. Race- and ethnicity-specific infant mortality per 1000 live births
2. Total deaths per 100,000 population
3. Motor vehicle crash deaths per 100,000 population
4. Work-related injury deaths per 100,000 population
5. Suicides per 100,000 population
6. Homicides per 100,000 population
7. Lung cancer deaths per 100,000 population
8. Female breast cancer deaths per 100,000 population
9. Cardiovascular disease deaths per 100,000 population
10. Reported incidence of acquired immunodeficiency syndrome per 100,000 population
11. Reported incidence of measles per 100,000 population
12. Reported incidence of tuberculosis per 100,000 population
13. Reported incidence of primary and secondary syphilis per 100,000 population
14. Percent of low birth weight as measured by the percentage of live-born infants weighing less than 2500 g at birth
15. Births to adolescents (aged 10–17 years) as a percentage of total live births
16. Prenatal care as measured by the percentage of mothers delivering live infants who did not receive care during the first trimester of pregnancy
17. Childhood poverty as measured by the proportion of children younger than 15 years of age living in families at or below the poverty level
18. Proportion of people living in counties exceeding US Environmental Protection Agency standards for air quality during the previous year

Source: Klein RJ, Hawk SA. Health status indicators: Definitions and national data. Healthy People Statistical Notes, *vol 1, No 3. Hyattsville, Md: National Center for Health Statistics; 1992.*

mortality, whereas the 2010 Leading Health Indicators were selected to reflect individual behaviors, physical and social environmental factors, and important health system issues that greatly affect the health of individuals and communities.[41,42]

Health Disparities

Racial and ethnic disparities in mortality, disability, and morbidity have existed for many years, and racial and ethnic minorities, with few exceptions, continue to experience higher rates of mortality, disability, and morbidity than nonminorities. In general, blacks or African Americans have worse health outcomes than any other race or ethnic group in the United States; American Indians or Alaska Natives and Hispanics often have worse health outcomes than whites; and Asians fare as well as, and sometimes better than, non-Hispanic whites. These racial dispar-

ities have been documented for decades and some have widened in recent years.

Mortality

Since the beginning of the 20th century, blacks or African Americans and other minorities have had a higher maternal mortality rate than whites (see Fig. A–3). In 2001, black or African American women who became pregnant had more than three times the risk of dying of pregnancy-related causes than white women. The maternal mortality rate was 6.5 per 100,000 live births for non-Hispanic whites, 24.7 per 100,000 live births for blacks or African Americans, and 9.5 for Hispanics.[3] Blacks or African Americans and other minorities have also always had a higher infant mortality rate than whites. In 2001, the infant mortality rate among blacks or African Americans was 14.0 infant deaths per 1000 live births compared with 5.7 among whites—2.5 times higher[3] (see Fig. A–4).

▶ **TABLE 1–2**. Healthy People 2010 Leading Health Indicators and Specific Objectives to Track Them

1. Physical Activity:
   - Increase the proportion of adolescents who engage in vigorous physical activity that promotes cardiorespiratory fitness 3 or more days per week for 20 or more minutes per occasion
   - Increase the proportion of adults who engage regularly, preferably daily, in moderate physical activity for at least 30 minutes per day
2. Overweight and Obesity:
   - Reduce the proportion of children and adolescents who are overweight or obese
   - Reduce the proportion of adults who are obese
3. Tobacco Use:
   - Reduce cigarette smoking by adolescents
   - Reduce cigarette smoking by adults
4. Substance Abuse:
   - Increase the proportion of adolescents not using alcohol or any illicit drugs during the past 30 days
   - Reduce the proportion of adults using any illicit drug during the past 30 days
   - Reduce the proportion of adults engaging in binge drinking of alcoholic beverages during the past month
5. Responsible Sexual Behavior:
   - Increase the proportion of adolescents who abstain from sexual intercourse or use condoms if currently sexually active
   - Increase the proportion of sexually active persons who use condoms
6. Mental Health:
   - Increase the proportion of adults with recognized depression who receive treatment
7. Injury and Violence:
   - Reduce deaths caused by motor vehicle crashes
   - Reduce homicides
8. Environmental Quality:
   - Reduce the proportion of people exposed to air that does not meet the US Environmental Protection Agency's health-based standards for ozone
   - Reduce the proportion of nonsmokers exposed to environmental tobacco smoke
9. Immunization:
   - Increase the proportion of young children who receive all vaccines recommended for universal administration for at least 5 years
   - Increase the proportion of noninstitutionalized adults who are vaccinated annually against influenza and ever vaccinated against pneumococcal disease
10. Access To Health Care:
    - Increase the proportion of people with health insurance
    - Increase the proportion of people who have a specific source of ongoing care
    - Increase the proportion of pregnant women who begin prenatal care in the first trimester of pregnancy

Source: Healthy People 2010: Leading Health Indicators. *Available at: http://www.healthypeople.gov/document/html/uih/ uih_4.htm.*

The gaps in maternal and infant mortality between blacks or African Americans and whites have widened over time. Neonatal and post-neonatal mortality rates were also higher among blacks or African Americans than among whites. Underlying the continuing higher infant mortality rate among blacks or African Americans are higher rates of low birth weight and preterm delivery: in 2002, the incidence of low birth weight among non-Hispanic whites was 5.02% of births compared with 11.44% among blacks or African Americans and 5.44% among Hispanics; the incidence of preterm delivery among blacks or African Americans was 15.98% compared with 9.07% for non-Hispanic whites and 10.63% among Hispanics.[43]

Since 1900, general and age-adjusted mortality rates have continued to be higher for blacks or African Americans than for whites.[3] Also since 1900, life expectancy at birth has continued to be better for whites than for blacks or African Americans.[3] In 2001, blacks or African Americans had an overall age-adjusted death rate that was 1.3 times higher than that of the white population. The overall death rates for all other minority populations were lower than that for whites (see Figs. A–5 through A–7).

In 2000, elevated mortality rates for blacks or African Americans compared with whites existed for eight of the leading causes of death.[5] Blacks or African Americans experienced the highest rates of mortality from heart disease, cancers (including breast and lung cancer), influenza and pneumonia, cerebrovascular disease (including stroke), HIV and AIDS, diabetes, and homicide of any racial or ethnic group.[5,44] Compared with whites, American Indians had lower death rates for cerebrovascular disease (including stroke), heart disease, and cancer (including breast and lung caner), but higher rates of death from motor vehicle crashes, diabetes, and cirrhosis of the liver. Hispanics had higher death rates than whites for diabetes, HIV and AIDS, and cirrhosis of the liver.[5,44] For all of the leading causes of death in the United States except for homicide, the Asian or Pacific Islander population had mortality rates considerably lower than those of whites[5,44] (Table 1–3).

Disability

The US Census Bureau reported that there were 49.7 million people with some type of long-lasting condition or disability in the United States in 2000, representing 19.3% of the population 5 years of age and older.[45] The incidence varied among the various racial and ethnic groups, ranging from 16.6% among Asians to 18.3% among whites, and 24.3% among blacks or African Americans and American Indians or Alaska Natives (see Fig. A–8). The incidence increased with age, but the differences held true for all age groups.[45] The incidence was much higher for adults aged 65 years and older but continued to be highest among the American Indian or Alaska Native population[45] (Table 1–4).

Morbidity and Health Status

When asked to assess their own health and the health of family members living in the same household, a much higher proportion of whites than blacks or African Americans or Hispanics assessed their health as excellent or very good[46] (Table 1–5). For selected morbidity measures, blacks or African Americans had higher reported incidence rates than whites for HIV and AIDS, tuberculosis, syphilis, diabetes, and childhood asthma[6,46] (see Table 1–5). High rates of tuberculosis were also reported among the other minority groups, with the highest rate of tuberculosis among the Asian or Pacific Islander population[6] (see Table 1–5). In 1998, it was estimated that the highest proportion of people living in counties with poor air quality was Hispanic and Asian or Pacific Islander (60%); obesity was most common among adolescent and adult male and female blacks or African Americans as well as among adolescent Hispanics[46,47] (see Table 1–5). Blacks or African Americans, Hispanics, and American Indians or Alaska Natives had higher rates of births among mothers aged 10 to 17 years than whites and Asians or Pacific Islanders[5] (see Table 1–5).

▶ **TABLE 1–3**. Mortality Rates by Leading Cause, Year, and Race or Ethnicity, United States

Indicator and Year[a] (Reference)	Race or Ethnicity				
	White	B/AA	H/L	AI/AN	A/PI
Age-adjusted mortality rate, 2001 (3)	836.5	1101.2	306.8	686.7	492.1
Diseases of the heart death rate, 2000 (5)	255.5	324.8	196.0	178.2	146.0
Malignant neoplasm death rate, 2000 (5)	200.6	248.5	134.9	127.8	121.9
Cerebrovascular disease death rate, 2000 (5)	59.0	81.9	46.4	45.0	52.9
Lung cancer death rate, 1998 (44)	38.3	46.0	13.6	25.1	17.2
Female breast cancer death rate, 2000 (5)	26.8	34.5	16.9	13.6	12.3
Influenza and pneumonia death rate, 2000 (5)	23.5	25.6	20.6	22.3	19.7
Stroke death rate, 1998 (44)	23.3	42.5	19.0	19.6	22.7
Diabetes mellitus death rate, 2000 (5)	21.8	49.5	36.9	41.5	16.4
Motor vehicle crash death rate, 2000 (5)	15.6	15.7	14.7	27.3	8.6
Suicide rate, 2000 (5)	12.0	5.5	5.9	9.8	5.5
Chronic liver disease and cirrhosis death rate, 2000 (5)	9.0	9.4	16.5	24.3	3.5
Work-related injury death rate, 2001 (5)	4.2	3.8	6.0	—	—
Homicide rate, 2000 (5)	2.8	20.5	7.5	6.8	3.0
HIV/AIDS death rate, 2000 (5)	2.2	23.3	6.7	2.2	0.6

B/AA, black or African American; H/L, Hispanic or Latino; AI/AN, American Indian or Alaska Native; A/PI, Asian or Pacific Islander; —, not available.

[a]Rates are per 100,000 people.

Source: Compiled from data in references 3, 5, and 44, as specified.

Other health status indicators were reported through the Behavioral Risk Factor Surveillance System (BRFSS).[48] The 1997 BRFSS reported that blacks or African Americans were most likely of all racial or ethnic groups to report that they were in fair or poor health and most likely to have been told by a health-care professional that their blood pressure was high.[48] American Indians or Alaska Natives were most likely to be obese; whites were most likely to have been told by a health-care professional that their blood cholesterol level was high; and blacks or African Americans and American Indians or Alaska Natives were most likely to have been told by a health-care professional that they had diabetes[48] (see Table 1–5).

▶ **TABLE 1–4**. Percent of Noninstitutionalized Population With Any Disability by Age and Race or Ethnicity, United States, 2000

Age	Race or Ethnicity					
	White	B/AA	H/L	AI/AN	Asian	NH/PI
≥ 5 years	18.3	24.3	20.9	24.3	16.6	19.0
5–15 years	5.7	7.0	5.4	7.7	2.9	5.1
16–64 years	16.2	26.4	24.0	27.0	16.9	21.0
≥ 65 years	40.4	52.5	48.5	57.6	40.8	48.5

B/AA, black or African American; H/L, Hispanic or Latino; AI/AN, American Indian or Alaska Native; NH/PI, Native Hawaiian or Other Pacific Islander.

Source: Disability Status: 2000. Census 2000 Brief. *Washington, DC: US Dept of Commerce, Economics and Statistics Administration, US Census Bureau; March 2003. Available at: http://www.census.gov/hhes/www/disability.html.*

▶ **TABLE 1–5**. Health Status and Morbidity Rates by Race and Ethnicity, United States

Indicator and Year (Reference)	Race or Ethnicity				
	White	B/AA	H/L	AI/AN	A/PI
% of persons of all ages whose health status was assessed as excellent or very good, 2003 (46)	71.0	57.2	58.2	—	—
% of children 0–14 years with at least one episode of asthma during the past 12 months, 2003 (46)	4.5	8.8	4.3	—	—
% people in counties with poor air quality, 1998 (44)	35.9	45.8	59.8	30.2	60.9
% of male adults obese, 2003 (46)	22.6	28.7	23.1	—	—
% of female adults obese, 2003 (46)	21.1	38.3	27.5	—	—
% <18 years living in poverty, 2001 (5)	9.5	30.2	28	—	11.5
% of children and adolescents overweight or obese, 2001 (47)	8.8	16	15.1	—	—
% of low birth weight, 2001 (5)	6.76	12.95	6.47	7.33	7.51
Incidence rate of AIDS, 2001 (6)[a]	6.67	60.45	9.72	9.10	3.80
% ≥18 years diagnosed with diabetes mellitus, 2003 (46)	5.7	10.1	8.3	—	—
Incidence rate of tuberculosis, 2001 (6)[a]	3.64	14.07	11.33	11.58	32.65
% of births to mothers 10–17 years, 2001 (5)	2.3	7.3	5.8	6.8	1.3
Incidence rate of syphilis, 2001 (6)[a]	0.67	10.59	2.05	4.08	0.48
Incidence rate of measles, 2001 (6)[a]	0.02	0.01	0.04	0.05	0.42

B/AA, black or African American; H/L, Hispanic or Latino; AI/AN, American Indian or Alaska Native; A/PI, Asian or Pacific Islander; —, not available.

[a] Rates are per 100,000 people.

Source: Compiled from data in references 5, 6, 44, 46, and 47.

Behavioral Risk Factors

Behavioral risk factor information is primarily derived from survey data and, in the absence of oversampling of small minority populations, no such information is available for several indicators for small minorities at the national level. Recent survey data indicate that white adolescents and adults were more likely to use tobacco products and consume alcohol than blacks or African Americans or Hispanics, but were more likely to engage in physical activity; Hispanic adolescents were least likely to abstain from sexual activity or use condoms.[5,46,47] Similar findings were reported through the BRFSS.[48] The 1997 BRFSS reported that black or African

American adults were least likely to be involved in leisure-time physical activity, adult whites were most likely to consume alcohol (at least one drink during last month), and American Indians or Alaska Natives were most likely to engage in binge drinking (five or more drinks at least on one occasion in the past month) or not use seat belts[48] (Table 1–6).

Health-Care Utilization and Access to Care

Rates of utilization of health care are different among the different minority populations. For example, in 2001, a higher proportion of white

▶ **TABLE 1–6**. Prevalence of Selected Behaviors by Race and Ethnicity, United States

Indicator, Year (Reference)	Race or Ethnicity				
	White	B/AA	H/L	AI/AN	A/PI
% of adolescents who abstain from sexual intercourse or use condoms, 2001 (47)	86.6	85.2	83.6	—	—
% of adolescents who engage in vigorous physical activity, 2001 (47)	66.5	59.7	60.5	—	—
% of adults (≥12 years) using alcohol (at least one drink in past 30 days), 2001 (5)	52.7	35.1	39.5	35.0	31.9 (AO)
% of adolescents using alcohol (at least one drink in past 30 days), 2001 (47)	50.4	32.7	49.2	—	—
% of adolescents who used tobacco at least once in past 30 days, 2001 (5)	37.7	19.4	29.4	—	—
% of adults who engage in moderate physical activity, 2003 (46)	36.2	26.1	25.2	—	—
% of adults (≥12 years) who used tobacco at least once in past 30 days, 2003 (5)	31.3	27.7	22.9	44.9	28.5
% of adults (≥12 years) engaging in binge drinking (*5 drinks or more in 1 day at least once in past year*), 2001 (5)	21.5	16.8	21.3	21.8	21.3
% of adults (≥12 years) using any illicit drugs in past 30 days, 2001 (5)	7.2	7.4	6.4	9.9	7.5

B/AA, black or African American; H/L, Hispanic or Latino; AI/AN, American Indian or Alaska Native; A/PI, Asian or Pacific Islander; AO, Asian Only; —, not available.
Source: Compiled from data in references 5, 46, and 47.

mothers received early prenatal care than mothers of other race or ethnicity; the lowest proportion of mothers receiving early prenatal care was among American Indians or Alaska Natives[5] (Table 1–7). Whites also had the highest proportion of children receiving all recommended vaccines, adults 65 years or older vaccinated against influenza, adults ever vaccinated against pneumococcal disease, persons having health insurance, and persons having a specific source of ongoing health care[5,46] (see Table 1–7). The 1997 BRFSS reported that Hispanics were least likely to seek preventive clinical services, including having had blood cholesterol checked within the past 5 years, having a Pap smear within the past 3 years, having a mammogram (for women older than 50) in the past 2 years, having a clinical breast exam (for women older than 50) in the past 2 years, having a home-kit fecal occult blood test (for people aged 50 or older), and having had a sigmoidoscopy (for people aged 50 or older).[48] In 1997, the highest prevalence of people with low educational attainment (less than high school education) was among the Hispanic population. Hispanics were also most likely to not have any health-care coverage, to not have a routine physical examination, and to report cost as a barrier to health care[48] (see Table 1–7).

Health-Care Disparity

Concern has grown that even at equivalent levels of access to care, racial and ethnic minorities experience a lower quality of health services and are less likely to receive routine medical procedures than white Americans. For example,

▶ **TABLE 1-7**. Health-Care Utilization and Health-Care Coverage by Race and Ethnicity, United States

Indicator, Year (Reference)	Race or Ethnicity				
	White	B/AA	H/L	AI/AN	A/PI
% of persons who have a specific source of ongoing care, 2003 (46)	90.4	86.4	78.1	—	—
% of mothers with first-trimester prenatal care, 2001 (5)	88.5	74.5	75.7	69.3	84.0
% of young children who receive all recommended vaccines, 2001 (5)	79	71	77	76	77
% of adults ≥ 65 years who were vaccinated against influenza in past 12 months, 1999–2001 (5)	66.7	48.8	54.8	—	62.6 (AO)
% of adults ≥ 65 ever vaccinated against pneumococcal disease, 1999–2001 (5)	56.0	32.4	30.8	—	36.4 (AO)
% of persons without health insurance, 2001 (5)	11.9	19.2	34.8	33.4	17.1 (AO)

B/AA, black or African American; H/L, Hispanic or Latino; AI/AN, American Indian or Alaska Native; A/PI, Asian or Pacific Islander; AO, Asians Only; —, not available.

Source: Compiled from data in references 5 and 46.

blacks or African Americans with end-stage renal disease were less likely to receive peritoneal dialysis and kidney transplantation,[49,50] blacks or African Americans and Hispanic patients with bone fractures seen in hospital emergency departments were less likely than whites to receive analgesia, and black or African American Medicare patients with congestive heart failure or pneumonia received poorer quality care than whites.[51,52] Moreover, a growing number of studies have found racial differences in the receipt of major therapeutic procedures for a broad range of conditions even after adjusting for insurance status and severity of disease, including situations in which differences in economic status and insurance coverage are minimized through the Veterans Health Administration System and the Medicare program.[53–56]

In 1999, concerned over increasing reports of disparities in health care, Congress directed the Institute of Medicine (IOM) to assess disparities in the types and quality of health care received by US racial and ethnic minorities and nonminorities. The IOM's Committee on Un-

derstanding and Eliminating Racial and Ethnic Disparities in Health Care defined health-care disparities as "racial and ethnic differences in the quality of health care that are not due to access-related factors of clinical needs, preferences, and appropriateness of intervention."[57] The committee examined many sources of data to assess the scope of disparities in health care, explore sources of these disparities, and generate strategies to eliminate them. Data sources included a review of the literature, commissioned papers, public testimony from professional societies and organizations, input from technical liaison panels, and focus group and roundtable input. The committee concluded that racial and ethnic disparities in health care are, with few exceptions, remarkably consistent across a range of illnesses and health-care services. These disparities are associated with socioeconomic differences and tend to diminish significantly, and in a few cases, disappear altogether when socioeconomic factors are controlled.[58] The majority of studies reviewed by the committee, however, found that racial and ethnic disparities remain even after adjustment for socioeconomic differences and other health-care access–related factors.[58–60]

▶ OTHER POPULATIONS

Although most attention and research has been directed toward health disparities among racial and ethnic minorities, recent statistics have documented serious health disparities among other segments of the population.

Persons With Disabilities

The US Census Bureau reported that in 2000, 49.7 million people with some type of long-lasting condition or disability lived in the United States.[45] Persons with disability are at risk of secondary conditions (preventable physical, mental, and social disorders) resulting directly or indirectly from an initial disabling condition.[61] Data from the National Health Interview Survey indicate that people with disabilities are more likely to smoke and to be overweight, and less likely to engage in moderate physical activity. Moreover, people with disabilities are more likely to report that their health is poor or fair (44.8%) compared with people without disabilities (9.4%); and people with disabilities are also less likely to become involved in physical activity.[62] In a survey conducted in Washington state, Kinne et al reported that the prevalence of each of 16 secondary conditions (eg, chronic pain, sleep problems, periods of depression, respiratory infections, falls or other injuries, lack of romantic relationships, problems making or seeing friends, asthma, etc) was two to three times higher among adults with disabilities than among adults without disabilities.[63] People with disabilities are also more likely to have smoked or to be current smokers.[64] Data from the National Health Interview Survey also indicate that people with disabilities are less likely to participate in social activities such as calling friends or relatives, get-

ting together with friends or relatives, or going to worship, to a restaurant, or to group events.[62] Furthermore, people with disabilities are less likely to be employed, and if employed, they are more likely to have lower income than people without disabilities.[62]

Geographic Location

Health disparities have also been observed among people living in rural areas. For example, adult men and women living in rural areas are less likely to use preventive services such as mammograms, Pap smears, proctosigmoidoscopy, and influenza and pneumococcal vaccinations.[2]

Socioeconomic Status

Another vulnerable segment of the US population are people classified as being of lower socioeconomic status (SES). This segment of the population also experiences worse health outcomes when compared with the higher SES group; for example, children from lower SES communities were found to have higher injury hospitalization and mortality rates[65]; and white, black or African American, and Mexican American men and women living in neighborhoods with lowest incomes were found to have two to four times higher mortality rates than those living in neighborhoods with the highest incomes.[66] Lower SES was also associated with lower reported health status and higher mortality.[67]

The Census Bureau reported that, in 2002, poor people were more likely to be without health insurance for the entire year independent of gender, race or ethnicity, or nativity.[68] Newacheck et al reported that, from 1979 to 2002, black or African American children experienced a higher prevalence of disability than white children. However, the investigators' multivariate analysis indicated that the difference in disability between blacks or African Americans and Whites could be explained entirely by differences in poverty status.[69]

▶ FACTORS CONTRIBUTING TO HEALTH DISPARITIES

Racial and ethnic variations in health result from variations in an individual's exposures or vulnerability and are a reflection of issues related to the health-care system. At the individual and community level, factors that contribute to variations in health include behavioral and psychosocial factors, material factors (education, occupation, and income), and environmental living conditions and resources. Health system factors include issues of access to health-care systems (physical, financial, and practical access [ie, customer friendliness]), access to services within the system (getting appointments, completing referrals to specialists, getting after-hours advice), health services utilization, healthcare quality, and the ability of the system and providers to effectively address patients' needs (awareness of patients' conditions and functional limitations, knowledge and clinical skills, and cultural competence). These factors are interdependent, affect one another to a large extent, and often are driven by socioeconomics.

Socioeconomics

Being in a lower socioeconomic class usually means having poorer housing conditions, fewer opportunities for higher education, less health insurance coverage, and lower access to health care. Environmental health risks—such as degradation; air, water and soil pollution; and other physical hazards—are more prevalent in low-income racial and ethnic minority communities. Individual risk factors for poor health are pronounced among many racial and ethnic minorities, and these risks are confounded by the disproportionate representation of minorities in the lower socioeconomic classes, as well as hazardous and low-paying occupations. For ex-

ample, in 1996 50% of all garbage collectors, over 33% of all elevator operators, and 33% of all nursing aides and orderlies were blacks or African Americans. Similarly, more than 75% of all miscellaneous woodworkers, 68% of all farm product graders and sorters, 37% of all farm workers, and 34% of all fabric machine operators were Latino.

Many classic case studies have documented differential exposure to work-related toxicants, resulting in disproportionately high rates of occupational diseases among miners, steelworkers, chemical-industry workers, rubber and textile workers, and others.[70,71] Moreover, SES, in and of itself, is correlated with health status independently of individual risk factors, because people in each ascending step along the socioeconomic gradient tend to have better health, even when individual health risk factors are accounted for.[72] Thus, research into the reasons for health differences between racial and ethnic groups has focused largely on differences in SES (income, wealth, unemployment, and social support) and the associated access to preventive health-care services, suggesting that inequalities in income and education underlie some health disparities.[73–75] Other factors, however, clearly enter the picture, as minorities with supposedly equal access to care through insurance coverage and those employed still suffer worse health outcomes when compared with whites.

During the past 40 years, major changes occurred that were expected to drastically reduce or eliminate socioeconomic differences in health: infectious disease has declined as a leading cause of morbidity and mortality; adequate nutrition, housing, water, and waste disposal have become available to most American families; and Medicaid and Medicare (federal health insurance for the poor and elderly) have put health care within the reach of many of the poor. Nevertheless, socioeconomic differences in health persist, and the traditional explanations alone have limited power to explain the continuing association between social stratification and health.[74,76]

Culture and Acculturation

Culture is defined as the integrated pattern of human knowledge, belief, and behavior that depends on the human capacity for learning and transmitting knowledge to succeeding generations.[77] That cultural factors—the customary beliefs, social forms, and material traits of a racial, religious, or social group[77]—also play a role in health disparities is demonstrated by differences in health status among different subpopulations in the United States. For example, among some immigrant Hispanic populations, birth outcomes have been found to be better than those of their US-born peers, suggesting that sociocultural risk increases with subsequent generations living in the United States.[78]

Data show that despite the fact that Mexican Americans tend to be poorer, less educated, and medically underserved compared with non-Hispanic whites, they are astonishingly healthy. Mexican American rates of infant mortality and low birth weight are equivalent to those for non-Hispanic whites and half those of blacks or African Americans, and overall mortality among Mexican Americans is lower than that among non-Hispanic whites.[5] Mexican Americans also have low rates of lung cancer, heart disease, and chronic respiratory disease.[79] These findings illustrate what researchers refer to as a paradox, because they are contrary to historical assumptions that increased risk associated with ethnicity can be explained in terms of genetic differences related to race or factors related to SES.[79]

In a 1989 study of low birth weight among Mexican Americans, Scribner and Dwyer proposed that factors associated with Mexican cultural orientation may be protective against the risk of low birth weight among Mexican Americans.[80] Scribner further suggests that this "acculturation" hypothesis explains the paradox in terms of cultural orientation linked to ethnicity.[79] Mexican American ethnicity is a marker of a Mexican cultural orientation that is defined by behavioral norms that can account for their favorable health status. Mexican Americans as a group smoke less, drink less, and eat a better diet than do non-Hispanic whites.[79] Over time, and once Mexican Americans have been fully acculturated in the high-risk environments of socioeconomically disadvantaged communities, their behavioral norms and health outcomes come to resemble those of other socioeconomically disadvantaged groups living in similar community environments.[79] Many studies have examined acculturation and reported that it does affect behaviors and the health status of immigrants. For example, recent adolescent immigrants were at lower risk than other students in relation to substance use,[81] greater acculturation was found to be associated with poorer childhood immunization status,[82] and Mexican American women had generally more undesirable behaviors and risk factors than Mexican immigrant women.[83] On the other hand, Mexican Americans who were born in the United States had a lower level of physical inactivity during leisure time[84]; older, US-born Hispanics were less likely to be current smokers[85]; and women who were more acculturated had significantly higher odds of ever and recently receiving a clinical breast examination and a mammogram than did less acculturated women.[86]

Racism and Discrimination

Racism is defined as "a belief that race is the primary determinant of human traits and capacities, and that racial differences produce an inherent superiority of a particular race."[77] Marx further proposes that, put into practice, racism refers to relationships in which one group, supposedly distinguished by physical differences, has more power (political, economic, military) than another, and can and does use that power to act on or against a similarly distinguished oppressed group. Racism is distinguished from prejudice, in that prejudice is a preconceived idea that is usually unfavorable but is not necessarily acted on with power and authority.[87]

Jones offers a basic framework for understanding racism and how it influences health outcomes. She proposes that racism exists at three levels: institutionalized, personally mediated, and internalized.[88] Institutionalized racism manifests itself both in material conditions (eg, differential access to quality education, sound housing, gainful employment, appropriate medical facilities, and a clean environment) and in access to power (eg, differential access to information, resources, and voice, including voting rights, representation in government, and control of the media). Institutionalized racism is often evident as inaction in the face of need.[88] Personally mediated racism is defined as prejudice (differential assumptions about the abilities, motives, and intentions of others based on their race) and discrimination (differential actions toward others based on race). Personally mediated racism can be intentional or unintentional and includes acts of commission as well as of omission. This form of racism manifests itself as lack of respect (poor or no service, failure to communicate options), suspicion (shopkeepers' vigilance; everyday avoidance, including street crossing, purse clutching, and standing when there are empty seats on public transportation), and devaluation (surprise at competence, stifling of aspirations, scapegoating, and dehumanization). Internalized racism is the acceptance by members of stigmatized races of negative messages about their own abilities and intrinsic worth, characterized by their not believing in others who look like them and not believing in themselves. Internalized racism manifests as an embracing of "whiteness," self-devaluation, resignation, helplessness, and hopelessness.[88]

Krieger et al and Williams et al suggest that discrimination and racism may create stress leading to poorer health among members of racial minority groups.[89,90] Research indicates that racial discrimination and racism have a significant impact on health and are important contributors to the racial and ethnic health disparities in the United States.[58,73,74,88–92] For example, Krieger and Sidney reported that systolic blood pressure was higher among black or African American adults who experienced racial discrimination and accepted unfair treatment, compared with those who experienced racial discrimination but reported that they challenged unfair treatment.[91] In a population-based survey of Chinese Americans living in Los Angeles, Gee reported that individual and institutional measures of racial discrimination were associated with health status of minority group members after controlling for acculturation, sex, age, social support, income, health insurance, employment status, education, neighborhood poverty, and housing value.[92]

Psychosocial Factors

Some researchers propose that psychosocial factors (health behaviors, stress in family, residential and occupational environments, social integration and support, perception of mastery and control, social ties, and attitudinal orientations) represent critical links between social structure and health status.[74,76] The social distribution of these factors represents the patterned response of social groups to the realities and constraints of the external environment imposed on them by social structure. Intervening mechanisms between social structure and health status are adaptive to the living and working conditions of the poor.[74] Accordingly, efforts to change the lifestyle of the poor without also altering social structure and life chances not only may be ineffective, but may do more harm than good. It has been reported that health education campaigns achieve only limited success and are more effective in producing behavior change in persons from higher socioeconomic levels than in their lower-level peers. For example, cigarettes are widely believed to alleviate stress and tension, and persons of lower SES face more stress and have fewer resources to cope with it than their better educated peers; thus strategies to promote smoking cessation could be much more complex among minority populations.[74]

Access to Care

Racial and ethnic minorities are less likely than whites to possess health insurance coverage and, even when insured, may face additional barriers to care because of other socioeconomic factors, such as high copayments, geographic factors, and insufficient transportation. For example, Newacheck et al found that minority children with special health care needs were more likely to be without both health insurance coverage and a usual source of care, and to report inability to obtain needed medical care.[93] Poverty appears to be a major factor affecting access to care; in 2002, the proportion of people without health insurance for the entire year was much higher for all racial and ethnic groups living in poverty, reaching 42.8% for poor Hispanics[67] (see Fig. A–9). Several other factors contributed to having health insurance: gender, age, nativity, household income, education, and work experience. In each case, people living in poverty were much more likely to have no health insurance for the entire year than the general public with similar characteristics.[67]

Health Care

Beyond access-related factors, the IOM's Committee on Understanding and Eliminating Racial and Ethnic Disparities in Health Care concluded that a range of patient-level, provider-level, and system-level factors may be involved in racial and ethnic health care disparities. At the patient level, minority patients are more likely to refuse recommended services, adhere poorly to treatment regimens, and delay seeking care.[94,95] However, the committee concluded that racial and ethnic differences in patient preferences, care-seeking behaviors, and attitudes are unlikely to be major sources of health-care disparities.

At the health systems level, the ways in which systems are organized and financed, and the availability of services, may exert differential effects on patient care, particularly for racial and ethnic minorities. Minority populations have less access to care independent of their insurance status because fewer physicians and clinics exist in their communities.[96] And where health facilities exist, they may be less well equipped or staffed, or be overcrowded. Moreover, people who are members of minority groups are less likely to be referred for tests, or to receive specialty care, mental health care, or needed procedures and surgery. Language barriers, for example, pose a problem for many patients in areas where health systems lack the resources, knowledge, or institutional priority to provide interpretation and translation services. Similarly, time pressures on physicians may hamper their ability to accurately assess presenting symptoms of minority patients, especially where cultural or linguistic barriers are present.

Several factors may contribute to disparities in health care at the provider level: greater clinical uncertainty when interacting with minority patients, bias or prejudice against minorities, and beliefs or stereotypes held by the provider about the behavior or health of minorities.[58] In deciding on a diagnosis and course of treatment, a physician must balance new information gained from a patient with his or her prior knowledge and expectations about the patient. If the physician has difficulty accurately assessing and understanding a patient's presenting symptoms and condition, he or she is likely to place greater weight on prior knowledge and expectations, resulting in an imbalance between treatment decisions and the patient's needs. Moreover, there is considerable empirical evidence that even well-meaning whites who are not overtly biased and who do not believe that they are prejudiced typically demonstrate unconscious implicit negative racial attitudes and stereotypes.[97] Survey research suggests that among white Americans, prejudicial attitudes toward minorities remain more common than not, as over half to three quarters believe that relative to whites, minorities—particularly blacks or African Americans—are less intelligent, more prone to violence, and prefer to live off of welfare.[98] The committee concluded that, while there is no direct evidence that provider biases affect the quality of care for minority patients, research suggests that health-care providers' diagnostic and treatment decisions, as well as their feelings about patients, are influenced by patients' race or ethnicity,[99–101] and, that the relationship between race or ethnicity and treatment decisions is complex and may also be influenced by providers' gender, perceptions, and attitudes toward patients, often in subtle ways.[58]

▶ PROGRAMS AND INTERVENTIONS

Over the past 20 years, health disparities have attracted the attention of many policy and program leaders at all levels. Programs have been developed, implemented, and evaluated at the local, state, and federal levels in an effort to "close the gap" in health disparities. Numerous recent federal initiatives were established both to draw attention to the problem of health disparities and to develop and implement concrete plans to address these disparities within the medical, academic, research, and public health communities. Programs have been initiated and supported technically and financially within all agencies of the federal DHHS to improve access to care, quality of care, workforce diversity, and cultural competence. During the 1990s, DHHS measured national trends in race- and ethnic-specific rates for 17 Health Status Indicators. All racial and ethnic groups experienced improvements in rates for 10 of the 17 indicators but, despite the overall improvements, in some areas racial and ethnic disparities remained the same or even increased.[102]

It is difficult to obtain a comprehensive inventory of federal programs, because almost every agency has initiated special projects to study the racial and ethnic disparity in health and to act to close the gap. Websites and publications of the various DHHS agencies list multiple projects ranging from presidential initiatives to department initiatives and agency projects. Following are some examples:

- The Health Resources and Services Administration's (HRSA) Minority Management Development Program is a public–private partnership initiative designed to enhance the representation of minority managers and administrators in the managed care industry. The program provides managerial training, work experience, and knowledge of the industry through focused didactic and interactive training opportunities. (For more information, see the department's website, at *http://www.hrsa.gov/OMH/OMH/main2_projects.htm#10.*)

- The Office of Management and Budget, Executive Office of the President, issued and modified Directive 15 (discussed earlier) to provide guidance on classification of race and ethnicity for use in civil rights monitoring and enforcement. (See *http://clinton4.nara.gov/OMB/fedreg/ombdir15.html.*)

- The Office of the Secretary of Health and Human Services prepares and monitors the Healthy People objectives discussed earlier (http://www.healthypeople.gov/) and created the "Cross Cultural Health Care Program" in 1992 to serve as a bridge between communities and health-care institutions to ensure access to health care that is culturally and linguistically appropriate. This program facilitates cultural competency training for providers and medical staff, interpreter training for community interpreters and bilingual health-care workers, outreach to underrepresented communities, community-based research, interpreter services, translation services, and publications and videos relating to cross-cultural health care. (See *http://www.xculture.org/.*)

- The Agency for Healthcare Research and Quality (AHRQ) has awarded grants to nine Excellence Centers to Eliminate Ethnic/Racial Disparities (EXCEED). Each center is investigating a different theme in an effort to understand causes of and factors influencing inequalities, and to identify and eliminate the causes of health disparities. (See *http://www.ahrq.gov/research/exceed.htm.*)

- The Centers for Medicare and Medicaid Services supports the Historically Black Colleges and Universities Grant Program (HBCUGP) and the Hispanic Health Services Research Grant Program (HHSRGP) to increase the pool of black or African American and Hispanic researchers available to carry out the research, demonstration, and evaluation activities of the center and to support governmental and foundation research in the health services area for the black or African American and Hispanic communities. Funding is provided to conduct research related to health-care delivery and health financing issues affecting minority populations, including issues of access to health care; utilization of health services; quality of services; health screening, prevention, and education; racial health disparities; social and economic differences; managed care systems; and costs of care. (See *http://www.cms.hhs.gov/researchers/priorities/grants.asp#HBCU.*)

- The National Institutes of Health (NIH) established the Trans-NIH Working Group to Develop a Strategic Research Agenda on Health Disparities, consisting of each NIH institute and center director. The goals of the working group are to develop a 5-year strategic research agenda; recruit and train minority investigators; form new and enhance current partnerships with minority and other organizations working to close health gaps; advance community outreach activities; define, code, track, analyze, and evaluate progress more uniformly across the agency; and enhance public awareness. (See *http://healthdisparities.nih.gov/working.html.*)

- The Centers for Disease Control and Prevention (CDC) implements the Racial and Ethnic Approaches to Community Health (REACH) project and supports many other projects targeted toward reducing and eliminating health disparities, such as the National Program for Cancer Registry, Alaska Native Colorectal Cancer Education Project, Hispanic Colorectal Cancer Outreach and Education Project, National Comprehensive Cancer Control Program, National Breast and Cervical Cancer Early Detection Program, National Training Center, and Research on Prostate Cancer Screening Behaviors. (See *http://www.cdc.gov/omh/AMH/AMH.htm.*) REACH 2010 is a federal project designed to eliminate disparities in six priority areas by the year 2010: cardiovascular disease, immunizations, breast and cervical cancer screening and management, diabetes, HIV and AIDS, and infant mortality. The racial and ethnic groups targeted by REACH 2010 are blacks or African Americans, American Indians, Alaska Natives, Asian Americans, Hispanic Americans, and Pacific Islanders. Local and community-based coalitions design, implement, and evaluate community-driven strategies to eliminate health disparities. (See *http://www.cdc.gov/reach2010.*)

State and local programs also play an integral role in reducing health disparities, and almost all states have initiated projects to narrow and eliminate health disparities. For example, in the state of California, the Healthy Start initiative sought to improve the lives of children, youth, and families. Healthy Start provided comprehensive services within the community, school, and home to produce measurable improvements in school readiness, educational success, physical health, emotional support, and family strength. In a 1997 statewide evaluation of Healthy Start Works, the California Department of Education reported that parents and students expressed strong support and guidance when needed as well as increased test scores and parent involvement in school activities. (For more information, see *http://www.cde.ca.gov/ls/pf/hs/facts.asp.*)

▶ EVALUATION

Most programs and initiatives developed to reduce or eliminate health disparities have yet to be evaluated using rigorous methodologies. Evaluation of such programs is complicated because of the multifactorial nature of disparities and the difficulty of having any one factor for reducing disparities emerge independent of others. Thus, in many cases when evaluation was conducted, it focused on process rather than outcome, because process is a more readily observable phenomenon.

The REACH 2010 evaluation model uses the following five stages to guide the collection of qualitative and quantitative data:

1. **Capacity building.** Community coalition actions to reduce disparities.
2. **Targeted actions.** Intervention activities believed to bring about a desired effect.
3. **Community and system changes.** Changes to the community environment and to the knowledge, attitudes, beliefs, and behaviors of influential individuals or groups.
4. **Widespread risk and protective behavior changes.** Changes in rates of risk-reduction behaviors among a significant percentage of community members.
5. **Health disparity reduction**. Narrowing gaps in health status.

Positive behavior changes that have reduced health risks among REACH 2010 communities to date include increases in the percentages of community members receiving mammograms, Pap smears, and cholesterol and glycosylated hemoglobin screenings. These changes have helped to reduce disparities in cholesterol and blood sugar screenings.

The Medical University of South Carolina at Charleston and the Georgetown REACH Diabetes Coalition have formed an urban–rural coalition to improve the health of more than 12,000 blacks or African Americans with diagnosed diabetes in Charleston and Georgetown counties. After 24 months of program participation, blacks or African Americans have more physical activity in their lives, healthier foods at group activities, and better diabetes care and control. Between 1999 and 2002, the gap between blacks or African Americans and whites in annual A_{1c} testing, which is used to measure blood glucose control, was virtually eliminated. The goal of the coalition is to eliminate all disparities in diabetes care and control in Charleston and Georgetown counties by 2007. (For further information, see *http://www.cdc.gov/nccdphp/aag/aag_reach.htm.*)

One of the most successful programs in eliminating health disparities has been the CDC efforts under the Childhood Immunization Initiative to eliminate disparities in vaccine coverage. During the 1989–1991 measles epidemic, which produced more than 55,000 cases of measles, the incidence of measles in minority children was four to seven times higher than that among white children.[103–105] As part of this initiative, a dual immunization strategy was developed with interventions likely to reach the majority of children (eg, increased funding for health departments and for vaccine programs, research, national public information campaigns, and annual state surveys of vaccine coverage). Additional interventions were designed to reach subgroups of the population with higher proportions of children from racial and ethnic minorities (eg, the Vaccine for Children program, free vaccines for uninsured or underinsured children, local immunization action plans, user-friendly hours for public clinics, special information campaigns).[103] As a result of these strategies, and in addition to dramatically improving vaccination coverage and eliminating measles in all racial and ethnic populations, the vaccination coverage gap between white and minority children was reduced from 15% in 1985 (49% among minorities and 64% among whites), to 6% in 1992 (78% among minorities and 84% among whites), and to 2% in 1997 (89% among blacks or African Americans, 88% among Hispanics, 92% among

American Indians or Alaska Natives, and 90% among whites).[104]

► SUMMARY AND RECOMMENDATIONS

Health disparities are the product of a multitude of factors, among them, racism; psychosocial, cultural, socioeconomic, and environmental factors; quality of care factors; and policy factors. Many of these factors fall outside the influence of the health-care system. Accordingly, the elimination of inequalities in health status ultimately may require changes not only in psychosocial factors (lifestyle characteristics and living conditions) and health-care delivery, but also in socioeconomic conditions.[74]

Health services interventions, alone or in collaboration with social and economic interventions, are likely to play a significant role in reducing racial and ethnic health disparities. The health-care system can contribute by addressing specific factors that have an impact on health disparities, such as understanding and targeting population-specific differences in risk factors for illness, developing prevention messages with a specific clinical or population focus, and promoting adequate utilization of self-care principles and health-promoting services by vulnerable populations. This will require enhanced data collection to define the various components of the problem (health indicators as well as access, utilization, workforce competence, health-care quality), develop targeted interventions to deal with each component, and implement these interventions in partnership with community-based organizations. The system should also intensify its efforts to ensure increasing use of services by underserved populations by making the system more accessible, responsive, and user-friendly. Steps in that direction include diversifying the health-care workforce and acting to improve the cultural competence of personnel. Above all, the health-care system must immediately deal with the issue of disparity in health care.[106] Over the past 20 years, numerous initiatives have been established both to draw attention to the problem of health disparities and to develop and implement concrete plans for addressing these disparities within the medical, academic, research, and public health communities. However, despite an overall improvement in health, in some areas racial and ethnic disparities remained the same or even increased.

The IOM Committee on Understanding and Eliminating Racial and Ethnic Disparities in Health Care recommended a comprehensive, multilevel strategy to eliminate health-care disparities. The committee recommended that all sectors involved in health-care delivery— including health-care providers, their patients, payers, health plan purchasers, and society at large—work together to ensure that all patients receive high-quality health care. The committee's first recommendation was to avoid fragmentation of health plans along socioeconomic lines. Racial and ethnic minorities are more likely than whites to be enrolled in "lower-end" health plans, which are characterized by higher per capita resource constraints and stricter limits on covered services.[107] The disproportionate presence of racial and ethnic minorities in lower-end health plans is a potential source of health-care disparities. Such socioeconomic fragmentation of health plans engenders different clinical cultures, with different practice norms, tied to varying per-capita resource constraints.[108] Equalizing access to high-quality plans can limit such fragmentation.

The committee further recommended strengthening the stability of patient–provider relationships in publicly funded health plans. Several lines of research suggest that the consistency and stability of the physician–patient relationship is an important determinant of patient satisfaction and access to care. Having a usual source of care is associated, for example, with use of preventive care services.[109]

The committee suggests that training and education of health-care providers are essential components of the proposed overall strategy. Educating health-care providers to make them aware of racial and ethnic disparities in health care, and the fact that these disparities often exist, despite providers' best intentions, can help alleviate stereotypes, bias, and clinical uncertainty that may influence clinicians' diagnostic and treatment decisions. Cross-cultural training of all current and future health-care providers can enhance their awareness of how cultural and social factors influence health care while providing methods to obtain, negotiate, and manage this information clinically once it is obtained. Cross-cultural education can be divided into three conceptual approaches focusing on *attitudes* (cultural sensitivity and awareness approach), *knowledge* (multicultural and categorical approach), and *skills* (cross-cultural approach).[58] It is also extremely important to intensify efforts to recruit and train more providers from disadvantaged minority backgrounds.

The IOM committee recommended increased efforts to collect data on patient and provider race and ethnicity to allow researchers to better disentangle factors associated with health-care disparities, help health plans monitor performance, ensure accountability to enrolled members and payers, improve patient choice, allow for evaluation of intervention programs, and help identify discriminatory practices.[58] The committee made further recommendations in conjunction with the training and educational strategies to eliminate racial and ethnic disparities in health care, including policy and regulatory strategies that address fragmentation of health plans along socioeconomic lines, and health systems interventions to the use of clinical practice guidelines and the use of interpretation services where community need exists.

There is an urgent need for the development of comprehensive programs that rely on evidence of successful interventions and avoid a one-size-fits-all approach. There is also a need for better coordination of initiatives and collaboration among public institutions, private foundations, and professional associations to achieve national health objectives. Health-care interventions should target high-risk populations; focus on the most important contributing factors for a given community, population, or disease condition; use culturally and linguistically appropriate methods; include measures of quality of care and health outcomes; and prioritize dissemination efforts.[75]

▶ REFERENCES

1. National Institutes of Health. *Addressing Health Disparities: The NIH Program of Action. What Are Health Disparities?* Available at: http://healthdisparities.nih.gov/whatare.html.

2. Casey MM, Thiede CK, Klingner JM. Are rural residents less likely to obtain recommended preventive health care services? *Am J Prev Med* 2001;21(3):182–188.

3. Arias E, Anderson RN, Hsiang-Ching K, et al. Deaths: Final data for 2001. *National Vital Statistics Reports,* vol 52, No. 3. Hyattsville, Md: National Center for Health Statistics; 2003.

4. Erickson P, Wilson R, Shannon I. Years of healthy life. *Healthy People 2000 Statistical Notes.* Atlanta, Ga, and Hyattsville, Md: Centers for Disease Control and Prevention, National Center for Health Statistics; 1997.

5. National Center for Health Statistics. *Health, United States, 2003.* Hyattsville, Md: NCHS; 2003.

6. Centers for Disease Control and Prevention. Summary of notifiable diseases, United States, 2001. *MMWR Morb Mortal Wkly Rep* 2001;50(53):1–22. Available at: http://www.edc.gov/mmwr/DPF/wk/mm 5033.pdf.

7. Shapiro MF, Morton SC, McCaffrey DF, et al. Variations in the care of HIV-infected adults in the United States: Results from the HIV Cost and Services Utilization Study. *JAMA* 1999;281(24):2305–2315.

8. Geronimus AT, Bound J, Waidmann TA, et al. Excess mortality among blacks and whites in the United States. *N Engl J Med* 1996;335(21):1552–1558.

9. Liao Y, Cooper RS, Cao G, et al. Mortality patterns among adult Hispanics: Findings from the NHIS, 1986 to 1990. *Am J Public Health* 1998;88(2):227–232.

10. Klatsky AL, Tekawa I, Armstrong MA, et al. The risk of hospitalization for ischemic heart disease among Asian Americans in northern California. *Am J Public Health* 1994;84(10):1672–1675.

11. Gibson C, Jung K. *Historical Census Statistics on Population Totals by Race, 1790 to 1990, and by Hispanic Origin, 1970 to 1990, for the United States, Regions, Divisions, and States*. Working Paper Series No. 56. Washington, DC: Population Division, US Census Bureau; 2002. Available at: http://www.census.gov/population/www/documentation/twps0056.html.

12. Overview of race and Hispanic origin. *US Census 2000 Brief*. Washington, DC: Dept of Commerce, Economics and Statistics Administration, US Census Bureau; 2001. Available at: http://www.census.gov/prod/2001pubs/c2kbr01-1.pdf.

13. *U.S. Interim Projections by Age, Sex, Race, and Hispanic Origin*. Washington, DC: US Census Bureau, Population Division, Population Projections Branch, US Dept of Commerce; 2004. Available at: http://www.census.gov/ipc/www/usinterimproj/.

14. Office of Management and Budget. Directive No. 15: Race and ethnic standards for federal statistics and administrative reporting. *Statistical Policy Handbook*. Washington, DC: US Dept of Commerce, Office of Federal Statistical Policy and Standards; 1978.

15. Office of Management and Budget. *Revisions to the Standards for the Classification of Federal Data on Race and Ethnicity*. Washington, DC: The White House; 1997. Available at: http://clinton4.nara.gov/OMB/fedreg/ombdir15.html.

16. The black population: 2000. *Census 2000 Brief*. Washington, DC: US Census Bureau, US Dept of Commerce, Economics and Statistics Administration; 2001.

17. The Hispanic population. *Census 2000 Brief*. Washington, DC: US Census Bureau, US Dept of Commerce, Economics and Statistics Administration; 2001. Available at: http://www.census.gov/prod/2001pubs/c2kbr01-3.pdf.

18. Rosenberg HM, Maurer JD, Sorlie PD, et al. Quality of death rates by race and Hispanic origin: A summary of current research, 1999. *Vital Health Statistics*, vol 2, No. 128. Hyattsville, Md: National Center for Health Statistics; 1999.

19. Centers for Disease Control and Prevention. Use of race and ethnicity in public health surveillance. Summary of the CDC/ATSDR Workshop. *MMWR Morb Mortal Wkly Rep* 1993;42(RR-10). Available at: http://www.census.gov/prod/2001pubs/c2kbr01-5.pdf.

20. Hetzel AM. *U.S. Vital Statistics System: Major Activities and Developments, 1950–1995*. Hyattsville, Md: National Center for Health Statistics; 1997.

21. Linder FE, Grove RD. *Vital Statistics Rates in the United States, 1900–1940*. Washington, DC: Federal Security Agency, US Public Health Service, National Office of Vital Statistics, Government Printing Office; 1947.

22. Grove RD, Hetzel AM. *Vital Statistics Rates in the United States 1940–1960*. Washington, DC: US Dept of Health, Education and Welfare, Public Health Service; 1968.

23. Anderson MJ. *The American Census: A Social History*. New Haven, Conn: Yale Univ Press; 1988.

24. *Report of the Vital and Social Statistics in the United States at the Eleventh Census: 1890. Part II—Vital Statistics*. Washington, DC: Dept of the Interior, Census Office, Government Printing Office; 1896.

25. *Census Reports Volume I: Twelfth Census of the United States, Taken in the Year 1900. Population, Part I*. Washington, DC: Dept of the Interior, Census Office, Government Printing Office; 1901.

26. *Mortality Statistics 1908. Ninth Annual Report*. Washington, DC: Dept of Commerce and labor, Bureau of the Census, Government Printing Office; 1910.

27. *Mortality Statistics 1923. Twenty-Fourth Annual Report*. Washington, DC: Dept of Commerce, Bureau of the Census, Government Printing Office; 1926.

28. *Vital Statistics of the United States 1975. Volume II: Mortality, Part A*. Hyattsville, Md: US Dept of Health, Education and Welfare, Public Health Service, National Center for Health Statistics; 1979.

29. *Mortality Statistics 1933. Thirty-Fourth Annual Report*. Washington, DC: Dept of Commerce, Bureau of the Census, Government Printing Office; 1936.

30. Williams DR. Race, socioeconomic status and health: The added effects of racism and discrimination. *Ann N Y Acad Sci* 1999;896:173–188.

31. Hahn R. The state of federal health statistics on racial and ethnic groups. *JAMA* 1992;267:268–271.

32. Sorlie PD, Rogot E, Johnson NJ. Validity of demographic characteristics on the death certificate. *Epidemiology* 1992;3(2):181–184.

33. Singh GK, Yu SM. Adverse pregnancy outcomes: Differences between US- and foreign-born women in major US racial and ethnic groups. *Am J Public Health* 1996;86(6):837–843.

34. Hambright TZ. Comparability of marital status, race, nativity, and country of origin on the death certificate and matching census record: United States, May–August 1960. *Vital Health Statistics*, vol 2, No. 34. Hyattsville, Md: National Center for Health Statistics; 1969.

35. National Center for Health Statistics. *Vital Statistics of the United States, Mortality. Technical Appendix 1995*. Washington, DC: Public Health Service; 1999.

36. US Public Health Service, Office of the Surgeon. *Healthy People: The Surgeon General's Report on Health Promotion and Disease Prevention*. DHEW (PHS) Publication No. 79-55071; 1979.

37. US Public Health Service. *Healthy People 2000: National Health Promotion and Disease Prevention Objectives*. Washington, DC: Dept of Health and Human Services, DHHS (PHS) Publication No. 91-50212; 1991.

38. US Dept of Health and Human Services. *Healthy People 2010*, 2nd ed. *With Understanding and Improving Health and Objectives for Improving Health*, 2 vols. Washington, DC: Government Printing Office; 2000.

39. National Center for Health Statistics. Recommendations from Committee 22.1. *Healthy People Statistics and Surveillance*, No. 4. Hyattsville, Md: Public Health Service; 1995.

40. Freedman MA. Health Status Indicators for the Year 2000. *Healthy People Statistical Notes*, vol 1, No. 1. Hyattsville, Md: National Center for Health Statistics; 1991.

41. Klein RJ, Hawk SA. Health status indicators: Definitions and national data. *Healthy People Statistical Notes*, vol 1, No. 3. Hyattsville, Md: National Center for Health Statistics; 1992.

42. *Healthy People 2010: Leading Health Indicators*. Available at: http://www.healthypeople.gov/document/html/uih/uih_4.html.

43. Martin JA, Hamilton BE, Sutton PD, et al. Births: Final data for 2002. *National Vital Statistics Reports*, vol 52, No. 10. Hyattsville, Md: National Center for Health Statistics; 2003.

44. Keppel KG, Pearcy JN, Wagener DK. Trends in racial and ethnic-specific rates for the health status indicators: United States, 1990–98. *Healthy People Statistical Notes*, No. 23. Hyattsville,

Md: National Center for Health Statistics; 2002.

45. Disability status: 2000. *Census 2000 Brief*. Washington, DC: US Dept of Commerce, Economics and Statistics Administration, US Census Bureau; 2003. Available at: http://www.census.gov/hhes/www/disability.html.

46. *Early Release of Selected Estimates Based on Data From the January–September 2003 National Health Interview Survey* (Released 03/24/04). Hyattsville, Md: National Center for Health Statistics. Available at: http://www.cdc.gov/nchs/about/major/nhis/released200403.html.

47. Grunbaum JA, Kann L, Kinchen S, et al. Youth risk behavior surveillance—United States, 2001. *MMWR Morb Mortal Wkly Rep* 2002;51(SS-4):4–68.

48. Bolen JC, Rhodes L, Powell-Griner EE, et al. State-specific prevalence of selected health behaviors, by race and ethnicity—behavioral risk factor surveillance system, 1997. *MMWR Morb Mortal Wkly Rep* 2000;49(SS02):1–60.

49. Kasiske BL. Race and socioeconomic factors influencing early placement on the kidney transplant waiting list. *J Am Soc Nephrol* 1998;9(11):2142–2147.

50. Barker-Cummings C, McClellan W, Soucie JM, et al. Ethnic differences in the use of peritoneal dialysis as initial treatment for end-stage renal disease. *JAMA* 1995;274:1858–1862.

51. Todd KH, Deaton C, D'Adamo AP, et al. Ethnicity and analgesic practice. *Ann Emerg Med* 2000;35(1):11–16.

52. Ayanian JZ, Weissman JS, Chasan-Taber S, et al. Quality of care by race and gender for congestive heart failure and pneumonia. *Med Care* 1999;37(12):1260–1269.

53. Harris DR, Andrews R, Elixhauser A. Racial and gender differences in use of procedures for black and white hospitalized adults. *Ethn Dis* 1997;7(2):91–105.

54. Wenneker MB, Epstein AM. Racial inequalities in the use of procedures for patients with ischemic heart disease in Massachusetts. *JAMA* 1989;261:253–257.

55. Whittle J, Conigliaro J, Good CB, et al. Racial differences in the use of invasive cardiovascular procedures in the Department of Veterans Affairs. *N Engl J Med* 1993;329(9):621–626.

56. McBean AM, Gornick M. Differences by race in the rates of procedures performed in hospitals

for Medicare beneficiaries. *Health Care Fin Rev* 1994;15(4):77–90.

57. Donaldson MS, ed. *Measuring the Quality of Health Care: A Statement by the National Roundtable on Health Care Quality.* Washington, DC: Division Of Health Care Services, Institute of Medicine, National Academy Press; 1999.

58. Smedley BD, Stith AY, Nelson AR, eds. *Unequal Treatment: Confronting Racial and Ethnic Disparities in Health Care.* Washington, DC: National Academies Press; 2002.

59. Kressin NR, Petersen LA. Racial differences in the use of invasive cardiovascular procedures: Review of the literature and prescription for future research. *Ann Intern Med* 2001;135(5):352–366.

60. Mayberry RM, Mili F, Ofili E. Racial and ethnic differences in access to medical care. *Med Care Res Rev* 2000;57(1):108–145.

61. Lollar DJ. Public health and disability: Emerging opportunities. *Public Health Rep* 2002;117:131–136.

62. *Healthy People 2010: Progress Review, Focus Area 6. Disability and Secondary Conditions.* Available at: http://www.cdc.gov/nchs/about/otheract/hpdata2010/focusareas/fa06-disability.html.

63. Kinne S, Patrick DL, Doyle DL. Prevalence of secondary conditions among people with disabilities. *Am J Public Health* 2004;94(3):443–445.

64. Brawarsky P, Brooks DR, Wilber N, et al. Tobacco use among adults with disabilities in Massachusetts. *Tob Control* 2002;11(suppl II):ii29–ii33.

65. Marcin JP, Schembri MS, He J, et al. A population-based analysis of socioeconomic status and insurance status and their relationship with pediatric trauma hospitalization and mortality rates. *Am J Public Health* 2003;93(3):461–466.

66. Winkleby MA, Cubbin C. Influence of individual and neighborhood socioeconomic status on mortality among black, Mexican-American, and white women and men in the United States. *J Epidemiol Community Health* 2003;57:444–452.

67. Franks P, Gold MR, Fiscella K. Sociodemographic, self-rated health, and mortality in the US. *Soc Sci Med* 2003;56:2505–2514.

68. *Health Insurance Coverage in the United States: 2002.* Washington, DC: US Census Bureau, US Dept of Commerce, Economics and Statistics Administration; 2003. Available at: http://www.census.gov/prod/2003pubs/p60-223.pdf.

69. Newacheck PW, Stein REK, Bauman L, et al. Disparities in the prevalence of disability between black and white children. *Arch Pediatr Adolesc Med* 2003;157:244–248.

70. Frumkin H, Walker ED, Friedman-Jimenez G. Minority workers and communities. *Occup Med* 1999;14(3):495–517.

71. Murray LR. Sick and tired of being sick and tired: Scientific evidence, methods, and research implications for racial and ethnic disparities in occupational health. *Am J Public Health* 2003;93(2):221–226.

72. Kaplan GA, Everson SA, Lynch JW. The contribution of social and behavioral research to an understanding of the distribution of disease: A multilevel approach. In: Smedley BD, Syme SL, eds. *Promoting Health: Intervention Strategies from Social and Behavioral Research.* Washington, DC: National Academy Press; 2000: 37–80.

73. House JS, Williams DR. Understanding and reducing socioeconomic and racial/ethnic disparities in health. In: Smedley BD, Syme SL, eds. *Promoting Health: Intervention Strategies from Social and Behavioral Research.* Washington, DC: National Academy Press; 2000:81–124.

74. Williams DR. Socioeconomic differentials in health: A review and redirection. *Soc Psychol Quart* 1990;53(2):81–99.

75. Cooper LA, Hill MN, Powe NR. Designing and evaluating interventions to eliminate racial and ethnic disparities in health care. *J Gen Intern Med* 2002;17(6):477–486.

76. Hogan VK, Njoroge T, Durant TM, et al. Eliminating disparities in perinatal outcomes—lessons learned. *Matern Child Health J* 2001;5(2):135–140.

77. *Merriam-Webster's Collegiate Dictionary,* 10th ed. Springfield, Mass: Merriam-Webster; 2002.

78. Korenbrot CC, Moss NE. Preconception, prenatal, perinatal, and postnatal influences on health. In: Smedley BD, Syme SL, eds. *Promoting Health: Intervention Strategies from Social and Behavioral Research.* Washington, DC: National Academy Press; 2000:125–169.

79. Scribner R. Paradox as paradigm—the health outcomes of Mexican Americans. *Am J Public Health* 1996;86(3):303–305.

80. Scribner R, Dwyer JH. Acculturation and low birthweight among Latinos in the Hispanic HANES. *Am J Public Health* 1989;79:1263–1267.

81. Blake SM, Ledsky R, Goodenow C, et al. Recency of immigration, substance use, and sexual behavior among Massachusetts adolescents. *Am J Public Health* 2001;91(5):794–798.

82. Anderson LM, Wood DL, Sherbourne CD. Maternal acculturation and childhood immunization levels among children in Latino families in Los Angeles. *Am J Public Health* 1997;87(12):2018–2021.

83. Zambrana RE, Scrimshaw SC, Collins N, et al. Prenatal health behaviors and psychosocial risk factors in pregnant women of Mexican origin: The role of acculturation. *Am J Public Health* 1997;87(6):1022–1026.

84. Crespo CJ, Smit E, Carter-Pokras O, et al. Acculturation and leisure-time physical inactivity in Mexican American adults: Results from NHANES III, 1988–1994. *Am J Public Health* 2001;91(8):1254–1257.

85. Perez-Stable EJ, Ramirez A, Villareal R, et al. Cigarette smoking behavior among US Latino men and women from different countries of origin. *Am J Public Health* 2001;91(9):1424–1430.

86. O'Malley AS, Kerner J, Johnson AE, et al. Acculturation and breast cancer screening among Hispanic women in New York City. *Am J Public Health* 1999;89(2):219–227.

87. Marx AW. Racial trends and scapegoating: Bringing in a comparative focus. In: Smelser NJ, Wilson WJ, Mitchell F, eds. *America Becoming: Racial Trends and Their Consequences.* Washington, DC: National Academy Press; 2001:302–317.

88. Jones CP. Levels of racism: A theoretical framework and a gardener's tale. *Am J Public Health* 2000;90(8):1212–1215.

89. Krieger N, Rowley DL, Herman AA, et al. Racism, sexism, and social class: Implications for studies of health, disease, and well-being. *Am J Prev Med* 1993;9(6 suppl):82–122.

90. Williams, DR, Risa LM, Rueben CW. The concept of race and health status in America. *Public Health Rep* 1994;109(1):26–41.

91. Krieger N, Sidney S. Racial discrimination and blood pressure: The CARDIA study of young black and white adults. *Am J Public Health* 1996;86(10):1370–1378.

92. Gee GC. A multilevel analysis of the relationship between institutional and individual racial discrimination and health status. *Am J Public Health* 2002;92(4):615–623.

93. Newacheck PW, Hung Y, Wright KK. Racial and ethnic disparities in access to care for children with special health care needs. *Ambulatory Pediatr* 2002;2:247–254.

94. Sedlis SP, Fisher VJ, Tice D, et al. Racial differences in performance of invasive cardiac procedures in a Department of Veterans Affairs Medical Center. *J Clin Epidemiol* 1997;50(8):899–901.

95. Mitchell JB, McCormack LA. Time trends in late-stage diagnosis of cervical cancer: Differences by race/ethnicity and income. *Med Care* 1997;35(12):1220–1224.

96. Kahn KL, Pearson ML, Harrison ER, et al. Health care for black and poor hospitalized Medicare patients. *JAMA* 1994;271(15):1169–1174.

97. Dovidio JF, Brigham JC, Johnson BT, et al. Stereotyping, prejudice, and discrimination: Another look. In: Macrae N, Stangor C, Hewstone M, eds. *Stereotypes and Stereotyping.* New York, NY: Guilford; 1996:276–319.

98. Bobo LD. Racial attitudes and relations at the close of the twentieth century. In: Smelser NJ, Wilson WJ, Mitchell F, eds. *America Becoming: Racial Trends and Their Consequences.* Washington, DC: National Academy Press; 2001:264–302.

99. Schulman KA, Berlin JA, Harless W, et al. The effect of race and sex on physicians' recommendations for cardiac catheterization. *N Engl J Med* 1999;340:618–626.

100. Weisse CS, Sorum PC, Sanders KN, et al. Do gender and race affect decisions about pain management? *J Gen Intern Med* 2001;16(4)211–217.

101. Van Ryn M, Burke J. The effect of patient race and socio-economic status on physician's perceptions of patients. *Soc Sci Med* 2000;50:813–828.

102. Campanelli RM. Addressing racial and ethnic health disparities. *Am J Public Health* 2003;93(10):1624–1626.

103. Atkinson W, et al. Measles. In: *Epidemiology, Control, and Prevention of Vaccine-Preventable Diseases,* 8th ed. 2004: Available at: http://www.cdc.gov/nip/publications/pink/default.htm.

104. Hutchins SS, Jiles R, Bernier R. Elimination of measles and of disparities in measles childhood

vaccine coverage among racial and ethnic minority populations in the United States. *J Invest Dermatol* 2004;189:146–152.

105. Flannery B, Schrag S, Bennett NM, et al. Impact of childhood vaccination on racial disparities in invasive *Streptococcus pneumoniae* infections. *JAMA* 2004;291:2197–2203.

106. Quill BE, DesVignes-Kendrick M. Reconsidering health disparities. *Public Health Rep* 2001;116(6):505–514.

107. Phillips KA, Mayer ML, Aday LA. Barriers to care among racial/ethnic groups under managed care. *Health Aff* 2000;19:65–75.

108. Bloche MG. Race and discretion in American medicine. *Yale J Health Pol Law Ethics* 2001;1:95–131.

109. Ettner SL. The timing of preventive services for women and children: The effect of having a usual source of care. *Am J Public Health* 1996;86(12):1748–1754.

CHAPTER 2

Geographic Studies of Black–White Mortality

ROBERT S. LEVINE, MD

NATHANIEL C. BRIGGS, MD, MSC

BAQAR A. HUSAINI, PhD

CHARLES H. HENNEKENS, MD, DrPH

▶ INTRODUCTION

No one would argue the existence of large health disparities in mortality by race in the United States.[1] It is more difficult, however, to quantify the magnitude of disparities in mortality for some racial and ethnic subgroups. Specifically, the available data on disparities in mortality among African Americans and Caucasians are the most widely, consistently, and longest studied and are considered to be the most reliable.[2] Data for other racial and ethnic subgroups are less consistently studied and only recently reported. As recently as 1979 to 1981, for example, only 21 states recorded Hispanic origin on the death certificate, and data from only 15 of these states were deemed of sufficient quality (at least 90% of deaths reported) to include in national reports.[2a]

In this chapter, we focus primarily on geographic studies of black–white differences in mortality, using the terms *black* and *white,* because that is how mortality data have been reported by the National Center for Health Statistics for most of the latter 20th century. Rather than excluding information on other racial and ethnic groups, however, these data are included as they occur in black–white investigations in order to present an accurate summary of the current literature. As will become apparent, geographic studies provide important relevant information that leads to proposals on how further research may identify modifiable determinants that could reduce observed disparities.

▶ GEOGRAPHIC STUDIES

Framework for Geographic Studies

The framework for studying the geographic distribution of disease is often ecologic, meaning that it focuses on comparisons between groups rather than individuals.[3] In ecologic studies, rates of disease are compared among many regions during the same period(s) of time. Frequently, they are used to identify spatial patterns consistent with an environmental effect.[4]

Advantages of ecologic studies include low cost and convenience; a capacity for providing estimates of exposures that may be difficult to obtain at the individual level; a further capacity for providing a wider range of exposures across groups than may be possible within a particular location; and a particular relevance to evaluating the impact of social processes or population interventions.[4] An important limitation of the ecologic approach is that group data may not reflect individual levels of exposure. Thus, for example, a correlation between the presence of certain industries and lung cancer across several counties might simply be due to a higher percentage of smokers in the counties in question.[4] Overestimating the importance of environmental factors in this way has become known as the "ecologic fallacy."[3] At the same time, recent studies have shown that important "area-level" or "contextual" determinants of disease may exist independently from individual-level factors. Moreover, area-level and individual-level factors can interact with each other to have synergistic or antagonistic effects.

Such studies, however, are complicated by two statistical problems. First, regions with smaller populations have unstable rates. Second, contiguous regions tend to be more alike than distant regions (autocorrelation).[4] Although statistical procedures can address autocorrelation,[4] another approach is to make comparisons that are transgeographic (ie, based on demographic comparability rather than geographic contiguity).[5,6] In most cases, this renders autocorrelation moot. Moreover, an exploratory focus in transgeographic study limits the need to include areas with unstable rates simply because they contribute to an understanding of spatial clustering. Finally, the study of variations in racial and ethnic disparities in contiguous or noncontiguous areas with similar demographic or risk characteristics is analogous to the approach used by Wennberg and Gittelsohn[7] in their studies of variations in health-care delivery in geographic areas of comparable demography and risk. It is possible that extension of the Wennberg–Gittelsohn

logic may be similarly productive in the area of research devoted to the reduction and elimination of health disparities.

Recent advances in ecologic research have also addressed the problem of including both individual-level and group-level measures in the same analysis. The most powerful of these methods, variously called *mixed-effects modeling, multilevel modeling,* or *hierarchical regression,*[4] permits an understanding of individual-level risk factors (biologic effects), ecologic factors (contextual effects), and their interactions. Comparative analyses of individual-ecologic–interactive effects could be used to compute attributable risk projections that identify the most efficient paths to racial equality. At the same time, this approach could assist in refining the meaning of "race" by identifying which individual–ecologic–interactive effects are needed to eliminate its influence on the occurrence of disease.

▶ NATIONAL STUDIES

Numerous investigations suggest that black race is primarily a surrogate for environmental exposures (eg, see Cooper and Freeman[7]; Jackson et al[8]; Schultz et al[9]; Williams et al[10]). The following section deals with health disparities in mortality between blacks and whites for the nation as a whole in terms of overall, infant, maternal, and childhood mortality, as well as mortality from selected causes of death.

Overall Mortality

Although black mortality in the United States began to decline at the beginning of the 20th century, Ewbank[11] was unable to find a single area or time when black mortality rates were close to white rates between 1850 and 1940. Tuberculosis was a major contributor to the difference during this period, but the problem extended to chronic diseases as well.[11] Figure 2–1A depicts the progress of overall age-adjusted

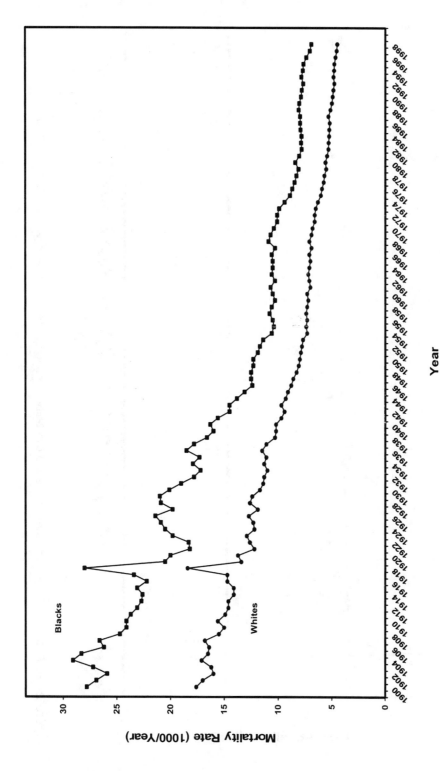

Figure 2-1A. US age-adjusted all-cause mortality rates for blacks and whites, 1900 to 1998. (Data from the National Center for Health Statistics and its predecessors.)

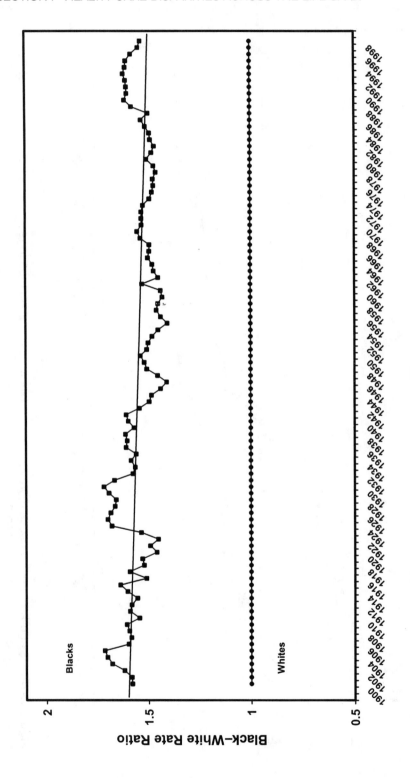

Figure 2-1B. Ratio of US age-adjusted all-cause mortality rates for blacks relative to whites, 1900 to 1998.

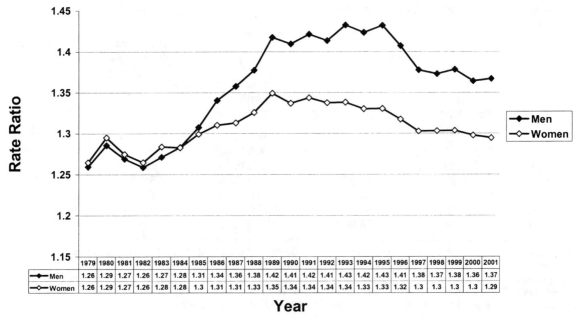

	1979	1980	1981	1982	1983	1984	1985	1986	1987	1988	1989	1990	1991	1992	1993	1994	1995	1996	1997	1998	1999	2000	2001
Men	1.26	1.29	1.27	1.26	1.27	1.28	1.31	1.34	1.36	1.38	1.42	1.41	1.42	1.41	1.43	1.42	1.43	1.41	1.38	1.37	1.38	1.36	1.37
Women	1.26	1.29	1.27	1.26	1.28	1.28	1.3	1.31	1.31	1.33	1.35	1.34	1.34	1.34	1.34	1.33	1.33	1.32	1.3	1.3	1.3	1.3	1.29

Figure 2–2. Gender-specific ratio of US age-adjusted all-cause mortality rates for blacks relative to whites, 1979–2001.

mortality rates among blacks and whites during the course of the 20th century as reported by the National Center for Health Statistics and its predecessors. Aside from the dramatic peak due to the influenza epidemic of 1918, progress in terms of declines in mortality rates and the absolute difference between the races was one of steady improvement for both races. Equality is a relative term, however, and as shown in Figure 2–1B, the relative position of blacks and whites, determined by mortality rate ratio, declined relatively little. Moreover, as shown in Figure 2–2, projections for black–white mortality based on national experience from 1945 to 1999 were for black–white mortality to increase.[1] During this period then, there was no evidence that any program produced a sustained decline in the relative position of black and white mortality rates. On the contrary, the record shows that the trend for the latter half of the 20th century was for the worse.[1]

These overall trends have been confirmed in a number of ways. For example, the esti-

mated life expectancy at birth for blacks in 1997 was 71.1 years overall, including 67.2 years for men and 74.7 years for women. These values approximate white values overall in 1966 (a 31-year lag), in men in 1957 (a 40-year lag), and in women in 1970 (a 27-year lag). Similar values for 1965 (the approximate midpoint between 1933 and 1997) were 22 years, 27 years, and 22 years, respectively. Age-adjusted all-cause mortality for blacks in 1998 was 6.9, which is the white value for 1969 (a 31-year gap). The corresponding figure for 1965 was 27 years.[1]

Another way of describing these patterns is shown in Table 2–1. This depicts the use of age-adjusted risk differences to estimate excess deaths among blacks. Based on the average of decennial values, plus that for 1998, it is estimated that there were 4,441,500 premature deaths among US blacks between 1940 and 1998 if the 1940 population standard is used and 4,158,900 if the year 2000 standard is used.[1] Since the start of the US *Healthy People* program, the average number of estimated excess deaths

▶ **TABLE 2–1.** Estimated Excess Deaths, African Americans Compared with Whites in the United States, 1940–1998

Year	White Population[a]	Black Population[a]	White–Black Mortality Rate Difference	Number of Excess Deaths (Mortality Rate Difference × Black Population)[b]	
				1940 Standard	Year 2000 Standard
1940	118,215	12,866	6.1/1000	78,500	66,700
1950	134,942	15,042	4.3/1000	66,700	52,200
1960	158,832	18,872	3.2/1000	60,400	50,200
1970	178,098	22,581	3.6/1000	81,300	73,300
1980	194,713	26,683	2.831/1000	75,500	80,600
1990	208,727	30,511	2.964/1000	90,400	103,900
2000	231,641	36,602	2.719/1000	—	99,520

[a]Population figures through 1990 are from the US Census Bureau, *Statistical Abstract of the United States*, Table 1412, 1999. Those for 2000 are from CDC Wonder System, 2004.

[b]The population at risk is taken to be the "black population" in column 3. For 1940–1990, these refer to data for the 1940 standard. For 2000, they refer to the year 2000 standard. Two estimates are provided, one that uses the 1940 population for age adjustment[6] and one that uses the year 2000 standard population for age adjustment.[35]

increased from 207 per day in 1980 (75,500) to 249 per day in 1998 (90,900), using the 1940 standard, and from 221 per day to 265 per day, using the year 2000 standard. In sum, although the estimated number of excess deaths per 1000 blacks declined during both periods, these gains were canceled by population growth so that the net effect was a steady increase in the number of excess deaths. In 1999 and 2000, the number of excess deaths using the year 2000 standard population was more than 100,000 per year.[12]

Studies seeking reasons for the national black–white gap have produced mixed results. The presence of the so-called crossover effect (ie, the lower mortality among blacks relative to whites after age 75)[13] suggested that if answers were to be found, they would have to be sought among younger age groups. Sorlie et al[14] therefore used data from the National Longitudinal Mortality Study to obtain information from about 500,000 whites and 50,000 blacks aged 25 years or older. In all, this translated into more than 2 million person-years of experience for whites and more than 200,000 person-years for blacks. There were 32,508 deaths in 7 years of follow up (1979 to 1985). Family income was used to investigate the extent to which excess mortality

among blacks could be explained as a function of their lower socioeconomic resources. First, it was found that low income was strongly associated with death among blacks and whites. Second, convergence between black and white mortality was noted at around 65 years of age, and was attributed to hardiness among survivors who had won through the excess mortality experiences of younger persons. Finally, family income only appeared to explain part of the excess risk among blacks younger than 65, accounting for 35% and 30% of excess all-cause mortality in men and women aged 25 to 44 years and 55% and 41% for men and women aged 45 to 64 years.

Initially, most studies of income inequality and mortality that followed this report focused on populations, with supporting data restricted primarily to ecologic correlations between indicators of income inequality and aggregate mortality or morbidity. This, however, led to criticisms about the validity of ecologic inferences, the measurement of income, the exclusion of covariates, and the applicability of the aggregate geographic unit.[15] From 1995 to 1998, however, these problems were addressed by research that included both aggregate and individual-level income information. Results were still unclear, however, leading LeClere and Soobader[15] to inquire about whether the apparent fragility of the income hypothesis could be explained, at least in part, by failure to include potential variations in income effects within subpopulations. They found that the morbidity of blacks of all ages, elderly whites, and middle-aged whites outside of the geographic areas of highest inequality were unaffected by income inequality when controls for individual characteristics and county-level poverty were in place. Mellor and Milyo,[16] who studied state-level mortality rates for 1960, 1970, 1980, and 1990, found that after controlling for regional variations in health outcomes, there was even less support for the hypothesis that income inequality is detrimental to either individual or population health. Their work is discussed in more detail later in this chapter, in the section on state-level investigations. As will be apparent from state and local area studies, the question of whether income inequality and racial composition produce independent effects is still controversial.

Another approach was taken by Hahn et al,[17] who conducted survival analysis to estimate the effect of poverty on mortality in a national sample of blacks and whites aged 25 to 74 years (the first National Health and Nutrition Examination Survey [NHANES I] and NHANES I Epidemiologic Follow-up Study). It was observed that in 1973, 6% of US mortality among black and white persons aged 25 to 74 years was attributable to poverty, and that in 1991, the corresponding figure was 5.9%. Rates of mortality attributable to poverty were lowest for white women, 2.2 times as high for white men, 3.6 times as high for black women, and 8.6 times as high for black men. After assessing confounding by known risk factors (eg, smoking, cholesterol levels, and physical inactivity), the effect of poverty on mortality among women was reduced by 42%, but there was little effect on the hazard ratio among men. It was concluded that commonly recognized risk factors did not explain the effect of poverty on mortality. Possible explanatory factors other than poverty or income-inequality have included differences in medical care, behavioral and lifestyle factors, and residential segregation[14]; failure to include prevention as a regular part of health care[1]; and social cohesion.[18]

In the United States since 1945 there has been no sustained, national improvement affecting black–white disparities in either overall age-adjusted mortality or overall life expectancy at birth. Forecasts based on total US experience since the end of World War II are poor regardless of whether inequality is measured by relative overall age-adjusted mortality, relative life expectancy, or gaps in either measure, and regardless of whether the 1940 or the year 2000 standard population is used for age adjustment.[1] Moreover, improvements in quality of life or other indicators would also fail to indicate success so long as disparities in mortality and life expectancy fail to improve. We have estimated that sustained disparities in health by race caused more than 4 million premature deaths among blacks during the 20th century.[1]

Changing a key national goal from "reducing" health disparities in *Healthy People 2000* to "eliminating" health disparities in *Healthy People 2010* signaled both a new level of determination to end these environmental barriers to health and tacit acknowledgment of disappointment.[1] In 1985, Margaret Heckler, then Secretary of the US Department of Health and Human Services, wrote: "There was a continual disparity in the burden of death and illness experienced by blacks and other minority Americans as compared with our Nation as a whole. That disparity began more than a generation ago and although our health charts do itemize steady gains in the health of minority Americans, the stubborn disparity remained . . . an affront to both [sic] our ideals and to the ongoing genius of American medicine."[19] Two decades later, little national progress has been made.

Infant Mortality

As was true for overall mortality, national trends for black–white infant mortality showed little evidence of relative improvement despite striking absolute declines. Analyzing race-specific infant mortality data for 1980 through 1999 and preliminary mortality data for 2000[20] the Centers for Disease Control and Prevention (CDC) found a greater decline among whites (from 10.9 per 1000 live births to 5.7 per 1000 live births, or 47.7%) than among blacks (from 22.2 to 14.0, or 36.9%). This was associated with an overall increase in the black–white mortality rate ratio from 2.0 to 2.5, although the bulk of the increase from 2.0 to 2.4 had occurred by 1990. The ratio remained stable at 2.4 for all years from 1990 to 1998, before increasing to 2.5 in 1999. The widening ratio was attributed to two main factors: (1) persistence of a two- to threefold risk for low birth weight (<2500 g) and very low birth weight (<1500 g) among black infants compared with white very-low-birth-weight infants; and (2) lower reductions in birth-weight-specific mortality rates among black very-low-birth-weight births compared with whites. Specifically, although 1990 to 2000 brought small improvements to black–white disparities in mortality from low birth weight (mortality rate ratio declined from 2.3 to 2.0) and very low birth weight (mortality rate ratio declined from 3.07 to 2.69), these were partly due to rising percentages of small infants (both low birth weight and very low birth weight) among whites rather than declines among blacks.[21,22]

Demissie et al,[22] who studied trends in preterm birth and neonatal mortality in the United States from 1989 to 1997, also commented on the rising percentage of low-birth-weight infants among whites. They noted that among whites, preterm births (<37 completed weeks of gestation) increased from 8.8% of live births in 1989 to 10.2% in 1997 (a 15.6% increase), while the corresponding figures for blacks were 19.0% and 17.5% (a 7.6% decrease). This, however, did not produce the anticipated mortality benefit because of suboptimal improvement in mortality among the remaining preterm infants. Specifically, neonatal mortality among preterm whites dropped 34% during the 8 years of observation, while the decrease was

only 24% among blacks. This meant that the percentage decline in neonatal mortality was similar for blacks and whites, with no benefit in disparities.

Interesting observations by Alexander et al[23] included the notation that among singleton live births to US resident mothers with a reported maternal ethnicity and race of non-Hispanic white, non-Hispanic black, or Hispanic in 1995 through 1997 (n = 10,610,715), blacks experienced lower risks of neonatal mortality for preterm and low-birth-weight infants, while having higher risks for mortality among term, postterm and normal, and macrosomic births.

Sources of the increased percentages of small infants among whites were attributed to "increases in pre-term delivery, changes in obstetrical practices, and induction of labor."[22] Changes in therapeutic practice that had a particular effect on whites included increased use of assisted reproductive therapies that were not only associated with low birth weight in singleton deliveries but also with small infants from increasing numbers of multiple birth pregnancies.[22] Causes of low and very low birth weight among blacks had a different profile from those affecting whites and could not be entirely explained by demographic risk factors such as maternal age, education, or income.[22,24] Instead, such factors as differences in medical history (including bacterial vaginosis, previous preterm birth, and other medical conditions), stress, social support, and unique life experiences may play a role.[22,25]

Beyond the frequency of low birth weight, a particular concern was that national advantages that low-birth-weight black infants had in the 1980s disappeared during the 1990s. As a result, the black–white mortality ratio for infants born at 1500 to 2499 g increased from 0.85 (26.6/31.4) in 1983 to 1.04 (16.5/15.9) in 1999, and the corresponding ratios for infants under 1500 g increased from 0.94 (378.4/404.0) to 1.15 (270.8/236.0).[20] These changes reflected disparities in mortality improvement that favored whites for specific medical disorders, such as respiratory distress syndrome[26,27–29] and may have been due to differential access to care that also favored whites.[26]

In addition to overall disparities, black–white disparities have been observed for twin births to teenagers born between 1995 and 1997.[28,30] Black rates, however, exceeded white rates only during the first 28 days of life (odds ratio [OR], adjusted for sibling correlations within twin pairs, 1.31; 95% confidence interval [CI], 1.11 to 1.54) and appeared to be more closely correlated with intrauterine growth retardation than with prematurity. After the neonatal period, black–white rates were comparable (adjusted OR, 0.86; 85% CI, 0.63 to 1.17).

As is true for overall mortality, there are many hypotheses about why national black–white differences in infant mortality exist, but none that have, to date, provided an answer that is likely to successfully eliminate the disadvantage experienced by black infants. However, a study by Vintzeleos et al[31] of 10,560,077 singleton births showed that disparities in fetal death were greater in the absence of prenatal care (17.2 versus 2.5 per 1000) than in the presence of prenatal care (4.2 versus 2.4 per 1000). They concluded that strategies to increase prenatal care participation, especially among blacks, are expected to decrease fetal death rates. Other studies indicating possible improvements may be found in more local studies, reviewed later in this chapter.

Maternal Mortality

National improvement in absolute maternal mortality has been far more dramatic than improvements in infant mortality, with a decline of over 100-fold from 0.85 per 1000 live births in 1900 to 0.0075 per 1000 live births in 1982. The overall decline halted in 1982, however, and black maternal mortality has been three to four times higher than white maternal mortality for over 60 years.[32] Optimism about overall progress is tempered somewhat by evidence that pregnancy-related mortality may be underreported by 30% to 150%.[32–36] In 1987, the CDC,

collaborating with state health departments and the American College of Obstetricians and Gynecologists Maternal Mortality Study Group, initiated a national Pregnancy Mortality Surveillance System. All 50 states, as well as the District of Columbia and New York City, provide the CDC with death certificates for all deaths occurring within 1 year of pregnancy termination, along with linked infant and fetal death certificates. These are supplemented by reports from state mortality review committees, the media, and individual providers. This information is systematically reviewed at the CDC to determine if the deaths are pregnancy related.

In a review of 4200 deaths incorporated within the Pregnancy Mortality Surveillance System between 1991 and 1999, Chang et al[32] found that the overall pregnancy-related mortality ratio (the number of deaths obtained by the surveillance system divided by the number of live births during the same period) increased from 10.3 to 13.2 during the period of observation ($P < .001$ for trend). Overall, the black–white pregnancy-related maternal mortality ratio was 3.7 times higher among blacks than whites (30.0 per 100,000 live births versus 8.1 per 100,000 live births; 95% CI, 2.9 to 4.7). Also, the black–white pregnancy-related maternal mortality ratio exceeded 1.00 for every leading characteristic examined, including whether prenatal care was absent, unknown, or initiated in the first, second, or third trimester; maternal age (<19 years, 20 to 24, 25 to 29, 30 to 34, 35 to 39 or >40); marital status (married or not married); and maternal education by age (<12 years, 12 years, or >12 years for mothers aged 20 to 24 years, 25 to 29, 30 to 34, 35 to 39 or >40).

For the most part, pregnancy outcomes associated with maternal mortality showed no statistically significant differences for blacks and whites, the sole exception being a twofold excess of ectopic pregnancy among blacks (8% versus 4%; $P < .001$). Although both black and white women experienced higher mortality associated with delivery of a fifth live birth as compared with a first live birth, black women had a three- to fourfold excess at each level of parity. The same pattern pertained for levels of education, where higher levels of education were protective for women older than 20 years of age, although levels for black women exceeded those for white women by three- to fourfold at every level. Similarly, although the leading causes of death for both black and white women were the same (embolism, hemorrhage, and pregnancy-induced hypertension), black women had a three- to fourfold greater chance of dying from these abnormalities and a sixfold greater risk of dying from cardiomyopathy and complications of anesthesia. Risk for black women was also particularly high among those older than 39 years, and unlike white women, mortality was higher among those who were married than those who were not. Additionally, the reduction in mortality among women receiving prenatal care compared with women receiving no prenatal care was higher among whites. Underlying reasons for the observed black–white differences cannot be obtained from existing surveillance data, in part because information about sociodemographic factors, family and community conditions, and other important items were not recorded on the certificates used for data collection. Similarly, detailed clinical data were not available, in part because the medical portion of the birth certificate (the lower section) was not consistently provided for inclusion in the surveillance database.

Childhood Mortality

DiLiberti[37] studied relationships between social stratification (measured by residential telephone availability) and all-cause mortality among children in the United States for the period 1968 through 1992. Although overall mortality rates declined, the differential affecting children living in the least advantaged counties worsened considerably between 1987 and 1992. These types of trends, however, were not found among black children, whose rates were far higher and slower to decline than those observed among whites.

Selected Causes

Age-adjusted black–white mortality ratios for most leading causes of death increased during the last two decades of the 20th century.[1] Overall in 1998, the life expectancy for blacks in the United States was 6 years lower than that for whites. Heart disease, cancer, and homicide were the top three contributors and account for most of the difference.[37a] Because 1998 was the last year during which the Ninth International Classification of Diseases (ICD-9) was used, comparisons beginning in 1999 were affected by limitations in comparability between the two systems at the time of this writing.

The following section deals with health disparities in mortality between blacks and whites for the nation as a whole for selected causes of death. These causes are presented in alphabetical order.

Acute Myocardial Infarction
Roig et al[38] used National Hospital Discharge Survey data for 1973 to 1984 to explore the observation of a crossover to lower mortality rates among blacks for mortality from coronary heart disease after age 70. In-hospital fatality rates were higher among nonwhites for each 20-year age group up to age 70, thereby duplicating the crossover observed in death certificate data. The age-specific trends in case-fatality were taken to support the hypothesis that cohort selection, in part, determines black–white disparities in coronary heart disease mortality. The authors cautioned against using age-adjusted rates, recommending instead age-specific rates for comparison of relative black–white risk.

Asthma
Several governmental and nongovernmental agencies have given asthma increased attention because of the increasing prominence of this

disease and because of its importance to the health of blacks. These include the CDC,[39] National Heart Lung and Blood Institute's National Asthma Education Prevention Program (NAEPP),[40] and the Pew Environmental Health Commission.[41]

The CDC's 2002 surveillance report for 1980 to 1999[39] shows that nationally, the age-adjusted black–white mortality rate ratio for asthma increased steadily, from 2.14 in 1980 to 2.23 in 1985, 2.34 in 1990, 2.46 in 1995, and 2.73 in 1999. Black mortality was 27.6 per 1 million population in 1980 and 38.7 per 1 million in 1999. Peak mortality among blacks during the period occurred in 1996 (48.0 per 1 million) with a decline to 44.7 per 1 million being observed in 1998. Data for 1999 are not directly comparable due in part to the 0.89 comparability ratio between ICD-9 and ICD-10 (with 0.89 meaning that 89% of deaths classified as being caused by asthma under the ICD-9 would be classified as asthma under the ICD-10). Even with the decline, however, black mortality from asthma increased 62% between 1980 (27.6 per 1 million) and 1998, while white mortality increased from 12.9 to 14.2 per 1 million (10%). During the same period, the estimated annual prevalence of asthma among blacks increased by 41% (from 33.1 to 46.7 per 1000 populations) while the corresponding figure for whites was 19% (from 31.4 to 37.5 per 1000 populations). CDC viewed adherence to published guidelines for asthma treatment as key to improvement.[39] Additional insight was provided by Grant et al,[41a] who used US mortality records for 1991 through 1996 to describe relations between socioeconomic factors and race or ethnicity as they pertained to national patterns of asthma mortality. They observed higher standardized mortality ratios for blacks versus whites (3.34 versus 0.65), low versus high educational level (1.51 versus 0.69) and low versus high income (1.46 versus 0.71). Although income and education were important, excess mortality for blacks was present in the highest and lowest quintiles of median county income and educational level.

Cancer

In 2003, an estimated 1.3 million Americans were diagnosed with cancer.[42] Among them, African Americans were expected to have a 10% higher incidence rate and a 30% higher death rate from all cancers combined than whites.[43] The US Surveillance Epidemiology and End Results (SEER) program collects cancer incidence and survival data on a routine basis from population-based cancer registries in various locations throughout the United States.[44] Among these, nine geographic areas (Connecticut; Hawaii; Iowa; New Mexico; Utah; Atlanta, Georgia; Detroit, Michigan; Seattle–Puget Sound, Washington; and San Francisco–Oakland, California) have participated since 1975. Based on 1990 census data, these nine SEER program areas comprise more than 9% of the US population, including 9% of non-Hispanic whites, 8% of Hispanic whites, 9% of African Americans, 29% of Asian Americans, 14% of American Indians, and 66% of Hawaiian natives.

Clegg et al[45] used this resource to assess cancer-specific survival rates for more than 1.78 million patients who resided in these areas between 1975 and 1997. Sex- and site-specific survival curves for patients diagnosed with cancer from 1988 to 1997 showed that male and female American Indians and Alaska Natives had the lowest survival rates for all cancers combined and for cancers of the breast, lung, and prostate. African Americans, however, had lower survival rates for colorectal, prostate, and breast cancer. Hispanic whites, non-Hispanic whites, and Asian Americans tended to have the best survival rates for these specific sites. Rates for Asian Americans, however, might have been affected by the inability to ascertain the outcome for those who may have returned to their homeland for family support or terminal care.[45] Although the authors suggested that differences in socioeconomic, medical, biologic, cultural, and other determinants could all play a role in explaining the observed differences, data from the SEER program itself could not provide differentiation.

Similar types of analyses have also been undertaken for the period 1995 through 1999.[43] They showed African American–white mortality rate ratios in excess of 1.0 among men and women for myeloma (2.0 in men; 2.5 in women), stomach (1.8; 2.2), esophagus (1.7; 2.2), larynx (1.7; 1.8), liver and intrahepatic bile duct (1.6; 1.6), pancreas (1.5; 1.6), kidney and renal pelvis (1.2; 1.3), and colon and rectum (1.1; 1.2 cancers). Values greater than 1.0 were found among men for cancers of the lung and bronchus (1.5), oral cavity and pharynx (1.3), and prostate (1.6). Corresponding values for women included small intestine (1.9), soft tissue (1.1), and uterine cervix (1.7). Notably absent from this list were female breast (0.9), female lung cancer (1.0), and non-Hodgkin lymphoma in both men and women (0.8; 0.7). The same authors reported lower 5-year survival rates for African Americans for 10 cancer sites, including prostate, female breast, urinary bladder, uterine cervix, colon and rectum, non-Hodgkin lymphoma, leukemia, oral cavity, lung and bronchus, and esophagus. Differences were not attributed to screening frequency, although the information cited did not address repeat screening. Economic disadvantage, higher prevalence of smoking in African American men, higher blood levels of cotinine, and greater consumption of heavily marketed cigarettes with higher levels of tar and nicotine among African American smokers in general, and lower levels of physical activity were also cited.

Additional SEER-based studies have addressed differential survival for breast cancer,[46,47] prostate cancer,[48] oral cancer,[49] and renal cancer.[50] National Cancer Institute studies have described patterns of occurrence of prostate cancer[51,52] and the leukemias.[53] The National Surgical Adjuvant Breast and Bowel project (NSABP), also sponsored by the National Cancer Institute, has investigated outcomes in colon cancer adjuvant therapy trials.[54]

Li et al[46] studied a cohort of 124,934 women diagnosed with a first primary invasive breast carcinoma between January 1, 1992 and December 31, 1998, including 97,999 non-Hispanic whites and 10,560 blacks. Blacks had a greater risk of presenting with stage 4 breast cancer than non-Hispanic whites and were also more likely to receive or elect a first course of surgical and radiation treatment not meeting the 2000 National Comprehensive Cancer Network standards. In addition, blacks had a greater risk of mortality than whites after a breast cancer diagnosis. Using breast cancer mortality rates for 1970 through 1995, SEER data for incidence rates from 1980 through 1995, and 3-year survival rates from 1980 through 1993, Chu et al[47] sought to learn why breast cancer mortality rates had decreased in the 1990s for white women but not for black women. They concluded that differential benefit from both early detection and treatment programs were of particular importance among women older than 40 years of age, and that declines in rates for women younger than 40 were most likely attributable to changes in risk factor status in that cohort.

Harlan et al's[48] study of prostate cancer documented a clear national trend toward more aggressive treatment, especially prostatectomy, during the study period (1984 to 1991). However, the proportion of black men receiving prostatectomy was substantially lower than among white men, and this disparity showed little change during the study period, even though rates among blacks increased. These results may, in part, explain the observations of Hsing and Devesa,[51] who used US mortality data from 1950 to 1989 to study prostate cancer mortality trends over time in whites, nonwhites, and black men. From 1950–1954 to 1985–1989, age-adjusted prostate cancer mortality rates increased slightly for whites (9%) but substantially for nonwhites (67%). Age-specific stratification showed increases among nonwhites were greatest among men 75 years of age and older, with lesser increases among those aged 65 to 74 years and declines among those younger than 65 years.

Chu et al[47] used both mortality data for 1969 to 1999 and SEER data for 1975 to 1999 to extend national studies of prostate cancer to more recent times. They observed declines in prostate cancer mortality rates for both black men and white men during the 1990s. The declines were attributable to declining distant disease mortality rates, coincident with declining distant disease incidence rates. Results were deemed consistent with the hypothesis of a stage shift resulting from earlier detection of cancer by prostate-specific antigen testing. Chu et al[52] also hinted that blacks and whites may not have received the benefits of this stage shift equally. Specifically, they noted without comment that the percent change in prostate cancer mortality rates from 1986 to 1999 were more favorable for white men than black men in all age groups studied. As such, the reader could calculate that the black–white mortality rate ratio also increased at all levels: from 2.66 to 3.28 for men aged 50 to 59 years, from 2.59 to 3.11 for those 60 to 69, from 2.32 to 2.69 for those 70 to 79, from 1.95 to 2.30 for those 80 to 84, and from 1.61 to 1.90 for those older than 85 years. Moreover, rates increased by 8% for whites older than 85 years and by 3.4% and 27.2% for blacks aged 80 to 84 years and 85-plus, respectively. Although rates for both blacks and whites were at their lowest rates in decades, black Americans, even in 1999, had the highest prostate cancer rates in the world.

Arbes et al[49] sought to identify factors that contributed to the poorer survival of blacks in the United States diagnosed with oral cancer. Data were reviewed from 6338 whites and 1165 blacks diagnosed from 1988 to 1993 with squamous cell carcinoma of the oral cavity and pharynx. When lower socioeconomic status, more advanced stage at diagnosis, and treatment variables were added to a model that accounted only for age and geographic area, the hazard ratio of death from oral cancer dropped from 1.7 (95% CI, 1.5 to 1.9) to 1.1 (95% CI, 0.9 to 1.4). In all, 86% of the excess hazard of death from oral cancer was accounted for by these three factors.

Chow et al[50] reviewed renal cancer data for 1975 through 1995 and found that age-adjusted (1970 US standard), sex-specific kidney cancer mortality rates for both black men and women were lower than those for whites during the 1970s. However, whereas white rates remained relatively stable during the 1980s and 1990s, rates for blacks not only increased but also surpassed those for whites. The increases were not explained by rising use of magnetic resonance imaging or improved subsite specification for kidney cancers. Nor did the well-recognized associations between kidney cancer, obesity, and hypertension explain the increase, since even though obesity and hypertension are more common in blacks, there was little correlation between the time course in the development of these factors and the rise in kidney cancer. On the other hand, given the long latency of tumor development, it was felt that differences in smoking habits might be part of the reason for the increasing disparity.

Finally, Groves et al[53] observed increasing incidence of acute myeloid leukemia among African American males, but once again, could not explain the increase in terms of known risk factors.

Outcomes investigation as to racial differences in mortality from colon cancer adjuvant therapy trials showed no statistically significant difference in colon cancer recurrence between African American and Caucasian patients treated in the NSABP. However, there was a statistically significant difference in survival, with blacks having a 21% greater increase in death (95% CI, 6% to 37%; $P = .004$). This suggests that while early detection and adjuvant therapy could improve colon cancer prognosis in African Americans, these measures would not completely eliminate the observed deficits.[54]

Cerebral Infarction

A biracial cohort of patients selected from a random 20% national sample of Medicare patients aged 65 and older hospitalized with cerebral infarction in 1991 was followed for a period of 3 years.[55] Compared with whites, African American patients were 6% more likely to die post–cerebral infarction. African Americans aged 65 to 74 years had much lower 3-year survival probabilities (15% to 20%) than their white counterparts.

Congenital Heart Disease

Multiple-cause mortality files compiled by the National Center for Health Statistics of the CDC from all US death certificates have been used to describe national trends in racial disparities associated with congenital heart disease mortality from 1979 to 1997.[56] Of the approximately 40.6 million deaths occurring during the study period, 124,832 (0.31%) were associated with a congenital heart defect. Mortality from congenital heart defects was higher and declined more slowly among blacks than among whites. Thus, from 1995 to 1997, infant mortality from congenital heart defects was found to be 19% higher among blacks than among whites (68.4 versus 55.5 per 100,000, respectively) and declined more slowly (2.1% versus 2.7% per year). This pattern recurred for most types of heart defects and throughout the study period. For several defects (eg, transposition of the great arteries, tetralogy of Fallot, and ventricular septal defects), blacks died at a much younger age, often about half the age of whites. Although these data could not specify the cause of these disparities, it was noted that reduced mortality is most likely attributable to improved diagnosis, better surgical techniques, and advances in intensive care.

Diabetes Mellitus

Valdez et al[57] used data from the National Mortality Followback Survey (1986) and the National Health Interview Survey (1987 to 1989) to study the impact of diabetes on mortality associated with pneumonia and influenza among non-Hispanic black and white US adults. They observed that for both blacks and whites, persons dying from pneumonia and influenza between 25 and 64 years of age were more likely to have diabetes mellitus (OR, 4.0; 95% CI, 2.3 to 7.7). However, among persons 65 years of age and older, the risk remained elevated among whites with diabetes (OR, 2.2; 95% CI, 1.7 to 2.7) but not among blacks with diabetes (OR, 1.0; 95% CI, 0.6 to 1.7). Although mortality studies of disparities in diabetes per se are sparse, the projected burden of diabetes mellitus among

the black population suggests that this will be a major source of disparity during the 21st century. The fastest growing ethnic group with diagnosed diabetes is expected to be black males (+336% between 2000 and 2050), followed by black females (+217%), white males (+148%), and white females (+107%).[57a]

Drowning

Waller et al,[58] in a study of injury mortality in the United States (1980 to 1985) observed that the drowning rate among whites was almost twice that of blacks for ages 1 to 4 years, but that in the 10- to 14-year-old group, the drowning rate for blacks was more than three times that of whites.

Homicide

Although rates of homicide were consistently observed to be higher among blacks, a study that linked eight consecutive years of the National Health Interview Survey (1987 to 1998) to the Multiple Cause of Death file through the National Death Index (1987 to 1997), noted that individual-level sociodemographic characteristics (age, sex, marital status, education, employment status, and geographic factors) explained about 35% of the racial differences in homicide mortality.[59] This is consistent with observations by Paulozzi et al[60] concerning homicide among intimate partners from 1981 to 1998, with a discussion by Onwuachi-Saunders and Hawkins[61] from the CDC, and with a notation by Centerwall[62] (see Appendix 2-A) that blacks and whites, given similar environments, had similar rates.

In an earlier study of 217,578 homicides occurring in the United States from 1979 to 1988, Hammett et al[63] noted that homicide was the most common cause of death among black males and black females 15 to 34 years of age during the study period. A 54% rise in homicide rates among 15- to 24-year-olds from 1985 to 1988 was accounted for by homicides in which the victim was killed with a firearm. Ikeda et al,[64] in a study that covered 1962 to 1993, observed that African American men had not only the highest rates but also the widest variation in total (unintentional, suicide, homicide, legal intervention, undetermined intention) firearm-related mortality. The prominence of firearms and observations of temporal fluctuations are also reflected in local studies (see Appendix 2-A).

Injury: Postneonatal Infants

Infant death certificate data have been used to investigate postneonatal mortality deaths due to injury in the United States for the period 1988 through 1998.[65] Overall, postneonatal mortality rates attributable to injury declined less among blacks (8.7%) than whites (13.6%), and rates among blacks (range, 2.4 to 3.0 per 1000 live births) averaged 2.6 times higher than whites. Black infants were more than three times as likely to die from homicide than white infants (range, 3.0 to 4.4), although the percent increase in blacks (9.9%) was slightly less than that for whites (10.6%). Regional differences adversely affecting black infants included motor vehicle crash-related deaths in the West and mechanical suffocation in the Midwest, and homicide in both these regions. Homicide rates increased among all infants regardless of race, except in the Northeast.

Legal Intervention

For the years 1979 through 1997, males accounted for almost all deaths of this type. Death rates for black males were several times higher than those for white males, with the highest rates among both blacks and whites occurring among 20- to 34-year-olds.[66]

Motor Vehicle Injury

Baker et al[67] added depth to mortality and census data from 1989 to 1993 by using travel data from the 1990 Nationwide Personal Transportation Survey to estimate mortality rates per billion miles traveled. They observed that although there were few differences in motor vehicle occupant death rates among children aged 5 to 12 years, according to population-based denominators for race and ethnicity, computation of mortality per billion vehicle-miles of travel revealed that non-Hispanic blacks had a rate of 14 compared with 8 for Hispanics and 5 for non-Hispanic whites. For teenagers (aged 13 to 19 years), rates per 100,000 persons were highest for non-Hispanic whites. However, rates per billion vehicle-miles were 45 for Hispanics, 34 for non-Hispanic blacks, and 30 for non-Hispanic whites. Black and Hispanic male teenagers were at particularly greater risk per billion vehicle-miles of travel than either white male teenagers or female teenagers in any racial or ethnic group. This interesting study showed some of the limits of population-based mortality data, as well as how mortality rates based on degree of exposure might overcome some of those limits.

Necrotizing Enterocolitis: Infant Mortality

Using US multiple cause of death records and linked birth–infant death data for 1979 through 1992, it was observed that low-birth-weight singleton infants who were black and male or born to a mother younger than 17 years were at increased risk. The introduction of surfactants in 1990 was coincident with an overall increase in mortality from this disease.[68]

Renal Disease

The US Renal Data System has been used to investigate human immunodeficiency virus/acquired immunodeficiency syndrome-associated nephropathy (HIVAN) in patients with end-stage renal disease (ESRD).[69] In all, 375,152 patients in this data system were initiated on ESRD therapy between January 1, 1992 and June 1997. Of these patients, 3653 had HIVAN, and 87.8% were African American. In these data, this meant that the odds of having this problem were more than 12 times higher for African Americans than for non–African Americans (OR, 12.2; 95% CI, 10.57 to 14.07). HIVAN, in turn, was associated with decreased patient survival. Moreover, the data appeared to indicate that HIVAN patients were being initiated on dialysis later and in poorer medical condition than other patients with ESRD, although there was no known clinical reason to support such a delay. Abbott et al[69] suggested that as yet undetermined and possibly familial factors might also play a role in the observed disparity.

In another national investigation, Owen et al[70] used a national hemodialysis database for 1994 that included 18,144 black and white patients receiving hemodialysis three times weekly who either lived the entire year receiving hemodialysis or died. After adjusting for age and diabetes, death probability curves were steepest for white women with urea reduction ratios of less than 60%. Death probability curves were least steep for black men.

Sepsis-associated Neonatal and Infant Deaths

Approximately 2260 infants (1521 newborns) died of sepsis per year from 1992 to 1994.[71] Sepsis-associated death was more likely to occur among infants who were male, black, preterm, or born in the South. Among blacks, the racial gap in sepsis-associated mortality was greater for term than for preterm infants.

Sudden Infant Death Syndrome

From 1980 to 1988, sudden infant death syndrome (SIDS) was the second leading cause of infant mortality in the United States. During this time, black infants were disproportionately affected, but rates among black infants were declining more rapidly than rates among whites, thereby narrowing the racial gap.[72] From 1991 to 1995, however, there was a significant increase in the black-to-nonblack postneonatal SIDS mortality ratio, from 2.00 to 2.28, reflecting a smaller decline in birth weight- and gestational age-specific mortality for blacks than for the nonblack population.[73]

▶ REGIONAL STUDIES

Regional studies of mortality have generally focused on the question of whether spatial clustering occurs, and if so, why. Cossman et al[74,75]

used death certificate data to study age-adjusted mortality patterns in 5-year blocks from 1968–1972 through 1993–1997. They observed four distinct clusters of high mortality, including (1) a belt across the southern United States, from the Piedmont areas of southeast Virginia, North Carolina, South Carolina, and Georgia, but not Alabama; (2) the Mississippi Delta region, centering on Louisiana, Mississippi, and Arkansas; (3) a portion of Appalachia, Kentucky, and West Virginia; and (4) a five-county group in Nevada. Three low-mortality clusters were identified: the first, including parts of Wisconsin, Iowa, Minnesota, and North and South Dakota; a second cluster to the southwest of the first, comprising parts of Nebraska, Kansas, and northeastern Colorado; and finally, a small cluster in northwest Oregon.

Despite being able to identify places with stable patterns of mortality over time, Cossman et al[75] caution that a question remains as to whether a particular place is unhealthy, whether the people living there are unhealthy, or both: "...as we hold the geography constant over time, is the population that we are observing permanent in that place, or is the population base constantly changing due to in- and out-migration? ... Once we have quantified the relative 'permanence,' we may begin to assess the relative role of 'place' versus 'population' characteristics."

In terms of black–white mortality, regional studies have focused on specific causes of death, including cancer, circulatory disease, coronary heart disease, diabetes mellitus, stroke, and Parkinson disease. A summary of recent investigations, showing cause of death studied, year of publication, author, period of observation, and major conclusions, is shown in Table 2–2. With few exceptions (eg, lung cancer in the northeastern United States[76] and recent transformations of the so-called stroke belt),[77] the southern United States, and particularly the Southeast, is identified as a particular problem. Not only is the risk of death from various causes elevated in the Southeast, but the burden of southeastern origins is transportable.[78–80] This

▶ **TABLE 2–2**. Recent Studies Oriented to Regional Differences in Black–White Mortality in the United States

Cause of Death	Year[a]	Author	Principal Observations
Cancer	1999	Devesa et al[76]	Rates of lung cancer among blacks were consistently elevated in northern areas of the United States and were low across the South from 1950–1994. Changes in mortality patterns generally coincided with regional trends in cigarette smoking.
	1997	Fang et al[79]	Analysis of death records for 1988–1992 in New York City linked with 2000 census data showed that cancer death rates for southern-born black males were substantially higher than those of black males born in the Northeast or the Caribbean. In general, Caribbean-born blacks had lower cancer mortality rates than other blacks and whites, but their advantage did not hold for prostate carcinoma, for which Caribbean-born men had the highest rates.
	1997	Tarone et al[133]	Breast cancer mortality data for 1969–1992, showed that rates among white women in the Northeast were significantly higher that in any other region on the United States, while rates for black women were not, thereby providing evidence against widespread environmental exposure as a cause. A marked moderation of risk by 4-year birth cohorts was observed for US white women born after 1950, whereas stable or slightly decreasing trends were observed for US black women. Black–white disparities were most likely due to earlier detection and increased use of adjuvant therapy.
	1995	Greenberg et al[134]	Southern-born black Americans, especially those who migrated to the Northeast and Midwest, had much higher cancer mortality rates during 1979–1991 than their counterparts who were born and died outside the South.
Cardiovascular disease	1996	Fang et al[114]	Analysis of mortality records from 1988–1992 in New York City linked with 2000 census data showed that mortality from cardiovascular disease among white and black New Yorkers born in the Northeast was similar, but that southern-born black men and women both had mortality from cardiovascular disease that was substantially higher than that of their counterparts born in either the Northeast or the Caribbean. Caribbean-born blacks had consistently lower rates death from coronary heart disease than whites.

(continued)

▶ **TABLE 2-2.** (Continued) Recent Studies Oriented to Regional Differences in Black–White Mortality in the United States

Cause of Death	Year[a]	Author	Principal Observations
Circulatory disease	1997	Schneider et al[135]	For both black males and black females, the highest rates for mortality from circulatory diseases during 1979–1991 occurred among those who were born in the South but died in the Midwest. Lowest rates were for those born in the West who died in the South. Excess mortality for both southern-born males and females began at ages 25–44.
Coronary heart disease (CHD)	2002	Halverson et al[138]	In comparison with the rest of the United States, the Appalachian region from 1980–1997 exhibited higher rates of heart disease (and stroke) mortality for all racial ethnic, gender, and age groups examined. Affected counties tended to be aggregated in particular areas rather than being dispersed regionwide. Counties designated as "economically distressed" were particularly vulnerable.
	2000	Barnett et al[136]	Within the Appalachian region, rates of decline in CHD mortality from 1980–1997 were slower in nonmetropolitan than in metropolitan areas, and among blacks as compared with whites, women compared with men, and older compared with younger adults.
	2000	Barnett et al[137]	For both black and white adults aged 35–64 years, the highest rates of premature CHD mortality and slowest mortality declines from 1985–1995 were observed in the rural South. Unexpectedly high rates of premature CHD mortality were observed for African Americans in major metropolitan areas outside the South despite favorable levels of socioeconomic resources.
Diabetes mellitus	1997	Schneider et al[135]	Mortality records for 1979–1991 were used to investigate combinations of five regions of birth and four regions of residence at time of death These records showed that southern-born African American males had significantly higher death rates from diabetes than did their counterparts who died in the same regions in 9 of 16 comparisons; for females, this was true in 15 of 16 comparisons. The results show that place of birth and early life experiences are associated with diabetes mortality among African Americans regardless of place of residence at time of death.

▶ **TABLE 2–2.** (Continued)

Cause of Death	Year[a]	Author	Principal Observations
Homicide	2002	Miller et al[88]	In 1988–1998, there was a robust correlation between household firearm ownership and the murder of women aged 5–14 years and 35 years of age and older in all regions of the country.
	2000	Cubbin et al[140]	Homicide data for 1988–1992 point to a strong association between homicide, urbanization, and sociocultural factors in all regions of the country for both black and white males
	1998	Kaplan and Geling[87]	There was no correlation between prevalence of firearm ownership and homicide mortality in blacks or whites.
	1997	Greenberg et al[139]	In 1979–1991, southern-born blacks had the highest homicide rates among the population 35+ years old in the Northeast, Midwest, South, and West. Yet nonmigrants had higher rates than their southern-born counterparts among the population aged 15–34 years. Long-distance migrants born in the Northeast or West, or outside the United States had the lowest homicide rates.
Infant mortality	1975	Shin[141]	When 10 selected southern states were compared with 7 selected northern states for the period from 1940–1970, no significant differences were observed. In both regions, the gaps between blacks and whites widened for both neonatal and postneonatal mortality.
Parkinson disease	1997	Lanska et al[142]	Reported rates among blacks in 1988 were significantly lower than among whites. There was no latitudinal or longitudinal gradient of underlying cause rates among blacks, and only a weak North-to-South decreasing gradient in total (underlying and contributing) rates. For whites, there was a strong North-South gradient, and the highest rates were found in the Northeast.
Stroke	2001	Howard et al[149]	Stroke mortality data for 1968–1996 suggest that the Deep South (Alabama and Mississippi) will fall from the stroke belt and be replaced by other regions (notably Oregon, Washington, and Arkansas, but also western Tennessee). New York City and southern Florida had low stroke mortality rates in 1968, particularly for whites, and experienced large declines that have further accentuated their heterogeneity as compared with the rest of the nation.

(*continued*)

▶ **TABLE 2-2**. (Continued) Recent Studies Oriented to Regional Differences in Black–White Mortality in the United States

Cause of Death	Year[a]	Author	Principal Observations
	2000	Obisesan et al[148]	In data from the NHANES III (1988–1994), southern residence was associated with increased hypertension prevalence among middle-aged, non-Hispanic white men, non-Hispanic black men and women, and older non-Hispanic white men.
	1999	Lackland et al[147]	Using mortality data for 1980–1996, it was observed that proportional mortality ratios for stroke in South Carolina were highest among persons born within the state, intermediate for those born in the Southeast other than South Carolina, and lowest for those born outside the Southeast. Lower ratios among persons born outside the Southeast were particularly striking for blacks, and the differences were not explained by gender, age, or markers of educational and socioeconomic status.
	1997	Lanska et al[146]	With few exceptions, mortality data for 1979–1981 showed that region-specific immigrant rates for whites and blacks were significantly lower than rates for ether US-born regional residents, US-born migrants to the regions, or US-born natives of the regions. The spatial pattern of immigrant rates did not parallel the patterns for US-born populations.
	1997	Pickle et al[145]	Mortality data for 1988–1992 showed persistence of previously described high mortality in the southeastern United States among black women and men, but compared with data for 1962–1988, there was a continuation of a previously described westward shift of high-rate areas to the Mississippi River valley. Areas of high stroke rates were more densely concentrated in the southeastern states in blacks. Although rates in the Pacific region were low overall, a surprising area of high rates was seen in southern California among women. An obvious black–white racial contrast was observed for all areas of Florida except the panhandle, likely driven by migration of affluent, elderly whites from northern states.

▶ **TABLE 2–2.** (Continued)

Cause of Death	Year[a]	Author	Principal Observations
	1996	Gillum et al[144]	NHANES I Epidemiologic Follow-up Study data (1971–1987) showed that some of the excess risk associated with residence in the Southeast compared with the Midwest could be explained by regional differences in known risk factors among white women, but this association was not evident for black men or women or for white men. However, there was a strong association between nonmetropolitan residence in blacks that was independent of region or other stroke risk factors.
	1993	Lanska et al[143]	From 1939–1941 to 1979–1981 for each racial–gender group, high age-adjusted stroke mortality rates were significantly clustered in the southeastern United States, particularly in the South Atlantic census division, with persistent extreme rates in Georgia and the Carolinas. The nonrandom distribution of stroke mortality across the United States, the large magnitude of the differences between high- and low-rate areas, the persistence of the pattern over more than four decades, the similarity of the distribution for different racial–gender groups, the lack of delimitation by administrative or political boundaries, and results of national cooperative studies completed in the late 1960s and 1970s together suggest that the pattern of excess stroke mortality is not an artifact of different diagnostic and reporting practices.

NHANES, National Health and Nutritional Examination Survey.
[a]Year listed is that of publication.

leads to elevated risk of death even when an individual leaves the South. Because there is considerable evidence that this is not an artifact,[81] and because more than 6 million southern-born blacks migrated to other sections of the United States during the 20th century (a trend that has been recently reversed), this has important implications.

First, it suggests that health planners and researchers alike need to consider region of birth and early life experiences as they devise community-based interventions and multilevel ecologic analyses. Second, because so many US blacks have a present or past residential connection to the South, it is unlikely that racial disparities in health in the United States will be eliminated unless problems found in the South (or among southerners) are solved. Third, and somewhat paradoxically, it suggests that some of the most valuable information about how to solve those problems is to be found outside the South. Fourth, it suggests that networks of defined populations in different parts of the nation, not simply defined local, populations may be needed to achieve internal validity for either evaluation or etiologic inquiry. Specifically, if there are regional effects tending to affect health and if the magnitude of those effects changes over time, then measurement of specific program or etiologic effects within that area would need to be able to account for regional influences, either by monitoring the degree of resistance to healthy change across different regions or by assuring simultaneous conduct of interventions in contrasting regions. Fifth, it may suggest ethical problems for community-based public health programs and community-based research alike. Specifically, if particular places or the people who live in particular places, or both, are associated with health choices that tend to harm present and future residents, is it still appropriate for community members to have primacy[82] with regard to decisions about health-care interventions? Should there be accountability beyond the capacity to make or break a "community" decision on the basis of what amounts to political strength? Why is it ethical for so-called grassroots (ie, political) entities to make decisions that affect the health of individuals who have never authorized those grassroots groups to speak for them? How does society outside a self-destructive community (and particularly the health professionals who are society's representatives) assure that they do not become enablers of unhealthy choices?

As far as the South is concerned, many questions about place versus person still remain unresolved. Hypotheses as to why the region appears to be in difficulty, not only in absolute terms but also with regard to relative racial differences, include lifestyle, local environment, medical care, and artifact resulting from inaccurate reporting.[81]

Concerning lifestyle, National Health Interview Survey data from 1991 suggested that the proportion of men and women who use salt, are overweight, report no leisure-time physical activity, and smoke cigarettes was generally highest in the Southeast,[81,83] but when risk factor data from the National Health Interview Survey for 1990 and NHANES data for 1988 through 1991 were analyzed for four age groups (18 to 29, 30 to 44, 45 to 64, and >65 years), southeastern dominance was not so clear.[81,84] Another factor, dietary potassium, has been noted to be lower in the Southeast than elsewhere, and it has been hypothesized that this may interact with high salt intake and obesity to lead to increased mortality from stroke in the southeast.[81] Additionally, the CARDIA study, initiated in 1985, followed more than 5000 young adult black and white men and women in four cities, including Birmingham, Alabama, and found lower intakes of fruits, vegetables, and antioxidants in the Birmingham contingent. It was suggested that this might contribute to a greater rise in blood pressure with age.[81,85] Finally, regarding the question of real versus apparent racial differences in the Southeast, a county-level study by Appel et al[86] found that racial differences dropped out of a multifactorial model entirely when obesity was considered. Further discussion of county-level inquiries is presented later in this chapter, in the section on smaller area studies.

In addition to risk factors for chronic disease, firearm ownership has also been studied in relation to regional differences. Results have been mixed. Kaplan[87] found that although there was a wide regional variation in prevalence of firearm ownership (from 39% in New England to 70% in the South Central United States), this did not correlate with homicide mortality in either blacks or whites. Miller et al[88] using data for 1988 to 1997, observed a robust correlation between household firearm ownership and the murder of women aged 5 to 14 years and 35 years and older in all regions, again failing to pinpoint a southeastern explanation.

Both specific genetic and environmental factors have also been discussed. It is speculated, for example, that differences in response to antihypertensive medications observed among blacks in the Southeast, as compared with blacks from other regions, might be genetically based, although the speculation was based on a nonrandomized study.[81,89] Possible environmental toxicities that have been suggested as part of the explanation for southeastern problems include soft water[90,91] and lead.[92] On a more general basis, Clark and Cushing[93] found that mortality from motor vehicle crashes was greater in the South than in other regions of the country, and that distance between hospitals appeared to contribute to some interregional differences within the United States. The applicability of such a model to other causes of death has not (to our knowledge) been reported.

► STATE STUDIES

A systematic, ongoing, state-based, national public heath review is conducted on a regular basis via collaboration between the United Health Foundation, the American Public Health Association, and the Partnership for Prevention.[94] This effort is primarily directed at summarizing the experience of an "average" state resident. However, some race- and ethnic-specific mortality information, including data for non-Hispanic whites and blacks, American Indians, and Asian and Pacific Islanders is also presented using the measure of years of potential life lost (YPLL) per 100,000 populations before age 75 years. To obtain this figure, the number of years of potential life lost is calculated for each individual by subtracting the age at death (if younger than 75) from 75 years, adding to find the total number of years lost, and then dividing that total by the population at risk. As is true for mortality, Asian and Pacific Islanders had the fewest years of potential life lost. Such results, however, must be interpreted in light of a National Center for Health Statistics disclaimer about all race-specific population data except that for blacks and whites.[94a] Table 2–3 shows black–white comparisons for each state and the District of Columbia. There is a wide range of values (1.22 to 3.48) but only two states (Alaska and Hawaii) have values of 1.25 or less. Overall, the national black–white YPLL (<75) ratio is 1.93 (13,424 YPLL per 100,000 in non-Hispanic blacks and 6961 in non-Hispanic whites). Notably, the highest

value for whites (9020 in Mississippi) is lower than the values for blacks in all but five states (Alaska, Hawaii, South Dakota, Vermont, and New Hampshire). The skewed nature of the black–white distribution is reflected in the fact that only 13 areas* have ratios equal to or higher than the national figure of 1.93. The absence of southern states from this list reflects relatively high YPLL levels among whites. In absolute terms, Louisiana (ranked 4th for YPLL/100,000 black, non-Hispanics), Mississippi (5th), Tennessee (7th), South Carolina (9th), Alabama (10th), North Carolina (13th), Florida (16th), and Georgia (20th) all have YPPL values that exceed the median value (12,602 YPLL <75 years per 100,000) for non-Hispanic blacks in the nation as a whole. The variations in state mortality noted in these data also are reflected in a comprehensive report by Oose[95] for the period from 1960 to 1990. The authors concluded that these observations offered "little support for the hypothesis that the levels of state mortality become more similar to each other over time."

In addition to this ongoing surveillance, state-level data have been used by several investigators to address the issues pertaining to relationships that may exist between income inequality and overall mortality. This is a controversial area, and an issue that has important ramifications for African American health. Specifically, if income inequality is associated with mortality, those who accept a "mirror-image" theory of risk versus protection (for a more complete discussion, see the later section on local area studies) are led to support social policies aimed at correcting that inequality (eg, Wilkinson).[96–98] At least two recent and comprehensive reviews of this subject have been published.[99,100] Macinko et al[100] noted that at least 33 studies show a significant association between income inequality and health outcomes (not exclusive to mortality), while at least 12 studies did not. Noting at least five

---

* These 13 areas were New York, Rhode Island, Missouri, Connecticut, Maryland, Minnesota, Nebraska, Pennsylvania, Wisconsin, Michigan, New Jersey, Illinois, and the District of Columbia.

▶ **TABLE 2–3**. Years of Potential Life Lost (YPLL) per 100,000 Population Before Age 75 Among Non-Hispanic Blacks and Whites, United States, 1998–2000[a]

State	YPLL per 100,000 Black Non-Hispanic	YPLL per 100,000 White Non-Hispanic	Black Non-Hispanic-to-White Non-Hispanic Ratio
District of Columbia	19,538	5613	3.48
Illinois	15,049	6643	2.32
New Jersey	13.869	6171	2.25
Michigan	15,048	6741	2.23
Wisconsin	13,689	6179	2.22
Pennsylvania	14,635	6778	2.16
Nebraska	13,160	6281	2.10
Maryland	13,430	6552	2.05
Minnesota	11,178	6552	2.05
Connecticut	11,471	5746	2.00
Missouri	14,747	7503	1.97
Rhode Island	11,547	5915	1.95
New York	11,719	6079	1.93
Iowa	11,865	6225	1.91
Indiana	14,152	7453	1.90
Kansas	13,098	6893	1.90
North Carolina	13,694	7293	1.88
California	12,552	6753	1.86
Virginia	11,836	6467	1.83
Louisiana	14,885	8191	1.82
South Carolina	14,397	7901	1.82
Colorado	11,269	6228	1.81
Ohio	12,599	7068	1.78
Delaware	12,474	7019	1.78
Wyoming	12,719	7247	1.76
Tennessee	14,668	8413	1.74
Florida	13,235	7631	1.73
Georgia	13,081	7561	1.73
Montana	11,486	6717	1.71
Massachusetts	9,939	5822	1.71
Texas	12,499	7349	1.70
Washington	10,600	6225	1.70
Arkansas	14,677	8703	1.69
Alabama	14,396	8685	1.66
Mississippi	14,818	9020	1.64
Arizona	11,704	7169	1.63
Idaho	10,539	6564	1.61
Oregon	10,830	6854	1.58
Utah	9,589	6144	1.56
Kentucky	12,602	8334	1.51
New Mexico	10,291	6885	1.49
West Virginia	12,895	8829	1.46
Oklahoma	13,039	9006	1.45

▶ **TABLE 2–3**. (Continued)

State	YPLL per 100,000 Black Non-Hispanic	YPLL per 100,000 White Non-Hispanic	Black Non-Hispanic-to-White Non-Hispanic Ratio
Nevada	12,763	8826	1.45
Maine	9,307	6470	1.44
New Hampshire	7,849	5485	1.43
Vermont	8,637	6358	1.36
South Dakota	8,520	6393	1.33
Hawaii	6,784	5416	1.25
Alaska	8,011	6577	1.22
North Dakota	—	5898	—
United States	13,424	6961	1.93

[a]Listed according to magnitude of black–white ratio.

[b] State values for YPLL per 100,000 Non-Hispanic blacks and whites are from United Health Foundation. Black–white ratios were derived from these values. YPLL for blacks in North Dakota is excluded because of small population size.

inconsistencies in this body of work (including different models of health determinants; inconsistent income inequality measures and data; use of different combinations of countries or states, or both; inconsistent time periods; and differing health outcome measures), these authors call for a more comprehensive model of health production that includes health system covariates, sufficient sample size, and adjustment for inconsistencies in income inequality data.

Lynch et al[99] reviewed 98 aggregate and multilevel studies of associations between income inequality and health, including aggregate multilevel international and within-country studies. They concluded that:

> . . . in aggregate level U.S. studies, the extent of income inequality across state and metropolitan areas seems reasonable robustly associated with a variety of health outcomes, especially when measured at the state level. In multilevel U.S. studies, using both individual and aggregate data, the evidence is more mixed, with state-level associations again being the most consistent. For other countries, the aggregate and multilevel evidence generally suggests little or no effect of income inequality on health indicators in rich countries such as Australia, Belgium, Canada, Denmark, Japan, New Zealand, Spain, and Sweden, but there may be some effects in the United Kingdom.[99]

It seemed then, that "the United States is somewhat exceptional in that it is the country where income inequality is the most consistently linked to population health."[99] Lynch et al went on to caution, however, that:

> . . . the largely negative findings for the direct health effects of income inequality in no way contradict the large body of evidence that at the individual level those people with higher incomes also are healthier. . . . . Although we found little evidence to support a direct effect of income inequality on health, this should not be interpreted to mean the factors that drive unequal income distribution at the system level are not important to individual and population health. Reducing income inequality by raising the incomes of more disadvantaged people will improve the health of poor individuals, help reduce health inequalities, and increase average population health.[99]

Several recent studies using statewide data pertaining to individual states within the United States have also addressed black–white disparities in mortality for specific causes of death. These studies, summarized in Table 2–4,

▶ **TABLE 2–4**. Recent Statewide Studies of Black–White Mortality Within the United States

Cause of Death	State and Period of Observation	Year[a]	Author	Principal Observations
All causes (**Note:** Although the outcome measure in this study was self-rated health, it is included both because of the pertinence of the material and the close relationship between self-rated health and mortality.)	50 states, 1995–1997	2003	Subramanian and Kawachi[50]	Analyses controlled for individual effects of age, sex, race (white, black, others), marital status (married or partnered; divorced or separated; widowed; single); education (graduate and above, college, high school/some college, 9th–12th grade, < 8th grade); income (>US$125,000, 75–125K, 50–75K, 30–50K, 15–30K, and <15 K, with household income divided by square root of the number of household members); health insurance coverage (yes or no), and employment status (employed; not employed, including those seeking work; retired; disabled; other residual groupings), Gini coefficient (a standard measure of income inequality) (state), proportion of black residents within each state. Sources of data included current population surveys (1995 and 1997) and state-level data from the 1990 US census. Conditioned on proportion black in a state, there remained an important association between state income inequality and individual self-rated poor health. For every 0.05-increase in the Gini coefficient the odds ratio (OR) of reporting poor health increased by 1.39 (95% CI 1.26–1.51). The focus of this research was to test specific claim made by Deaton and Lubotsky (2003; see Appendix 2-A) that the observed association between state income inequality and health can be explained by racial composition within states. The findings demonstrate that neither race, at the individual level, nor racial composition, as measured at the state level, explain away the previously reported association between income inequality and poorer health status in the United States.

▶ **TABLE 2–4**. (Continued)

Cause of Death	State and Period of Observation	Year[a]	Author	Principal Observations
	Texas, 1989–1991	2001	Franzini et al[151]	Among counties with populations >150,000, the risk of death was lower in counties with more equal income distribution than in counties with less equal income distribution. Among counties with population <150,000, median income affected relative risk in counties with <30% Hispanics, but not in those with >30% Hispanics. The results support the hypothesis that income inequality at the county level is associated with higher mortality.
	39 states, 1990	1997	Kennedy et al[152]	Collective disrespect for African Americans was measured by weighted responses to a national survey, which asked for yes or no answers to each of four questions: "On the average, blacks have worse jobs, income, and housing than white people. Do you think the differences are: (A) Mainly due to discrimination? (B) Because most blacks have less in-born ability to learn? (C) Because most blacks don't have the chance for education that it takes to rise out of poverty? (D) Because most blacks just don't have the motivation or will power to pull themselves up out of poverty?" The percentage of respondents who answered in the affirmative to these was calculated for each state and correlated with age-standardized total and cause-specific mortality rates. Collective disrespect had a positive and statistically significant correlation with both black mortality and white mortality. A 1% increase in the prevalence of those who believed that blacks lacked innate ability was associated with an increase in age-adjusted black mortality rate of 359.8/100,000 (95% CI, 187.5–532.1 deaths per 100,000).

▶ **TABLE 2–4.** (Continued) Recent Statewide Studies of Black–White Mortality Within the United States

Cause of Death	State and Period of Observation	Year[a]	Author	Principal Observations
	Michigan, 1989–1991	1995	Christianson and Johnson[153]	Reduced black mortality relative to whites was associated with moving from secondary to postsecondary level of education but there was less reduction among blacks than whites associated with moving from primary to secondary level of education.
Acquired immunodeficiency syndrome	Alabama, 1981–1985, 1986–1990, 1991–1995	1997	Holmes et al[154]	Surveillance data showed that rates for black women and white women increased 170-fold and 23-fold, respectively, from 1981–1985 to 1991–1995. For the same periods, rates for black men and white men increased >80-fold and 50-fold, respectively. HIV infection was found to be increasingly prevalent in rural and small-town communities, with more frequent heterosexual transmission placing black women at disproportionately high risk.
Asthma	California, 1981–1995	2000	Schleicher et al[155]	Among youths aged 5–17 years, there was little change in frequency over time and no spatial clustering. Being African American (twofold increase relative to white) and having low income (below statewide median) were associated with increased risk of death.
Breast cancer	Connecticut, 1988–1995	2002	Polednak[156]	Among 16,931 women, risk of death was elevated for blacks, nonmarried, and low socioeconomic status, independent from stage at diagnosis especially <65 years. Health access was not independently associated with survival.

▶ **TABLE 2–4.** (Continued)

Cause of Death	State and Period of Observation	Year[a]	Author	Principal Observations
	Upstate New York, 1976–1981	1988	Polednak[157]	Using data on passive follow-up to the New York State Cancer Registry for 890 black and 24,372 white female breast cancer patients, there were nearly identical survival rates for blacks and whites diagnosed at stage 1 (local disease). Within clinical stage 3 (metastatic) cases, however, survival tended to be poorer in younger (<60 years) black versus white patients. The data suggested the need for programs aimed at early detection of breast cancer among black women at younger ages.
Cerebrovascular disease	North Carolina, 1984–1993	1997	Casper et al[158]	For black men and white men aged 35–54 years, the highest rates of premature stroke mortality were observed among the lowest social classes. Within each social class, black men had substantially higher rates of premature stroke mortality than white men (black–white rate ratios ranged from 4.0–4.9).
Heart disease	New York, 1988–1992	2003	Armstrong et al[159]	In upstate New York (57 counties), the lowest coronary heart disease mortality among 35–64-year-old men was found among white men residing in counties with the highest percentages of white-collar workers (135/100,000). Among blue-collar workers, mortality was 1.3–1.8 times higher among black compared with white, blue-collar workers. Highest mortality (689/100,000) was found among black, blue-collar workers.

(*continued*)

▶ **TABLE 2–4**. (Continued) Recent Statewide Studies of Black–White Mortality Within the United States

Cause of Death	State and Period of Observation	Year[a]	Author	Principal Observations
	Texas, 1991	2003	Franzini et al[151]	Being female, having more education, and residing in areas with higher median house value were associated with less premature mortality. Block-group level wealth, census-tract level "own-group" racial or ethnic density, and county-level social capital (homeownership and lower crime) had a significant influence on years of life lost to heart disease, although blacks and Hispanics lost more years of life to heart disease. Inequality, economic conditions, human capital, and demographic characteristics at the county level did not have an effect on premature heart disease mortality.
	North Carolina, 1984–1993	1999	Barnett et al[160]	Analyses of coronary heart disease mortality among 35–54-years-olds, showed that blacks in the highest social class (primary white collar) experienced a 33% decline in coronary heart disease mortality, while black men in secondary white-collar, primary blue-collar, and secondary blue-collar jobs had increases of 18%, 2%, and 6% respectively. Rates for whites declined in all social classes over the 10-year study period.
	North Carolina, 1986–1994	1999	Corti et al[161]	Among 1875 whites and 2261 blacks, blacks aged 80 years or older had significantly lower risk of all-cause (HR, 0.75; 95% CI 0.62–0.90) and coronary heart disease (HR, 0.44; 95% CI, 0.30–0.66). This was not observed for other causes of death, leading to the conclusion that the observation was less likely to be an artifact.
Homicide	Delaware	1994	Cannon[162]	Rates among black males were noted to be significantly lower than US rates.

► **TABLE 2–4**. (Continued)

Cause of Death	State and Period of Observation	Year[a]	Author	Principal Observations
Infant mortality	Wisconsin, 1980–1999	2003	Hagen and Andrade[163]	The rate for black infants was 19.4/1000 live births in 1980–1984 and 17.8/1000 in 1995–1999. Disparity between blacks and whites remained large and continued to increase. Death rates due to prematurity increased almost 82% between 1980 and 1999, while deaths from congenital anomalies declined.
	Louisiana, 1990–1998	2001	Jooma et al[164]	Extremes of maternal age, maternal black race, being unmarried, and having less education and prenatal care were associated with increased risk of infant death.
	California, 1994–1995	2001	Pearl et al[105]	Using birth records linked to census block-group data for 22,304 women delivering infants at 18 California hospitals and a surveyed subset of 8457 women, less-favorable neighborhood socioeconomic characteristics were associated with lower birth weight among blacks and Asians. Neighborhood socioeconomic characteristics were not associated with birth weight among whites or US- or foreign-born Latinas, but birth weight increased with less-favorable neighborhood socioeconomic characteristics among foreign-born Latinas in high-poverty or high-unemployment neighborhoods, independent from measured behavioral or cultural factors.
	Connecticut, 1981–1992	1997	Roberts et al[165]	Although overall rates declined from, 12.2/1000 live births to 7.3/1000 live births, differential declines produced an increased relative risk of infant death over time for infants of black women compared with infants of white women.

(continued)

▶ **TABLE 2–4.** (Continued) Recent Statewide Studies of Black–White Mortality Within the United States

Cause of Death	State and Period of Observation	Year[a]	Author	Principal Observations
	Michigan, 1989	1996	Geronimus[125]	Linked live birth and infant death information and census data showed that among blacks, but not whites, advancing maternal age >15 years was associated with increased odds of low birth weight and very low birth weight. Among blacks in low-income areas, odds of low birth weight increased 3-fold and of very low birth weight four-fold between maternal ages 15 and 34 years. African American women, on average, and those residing in low-income areas, in particular, experience worsening health profiles between their teens and young adulthood, contributing to their risk of low birth weight and very low birth weight with advancing maternal age and to the black–white gap in this risk. Of interest, among other populations in which early births are most common are those in which early births are the lowest risk, raising questions about the social construction of teenage childbearing as a universally deleterious behavior.
	Texas, 1989–1991	1995	Kerr et al[166]	Infant mortality rates for 30 of the top 59 causes of death were at least 1.5 times higher in African American than in Anglo and Hispanic infants, while a comparable excess in Hispanic infants was noted only for anencephaly. Anglo infants did not have an excessive mortality rate for any of the 59 causes. About 37% of all infant deaths (but 48% of African American infant deaths) were associated with adverse pregnancy outcomes. Reduction of the racial infant mortality rate

▶ **TABLE 2–4.** (Continued)

Cause of Death	State and Period of Observation	Year[a]	Author	Principal Observations
				discrepancy in Texas will therefore require clarification and correction of factors that place pregnancies of African American women at increased risk for adverse pregnancy outcomes and those that place their infants at increased risk for death from a wide range of causes.
	North Carolina, 1993–1997	2003	Leslie et al[102]	Linked birth and infant death certificates showed that among Hispanic women, low birth weight and prematurity rates were similar to those of infants born to white women and lower than those of infants born to African American women. Hispanics also had the lowest infant mortality rate. This occurred even though use of prenatal care and socioeconomic characteristics of Hispanic and African American women were similar.
	Wisconsin, 1980–1998	2000	Kvale et al[167]	White infant mortality declined from 9.6/1000 live births in 1980 to 7.2/1000 in 1998, but African American infant mortality remained at about 18/1000 live births throughout the same period. The black–white ratio increased from 2:1 to 3.2:1. In 1998, the Wisconsin African American rate (17.9) surpassed the national African American rate of 14.1/1000.
	All states, 1988	1998	Bird and Bauman[168]	Twenty-three of the 50 states had a black infant mortality rate that was more than twice as large as its white infant mortality rate. Proportion black, percent with bachelor's degree or higher, percent below poverty, and index of black–white dissimilarity each made a unique contribution to the black infant mortality model.

(continued)

▶ **TABLE 2–4.** (Continued) Recent Statewide Studies of Black–White Mortality Within the United States

Cause of Death	State and Period of Observation	Year[a]	Author	Principal Observations
				Percent with bachelor's degree or higher was the only measure that made a significant contribution to white infant mortality. State-level structural variables therefore related differentially to states' black and white infant mortality rates and supported the need for race-specific models of infant mortality.
Parkinson disease	California, 1984–1994	2000	Ritz and Yu[169]	After controlling for age, gender, race, birthplace, year of death, and education, mortality from Parkinson disease was higher in counties with agricultural pesticide use than in nonuse counties. The risk of death associated with Parkinson disease was greater among whites than among African Americans.
Sickle cell disease	US states, cities, and counties, 1968–1992	1997	Davis et al[170]	A range of values was found. One-through four-year-old children with the disease in 1968–1980 and 1981–1992 had a markedly higher risk of dying in Florida and a markedly lower risk of dying in Pennsylvania. For 1981–1992, Maryland had the lowest mortality rate in the nation, with no cases recorded in Baltimore; an especially high risk was noted for five Florida counties.
Sudden infant death syndrome (SIDS)	California, 1990–1995	1998	Adams et al[171]	California SIDS deaths declined 20% for blacks (2.69/1000 live births to 2.15) and 41% for others (1.04 to 0.61). Declines coincided with campaigns to reduce environmental risk factors, but the net effect was to widen the racial disparity from a black–nonblack rate ratio of 2.59 to 3.52.

▶ **TABLE 2–4.** (Continued)

Cause of Death	State and Period of Observation	Year[a]	Author	Principal Observations
Temperature-related deaths	Alabama, 1987–19989	2000	Taylor and Mcgwin[172]	Highest rates of hyperthermia- and hypothermia-related deaths were reported among black males. Mortality rates increased with age (a sharp increase began at ages 50–59 years for heat-related deaths) for both causes of death. The death rate from hypothermia was twice as high as that for hyperthermia, but this may have reflected underreporting of hyperthermia-related deaths. It was noted that adequacy of home heating may be related to socioeconomic status.

CI, confidence interval; HIV, human immunodeficiency virus; HR, hazard ratio.

[a] Year listed is that of publication.

corroborate the intrastate heterogeneity suggested by national surveillance.[94] Access to and use of health care was studied (for breast cancer[101] and infant mortality[102]), and did not appear to be important. One particularly novel finding is the observation by Franzini et al[103] that residence in a racially or ethnically segregated area appeared to improve heart disease mortality among Hispanics and blacks, but particularly among Hispanics (also supported in a New York study by Fang et al[104]). Pearl et al[105] also noted that Latina women residing in neighborhoods with less-favorable socioeconomic characteristics had infants with higher birth weights. Another set of observations that challenges traditional wisdom is found in the work of Geronimus,[106] who suggests that teenage pregnancy may constitute a positive survival mechanism for urban blacks. These types of evidence, in particular, pose a challenge to the "mirror-image" theory of risk and protection, whether at the aggregate or individual levels. If low-income persons living in low-income, highly segregated areas are able to find

a pathway to health, it suggests that reduction of factors such as income inequality and segregation, although important, are not the only pathways to success. A focus on determinants of success within and outside of adverse circumstances might also yield important insights to inform social policy on ways to decrease disparities in mortality.

State Data and *Healthy People* Programs

State-specific data have also been used by the US Office of Minority Health to track progress toward the goals of the *Healthy People* program.[107,108] Four states and one district with the largest percentage of blacks (District of Columbia, Mississippi, Louisiana, South Carolina, and Georgia) and five with large concentrations of blacks in urban areas (New York, Illinois, Florida, Texas, and California) were included in a presentation that focused on the six health priority areas identified in the President's

Race Initiative—coronary heart disease, diabetes, cancer, infant mortality, acquired immunodeficiency syndrome (AIDS), immunization—and two additional health areas of particular importance to blacks—homicide and stroke.

For coronary heart disease, age-adjusted death rates were identical for blacks and whites in 1980, but due to a slower rate of decline for blacks, rates in blacks were 34% higher than those for whites by 1994,[109] and this pattern is reflected in most of the 10 profile states. Illinois was an exception in that it experienced increases in age-adjusted deaths for blacks. Rates in New York, Mississippi, and California were above the rate for US blacks, whereas rates in Georgia, South Carolina, and the District of Columbia were lower. For stroke, progress toward *Healthy People* goals was noted for New York, but rates for South Carolina and Georgia remained above the age-adjusted death rate for US blacks.

Diabetes mortality presented particularly discouraging patterns, with a lack of progress towards the *Healthy People 2000* objective of 58 deaths per 100,000 for the black population. Nor did state profiles show progress toward closing the gap between blacks and total population deaths. As a 1997 review of progress in meeting these goals noted: "Unless decisive action is undertaken by federal, state and local health officials to curtail the human suffering from this chronic and disabling condition, the burden of diabetes on the Black population and the country will continue to increase."[109]

Cancer, in contrast, presented some areas of improvement, with declines in New York, where death rates for blacks were lower than the rate for blacks nationally. Blacks in the District of Columbia, Louisiana, and Illinois, however, had excess mortality compared with their respective states and the US total population.

Infant mortality, as reflected in national, regional, and local research cited elsewhere in this chapter, was a continuing problem. For all 10 states in the profile, black infant mortality was double or more than double the white infant mortality rate. There were huge differences in the profile states with respect to differences between total state population and black population rates in every state, and the differences were increasing.

Finally, concerning homicide, only Mississippi men and women, Texas men and women, Georgia women, New York men, and Florida men had either reached or were moving at a rate that was projected to meet the year 2000 goal.

▶ LIMITED AREA STUDIES (COUNTIES, STANDARD METROPOLITAN STATISTICAL AREAS, ZIP CODES, CENSUS TRACTS)

These investigations comprise the majority of peer-reviewed geographic studies cited herein. Two areas of inquiry that have received most attention are all-cause mortality and infant mortality, perhaps reflecting the relative validity of death certificate information on mortality, in contrast to that for specific causes of death.[3] Two general tables trace the development of research in racial disparities affecting all-cause mortality (Table 2–5) and infant mortality (Table 2–6) as performed in smaller geographic areas. Appendix 2-A, at the end of this chapter, presents a more detailed summary of results from small area studies, including all-cause mortality, infant mortality, and selected causes of death.

All-cause Mortality Research: Tracing Research Development

Table 2–5 traces the development of research ideas on factors that contribute to increased and decreased risk of black–white disparities in all-cause mortality retrospectively, starting with the year 2003 through the decade of the 1990s. Taking factors associated with increased disparities in mortality as a composite, it would be expected that they would comprise communities

▶ **TABLE 2–5.** Tracing the Development of Conclusions About Contributors to Increased and Decreased Risk of Black–White Disparities for All-Cause Mortality in State and Local Area Studies, United States, 2003–1985[a]

Increased Risk	No Increased Risk	Decreased Risk	No Decreased Risk
Percent black population (Deaton, 2003[111]; Singh, 2003[173]; Kindig, 2002[175]; McLaughlin, 2002[112]; Cooper, 2001[174]; LeClere, 1997[15])	Income inequality (Deaton, 2003[111]; Singh, 2003[173]; McLaughlin, 2002—income inequality becomes less of a risk factor as percent black increases[112])		
Larger numbers of black residents (Mansfield, 1999[176])			
Low level of formal education (Singh, 2003[173]; Kindig, 2002[175])			
Rural residence (Singh, 2003[173]; Mansfield, 1999[176])			
Western or southern residence (Singh, 2003[173]; Kindig, 2002[175]; Cooper, 2002[177]; Mansfield, 1999[176])			
Residence in selected urban northern communities (Geronimus 1999[110])			
High Medicare expenditures (Kindig, 2002[175])		Employment in agriculture and forestry (Kindig, 2002[175])	
Primary care physician availability in rural counties (Mansfield, 1999[176])			
Income inequality (McLaughlin, 2002[112]; Cooper 2001[174]; Shi, 2001[119];			
Low income (Kindig, 2002[175]; Silva, 2001[180])			
Residential segregation (Cooper, 2001[174]; Polednak, 1998—men and women, aged 15–44 years[183]; Hart, 1998[181])		Residence in rural high poverty areas (Geronimus, 2001[178]; 1999[110])	

(*continued*)

► **TABLE 2–5.** (Continued) Tracing the Development of Conclusions About Contributors to Increased and Decreased Risk of Black–White Disparities for All-Cause Mortality in State and Local Area Studies, United States, 2003–1985[a]

Increased Risk	No Increased Risk	Decreased Risk	No Decreased Risk
		Primary care physician supply (Shi, 2001—white mortality only[119]) Primary care physician availability in metropolitan counties (Mansfield, 1999[176]) Specialist physician availability in rural counties (Mansfield, 1999[176])	
Residence in a census tract with large housing projects—black men only (Polednak 2000[182]) Female-headed households (Mansfield, 1999[176])		Teenage pregnancy (Geronimus, 1999[125])—Improved odds of maternal survival sufficient to raise newborn to adulthood	
Chronic unemployment (Mansfield, 1999[176]) Circulatory diseases (Geronimus 1999[110]—high poverty areas; Polednak, 1998—Blacks[183]; McCord, 1990[184]) Cancer (Polenak, 1998—blacks[183]; McCord, 1990[184]) Cirrhosis and homicide (McCord, 1990[184])	Homicide and AIDS in high poverty areas (Geronimus, 1999[110])		
		Residence within racially segregated areas (and in comparison to members of the same race residing in other areas); membership in the majority racial group for whites of all ages and for elderly blacks (Fang, 1998[104])	

▶ **TABLE 2–5.** (Continued)

Increased Risk	No Increased Risk	Decreased Risk	No Decreased Risk
		Metropolitanized local government—for black males and females and for white females (Hart, 1998[181])	
			Medicare (Gornick, 1996— persons 65 and older[113])
		Residence in an area with relatively low black–white MRR (Polednak, 1993[179])	
Membership in younger cohorts (Wing, 1990[185]; McCord, 1990[184]) Younger age—35–64 years for all causes, cerebrovascular disease, and diabetes; 35–64 years for ischemic heart disease in women (Polednak, 1990[186])		Older age (≥75 and older for all causes among black males and females (Polednak, 1990[186]); ≥73 for all causes among black males and ≥85 for all causes among black famales (Wing, 1985[116])	Older age in African Americans (Preston, 1996[117])

AIDS, acquired immunodeficiency syndrome; MRR, mortality rate ratio.

[a] References are to first author, only.

with high percentages of black residents, female-headed households, residential segregation, income inequality, and the presence of large housing projects. Residents of high-disparity communities would tend to have low levels of education, and would face both chronic unemployment and a disproportionate burden of cardiovascular disease, cancer, cirrhosis, and homicide. HIV and AIDS, although a problem, would not occur with sufficient frequency to drive all-cause disparities in high poverty areas.[110] Blacks of middle age and younger would be particularly at risk, especially men. Both urban and rural areas would be affected, but the South and West seem particularly vulnerable.

A controversy exists with respect to the relative importance of percent black versus income inequality. Deaton and Lubotsky[111] suggest that income inequality may be a mask for the effects of racial composition. Others (eg, McLaughlin et al[112]) suggest an interaction between the two, pointing out that confounding should not be confused with effect modification. Medicare did not appear to have had a significant impact on disparities,[113] and primary care physician supply is noted to be associated with higher mortality in rural areas.

▶ **TABLE 2–6.** Tracing the Development of Conclusions About Contributors to Increased and Decreased Risk of Black–White Disparities for Infant Mortality in State and Local Area Studies, United States, 2003–1985[a]

Increased Risk	No Increased Risk	Decreased Risk
Higher proportion of black births (Haynatzka, 2002[120])		
Residence in *non*impoverished neighborhood for postneonatal mortality (Papacek, 2002[187])		
Residence in *less* socioeconomically favorable neighborhood for infant mortality (Sims, 2002[121]; Pearl, 2001[105]; (Laveist, 1993[12])		
US-born, non-Hispanic African American maternal birth (Rosenberg, 2002[123])		
Residential segregation (Sims, 2002[121]; Laveist, 1993[124]; Polednak, 1991[188])		
Inadequate prenatal care (Sims, 2002[121])		
College education (Scott-Wright, 1998[189])		
	Residence in a nonmetropolitan county (Larson, 1997[126])	
Maternal age > 15 years (Geronimus, 1996[125])	Income status in nonwhites (Stockwell, 1996[127])	
	Economic or family life characteristics at the census tract level (Creighton-Zollar, 1990[128])	
Percent black, percent below poverty, and black–white income inequality at the state level (Bird, 1995[122])		College education or higher at the state level (Bird, 1995[122]); county level (Scott-Wright, 1998[189]); Army community (Rawlings, 1992[190])
		Black political empowerment (Laveist, 1993[124])
		Guaranteed access to health care (Rawlings, 1992[190])

[a] References are to first author, only.

To some extent, protective factors simply mirror risk factors. However, not all results follow this pattern, making the composite of protective factors quite different from what might be expected on the basis of risk factor identification alone. Fang et al[114] observed that within highly segregated, low-income areas, black or white elderly members of the majority group within the segregated area did better than their race- and age-group peers living in less segregated areas where they were in the minority. The fact that some high-poverty rural areas appear to have an advantage[110,115] also suggests that teenage pregnancy may be protective to the community in the sense that it may increase the likelihood that a mother will survive to raise her child to adulthood. Old age, in addition, may be associated with less disparity and the crossover effect,[116] although this is still a matter of debate.[117]

Analyses of health care produced mixed results. Neither Mansfield et al[118] nor Shi et al[119] were able to show that availability of primary care physicians helped blacks in rural areas, although Shi et al[119] reported that increased primary care physician supply helped whites, and Mansfield et al[118] noted that the primary care physician supply helped disparities in metropolitan areas while specialty physician supply improved mortality disparity in rural areas.

Infant Mortality: Tracing Research Development

Disparities in infant mortality are summarized in Table 2–6. Residence in a nonimpoverished neighborhood appeared to increase black–white disparities in postneonatal mortality,[120] while the reverse was true for infant mortality as a whole.[121,122] Other factors favoring widened black–white disparity included populations with a higher proportion of foreign-born, non-Hispanic African Americans,[123] residential segregation,[120,124] inadequate prenatal care,[120] and maternal age greater than 15 years

(Geronimus[125] pointed out that this observation was consistent with a need to reconsider blanket policies targeting all teenage pregnancies as high risk). Residence in a nonmetropolitan county was not associated with increased disparity in the study by Larson et al,[126] and at least two studies have challenged the importance of income status, especially for nonwhites.[127,128]

Specific Causes of Death and a New Pathway

As is true for other geographic research, most small area studies have focused on identifying determinants of increased risk. Results from small area studies are summarized in Appendix 2-A. As discussed in the section on overall mortality, earlier in this chapter, a basic problem is that despite decades of intensive inquiry and the development of many important clues from national, regional, state, and small area studies, "risk factor" research has failed to produce sustained reversal of the secular national trends adversely affecting American blacks since the end of World War II. We[129] have sought to apply a mirror of the Wennberg–Gittelsohn[130] model (see "Framework for Geographic Studies," earlier) in order to define a new pathway.

To investigate mortality rates for blacks and whites in comparable geographic regions, US census 2000 data[131] were used to define a 41-county cohort comprising all US counties with populations of 500,000 to 749,999 and with 15,000 or more residents reporting race as black only. Considerable variability in black–white mortality rate ratios was found within substrata of counties comprising high as well as low black–white poverty rate ratios. In the low black–white poverty rate ratio substratum, ratios ranged from 0.87 (Norfolk, Massachusetts) to 1.43 (San Mateo, California), with two counties revealing mortality rates for blacks that were lower than those for whites and three for which rates for blacks exceeded those for whites by less than 10%. In the high black–white poverty rate ratio substratum, ratios ranged from 0.69 (Essex, Massachusetts) to 1.85 (Washington, DC), with one county in which black rates exceeded those for whites by less than 10%. An unhealthy regional equality, or pseudoequality, was evident for some counties in each stratum, characterized by mortality rates for both blacks and whites that were much higher than mortality rates for their race-specific counterparts in other counties. A third pattern was characterized by high black–white mortality rate ratios as a result of high mortality rates among blacks and low mortality rates among whites. The key observation, however, was that inequality in black–white mortality is not inevitable in the United States, even in places with relatively high black–white poverty rate ratios. By identifying geographic areas that achieve relative equality despite unpromising demographic profiles, it may be possible to discover pathways that lead to success.

▶ SUMMARY AND RECOMMENDATIONS

For almost 60 years, there has been no sustained decrease in mortality among blacks relative

▶ **TABLE 2–7.** Summary of Major Findings Regarding Disparities in Black–White Mortality

- There is little disagreement regarding the existence of large health disparities between minority and majority populations in the United States
- Blacks and whites have been the most widely, consistently, and longest studied, with most reliable data available
- The Wennberg–Gittelsohn logic model can be extended to identify geographic locations with similar demographic and risk profiles but different levels of inequality
- No sustained improvement in overall, age-adjusted black–white mortality has been seen nationally since the end of World War II; more than 4 million excess deaths among blacks occurred during this time
- Disparities are present across a wide range of causes
- Regional and state studies show that place matters; where people were born and where they reside make a difference in differential survival by race and ethnicity
- The southeastern United States is especially unhealthy; the problems of the Southeast must be solved if national disparities are to be reversed, but solutions are more likely to be found in other parts of the country
- Small area studies have provided a surfeit of data on risk factors associated with adverse outcomes; however, there has been little emphasis on factors associated with success
- These studies demonstrate that black–white disparities in mortality are not inevitable in the United States
- Current research has failed to produce sustained improvements in national black–white mortality
- Investigation of geographic regions with comparable demographic characteristics with a spectrum of black–white mortality rate ratios ranging from equality to inequality could provide a powerful vehicle for the identification of modifiable determinants of the black–white mortality gap
- Equality may have existed in some of regions because of factors protective for both blacks and whites, and not simply because of risk reduction among blacks; this provides further evidence against the theory that protection mirrors risk
- A closer focus on modifiable determinants, guided, in part, by the identification of areas in the United States where black–white rate ratios already approach or equal unity, offers the promise of future analytic epidemiologic studies to identify new ways to decrease racial mortality disparities

to whites at the national level, despite absolute declines in mortality rates for both races.[1] Geographic studies have tended to focus largely on risk factors for inequality based on analysis of health disparities in contiguous geographic areas. Moreover, calls for investigation of non-contiguous (or transgeographic) counties with comparable characteristics[5,6] have largely been ignored, and a suggestion to search for areas of regional equality as opposed to inequality[132] has been neglected. However, investigation of geographic regions having comparable demographic characteristics and a spectrum of black–white mortality rate ratios ranging from equality to inequality could provide a powerful vehicle for the identification of modifiable determinants of the black–white mortality gap. Moreover, the finding that regional equality was evident in transgeographic regions with comparable population sizes, regardless of black–white poverty rate ratios, is consistent with the hypothesis that equality may have existed in some regions because of factors protective for both blacks and whites, and not simply because of risk reduction among blacks.

Two specific scenarios illustrate the complexity of this topic:

1. **Traditional "risk factor" epidemiology versus building from success.** Based on risk factor analysis, public health officers have generally recommended against teenage pregnancy. On the other hand, substantial data exist to suggest that black teenagers who give birth are more likely to survive to see that child reach the age of 20.[106] Thus, what traditionalists view as a risk factor may actually be a means for improving the overall health of the black population. Health promotion, in other words, may not be the simple opposite of risk reduction.
2. **National data may obscure local success.** Although national data about black–white

mortality are almost uniformly grim, there are local areas in the United States where black mortality is equal to or lower than that of white mortality, even when the black poverty level is relatively high. By continuously focusing on the negative (ie, situations in which blacks do worse relative to other groups), we may miss the opportunity to learn about what works.

In summary, the descriptive data provided by geographic studies of disparities in black–white mortality are useful to formulate hypotheses concerning the disparities in black–white mortality ratios, including regions of success. A closer focus on modifiable determinants, guided in part by the identification of areas in the United States where black–white rate ratios already approach or equal parity, offers the promise of future analytic epidemiologic studies to identify new ways to decrease racial mortality disparities. Summaries of the findings discussed in this chapter and recommendations to help ameliorate disparities in black–white mortality appear in Tables 2–7 and 2–8.

▶ **TABLE 2–8.** Summary of Recommendations

- **Acknowledge.** Recognize that no scientific, social, or political program since the end of World War II has demonstrated the capability of producing sustained improvement in overall black–white mortality at the national level
- **Ask.** Ask policy makers, legislators, and scientists why more than 100,000 premature deaths per year has become the quiet norm for blacks; ask if they are ready for this to change
- **Assist.** Learn that racial inequality in mortality is not inevitable in the United States
- **Advise.** Quantify probabilities for success, not simply risk factors for failure

▶ **APPENDIX 2-A.** Recent Local Area Studies of Black–White Mortality Within the United States[a]

Cause of Death	Region and Period of Observation	Year[b]	Author	Primary Observations and Methodologic Considerations
All causes	287 metropolitan statistical areas (MSAs) in the United States, excluding Alaska, 1980 and 1990	2003	Deaton and Lubotsky[111]	Mortality from Compressed Mortality Files (National Center for Health Statistics). Counties were mapped to MSAs except in New England, where New England county metropolitan areas were used. The same counties comprised 237 of 287 MSAs in 1980 and 1990. Differences in the remaining 50, however, were slight. Gini coefficient was the primary measure of income inequality; level of education (five categories) was also used. Results showed that after controlling for the fraction of the population that is black, there was no relationship in 1980 or in 1990 between income inequality and mortality across either states or cities. The fraction of the population that is black was *positively* correlated with average white incomes and *negatively* correlated with average black incomes. Between-group income inequality was therefore higher where the fraction black was higher, as is true of income inequality in general. Mortality rates were higher where the fraction black was higher, not only because of the mechanical effect of higher black mortality rates and lower black incomes, but also because *white* mortality rates were higher in places where the fraction black was higher. This was robust to conditioning on income, education, and (in MSAs) on state fixed effects. People with higher education had lower mortality rates, but this did nothing to moderate the estimated effect of the fraction black on white mortality rates. Results were not explained by provision of public services, regional differences, or differences in age composition. The hypothesis that high fraction black generates psychosocial stress that is directly harmful to health is plausible, and if verified, would reconcile Canadian evidence to showing no correlation between income inequality in Canadian provinces or cities; this would be expected if income inequality is a mask for the effects of racial composition on trust, because race lacks the social salience in Canada that it does in the United States.

Massachusetts and Rhode Island block group, census tract, and zip code areas, 1990	2003	Krieger et al[191]	Measures of economic deprivation such as percent below poverty were most sensitive to socioeconomic gradients in health regardless of race or ethnicity. The most consistent results and maximal geocoding linkage were evident for analyses at the census-tract level.
US counties, 1969–1998	2003	Singh[173]	This study analyzed area variations in mortality as a function of an ecologic variable, area deprivation. Twenty-one ecologically defined socioeconomic indicators were used to formulate an index of deprivation. Area deprivation gradients in US mortality increased during the study period. Area inequalities in mortality widened because of slower mortality declines in more deprived areas. Area gradients among black men followed the overall pattern, and were comparable to those for white men. Area gradients for black women remained generally stable over time. More deprived areas had substantially higher proportions of black and rural residents. Moreover, 62% of the population in the most deprived areas was located in the South, in contrast to only 19% of the population of the least deprived areas. Caution was advised when comparing area variations in mortality with individual-level socioeconomic differentials.
320 primary MSAs and 46 nonmetropolitan counties within state boundaries, 1990–1992	2002	Kindig et al[175]	Differences in death rates were analyzed in this cross-sectional study using racial and ethnic identity, socioeconomic composition, rural and urban differences, medical services, and geographic region. The strongest association of age-adjusted death rate was with the percentage of the population that was African American, and this association was independent of income, education, physician supply, and region. Other strong, independent, positive correlates of mortality were having < high school education, high Medicare expenditures, and location in western or southern regions. Factors with the strongest independent negative association were employment in agriculture and forestry, Hispanic ethnicity, and per capita income.

(continued)

▶ **APPENDIX 2-A.** (Continued) Recent Local Area Studies of Black–White Mortality Within the United States[a]

Cause of Death	Region and Period of Observation	Year[b]	Author	Primary Observations and Methodologic Considerations
	US counties, 1988–1992	2002	McLaughlin and Stokes[112]	Higher income inequality at the county level was significantly associated with higher total mortality. Higher minority racial concentration was also significantly related to higher mortality and interacted with income inequality, with the influence of inequality declining as the percent black increased. Among counties with relatively high minority concentration, those with low levels of income inequality had the highest mortality rates, while counties with the highest levels of income inequality had the lowest mortality rates. Each percentage point increase in the percentage of blacks corresponded to 3.8 additional deaths per 100,000 people per year.
	267 US metropolitan areas, 1989–1991	2001	Cooper et al[174]	Among persons < 65 years, age-adjusted premature mortality was 81% higher in blacks than in whites, and median household income was 40% lower. The percentage of the population that is black and income inequality (r = 0.26, black; r = 0.20 white) were significant predictors of premature mortality, and residential segregation was associated with premature mortality in blacks (r = 0.38). The association of segregation with premature mortality was much more pronounced in the southern United States and in areas with larger black populations.
	23 diverse local areas, 1990	2001	Geronimus et al[178]	Rural residents outlive urban residents, but their additional years are primarily inactive. Among urban residents, those in more affluent areas outlive those in high-poverty areas. For both blacks and whites, these gains represent increases in active years. For whites alone, they also reflect reductions in years spent in poor health.
	273 US metropolitan areas, 1990	2001	Shi and Starfield[119]	Both income inequality and primary care physician supply were significantly associated with white mortality (P < .10). After inclusion of socioeconomic status covariates, the effect of income inequality on black mortality remained significant (P < .01) but the effect of primary care physician supply was no longer significant (P > .10), particularly in areas with high income inequality.

Chicago, Ill, 1979–1991, 1991–1993, 1996–1998	2001	Silva et al[180]	Black–white rate ratios increased for virtually all measures of mortality and morbidity. From 1980–1998, the black–white ratio for all-cause mortality increased by 57% to 2.03. From 1979–1981 to 1996–1998, the low-income–high income rate ratio for all-cause mortality increased by 56% to 2.68. The fact that the *Healthy People 2000* campaign to reduce and then eliminate health disparities was not effective must serve as a stimulus for improved strategies.
US counties, 1990–1992	1999	Mansfield et al[176]	Age-adjusted years of life lost before age 75 were calculated and mapped by county. Premature mortality was greatest in rural counties in the Southeast and Southwest. Ecologic measures of community structure included age, race, per capita income education (proportion 25 years or older with < 9 years of education in 1980), chronic unemployment, vacant housing, per capita local government spending and local welfare spending, and proportion of households headed by women with children (no spouse present). There were slightly more years of life lost in rural areas than in urban or metropolitan areas, with southeastern and southwestern states bearing a disproportionate burden. The predictive power of larger black populations held across geographic groupings. The strong association between proportion of female-headed households and premature mortality held across the metropolitan–urban–rural continuum. In rural counties with high proportions of black population and female-headed households, Chronic interaction predicted additional premature mortality. Chronic unemployment was a predictor. Analyses showed little relationship between greater availability of medical care and years of potential life lost, although availability of specialist physicians appeared to help in rural areas and availability of generalist physicians predicted fewer years of life lost in metropolitan counties but more in rural counties.

(continued)

▶ **APPENDIX 2-A.** (Continued) Recent Local Area Studies of Black–White Mortality Within the United States[a]

Cause of Death	Region and Period of Observation	Year[b]	Author	Primary Observations and Methodologic Considerations
	Black women residing in four geographic aggregates of impoverished census tracts or zip codes—Harlem (New York City), Detroit (central city), Chicago (south side), and Los Angeles (Watts area), 1989–1991	1999	Geronimus et al[115]	The probability that a 15-year old mother in one of the study populations would survive to her child's 20th birthday was about the same as that for a typical 30-year-old white mother in the nation as a whole. Twenty-through 30-year-old mothers in the study areas had lower rates of survival to their children's 20th birthdays than mothers of any age nationwide, and they experienced a 6–10% reduction in their probability of survival if they postponed childbirth from age 15 to age 30. Ten to 15% of 30-year-old mothers in the study populations could not expect to survive until their child's 20th birthday, compared with 3% of white and 6% of black 30-year-old mothers nationwide. Fifteen-year-old fathers in the study areas had less chance of surviving to their child's 20th birthday than the typical 30-year-old white father nationwide, and those waiting until 20 to become fathers had a lower chance than typical black fathers nationwide. Over 30% of Harlem men who waited to father a child until age 30 were not likely to survive to that child's 20th birthday. This was a 21% reduction compared to a Harlem man who was 15 at the child's birth and a 26% lower probability than the typical white counterpart nationwide. If black parents residing in the study areas survived, their rates of disability were 1.5 times higher than blacks nationwide and three times higher than whites nationwide. About one third of mothers or fathers in Watts who survived to age 25 or 30 and postponed childbearing until then could have expected to be disabled by their child's 20th birthday. Less than 75% of blacks nationwide who postponed childbirth until age 30 could have expected to survive and be able-bodied at the child's 20th birthday. Fathers in the study areas who waited until age 30 to become fathers had about a 50% chance of surviving able-bodied to their child's 20th birthday, and the probability for mothers was about 60%.

Reference	Year	Population/period	Findings
			Only 75% of teenage mothers in the study areas could have expected their own mothers to survive able-bodied until their children reach age 5 years (slightly lower than typical 30-year-old mothers nationwide). For 30-year-olds in the study areas, this figure was 25% versus 58% for whites nationwide. Early fertility in this population may express the attempt to embrace the widely shared value that responsible parents strive to bring children into the world when they are most prepared to provide for their children's well-being.
Geronimus et al[110]	1999	Selected high-poverty areas (African American and white), 1979–1981 and 1989–1991	Substantial variability was found in levels, trends, and causes of excess mortality in poor populations. African American residents of urban and northern communities suffer extremely high and growing rates of excess mortality. Rural residents had an important advantage that widened over the period of observation. Circulatory diseases were the leading cause of excess mortality in most locations. Neither homicide nor AIDS contributed a great deal to the excess, outside of a few local effects for AIDS.
Hart et al[181]	1998	114 US standard MSAs, 1990–1991	Lower mortality rates for African Americans were associated with metropolitanized local governments and lower levels of residential segregation. Mortality for male and female whites was not associated in either direction with residential segregation. White male mortality was not associated with level of metropolitanization, but lower female white mortality rates were associated with less metropolitanization.
LeClere	1997	US census tracts	The mortality of men and women of all races is higher when the census tract in which they live has a larger fraction of African Americans (cited by Deaton and Lubotsky, 2003[111])
Preston et al[117]	1996	1985	Linkage of death certificate, social security, and census information showed that ages at death reported on death certificates are too young on average, with errors being greater for women than men. When corrected ages at death are used to estimate age-specific death rates, African American mortality rates increase substantially above age 85 and the racial crossover in mortality disappears. Uncertainty about white rates at ages 95+, however, prevents a decisive racial comparison at the very oldest ages.

(*continued*)

▶ **APPENDIX 2–A.** (Continued) Recent Local Area Studies of Black–White Mortality Within the United States[a]

Cause of Death	Region and Period of Observation	Year[b]	Author	Primary Observations and Methodologic Considerations
	Evans County, Georgia, 1960–1980	1985	Wing et al[192]	A statistically significant black–white mortality crossover for both men (at age 73) and women (at age 85) was found in this longitudinally followed population. Because the analyses did not rely on age reporting either in census data or on the death certificate, it suggests that crossover observations based on vital statistics are not artifacts. In addition to gene–environment interaction, the authors suggested that social support is a factor.
All causes/ specific causes (sentinel causes of death)	60 US counties located in large metropolitan areas, 1979–1981 and 1994–1996	2000	Polednak[182]	The black–white ratio of death rates before age 65 years for causes regarded as preventable by medical treatment and as useful in assessing overall quality of health care showed that counties with the highest black–white death rate ratios (> 3.5) and the highest death rates for blacks included the District of Columbia, Essex (Newark), NJ; Coo (Chicago), Illinois; Wayne (Detroit), Michigan; and Dade (Miami) Florida. In contrast with the rest of the United States, the death rate from the sentinel causes for blacks had not declined from 1979–1981 to 1994–1996, suggesting that racial inequalities in health care may be unusually great in certain counties in large metropolitan areas.
All causes/ specific causes	Hartford, Connecticut, census tracts with large public housing projects, 1988–1991	1998	Polednak[183]	Ratios of observed (based on housing project census tracts) to expected (based on age-specific death rates for all blacks in the city) numbers of deaths showed that all causes of death were statistically higher for black male (but not black female) residents living in census tracts with large housing projects, due, in part, to statistically significant elevations in both cancer and cardiovascular diseases, and for the subcategory of coronary heart disease. Poverty alone did not explain the results, leading to a call for research on quality of life and health care among residents of housing projects in Hartford and, by extension, to other US cities.

| All causes/selected causes (cardiovascular disease, coronary heart disease, myocardial infarction, stroke, hypertension) | New York City zip codes, 1998–1994 | 1998 | Fang et al[78] | This cross-sectional study linked mortality records with 1990 census data. Zip codes were aggregated by level of residential segregation (predominantly $\geq$ 75% white and black). Segregation was associated with mortality, independent from other relevant socioeconomic and demographic characteristics, but its impact was discrete, being associated with increased mortality for some diseases (eg, coronary heart disease) and not others (eg, stroke or hypertension). The authors suggest that this was possibly due to diminished impact of place when genetic factors were more powerful. In addition, within racially segregated areas, members of the dominant group, for all ages, among whites and elderly blacks enjoyed outcomes superior both to members of the minority racial group of their community and to members of the same race residing in other areas, where they are in the minority, independent of socioeconomic status. Thus, whites living in higher (and mainly white) socioeconomic areas had lower mortality rates than whites living in predominantly black areas (1473.7 versus 1934.1 for males, and 909 versus 1414.7 for females for all-cause mortality). This was true for all ages. In contrast, elderly blacks living in black areas, despite their less-favorable socioeconomic status, had lower mortality rates for all-cause, total cardiovascular disease, and coronary heart disease, than did those living in white areas, even after adjusting for available socioeconomic variables. Harlem was studied separately, because its mortality experience was previously reported to highlight the health disadvantage of blacks (McCord and Freeman, 1990[184]). |

(continued)

▶ **APPENDIX 2-A.** (Continued) Recent Local Area Studies of Black–White Mortality Within the United States[a]

Cause of Death	Region and Period of Observation	Year[b]	Author	Primary Observations and Methodologic Considerations
	US zip code areas, 1993	1996	Gornick et al[113]	Harlem had a more disadvantaged socioeconomic status and mortality. Nevertheless, elderly blacks living in Harlem still enjoyed an advantage in terms of coronary heart disease mortality compared with black residents in white areas. Suggestions as to other possible reasons for the observations included poorer social support among minorities regardless of race, worse physical environments, more tension and social unrest in black-segregated neighborhoods, the likelihood that southern blacks emigrating to New York tended to reside in low-socioeconomic, black-segregated areas, and that poor health was a cause of residence in more segregated areas rather than an effect of living in such places.
				Among 26.3 million Medicare beneficiaries ≥ 65 years of age (24.2 million whites and 2.1 million blacks) black–white mortality rate ratios were 1.19 for men and 1.16 for women ($P < .001$ for both). For every 100 women, there were 26.0 mammograms among whites and 17.1 among blacks. Rates in the least affluent zip code areas (compared with those in the most affluent areas) were 33% lower among whites and 22% lower among blacks. For every 1000 beneficiaries, there were 515 influenza immunizations among whites and 313 among blacks. As compared with the most affluent group, immunization rates were 26% lower in whites and 39% lower in blacks. Adjustment for differences in income had a relatively small effect on the racial differences. It was concluded that provision of health insurance alone is insufficient to ensure effective and equitable use of Medicare by all beneficiaries.
	38 MSAs with populations >1 million in 1980, 1982–1986	1993	Polednak[179]	The black–white poverty rate ratio was a stronger predictor of variation in the black–white mortality ratio for men than for women. For both men and women aged 15–44 years, the level of black–white segregation was a significant (positive) predictor of the black–white ratio of the age-standardized death rate. This analysis also identifies MSAs containing geographic areas with unusually high or low black–white mortality ratios, and indicates the need for more detailed studies of explanations for such variation.

All cause/specific cause (cardio-vascular disease)	1990	Wing et al[185]	US counties, 1962–1982	This study focused on trends in the coefficient of variation (defined as the standard deviation of rates divided by the mean) rather than the mean of the distribution of local rates to measure changes in geographic inequality of mortality. The trend of geographic inequality was broadly similar between race and sex groups for each cause, with an upward trend of relative inequality at younger ages and downward trend at older ages. However, the trend of inequality tended to be more favorable for white women than for white men and somewhat more favorable for black men than for black women, with the exception of stroke mortality, where increases of geographic inequality were greater for white women than white men at ages < 65 and about twice as great in black women as in black men at those ages. Because increases in relative inequality were strongest in the younger age groups, the pattern of inequality may be accentuated as these cohorts move into ages of higher mortality. If these trends continue, geographic inequality in cardiovascular disease mortality will increase rapidly as younger cohorts move into ages of higher mortality.
All cause/specific causes (cardio-vascular disease, cirrhosis, homicide, neo-plasm)	1990	McCord and Freeman[184]	Central Harlem Health District, New York City, 1979–1981	According to the 1980 census, 96% of Harlem residents were black, and 41% lived below the poverty level. The age-adjusted all-cause mortality rate was the highest in New York City, more than double that of US whites and 50% higher than that of US blacks. Almost all the excess mortality was among those < 65 years of age. Chief causes of the excess were cardiovascular disease (23.5% of excess deaths), cirrhosis (17.9%), homicide (14.98%), and neoplasm (12.6%). Survival analysis showed that black men in Harlem were less likely to reach the age of 65 than men in Bangladesh.

(continued)

▶ APPENDIX 2–A. (Continued) Recent Local Area Studies of Black–White Mortality Within the United States[a]

Cause of Death	Region and Period of Observation	Year[b]	Author	Primary Observations and Methodologic Considerations
All causes/specific causes (diabetes mellitus, ischemic heart disease, and cerebrovascular disease)	Suffolk County, New York, 1979–1983	1990	Polednak[186]	In this higher income area, where blacks had a median family income of almost $20,000 versus $12,618 for blacks in the entire United States, black–white ratios of age-specific death rates were elevated for all causes for men and women aged 35–44 through 55–64 years (but not for those 75 years or older), for ischemic heart disease for women (but not men) aged 35–44 through 55–64, for diabetes mellitus for most ages (especially for women), and for cerebrovascular disease for both men and women aged 35–44 through 65–74 years.
All causes, children	US counties, 1968–1992	2000	DeLiberti[37]	Social stratification was represented by the proportion of occupied housing units having a telephone. Counties were stratified into quintiles. Although there was an overall correlation between early childhood poverty and all-cause mortality, taking into account an apparent 9-year lag among black children, there was no consistent association between mortality rates (either age-adjusted or individual age group rates) and social stratification. However, age-adjusted mortality rates for black children living in the most advantaged counties almost uniformly exceeded the rates for the white population living in the least disadvantaged.
Cancer (all types)	Metropolitan Atlanta, Georgia, 1980–1987	1990	Murphy et al[193]	In a pilot study, the proportion of cancer mortality among 110 black Seventh-Day Adventists was observed to be lower than expected.
Cardiovascular disease	Metropolitan Atlanta, Georgia, 1979–1985	1992	Sung et al[194]	Deaths from hypertension, stroke, ischemic heart disease, and atherosclerosis were reviewed. The greatest black–white disparities were found for hypertension (excesses after age-adjustment of more than 200% for both men and women, and a 10-fold excess among 30–49-year-olds). An excess of stroke was observed among blacks

Cerebro-vascular disease	Anderson and Pee Dee areas of South Carolina, 1990	1998	Lackland et al[195]	< age 75, with whites having greater risk thereafter. Similar crossovers were observed for ischemic heart disease (30–59 for men), atherosclerosis (40–59 for men) and for all causes (75+ among women). Blacks were at higher risks for all four causes at younger age groups.
				All hospitalized and out-of-hospital deaths occurring among residents of these two areas were included. Incidence rates for blacks were nearly twice the rates for whites. However, rates among blacks for both of these predominantly rural sites were similar, while rates for white males were higher in Pee Dee, causing overall rates in Pee Dee to be 40% higher than Anderson ($P < .05$). Both area were regarded as similar with respect to medical care facilities and manpower, profiles of stroke subtypes, stroke case-fatality rates, and population-based estimates of education and socioeconomic status, hypertension, smoking, obesity, and percentage of Medicaid admissions for stroke.
	153 coastal plain ("south-eastern stroke belt") counties compared with the rest of the United States, 1968–1991	1995	Howard et al[196]	Among persons ≥ 45 years, excess stroke mortality was slightly greater in black men (ranging from 1.43–1.50 across 4-year intervals throughout the period of observation) than in white men and black women (1.33–1.43, and 1.32–1.42, respectively) and was lowest in white women (1.27–1.33). This translates to a greater than 40% excess risk of stroke mortality and more than 1200 excess stroke deaths annually.
Colorectal cancer	329 most populous US counties, 1989–1991	1997	Cooper et al[177]	Counties were divided into quartiles based on proportion of blacks in the population, and aggregate incidence and 2-year case-fatality rates were compared within and between quartiles. Within each quartile, the adjusted incidence rate for whites was consistently higher than that for blacks ($P < .001$), and case-fatality rates were consistently lower among whites ($P < .001$) for all but the quartile with the lowest proportion of blacks. Among both blacks and whites, incidence rates increased and case fatality decreased as the percentage of blacks increased
Diabetes	Allegheny County, Pennsylvania, 1965–1999	2001	Nishimura et al[197]	Mortality status in 1999 was confirmed for 972 of 1075 cases of type 1 diabetes mellitus diagnosed between January 1, 1965 and December 31, 1979. The mortality rate for African Americans (1388/100,000 person-years) was greater than that for whites (57/100,000 person-years)

(continued)

▶ **APPENDIX 2-A.** (Continued) Recent Local Area Studies of Black-White Mortality Within the United States[a]

Cause of Death	Region and Period of Observation	Year[b]	Author	Primary Observations and Methodologic Considerations
				($P < .05$). Mortality rates declined, but trends were not statistically significant for either race. Survival curves were worse for African Americans, and older age at diagnosis was associated wit higher risk of death.
Heart disease	Forsyth County, North Carolina; city of Jackson, Mississippi; eight suburbs of Minneapolis, Minnesota; Washington County, Maryland, 1987–1996	2001	Rosamond et al[198]	Surveillance included > 360,000 men and women. Admission to acute care hospitals and deaths due to coronary heart disease among all residents aged 35–74 years were monitored. Age-adjusted coronary heart disease mortality was highest among black men (2.7/1000) followed by white men (2.0/1000), black women (1.5/1000) and white women (0.6/1000). The same pattern occurred for average annual rate of decline in incidence. Black men also had the highest age-adjusted hospitalized myocardial infarction incidence rate in 1996.
	Los Angeles, California, 1993–1998; prospective, multiethnic cohort	2001	Henderson et al[199]	Despite appearing to have similar socioeconomic profiles and similar accesses to health care, African Americans bore a greater burden of cardiovascular disease. After adjustment for potential risk modifiers such as age, smoking, body mass index, and presence of hypertension, African Americans remained with an adjusted relative risk of cardiovascular mortality higher than that of Hispanics.
	313 US areas, 1990	2001	Fuchs et al[200]	Among whites aged 65–84 years, mortality is positively correlated to utilization of in-patient care, cigarette sales, obesity, air pollution, and percent black. Florida is an outlier for both utilization (very high) and mortality (very low).

State Economic Areas (SEAs) surrounding ARIC (Atherosclerosis Risk in Communities) study	1999	Williams et al[201]	Racial variations were noted in coronary heart disease mortality rates (1968–1992) of residents aged 35–84 years. The black–white mortality rate ratio increased over time regardless of gender. The black disadvantage in coronary heart disease mortality was increasingly greater in ARIC SEAs than in the United States as a whole. These differences were concurrent with racial differences in risk factors, the incidence of myocardial infarction, and case fatality rates.
All counties in US South, 1968–1986	1999	Barnett et al[160]	For African Americans aged 35–74 years and living in a greater metropolitan area in 1968, there was a 29% excess in coronary heart disease mortality compared with isolated rural areas, while for African American women there was a 45% excess. By 1986, thanks to greater declines in metropolitan than rural areas, the corresponding excesses were 3% and 11%.
All US counties, 1980–1988	1998	Armstrong et al[159]	Among blacks aged 35–64 years, coronary heart disease rates were highest in counties with intermediate percentages of white-collar workers, while rates for whites were highest in counties with the smallest percentages of white-collar workers. Per capita levels of income and numbers of medical-care providers were positively associated with the percentage of white-collar workers.
Charleston, South Carolina, 1960–1990	1993	Keil et al[202]	Rates of death from coronary disease in a small cohort of participants (653 white men, 333 black men, 741 white women, and 454 black women at baseline in 1960–1961) followed for 30 years were somewhat lower among black men than white men and higher among black women than white women. The black–white mortality rate ratios were not statistically significant, and the major risk factors for mortality from coronary disease were similar in blacks and whites.
Homicide US counties, 1987–1995	1998	Fingerhut et al[203]	For black males aged 15–24 years in 1995, firearms were the mechanism in 92% of all homicides versus 82% for white males, 70% for black females and 56% for white females. The black male firearm homicide rate in core metropolitan areas was 174.5 deaths per 100,000 populations, versus 29.8 for white males, 14.2 for black females, and 3.5 for white females. Differences between core (highly urban) areas and nonmetropolitan areas were more marked for blacks than whites.

(continued)

▶ **APPENDIX 2-A.** (Continued) Recent Local Area Studies of Black–White Mortality Within the United States[a]

Cause of Death	Region and Period of Observation	Year[b]	Author	Primary Observations and Methodologic Considerations
	Allegheny County, Pennsylvania, 1966–1974, 1984–1993, and 1996	1998	Smith et al[204]	Two separate homicide epidemics occurred between 1966 and 1993: one between 1966 and 1976, the other between 1990 and 1993. Black males aged 15–24 years were particularly affected, with rates of 275/100,000 being recorded in 1992–1993. Although each epidemic had different characteristics (eg, more homicides out of home, among strangers; less association with alcohol and more association with drug use; and multiple perpetrators in the second epidemic), guns were consistent as primary agents.
	Jefferson County, Alabama, 1978–1989	1994	Fine et al[205]	Using data from the coroner or medical examiner's office, it was observed that the highest annual race-specific homicide rate was in black males (75.9) followed by black females (12.4), white males (10.4), and white females (4.1). Age and race-specific rates for black males according to rank were 25–34 (159.7), 35–44 (151.7), and 14–24 (96.2). Among black males, key factors were black male-on-male violence, acquaintance of the victim and perpetrator, and the importance of arguments as the inciting event. Rates in black males, however, were declining at a greater rate than for all other race–sex groups, and among 15–24-year-olds such factors as drug use, increased availability of firearms, and child abuse were not major determinants of change.
	22 heavily urbanized US counties, 1979–1985	1991	Greenberg et al[206]	Among white males aged 15–24 years, significant excesses were observed on weekends and on national holidays. Among black males of the same age, deaths were disproportionately likely to occur in a pattern of single days with multiple homicides as well as in periodic spikes lasting less than 1 week.
	Atlanta, Georgia, 1971–1972	1984	Centerwall[62]	In a study of domestic homicide (defined as a criminal homicide committed in a residence by a relative or acquaintance of the victim), it was observed that when black and white populations were matched for rates of household crowding, the relative risk of intraracial domestic homicide in black populations was comparable to that for white populations (RR, 1.2; 95% CI, 10.7–2.0).

Infant mortality	New York City—156 zip code regions (97% of live births and 96% of infant deaths), 1988–1989 and 1992–1993	Sohler et al[207]	2003	Analyses addressed per capita income and income inequality (percent of income received by the least well-off 50% of households—method of Kaplan et al, 1996). An increase of one standard deviation in income inequality was associated with an increase of 0.80 deaths per 1000 live births ($P < .001$), controlling for other socioeconomic factors (including percent black, percent with high school education, and percent unemployed).
	60 largest US cities, 1995–1998	Haynatzka et al[120]	2002	Cities with the highest rates tended to have a larger proportion of black births and a smaller proportion of Hispanic births, while the reverse was true for cities with the lowest rates. Highest-quartile cities had more very-low- and moderately-low-birth-weight infants, more births to teenage mothers, more late or absent prenatal care, and more racial segregation. Education of the mother did not confer the same protection among infants of black women as it did among whites. Cities with higher rates were more common in the Midwest, Southeast, and Northeast, and those with lower rates were clustered in the Pacific West and West Central regions. Despite higher poverty and lower education rates, Hispanic infants had higher birth weights, and their rates approximated those of non-Hispanic whites. The wide differences both within and among racial and ethnic groups suggest that rates can be reduced further.
	Chicago, Illinois, 1992–1995	Papacek et al[187]	2002	The postneonatal infant mortality rate for African Americans was 7.5/1000 live births, compared with 2.7 for whites (RR, 2.8; 95% CI, 2.3–3.3). Although 79% of African American infants (compared with 9% for whites) lived in impoverished neighborhoods, the adjusted odds ratio (OR; controlling for infant and maternal individual-level risk factors) for African Americans in impoverished neighborhoods was 1.5 (95% CI, 0.5–4.2), while that for African American infants in nonimpoverished neighborhoods was 1.8 (95% CI, 1.1–2.9)

(continued)

▶ **APPENDIX 2–A.** (Continued) Recent Local Area Studies of Black–White Mortality Within the United States[a]

Cause of Death	Region and Period of Observation	Author	Year[b]	Primary Observations and Methodologic Considerations
	New York City, 1988–1992	Rosenberg et al[123]	2002	After controlling for potential confounders, infants of native-born non-Hispanic black women had a greater risk of death than infants of foreign-born, non-Hispanic, black women (OR, 1.32; 95% CI, 1.21–1.43).
	Census blocks in Milwaukee, Wisconsin, 1992–1994	Sims and Rainge[121]	2002	African American infant, neonatal, and postneonatal mortality rates were 2.3, 2.0, and 3.0 times higher than corresponding rates for whites. African American mothers lived in less-desirable, more segregated neighborhoods and were eight times as likely as all white mothers to have inadequate prenatal care. Poor African American mothers were three times more likely to have inadequate prenatal care than poor white mothers.
	Davidson County, Tennessee, 1990–1994	Scott-Wright et al[189]	1998	Linked birth and death data showed that among infants born to college-educated white and black women, black race was not identified as a significant predictor of infant mortality. The most significant predictor was gestational age < 28 weeks.
	Chicago, Illinois, 1982–1983	Collins and Hawkes[208]	1997	Four environmental predictors of postneonatal death were studied: median family income of < $10,000/year; poverty prevalence of > 50%; violent crime rates of > 11/1000 population, and limited community access to primary medical care based on physician supply ratios. Postneonatal black mortality exceeded that for whites by more than threefold (10/1000 live births versus 3/1000 live births). Accounting for these risk factors reduced the OR for black infants from 3.0 (95% CI, 2.5–3.6) to 1.7 (95% CI, 1.5–1.9). Accounting for differences in maternal age, education martial status, and infant birth weight reduced the OR to 1.5 (95% CI, 1.3–1.7)
	US counties, 1985–1987	Larson et al[126]	1997	Residence in a nonmetropolitan county was not found to be associated with increased risk of adverse birth outcome, low birth weight, or neonatal mortality at the national level or in most states, after controlling for relevant demographic and biologic risk factors. Nonmetropolitan residence may be associated with problems of access to routine care, as exemplified by its association with greater risk of postneonatal mortality at the national level, and with late institution of prenatal care at both national in most states.

Metropolitan Ohio, 1960, 1970, 1980, 1990	1996	Stockwell and Goza[127]	A pronounced inverse association was found between income status and infant mortality for whites, but not for nonwhites. Nonwhite postneonatal death rates were higher for the lowest income areas, but for neonatal mortality, total infant deaths, and exogenous and endogenous cause-specific death rates, there was no discernible socioeconomic differential.
US cities with population of 50,000 at least 10% of which is black	1993	Laveist[124]	Racial residential segregation, black political empowerment, and black and white poverty were the characteristics that distinguished cities with a high degree of disparity in black–white infant mortality from cities that did not.
Madigan Army Medical Center Tacoma, Washington, 1985–1990 (in this case, the hospital is taken to represent the experience of a military community)	1992	Rawlings and Weir[190]	The mortality rate among black infants was 11.1/1000 live births compared with 17.9/1000 live births among all black Americans in 1987. There were no significant differences by military rank. The authors suggested that the lower rates among black infants might be due to guaranteed access to health care and higher levels of family education and income in the multiracial subpopulation served by this medical center.
38 standard MSAs with populations > 1,000,000 in 1980, 1982–1986	1991	Polednak[188]	Black–white difference in infant mortality varied by a factor of almost seven. The most important predictor of the black–white difference was the segregation index, independent of median family income and poverty prevalence.
Richmond, Virginia, 1979–1981	1990	Creighton-Zollar[128]	An inverse relationship was found between socioeconomic status and infant mortality for the total white and black population. For the black population alone, however, there did not appear to be any relationship between the economic or family life characteristics of census-tract population and their level of infant mortality.

(continued)

▶ **APPENDIX 2-A.** (Continued) Recent Local Area Studies of Black–White Mortality Within the United States[a]

Cause of Death	Region and Period of Observation	Year[b]	Author	Primary Observations and Methodologic Considerations
Preventable causes	107 US cities with a central city population of at least 100,000 and an African American population of at least 10%, 1989–1991	1999	Collins[209]	Basing classification of segregation on block-group measures of racial isolation, mortality amenable to prevention (including infections and parasitic diseases, specific cancers, anemia, pneumonia and influenza, appendicitis, heart diseases, viral hepatitis, diabetes, ulcers, and congenital anomalies) showed that such mortality was significantly associated with segregation, particularly in the Midwest for African American (marginally significant) and white males. Black social isolation was positively related to elevated mortality in the Northeast, but only for African American men (marginally significant) and women. In the South, residential segregation was significantly associated with causes of death amenable to medical intervention among African Americans and white men and white women.
Prostate cancer	Wayne County, Michigan (Allen Part Veterans Affairs Medical Center), 1973–1992	1995	Powell et al[210]	SEER-trained abstractors determined stage at diagnosis for all prostate cancers diagnosed during the period. Ages of black and white patients were comparable, and the proportion of whites and blacks presenting with localized disease was similar (57% and 54%, respectively), but a greater proportion of blacks presented with distant disease (25% versus 19%; $P = .45$), and survival among blacks was poorer than found among whites until age 70. The results suggested that removal of financial barriers to care within this system did not influence the higher proportion of distant disease or poorer survival of African American patients.
Systemic lupus erythematosus	All US counties	2001	Walsh and Fenster[211]	Comparisons between geographic clusters of high (Alabama, Arkansas, Louisiana, New Mexico) and low (Minnesota, Vermont, Virginia, Washington) mortality showed relative risks of 3.2, 3.4, and 5.9 for white, black, and "other" race women. Clusters with elevated mortality had higher poverty rates or greater percentages of ethnic Hispanic (or both) than those with lower mortality.
Systemic sclerosis	955 counties in 12 southeastern states, 1981–1990	1997	Walsh and DeChello[212]	From 1989–1990 significant excess mortality from systemic sclerosis occurred among white and black males, but not among white or black females. Clusters among white males were centered in Coffee County, Tennessee; Calhoun, Alabama; and Chattoga, Georgia. A single

	Local areas[a]	Year[b]	Authors	
Sudden infant death syndrome (SIDS)	Chicago, Illinois, 1993–1996	2002, 2003	Hauck et al[213,214]	significant cluster was found for black males, centered at Northampton, North Carolina. Cluster areas accounted for 79% and 66% of excess deaths among white and black males across the Southeast. In a population-based, case-control study of 260 SIDS deaths and an equal number of matched living controls (75% black, 13.1% Hispanic white, and 11.9% non-Hispanic white), prone sleeping, use of soft bedding and pillows, and bed sharing were all important factors in this population, and prone sleeping was found to account for about one third of SIDS deaths.
Suicide	38 US cities, 1970	2000	Lester[215]	An index of residential segregation in 1960 did not predict the 1970 African American suicide rates.
Trauma	Los Angeles County, 1996	1998	Demetriades et al[216]	Mortality from homicide was 40.4/100,000 among African Americans, 18.7/100,000 among Hispanics, 4.0/100,000 among Caucasians, and 3.7/100,000 among Asians. African American males were at very high risk (73.3/100,000), particularly those aged 15–34 years (164.2/100,000). African American and Hispanic males > 55 years had the highest rates of death from traffic accidents, and pedestrian deaths were more common in African Americans and Hispanics. Caucasians, particularly males > 65, had the highest rates of suicide. No suicides attributable to penetrating injury occurred among African Americans.
	Hinds County, Mississippi (a "dry" [alcohol] area) and Contra Costa County, California ("wet"), 1995–1997	1996	Cherpitel[217]	Fatal injuries during a 1-year period among persons ≥ 18 years of age were more likely to involve alcohol in the "dry" county (57%) than in the "wet" county (40%). Across both counties, younger age and black race predicted homicide. Nonblacks with positive drug screenings were more likely to die from suicide, and nonblacks with a positive blood alcohol concentration and negative drug screening were more likely to die from motor vehicle accidents.

AIDS, acquired immunodeficiency syndrome; CI, confidence interval; OR, odds ratio; RR, relative risk; SEER, Surveillance Epidemiology and End Results Program.

[a] Local areas include city, county, census tract, zip code, and neighborhood areas.

[b] Year listed is that of publication.

▶ REFERENCES

1. Levine RS, Foster JE, Fullilove RE, et al Black–white inequalities in mortality and life expectancy from 1933–1999: Implications for Healthy People 2010. *Public Hltb Rep* 2001;116:474–483.

2. Rosenberg HM, Maurer JD, Sorlie PD, et al. Quality of death rates by race and Hispanic origin: A summary of current research. *Vital Health Stat 2* 1999;128:1–13.

2a. Maurer JD, Rosenberg H, Keemer JB. Deaths of Hispanic origin. 15 reporting states. 1079–1981. *Vital Health Stat Ser* 1980;20(13).

3. Hennekens CH, Buring JE. *Epidemiology in Medicine.* Boston, Mass: Little Brown; 1987.

4. Morgenstern H. Ecologic studies. In: Rothman KJ, Greenland S. *Modern Epidemiology,* 2nd ed. Philadelphia, PA: Lippincott-Raven; 1998:459–480.

5. Community Health Status Indicators Project Team. *Community Health Status Report: Data Sources, Definitions, and Notes.* Washington, DC: July 2000.

6. Kanarek NF, Sockwell DC, Bialek R, et al. Use of peer counties: The community health status indicators project status reports. Abstract No. 6616. 128th meeting of the American Public Health Association; 2000. Available at: http://apha.confex.com/apha/128am/techprogram/paper_6616.htm. Accessed January 27, 2004.

7. Cooper RS, Freeman VL. Limitations in the use of race in the study of disease causation. *J Natl Med Assoc* 1999;91:378–383.

8. Jackson SA, Anderson RT, Johnson NJ, Sorlie PD. The relation of residential segregation to all-cause mortality: A study in black and white. *Am J Public Health* 2000;90:615–617.

9. Schultz AG, Williams DR, Israel BA, Lempert LB. Racial and spatial relations as fundamental determinants of health in Detroit. *Milbank Q* 2002;80:677–707.

10. Williams DR, Neighbors HW, Jackson JS. Racial/ethnic discrimination and health: Findings from community studies. *Am J Public Health* 2003;93:200–208.

11. Ewbank DC. History of black mortality and health before 1940. *Milbank Q* 1987;65(suppl 1):100–128.

12. CDC Wonder System. 2004. Available at: http:/wonder.cdc.gov/. Accessed March 1, 2004.

13. National Center for Health Statistics, Public Health Service. *Health, United States, 1988.* (DHHS Publication No. PHS 89-1232.) Washington, DC: US Government Printing Office; 1989.

14. Sorlie PD, Backlund E, Keller JB. US mortality by economic, demographic, and social characteristics: The National Longitudinal Mortality Study. *Am J Public Health* 1995;85(7):949–956.

15. LeClere FB, Soobader M-J. The effect of income inequality on the health of selected US demographic groups. *Am J Public Health* 2000;90:1.892–897.

16. Mellor JM, Milyo J. Is exposure to income inequality a public health concern? Lagged effects of income inequality on individual and population health. *Health Serv Res* 2003;38:137–151.

17. Hahn RA, Eaker ED, Barker ND, et al. Poverty and death in the United States. *Int J Health Serv* 1996;26(4):673–690.

18. Reidpath DD. "Love thy neighbour"—it's good for your health: A study of racial homogeneity, mortality and social cohesion in the United States. *Soc Sci Med* 2003;57:253–261.

19. US Dept of Health and Human Services (DHHS) Task Force on Black and Minority Health. *Report of the Secretary's Task Force on Black and Minority Health* (Vol 1, Executive Summary). Washington, DC: US Government Printing Office; 1985.

20. Iyasu S, Tomashek K, Barfield W. Infant mortality and low birth weight among black and white infants—United States, 1980–2000. *MMWR Morb Mortal Wkly Rep* 2002;51:589–592.

21. CDC's campaign to prevent antimicrobial resistance in health-care settings. *MMWR Morb Mortal Wkly Rep* 2002;51(15):343

22. Demissie K, Rhoads GG, Ananth CV, et al. Trends in preterm birth and neonatal mortality among blacks and whites in the United States from 1989 to 1997. *Am J Epidemiol* 2001;154:307–315.

23. Alexander GR, Kogan M, Bader D, et al. US birth weight/gestational age-specific neonatal mortality: 1995–1997 rates for whites, Hispanics, and blacks. *Pediatrics* 2003;111(1):e61–66.

24. Schoendorf K, Hogue CJ, Kleinman J, Rowley DL. Mortality among infants of black as compared to white college graduates. *N Engl J Med* 1992;326:1522–1526.

25. Hogan VK, Richardson JL, Ferre CD, et al. A public health framework for addressing black and

white disparities in preterm delivery. *J Am Med Womens Assoc* 2000;56:177–180.

26. Editorial note. *MMWR Morb Mortal Wkly Rep* 2002;57:590–591.

27. Carmichael SL, Iyasu S, Hatfield-Timajchy K. Cause-specific trends in neonatal mortality among black and white infants, United States, 1980–1995. *Matern Child Health J* 1998;2:67–76.

28. Carmichael SL, Iyasu S. Changes in the black–white infant mortality gap from 1983 to 1991 in the United States. *Am J Prev Med* 1998;15:220–227.

29. Carmichael SL, Iyasu S. Hatfield-Timajchy K. Cause-specific trends in neonatal mortality among black and white infants, United States, 1980–1995. *Matern Child Health J* 1998;2:67–76.

30. Salihu HM, Alexander MR, Shumpert MN, et al. Infant mortality among twins born to teenagers in the United States. Black–white disparity. *J Reprod Med* 2003;48:257–267.

31. Vintzeleos AM, Ananth CV, Sumulia JC, et al. Prenatal care and black–white fetal death disparity in the United States: Heterogeneity by high-risk conditions. *Obstet Gynecol* 2002;99:483–489.

32. Chang J, Elam-Evans LD, Berg CJ, et al. Pregnancy-related mortality surveillance—United States, 1991–1999. *MMWR CDC Surveill Summ* 2003;52(2):1–8.

33. Centers for Disease Control and Prevention. Perspectives in disease prevention and health promotion enhanced maternal mortality surveillance—North Carolina, 1988 and 1989. *MMWR Morb Mortal Wkly Rep* 1991;40:469–471.

34. Centers for Disease Control and Prevention. Pregnancy-related mortality—Georgia, 1990–1992. *MMWR Morb Mortal Wkly Rep* 1995;44:93–96.

35. Centers for Disease Control and Prevention. Misclassification of maternal deaths—Washington state. *MMWR Morb Mortal Wkly Rep* 1986;35:621–623.

36. Allen MH, Chavkin W, Marinoff J. Ascertainment of maternal deaths in New York City. *Am J Public Health* 1991;81:380–382.

37. DiLiberti JH. The relationship between social stratification and all-cause mortality among children in the United States: 1968–1992. *Pediatrics* 2000;105:e2. Available at: http://www.pediatrics.org/cgi/content/full/105/1/e2.

37a. Centers for Disease Control and Prevention. Influence of homicide on racial disparity in life expectancy—United States, 1998. *MMWR Morb Mortal Wkly Rep* 2001;50:780–783.

38. Roig E, Castaner A. Simmons B, et al. In-hospital mortality rates from acute myocardial infarction by race in U.S. hospitals: Findings from the National Hospital Discharge Survey. *Circulation* 1987;76:280–288.

39. Mannino DM, Homa DM, Akinbami LJ, et al. Surveillance for asthma—United States, 1980–1999. *MMWR CDC Surveill Summ* 2002;51(1):1–13.

40. Sheffer AL, Taggart VS. National Asthma Education Program. Expert panel report guidelines for the diagnosis and management of asthma. National Heart, Lung, and Blood Institute. *Med Care* 1993;31(3 suppl):MS20–28.

41. Pew Environmental Health Commission. *Attack Asthma: Why America Needs a Public Health Defense System to Battle Environmental Threats.* Baltimore, Md: John Hopkins School of Public Health, Pew Environmental Health Commissions; 2001.

41a. Grant EN, Lyttle CS, Weiss KB. The relation of socioeconomic factors and racial/ethnic differences in US asthma mortality. *Am J Public Health* 2000;90(12):1923–1925.

42. American Cancer Society. *Cancer Facts and Figures 2003.* Atlanta, Ga: American Cancer Society; 2003.

43. Ghafoor A, Jemal A, Cokkinides V, et al. Cancer statistics for African Americans. *CA Cancer J Clin* 2002;52(6):326–341.

44. Cancer Statistics Branch, National Cancer Institute. *SEER Extent of Disease.* Bethesda, Md: National Cancer Institute; 1988.

45. Clegg LX, Li FP, Hankey BF, et al. Cancer survival among US whites and minorities: A SEER (Surveillance, Epidemiology, and End Results) Program population-based study. *Arch Int Med* 2002;162:1985–1993.

46. Li CI, Malone KE, Daling JR. Differences in breast cancer stage, treatment, and survival by race and ethnicity. *Arch Intern Med* 2003;13;163(1):49–56.

47. Chu KC, Tarone RE, Brawley OW. Breast cancer trends of black women compared with white women. *Arch Fam Med* 1999;8:521–528.

48. Harlan L, Brawley O, Pommerenke F, et al. Geographic, age, and racial variation in the treatment of local/regional carcinoma of the prostate. *J Clin Oncol* 1995;13:93–100.

49. Arbes SJ Jr, Olshan AF, Caplan DJ, et al. Factors contributing to the poorer survival of black Americans diagnosed with oral cancer (United States). *Cancer Causes Control* 1999;10:513–523.

50. Chow WH, Devesa SS, Warren JL, Fraumeni JF Jr. Rising incidence of renal cell cancer in the United States. *JAMA* 1999;281:1628–1631.

51. Hsing AW, Devesa SS. Prostate cancer mortality in the United States by cohort year of birth, 1865–1940. *Cancer Epidemiol Biomarkers Prev* 1994;3(7):527–530.

52. Chu KC, Tarone RE, Freeman HP. Trends in prostate cancer mortality among black men and white men in the United States. *Cancer* 2003;97:1507–1516.

53. Groves FD, Linet MS, Devesa SS. Patterns of occurrence of the leukaemias. *Eur J Cancer* 1995;31A(6):941–949. Erratum in *Eur J Cancer* 1995;31A(11):1903.

54. Dignam JJ, Colangelo L, Tian W, et al. Outcomes among African-Americans and Caucasians in colon cancer adjuvant therapy trials: Findings from the National Surgical Adjuvant Breast and Bowel projects. *J Natl Cancer Inst* 1999;91:1933–1940.

55. Bian J, Oddone EZ, Samsa GP, et al. Racial differences in survival post cerebral infarction among the elderly. *Neurology* 2003;60:285–290.

56. Boneva RS, Botto LD, Moore CA, et al. Mortality associated with congenital heart defects in the United States: Trends in racial disparities, 1979–1997. *Circulation* 2001;103:2376–2381.

57. Valdez R, Narayan KM, Geiss LS, Engelgau MM. Impact of diabetes mellitus on mortality associated with pneumonia and influenza among non-Hispanic black and white US adults. *Am J Public Health* 1999;89(11):1715–1721.

57a. Boyle JR, Honeycutt AA, Narayan KMV, et al. Projection of diabetes burden through 2050. *Diabetes Care* 2001;24:1936–1940.

58. Waller AE, Baker SP, Szocka A. Childhood injury deaths: National analysis and geographic variations. *Am J Public Health* 1989;79:310–315.

59. Rogers RG, Rosenblatt R, Hummer RA, Krueger PM. Black–white differentials in adult homicide mortality in the United States. *Soc Sci Q* 2001;82:435–452.

60. Paulozzi LJ, Saltzman LE, Thompson MP, Holmgreen P. Surveillance for homicide among intimate partners—United States, 1981–1998. *MMWR CDC Surveill Summ* 2001;12:1–15.

61. Onwuachi-Saunders C, Hawkins DF. Black–white differences in injury. Race or social class? *Ann Epidemiol* 1993;3:150–153.

62. Centerwall BS. Race, socioeconomic status, and domestic homicide, Atlanta, 1971–72. *Am J Public Health* 1984;74:813–815.

63. Hammett M, Powell KE, O'Carroll PW, Clanton ST. Homicide surveillance—United States, 1979–1988. *MMWR CDC Surveill Summ* 1992;41(3):1–33.

64. Ikeda RM, Gorwitz R, James SP, et al. Trends in fatal firearm-related injuries, United States, 1962–1993. *Am J Prev Med* 1997;13:396–400.

65. Tomashek KM, Hsia J, Iyasu S. Trends in postneonatal mortality attributable to injury, United States, 1988–1998. *Pediatrics* 2003;111:1219–1225.

66. Sikora AG, Mulvihill M. Trends in mortality due to legal intervention in the United States, 1979 through 1997. *Am J Public Health* 2002;92(5):841–843.

67. Baker SP, Braver ER, Chen LH, et al. Motor vehicle occupant deaths among Hispanic and black children and teenagers. *Arch Pediatr Adolesc Med* 1998;152:1209–1212.

68. Holman RC, Stoll BJ, Clarke MJ, Glass RI. The epidemiology of necrotizing enterocolitis infant mortality in the United States. *Am J Public Health* 1997;87:2026–2031.

69. Abbott KC, Hypolite I, Welch PG, Agodoa LYC. Human immunodeficiency virus/acquired immunodeficiency syndrome–associated nephropathy at end-stage renal disease in the United States: Patient characteristics and survival in the pre highly active antiretroviral therapy era. *J Nephrol* 2001;14:377–383.

70. Owen WF Jr, Chertow GM, Lazarus JM, Lowrie EG. Dose of hemodialysis and survival: Differences by race and sex. *JAMA* 1998;280(20):1764–1768.

71. Stoll BJ, Holman RC, Schuchat A. Decline in sepsis-associated neonatal and infant deaths in the United States, 1979 through 1994. *Pediatrics* 1998;102:e18

72. Variations in the incidence of sudden infant death syndrome (SIDS), United States, 1980–1988. *Stat Bull Metrop Insur Co* 1993;74:10–18.

73. Malloy MH, Freeman DH Jr. Birth weight- and gestational age-specific sudden infant death syndrome mortality: United States, 1991 versus 1995. *Pediatrics* 2000;105:1227–1231.

74. Cossman RE, Cossman JS, Jackson R, Cosby A. Mapping high or low mortality places across time in the United States: A research note on a health visualization and analysis project. *Health Place* 2003;9:361–369.

75. Cossman R, Blanchard T, James W, et al. Healthy and unhealthy places in America: Are these really spatial clusters? Available at: http://gis.esri.com/library/userconf/proc02/pap1064.htm. Accessed March, 2004.

76. Devesa SS, Grauman DJ, Blot WJ, Fraumeni JF Jr. Cancer surveillance series: Changing geographic patterns of lung cancer mortality in the United States, 1950 through 1994. *J Natl Cancer Instit* 1999;91:1040–1050.

77. Howard G, Howard VJ, Katholi C, et al. Decline in US stroke mortality: An analysis of temporal patterns by sex, race, and geographic region. *Stroke* 2001;32:2213–2220.

78. Fang J, Madhavan S, Bosworth W, Alderman MH. Residential segregation and mortality in New York City. *Soc Sci Med* 1998;47:469–476.

79. Fang J, Madhavan S, Alderman MH. Influence of nativity on cancer mortality among black New Yorkers. *Cancer* 1997;80:129–135.

80. Schneider D, Greenberg M, Lu L. Early life experiences linked to diabetes mellitus: A study of African American migration. *J Natl Med Assoc* 1997;89:29–34.

81. Perry HM, Roccella EJ. Conference report on stroke mortality in the southeastern United States. *Hypertension* 1998;31:1206–1215.

82. Israel BA, Schulz AJ, Parker EA, Becker AB. Community-based participatory research: Policy recommendations for promoting a partnership approach in health research. *Educ Health (Abingdon)* 2001;14:1820–1897.

83. Adams PF, Benson V. Current estimates from the National Health Interview Survey, 1991. National Center for Health Statistics. *Vital Health Stat* 1992;Dec(184):1–232.

84. Adams PF, Benson V. Current estimates from the National Health Interview Survey, 1990. National Center for Health Statistics. *Vital Health Stat* 1991;Dec(181):1–212.

85. McDonald A, Van Horn L, Slatter ML, et al. The CARDIA diet history: Development and implementation. *J Am Diet Assoc* 1991;91:1104–1112.

86. Appel SJ, Harrell JS, Deng S. Racial and socioeconomic differences in risk factors for cardiovascular disease among Southern rural women. *Nurs Res* 2002;51(3):140–147.

87. Kaplan MS, Geling O. Firearm suicides and homicides in the United States: Regional variations and patterns of gun ownership. *Soc Sci Med* 1998;46:1227–1233.

88. Miller M, Azrael D, Hemenway D. Rates of household firearm ownership and homicide across US regions and states, 1988–1997. *Am J Public Health* 2002;92:1988–1993.

89. Cushman WC, Reda DJ, Materson BJ, Perry HM for the Department of Veterans Affairs Cooperative Study Group in Antihypertensive Agents. Stroke Belt as a predictor of antihypertensive efficacy with single-drug therapy. *Am J Hypertens* 1995;8:34A.

90. Schroeder HA. Municipal drinking water and cardiovascular death rates. *JAMA* 1966;195:81–85.

91. Morris JN, Crawford MD, Heady JA. Hardness of local water supplies and mortality from cardiovascular disease. *Lancet* 1961;1:860–862.

92. Perry HM, Erlanger MS, Perry EF. Increase in blood pressure of rats chronically fed low levels of lead. *Environ Health Perspect* 1988;78:107–111.

93. Clark DE, Cushing BM. Predicting regional variations in mortality from motor vehicle crashes. *Acad Emerg Med* 1999;6(2):125–130.

94. United Health Foundation. *America's Health: State Health Rankings—2003 Edition*. Minnetonka, Minn: United Health Foundation; 2003.

94a. Rosenberg HM, Maurer JD, Sorlie PD, et al. Quality of death rates by race and Hispanic origin: A summary of current research, 1999. National Center for Health Statistics. *Vital Health Stat* 1999;2:128.

95. Oose M. Variations in state mortality from 1960 to 1990. Population Division, US Census Bureau. Population Division Working Paper Series No. 49; May 2003.

96. Wilkinson RG. *Unhealthy Societies: The Affliction of Inequality*. London, England: Routledge; 1996.

97. Daniels N, Kennedy BP, Kawachi I. Why justice is good for our health: The social determinants of health inequalities. *Daedalus* 1999;128(4):215–251.

98. Lochner K, Pamuk E, Makuc D, et al. State-level income inequality and individual mortality risk: A prospective, multilevel study. *Am J Public Health* 2001;91:385–391.

99. Lynch JW, Kaplan GA, Pamuk ER, et al. Income inequality and mortality in metropolitan areas of the United States. *Am J Public Health* 1998;88:1074–1080.

100. Macinko JA, Shi L, Starfield B, Wulu JT Jr. Income inequality and health: A critical review of the literature. *Med Care Res Rev* 2003;60:407–452.

101. Polednak AP. Survival of breast cancer patients in Connecticut in relation to socioeconomic and health care access indicators. *J Urban Health* 2002;79:211–218.

102. Leslie JC, Galvin SL, Diehl SJ, et al. Infant mortality, low birth weight, and prematurity among Hispanic, white, and African American women in North Carolina. *Am J Obstet Gynecol* 2003;188:1238–1240.

103. Franzini L and Spears W. Contributions of social context to inequalities in years of life lost to heart disease in Texas, USA. *Soc Sci Med* 2003;57:1847–1861.

104. Fang J, Madhavan S, Bosworth W, Alderman MH. Residential segregation and mortality in New York City. *Soc Sci Med* 1998;47(4):469–476.

105. Pearl M, Braveman P, Abrams B. The relationship of neighborhood socioeconomic characteristics to birthweight among 5 ethnic groups in California. *Am J Public Health* 2001;91:1808–1814.

106. Geronimus AT. Black/white differences in the relationship of maternal age to birthweight: A population-based test of the weathering hypothesis. *Soc Sci Med* 1996;42(4):589–597.

107. US Dept of Health and Human Services. *Healthy People 2000.* (DHHS Publication No. PHS 91-50212.) Hyattsville, Md: DHHS; 1991.

108. US Dept of Health and Human Services. *Healthy People 2010.* (DHHS Publication No. 017-001-00543-6.) Hyattsville, Md: DHHS; 2000.

109. US Dept of Health and Human Services. Healthy People 2000 progress review for black Americans. *Healthy People 2000 Review 1997.* Hyattsville, Md: DHHS; 1997.

110. Geronimus AT, Bound J, Waidmann TA. Poverty, time, and place; variation in excess mortality across selected US populations, 1980–1990. *J Epidemiol Community Health* 1999;53:325–334.

111. Deaton A, Lubotsky D. Mortality, equality and race in American cities and states. *Soc Sci Med* 2003;56:1139–1153.

112. McLaughlin DK, Stokes CS. Income inequality and mortality in US counties: Does minority racial concentration matter? *Am J Public Health* 2002;92:99–104.

113. Gornick ME, Eggers PW, Reilly TW, et al. Effects of race and income on mortality and use of services among Medicare beneficiaries. *N Engl J Med* 1996;335:791–799.

114. Fang J, Madhavan S, Alderman MH. The association between birthplace and mortality form cardiovascular causes among black and white residents of New York City. *N Engl J Med* 1996;335:1545–1551.

115. Geronimus AT, Bound J, Waidmann A. Health inequality and population variation in fertility timing. *Soc Sci Med* 1999;49:1623–1636.

116. Wing S, Mmanton KG, Stallard E, et al. The black/white mortality crossover: Investigation in a community-based study. *J Gerontol* 1985;40:78–84.

117. Preston SH, Elo IT, Rosenwaike I, Hill M. African-American mortality at older ages: Results of a matching study. *Demography* 1996;33:193–209.

118. Mansfield CJ, Wilson JL, Kobrinski MA, Mitchell J. Premature mortality in the United States: The roles of geographic area, socioeconomic status, household type, and availability of medical care. *Am J Public Health* 1999;89:893–898.

119. Shi L, Starfield B. The effect of primary care physician supply and income inequality on mortality among blacks and whites in US metropolitan areas. *Am J Public Health* 2001;91:1246–1250.

120. Haynatzka V, Peck M, CityMat CH, et al. Racial and ethnic disparities in infant mortality rates—60 largest U.S. cities, 1995–1998. *MMWR Morb Mortal Wkly Rep* 2002;51:329–332.

121. Sims M, Rainge Y. Urban poverty and infant-health disparities among African American and whites in Milwaukee. *J Natl Med Assoc* 2002;94:472–479.

122. Bird ST. Separate black and white infant mortality models: Differences in the importance of structural variables. *Soc Sci Med* 1995;41:1507–1512.

123. Rosenberg KD, Desai RA, Kan J. Why do foreign-born blacks have lower infant mortality than native-born blacks? New directions in African-American infant mortality research. *J Natl Med Assoc* 2002;94:770–778.

124. Laveist TA. Segregation, poverty, and empowerment: Health consequences for African Americans. *Milbank Q* 1993;71:41–64.

125. Geronimus AT. Black/white differences in the relationship of maternal age to birthweight: A population-based test of the weathering hypothesis. *Soc Sci Med* 1996;42(4):589–597.

126. Larson EH, Hart LG, Rosenblatt RA. Is non-metropolitan residence a risk factor for poor birth outcome in the U.S.? *Soc Sci Med* 1997;45:171–188.

127. Stockwell EG, Goza FW. Racial differences in the relationship between infant mortality and socioeconomic status. *J Biosoc Sci* 1996;28(1):73–84.

128. Creighton-Zollar A. Infant mortality by socioeconomic status and race in Richmond, Virginia 1979–1981: A research note. *Sociol Spectr* 1990;10:133–142.

129. Levine RS, Briggs NC, Husaini BA, Hennekens CH. A new pathway to decrease black:white differences in mortality. *Am J Epidemiol* 2004;159:S65.

130. Wennberg J, Gittelsohn. Small area variations in health care delivery. *Science* 1973;182(117):1102–1108.

131. US Census 2000 Summary File 3 (SF 3). Tables P160A and P160B. Available at: http://factfinder.census.gov.home. Accessed February 27, 2004.

132. Polednak AP. Poverty, residential segregation, and black/white mortality ratios in urban areas. *J Health Care Poor Underserved* 1993;4:363–373.

133. Tarone RE, Chu KC, Gaudette LA. Birth cohort and calendar period trends in breast cancer mortality in the United States and Canada. *J Natl Cancer Inst* 1997;5:251–256.

134. Greenberg M, Schneider D. The cancer burden of southern-born African Americans: Analysis of social-geographic legacy. *Milbank Q* 1995;73:599–620

135. Schneider D, Greenberg MR, Lu LL. Region of birth and mortality from circulatory diseases among black Americans. *Am J Public Health* 1997;87:800–804.

136. Barnett E, Halverson JA, Elmes GA, Braham VE. Metropolitan and non-metropolitan trends in coronary heart disease mortality within Appalachia, 1980–1997. *Ann Epidemiol* 2000:10:370–379.

137. Barnett E, Halverson J. Disparities in premature coronary heart disease mortality by region and urbanicity among black and white adults ages 35–64, 1985–1995. *Public Health Rep* 2000;115:52–64.

138. Halverson JA, Barnett E, Casper M. Geographic disparities in heart disease and stroke mortality among black and white populations in the Appalachian region. *Ethn Dis* 2002;12:S3-82–91.

139. Greenberg M, Schneider D. Region of birth, migration and homicide rates of African Americans. *Ethn Health* 1997;2:197–207.

140. Cubbin C, Pickle LW, Fingerhut L. Social context and geographic patterns of homicide among US black and white males. *Am J Public Health* 2000;90:579–587.

141. Shin EH. Black–white differentials in infant mortality in the South, 1940–1970. *Demography* 1975;12:1–19.

142. Lanska DJ. The geographic distribution of Parkinson's disease mortality in the United States. *J Neurol Sci* 1997;150:63–70.

143. Lanska DJ. Geographic distribution of stroke mortality in the United States 1939–1941 to 1979–1981. *Neurology* 1993;43:1839–1851.

144. Gillum RF, Ingram DD. Relation between residence in the southeast region of the United States and stroke incidence. The NHANES I Epidemiologic Followup Study. *Am J Epidemiol* 1996;144(7):665–673.

145. Pickle LW, Mungiole M, Gillum RF. Geographic variation in stroke mortality in blacks and whites in the United States. *Stroke* 1997;28:1639–1647.

146. Lanska DJ. Geographic distribution of stroke mortality among immigrants to the United States. *Stroke* 1997;28:53–57.

147. Lackland DT, Egan BM, Jones PJ. Impact of nativity and race on "stroke belt" mortality. *Hypertension* 1999;34:57–62.

148. Obisesan TO, Vargas CM, Gillum RF. Geographic variation in stroke risk in the United States: Region, urbanization and hypertension in the Third National Health and Nutrition Examination Survey. *Stroke* 2000;31:19–25.

149. Howard G, Howard VJ, Katholi C, et al. Decline in US stroke mortality: An analysis of temporal patterns by sex, race, and geographic region. *Stroke* 2001;32:2213–2220.

150. Subramanian SV, Kawachi I. The association between state income inequality and worse health is not confounded by race. *Int J Epidemiol* 2003;32:1022–1028.

151. Franzini L, Ribble, Spears W. The effects of income inequality and income level on mortality vary by population size in Texas Counties. *J Health Social Behavior* 2001;42:373–387.

152. Kennedy BP, Kawachi I, Lochner K, et al. (Dis)respect and black mortality. *Ethn Dis* 1997;7:207–214.

153. Christianson BA, Johnson NE. Educational inequality in adult mortality: An assessment with death certificate data from Michigan. *Demography* 1995;32:215–229.

154. Holmes R, Fawal H, Moon TD, et al. Acquired immunodeficiency syndrome in Alabama: Special concerns for black women. *South Med J* 1997;90:697–701.

155. Schleicher NC, Koziol JA, Christiansen SC. Asthma mortality rates among California youths. *J Asthma* 2000;37:259–265.

156. Polednak AP. Survival of breast cancer patients in Connecticut in relation to socioeconomic and health care access indicators. *J Urban Health* 2002;79(2):211–218.

157. Polednak AP. A comparison of survival of black and white female breast cancer cases in Upstate New York. *Cancer Detect Prev* 1988;11(3–6): 245–249.

158. Casper ML, Barnett EB, Armstron DL, et al. Social class and race disparities in premature stroke mortality among men in North Carolina. *Ann Epidemiol* 1997;146–153.

159. Armstrong D, Barnett E, Casper M, Wing S. Community occupational structure, medical and economic resources, and coronary mortality among U.S. blacks and whites, 1980–1988. *Ann Epidemiol* 1998;8:184–191.

160. Barnett E, Armstrong DL, Casper ML. Evidence of increasing coronary heart disease mortality among black men of lower social class. *Ann Epidemiol* 1999;9:464–471.

161. Corti MC, Guralnik JM, Ferrucci L, et al. Evidence for a black–white crossover in all-cause and coronary heart disease mortality in an older population: The North Carolina EPESE. *Am J Public Health* 1999;89:308–314.

162. Cannon ME. Homicide mortality in Delaware: Variations by age, race and sex. *Del Med J* 1994;66:591–597.

163. Hagen EW, Andrade FC. Monitoring infant mortality trends in Wisconsin, 1980 to 1999. *WMJ* 2003;102:27–30.

164. Jooma N, Borstell J, Yu S, et al. Infant mortality in Louisiana—identifying the risks. *J La State Med Soc* 2001;153:85–91.

165. Roberts CL, Algert C, Mueller L, Nadler JL. Trends in infant mortality in Connecticut, 1981–1992. *J Public Health Manag Pract* 1997;3: 50–57.

166. Kerr GR, Ying J, Spears W. Ethnic differences in causes of infant mortality: Texas births, 1989 through 1991. *Tex Med* 1995;91:50–56.

167. Kvale K, Cronk C, Blysch R, Aronson R. Racial disparities in African American and white infant mortality United States and Wisconsin, 1980 to 1998. *WMJ* 2000;99:52–54.

168. Bird ST, Bauman KE. State-level infant, neonatal, and postneonatal mortality: The contribution of selected structural socioeconomic variables. *Int J Health Serv* 1998;28:13–27.

169. Ritz R, Yu F. Parkinson's disease mortality and pesticide exposure in California, 1984–1994. *Int J Epidemiol* 2000;29:323–329.

170. Davis H, Gergen PJ, Moore RM JR. Geographic differences in mortality of young children with sickle cell disease in the United States. *Public Health Rep* 1997;112:52–58. Erratum in *Public Health Rep* 1997;112:89.

171. Adams EJ, Chavez GF, Steen D, et al. Changes in the epidemiologic profile of sudden infant death syndrome as rates decline among California infants: 1990–1995. *Pediatrics* 1998;102(6):1445–1451.

172. Taylor AL, Mcgwin D Jr. Temperature-related deaths in Alabama. *South Med J* 2000;93:787–792.

173. Singh GK. Area deprivation and widening inequalities in US mortality, 1969–1998. *Am J Public Health* 2003;93:1137–1143.

174. Cooper RS, Kennelly JF, Durazo-Arvizu R, et al. Relationship between premature mortality and socioeconomic factors in black and white populations of US metropolitan areas. *Pub Health Rep* 2001;116:464–473.

175. Kindig DA, Seplaki CL, Libby DL. Death rate variation in US subpopulations. *Bull World Health Organ* 2002;80(1):9–15.

176. Mansfield CJ, Wilson JL, Kobrinski EJ, Mitchell J. Premature mortality in the United States: The roles of geographic area, socioeconomic status, household type, and availability of medical care. *Am J Public Health* 1999;89(6):893–898.

177. Cooper GS, Yuan Z, Rimm AA. Racial disparity in the incidence and case-fatality of colorectal cancer: Analysis of 329 United States counties. *Cancer Epidemiol Biomarkers Prev* 1997;6(4):283–285.

178. Geronimus AT, Bound J, Waidmann TA, et al. Inequality in life expectancy, functional status, and active life expectancy across selected black and white populations in the United States. *Demography* 2001;38:227–251.

179. Polednak AP. Poverty, residential segregation, and black/white mortality ratios in urban areas. *J Health Care Poor Underserved* 1993;4:363–373.

180. Silva A, Whitman S, Margellos H, Ansell D. Evaluating Chicago's success in reaching the Healthy People 2000 goal of reducing health disparities. *Public Health Rep* 2001;116:484–494.

181. Hart KD, Kunitz SJ, Sell RR, Mukamel DB. Metropolitan governance, residential segregation, and mortality among African Americans. *Am J Public Health* 1998;88:434–438.

182. Polednak AP. Black–white differences in sentinel causes of death: Counties in large metropolitan areas. *J Urban Health* 2000;77:501–507.

183. Polednak AP. Mortality among blacks living in census tracts with public housing projects in Hartford, Connecticut. *Ethn Dis* 1998;8:36–42.

184. McCord C, Freeman HP. Excess mortality in Harlem. *N Engl J Med* 1990;322:173–177.

185. Wing S, Casper M, Davis W, et al. Trends in the geographic inequality of cardiovascular disease mortality in the United States, 1962–1982. *Soc Sci Med* 1990;30:261–266.

186. Polednak AP. Mortality from diabetes mellitus, ischemic heart disease, and cerebrovascular disease among blacks in a higher income area. *Public Health Rep* 1990;105(4):393–399.

187. Papacek EM, Collins JW Jr, Schulte NF, et al. Differing postneonatal mortality rates of African-American and white infants in Chicago: An ecologic study. *Matern Child Health J* 2002;6(2):99–105.

188. Polednak AP. Black–white differences in infant mortality in 38 standard metropolitan statistical areas. *Am J Public Health* 1991;81:1480–1482.

189. Scott-Wright AO, Wrona RM, Flanagan TM. Predictors of infant mortality among college-educated black and white women, Davidson County, Tennessee, 1990–1994. *J Natl Med Assoc* 1998;90(8):477–483.

190. Rawlings JS, Weir MR. Race- and rank-specific infant mortality in a US military population. *Am J Dis Child* 1992;146:313–316.

191. Krieger N, Chen JT, Waterman PC, et al. Race/ethnicity, gender, and monitoring socioeconomic gradients in health: A comparison of area-based socioeconomic measures—the public health disparities geocoding project. *Am J Public Health* 2003;93:1655–1671.

192. Wing S, Manton KG, Stallard E, et al. The black/white mortality crossover: Investigation in a community-based study. *J Gerontol* 1985;40(1):78–84.

193. Murphy FG, Blumenthal DS, Dickson-Smith J, Peay RP. The mortality profile of black Seventh-Day Adventists residing in metropolitan Atlanta: A pilot study. *Am J Public Health* 1990;80:984–985.

194. Sung JF, Harris-Hooker SA, Schmid G, et al. Racial differences in mortality from cardiovascular disease in Atlanta, 1979–1985. *J Natl Med Assoc* 1992;84(3):259–263.

195. Lackland DT, Bachman DL, Carter TD, et al. The geographic variation in stroke incidence in two areas of the southeastern stroke belt: The Anderson and Pee Dee Stroke Study. *Stroke* 1998;29:2061–2068.

196. Howard G, Russell GB, Anderson R, et al. Role of social class in excess black stroke mortality. *Stroke* 1995;26(10):1759–1763.

197. Nishimura R, LaPorte RE, Dorman JS, et al. Mortality trends in type 1 diabetes: The Allegheny County (Pennsylvania) Registry 1965–1999. *Diabetes Care* 2001;24(5):823–827.

198. Rosamond WE, Folsom AR, Chambless LE, Wang C–H for the ARIC Investigators. Coronary heart disease trend in four United States communities. The Atherosclerosis Risk in Communities (ARIC) study, 1987–1996. *Int J Epidemiol* 2001;30:517–522.

199. Henderson SO, Bretsky P, Henderson BE, Stram DO. Risk factors for cardiovascular and cerebrovascular death among African Americans and Hispanics in Los Angeles, California. *Acad Emerg Med* 2001;8:1163–1172.

200. Fuchs VR, McClellan M, Skinner J., Area Differences in Utilization of Medical Care and Mortality among U.S. Elderly. NBER Working Paper No. 8628; December 2001.

201. Williams JE, Massing M, Rosamond WD, et al. Racial disparities in CHD mortality from 1968–1992 in the state economic areas surrounding the ARIC study communities. Atherosclerosis

Risk in Communities. *Ann Epidemiol* 1999;9(8): 472–480.

202. Keil JE, Sutherland SE, Knapp RG, et al. Mortality rates and risk factors for coronary disease in black as compared with white men and women. *N Engl J Med* 1993;329:73–78

203. Fingerhut LA, Ingram DD, Feldman JJ. Homicide rates among US teenagers and young adults; Differences by mechanism, level of urbanization, race and sex, 1987 through 1995. *JAMA* 1998;280:423–427.

204. Smith AT Jr, Kuller LH, Perper JA, et al. Epidemiology of homicide in Allegheny County, Pennsylvania, between 1966–1974 and 1984–1993. *Prev Med* 1998;27:452–460.

205. Fine PR, Roseman JM, Constandinou CM, et al. Homicide among black males in Jefferson County, Alabama, 1978–1989. *J Forensic Sci* 1994;39:674–684.

206. Greenberg M, Naus J, Schneider D, Wartenberg D. Temporal clustering of homicide among urban 15- to 24-year-old white and black Americans. *Ethn Dis* 1991;1:342–350.

207. Sohler NL, Arno PS, Chang CJ, et al. Income inequality and infant mortality in New York City. *J Urban Health* 2003;80(4):650–657.

208. Collins JW Jr, Hawkes EK. Racial differences in post-neonatal mortality in Chicago: What risk factors explain the black infant's disadvantage? *Ethn Health* 1997;2:117–125.

209. Collins CA. Racism and health: Segregation and causes of death amenable to medical intervention in major U.S. cities. *Ann N Y Acad Sci* 1999;896:396–398.

210. Powell IJ, Schwartz K, Hussain M. Removal of the financial barrier to health care: Does it impact on prostate cancer at presentation and survival? A comparative study between blacks and white men in a Veterans Affairs system. *Urology* 1995;46(6):825—830.

211. Walsh SJ, Fenster JR. Geographical clustering of mortality from systemic sclerosis in the Southeastern United States, 1981–90 *J Rheumatol* 24(12):2348–2352.

212. Walsh SJ, DeChello LM. Geographical variation in mortality from systemic lupus erythematosus in the United States. *Lupus* 2001;10:637–646.

213. Hauck FR, Moore CM, Herman SM, et al. The contribution of prone sleeping position to the racial disparity in sudden infant death syndrome: The Chicago Infant Mortality Study. *Pediatrics* 2002;110:772–780.

214. Hauck FR, Herman SM, Donovan M, et al. Sleep environment and the risk of sudden infant death syndrome in an urban population: The Chicago Infant Mortality Study. *Pediatrics* 2003;111:1207–1214.

215. Lester D. Does residential segregation in cities predict African-American suicide rates? *Percept Mot Skills* 2000;91:870.

216. Demetriades D, Murray J, Sinz B, et al. Epidemiology of major trauma and trauma deaths in Los Angeles County. *J Am Coll Surg* 1998;187:373–383.

217. Cherpitel CJ. Regional differences in alcohol and fatal injury: A comparison of data from two county coroners. *J Stud Alcohol* 1996;57:244–248.

CHAPTER 3

Pregnancy and Women's Health

KIMBERLY D. GREGORY, MD, MPH

MAGDA G. PECK, SCD

EZRA C. DAVIDSON JR, MD

▶ INTRODUCTION

Pregnancy is a significant event in most women's lives and has a profound impact on their health and well-being. More importantly, emerging data suggest that the health and well-being of a woman sets the stage for the health and well-being of her offspring, and ultimately her family.[1-3] Further, representative indicators specific to women's health are widely used to reflect the health of a population. For example, both maternal mortality and infant mortality are actively monitored across local, national, and international regions and comparisons reveal disparate results in both developing and developed countries. Third-world countries have maternal and neonatal mortality rates that are 10-fold that of developed countries, reflecting lack of health-care access, limited resources, and impoverished nutritional, social, and economic conditions.[4] The United States, considered an international leader, has a remarkably low maternal mortality ratio (0.115 per 1000), yet its infant mortality rate is 6.9 per 1000 live births—surprisingly high and ranked 25th among developed countries.[5-7] Attempts to explain this apparent discrepancy have led to stratified analyses by race and ethnicity, and socioeconomic

status (SES). Caucasian women and women with high SES status have enviable maternal and infant mortality rates (6.0 and 5.7, respectively), whereas rates for women who are nonwhite and have low SES are approximately three- to fourfold that of Caucasian women.[8] Recognizing that nonwhite women account for one third of the US population, their health and reproductive outcomes significantly influence and reflect the health of the nation.[9]

Because addressing these long-standing racial and ethnic gaps in health risks and health status among the most vulnerable segments of the population—newborns and their mothers—is of utmost importance, the national blueprint for action, *Healthy People 2010,* includes among its leading goals for this decade the elimination of health disparities in infant mortality and five other major areas of women's health.[10] In this chapter, we describe recognized disparities in pregnancy and women's health related primarily to reproductive health conditions. Framing the discussion of women's health within the context of a woman's reproductive life span provides opportunities to identify the gaps in knowledge about women's health outcomes, and to develop potential solutions. Also in this chapter, we provide an overview of the public health implications of persistent disparities in pregnancy and women's health for individuals and their families, as well as for health-care providers and for the communities in which these individuals live. Strategic challenges and opportunities for strengthening knowledge and promoting evidenced-based action for this vulnerable population are described.

Given the complexity and breadth of the subject, we have utilized three conceptual frameworks to organize this chapter to enhance readers' consideration of health disparities in pregnancy and women's health. The three conceptual frameworks include the Institute of Medicine's (IOM) definition of health,[11] the IOM model of determinants of population health,[12] and a model of women's health focused on the reproductive life span, described here as the Women's Health Continuum.[13] A brief description of each of these models is provided next.

Definition of Health

Each year in the United States, approximately 4 million live births occur, and an estimated 60% or more additional pregnancies result in spontaneous or induced abortions or stillbirths.[14] Multiple and complex pathways lead to adverse reproductive outcomes for both mother and infant, requiring a broad approach to optimal pregnancy and women's health. The IOM's encompassing definition of health acknowledges "the important contributions to health that are made outside the formal medical care and public health systems," such as an individual's biology, behavior, genetic endowment, and physical and social environment. Its holistic definition of health—"a state of well-being and the capability to function in the face of changing circumstances"[11] which emphasizes social and personal resources as well as physical capabilities, provides an inclusive context for the challenge of persistent disparities in reproductive health outcome.

Determinants of Population Health

Eliminating health disparities in pregnancy and women's health requires strategic action at multiple levels; individual behavioral change and clinical interventions are necessary but insufficient to address larger community and societal forces, which underlie persistent racial and socioeconomic differences. A recent IOM study, which focused on "Assuring the Health of the Public in the 21st Century," offers an organizing construct for understanding risk and outcomes at multiple levels and for crafting integrated solutions that reflect the synergy among these levels. This "guide to thinking about the determinants of population health" through the life span acknowledges that individual traits and the biology of disease are at the core, surrounded by increasing layers of influence: individual behaviors; social, family, and community networks; living and working conditions; and broad social, economic, cultural, health, and environmental conditions and policies at the global, national, state, and local levels.[12] This model can help the broad range of health professionals who serve varied roles in addressing disparities better understand how each can and must be part of narrowing racial and socioeconomic gaps at all levels.

A Life Span Approach: "The Women's Health Continuum"

Focusing women's health within the context of her life span has been suggested by numerous investigators.[13,15-18] We describe recognized disparities in pregnancy and women's health related primarily to reproductive health conditions. Indicators of reproductive health have been limited to a traditional set of measures, including fertility, maternal mortality, onset and adequacy of prenatal care, fetal and infant mortality, prematurity, and low birth weight. However, the definition of prenatal care, as espoused by both the American Academy of

Pediatrics (AAP) and the American College of Obstetricians and Gynecologists (ACOG)—*care of women, their newborns, and family through the first year of life*—necessitates a more broadly defined set of outcomes.[2,19] Accordingly, we include a description of disparities in other health outcomes based on the continuum of a woman's life span before, during, and after conception and pregnancy. Focusing on reproductive health in the broader context of health and a woman's life course allows for the opportunity to consider mediating factors and potential intervention strategies.

► RECOGNIZED DISPARITIES THROUGHOUT THE WOMEN'S HEALTH CONTINUUM

Using the Life Span Approach

Protective behaviors and risk factors throughout the course of a woman's life influence her health during pregnancy, and recent studies suggest that these influences start in utero.[17,20–22] Hence, the health of any woman is influenced by her genetic makeup, her own in utero exposures, the effect of her health during childhood and adolescence, and her behaviors prior to pregnancy. Additional environmental stressors, such as early infant experiences and social conditions (eg, race, ethnicity, poverty, stress), all have a cumulative impact on the course of an individual's health from adolescence to death.[1,17,22–27] The Women's Health Continuum illustrates how multiple factors have an impact the health of a woman over time.[13] Reproductive health outcomes therefore include factors pertinent to multiple time periods: puberty, preconception, pregnancy, postpartum and newborn, interconception, menopause, and postreproduction. Eliminating disparities in risks and outcomes corresponding to each of these time periods will require targeted strategies for prevention, screening, and intervention.

Tables 3–1 through 3–5 list representative indicators of pregnancy and women's health outcomes for each phase of the Women's Health Continuum and indicate differences by race and ethnicity.[6–8] Neither the tables nor the summary comments for each of the reproductive phases is meant to be exhaustive or exclusive but are put forth as a stimulus for discussions related to pregnancy, women's health, population health, and strategies to decrease health disparities and thereby increase the health all people. Categorization of selected conditions, which can manifest in multiple time periods, is somewhat arbitrary and there is the potential for overlap. For example, infertility is placed in the puberty and preconception period, but it is equally appropriate in the postpartum or interconception period. Likewise, gynecologic conditions such as pelvic prolapse, incontinence, and cancer are categorized in the postreproduction period but are equally applicable to the postpartum and interconception period.

Race and ethnicity data are limited to those reported at the national level, and to those population groups for which there are adequate numbers of events to be reliable in reporting. Accordingly, data for Hispanic, Native American, and Asian and Pacific Islander subgroups are provided when sufficient and available. Recognizing that one third of the US population is composed of minority women and that most of these women are Hispanic or Asian and Pacific Islanders, focusing on black–white disparities may be misleading. Future data, stratified by subgroups, are needed on these other racial and ethnic populations as the limited data available suggest different health outcomes within subgroups. Puerto Rican, Native American, and specific subgroups of Asian and Pacific Islanders have particularly adverse outcomes, likely due to the same multifactorial mechanisms underlying poor health and reproductive outcomes for poor or African American women.

Additionally, the Women's Health Continuum, with its life span emphasis, has the potential to be all-encompassing; however, our focus on conditions specific to the reproductive system limits its widespread applicability. For example, it should be noted that we have not mentioned chronic diseases such as obesity, diabetes, hypertension, or heart disease—but it is well known that poor and minority women are at higher risk for these disorders. Emerging data suggest that some of these conditions may in fact be preprogrammed in utero due to genetics, or exacerbated by life circumstances related to personal, nutritional, occupational, or environmental stressors, and personal behaviors. Adverse health can emerge in childhood or adolescence, and these conditions frequently coexist or complicate pregnancy and affect management decisions later in the reproductive life span. For example, obese and diabetic patients are not considered good surgical candidates for elective procedures such as myomectomy. This could lead to delayed treatment for symptoms caused by fibroids, or to radical, definitive procedures such as hysterectomy, resulting in surgical sterilization instead of temporizing, fertility preserving, conservative treatments such as hysteroscopic ablative techniques or laparoscopic extirpation. Likewise this chapter does not address rheumatologic, immunologic, or neurologic diseases that may have a female preponderance. Finally, women in general, and poor and minority women in particular, are at increased risk for domestic violence and injury, both of which can occur throughout the life course. However, neither is specific to reproductive conditions; hence these topics are not discussed in this chapter. Instead we refer the reader to the appropriate chapters within this textbook for more in-depth consideration of chronic medical conditions that affect health but are not unique to women or pregnancy.

Puberty and Preconception

Table 3–1 lists disparities in reproductive health conditions that can occur during puberty and the preconception period. Population-based studies within the United States have found a consistent trend toward earlier maturation in African American girls as compared with Caucasian girls.[28–30] African American girls enter puberty 1 to 1.5 years earlier (aged 8 to 9 years) and start menses 8.5 months earlier (aged 12.1 years) than Caucasian girls. Anecdotal reports suggest the onset of puberty among Asians and American Indians is comparable to (or later than) Caucasians, but this has not been formally studied.[31] Although global statements about Hispanic maturation cannot be made due

► **TABLE 3–1.** Reproductive Health Conditions Along the Women's Health Continuum: Puberty and Preconception

Condition	Total	White	Black	Hispanic	Asian	Other	Reference
1. Puberty (mean age, years)		12.7	12.0	—	Same as white or later	Same as white or later	28, 30
2. Contraception use[a] (current)	46.6	66.6	62.2	58.9	—	—	39
3. Sexually transmitted disease (PID)[a]	8.0	11.0	8.0	—	—	—	39
4. Teen pregnancy[a]	45.9	28.5	68.3	83.4	18.3	53.8 NA[b]	14
5. Abortion (per 100 live births)	25.6	17.7	52.9	26.1			14

PID, pelvic inflammatory disease.

[a] *Healthy People 2010* indicator.

[b] NA, Native American.

to likely variation in subtypes, data from the National Hispanic Health and Examination Survey (NHANES) suggest that Mexican American girls enter puberty at the same time as Caucasian girls, but have a delayed maturation process such that they reach the adult stages later.[32]

One could argue that these findings are just "differences" and not necessarily disparities; however, other studies suggest environmental factors such as lead, nutrition, and obesity may influence maturation, and these risk factors are disproportionately distributed.[30,33,34] Moreover, understanding when differences in sexual maturation occur has important clinical, educational, and social implications related to the following: (1) timing of referrals for precocious or delayed puberty, (2) providing anticipatory guidance to parents and children regarding what to expect and when, and (3) determining the time and content of age-appropriate sex education and rape and violence prevention programs.[28]

It is widely held that maternal health during pregnancy is directly related to maternal health prior to pregnancy; hence the emerging emphasis on preconception care and health maintenance. Women cared for during the prepregnancy planning period should be considered at risk for conception. Interactions with health-care workers can be viewed as contraception or preconception visits, providing an opportunity for health promotion and primary preventive health activities. With regard to primary prevention, use of contraception (condoms) can directly prevent sexually transmitted diseases (STDs), as well as teen pregnancies and unintended pregnancies among adults. Unfortunately, only 2% of women obtain preconceptional care.[35] The low rate of preconceptional care places women at risk for unintended pregnancies, which nationally approaches 50% of all births.[36] International data espoused by the World Health Organization (WHO) emphasize the importance of contraception as an opportunity not only to delay first births but also to promote birth spacing by at least 2 years in order to decrease infant deaths and promote improved maternal nutrition and family health.[37]

As noted in Table 3–1, rates of contraceptive use, STDs, and pregnancy termination vary by race and ethnicity. Currently, there are 25 recognized STDs.[10] Increased rates of STDs among African American women are particularly noteworthy because there are significant downstream sequelae associated with these diseases, such as increased risk of ectopic pregnancy and associated complications, including but not limited to infertility and maternal death from hemorrhage. Likewise, some pathogens such as bacterial vaginosis have been implicated in an increased risk for preterm birth.[38] African Americans are at increased risk for both conditions, and little data exist to explain these disparities. Because preterm birth is the leading contributor to infant mortality and neonatal health-care costs, considerable effort needs to be directed toward understanding and eliminating the gap in preterm birth rates.

Pregnancy

It has been estimated that over 90% of US women expect to give birth at least once during their lifetimes.[39] Hence, pregnancy is another ideal opportunity for health promotion and primary preventive health activities for three reasons: (1) this time period may be the only opportunity that some women have to interact with the health-care system due to financial or other access issues; (2) it is a time that most women are motivated to change behaviors in order to optimize pregnancy outcome; and (3) studies suggest that women who seek prenatal care also sustain interactions with the health-care system for their newborn.[40] Table 3–2 lists the selected reproductive health conditions that can occur during the pregnancy period. Prenatal care, a frequently reported reproductive health indicator, varies by race and ethnicity. African American, Hispanic, and Native American women have lower prenatal care rates than Caucasian and Asian women.

The fertility rate, a more global indicator of reproductive health, also varies by race and

► TABLE 3-2. Reproductive Health Conditions Along the Women's Health Continuum: Pregnancy

Condition	Total	White	Black	Hispanic[b]	Asian[c]	Other[d]	Reference
1. Fertility rate (per 1000 aged 15–44)	67.5	58.0	69.3	107.4	69.4	70.4 NA	8
2. Birth rate (per 1000 population)	—	66.5	71.7	105.9 115.1 MA 84.3 PR 57.3 CU 94.3 CA	70.7	71.9 NA	8
3. Miscarriages (% of clinically recognized pregnancies)	13.8	13.8	13.5	—	—	—	
4. Ectopics (% of clinically recognized pregnancies)	1.3	1.2	1.6	—	—	—	
5. Prenatal care first trimester[a]	83.2[14]	85.0[14]	74.3[14]	74.4[14] 74.6 MA[6] 79.1 PR[6] 91.8 CU[6] 77.4 CA[6]	84.0[14] 90.1 JA[6] 87.0 CH[6] 85.0 FIL[6] 82.7 OTH[6] 79.1 HA[6]	69.3 NA[6]	6, 14 (as specified in columns 2–7)
6. No prenatal care[a]	3.7[14]	3.2[14]	6.5[14]	5.9[14] 6.2 MA[6] 4.6 PR[6] 4.3 CU[6] 5.7 CA[6]	8.2[14] 2.0 JA[6] 3.4 CH[6] 3.0 FIL[6] 3.8 OTH[6] 4.8 HA[6]	6.5 NA[14]	6, 14 (as specified in columns 2–7)

	Col 1	Col 2	Col 3	Col 4[c]	Col 5[d]	Col 6[b]	Ref
7. Maternal mortality[a]	11.5[5]	6.0[8]	25.1[8]	10.3[8] 9.7 MA[14] 13.4 PR[14] 7.8 CU[14]	11.3[5]	12.2 NA[5]	5, 8, 14 (as specified in columns 2–7)
8. Pregnancy complications[a]	GD 2.9 HTN 3.9	GD 2.7 HTN 4.2	GD 2.8 HTN 2.8	DM 2.9 HTN 3.9	—	—	8, 14
9. Cesarean rate[a]	26.1	25.9	27.6	25.2 24.5 MA 22.2 PR 36.9 CU 27.0 CA	25.0 20.8 JA 23.9 CH 28.5 FIL 24.8 OTH 22.4 HA	23.1	14
10. Delayed childbearing ≥ 35 years	48.3	48.5	39.4	60.3 62.9 MA 40.8 PR 50.5 CU 62.6 CA	73.1	39.8 NA	8
11. Infertility[a] (% reproductive-age women)	15.0	—	—	—	—	—	39
Primary etiology (%)	Ovarian 46.5 Male function 24.5 Other 15.3 Tubal 13.8 Unknown 11.0 Endometrial 4.7 Sterilized 4.6	14.0 11.5 3.6 41.0 12.8 2.6 25.6					41

GD, gestational diabetes; HTN, hypertension.

[a] *Healthy People 2010* indicator.

[b] NA, Native American.

[c] MA, Mexican American; CA, Central American; CU, Cuban; PR, Puerto Rican.

[d] CH, Chinese; FIL, Filipino; HA, Hawaiian; JA, Japanese American; OTH, Other Asian and Pacific Island heritage.

ethnicity. The fertility rate for the US population in 2001–2002 was 67.5 per 1000 women aged 15–44 years.[7,8] All racial and ethnic groups had a higher birth rate than Caucasian women; and Hispanic women have the highest birth rate of all ethnic groups. Delayed childbearing (maternal age older than age 35 at delivery) was more common among Caucasian and Asian American women. The 1995 National Survey of Family Growth estimated that 15% of reproductive-age women have used infertility services, including seeking medical advice, diagnostic tests and procedures, drugs, or other treatments.[39] Although little data are available regarding differences in rates of infertility by ethnicity, one urban practice-based study showed the proportion of new patient referrals mirrored the ethnic distribution of the city's population.[41] However, when analyzed at the patient level by cause of infertility, there were significant differences by ethnicity, with African American women having more tubal factor disorders as compared with Caucasian women who had more ovarian disorders as the primary cause of infertility.[41]

US women are delaying childbearing into middle age (40s and 50s), and this trend is more prevalent among white women.[7] The use of assisted reproductive technologies varies by race and ethnicity and is associated with specific reproductive health consequences, some of which are clear (eg, multiple gestation and associated costs and sequelae of preterm birth) and others which are still being debated (eg, increased cancer risks, increased birth defects).[42–44]

Newborn

The most widely recognized reproductive health disparity, infant mortality, is related to the newborn period Table 3–3. African Americans have significantly higher rates of preterm birth; low birth weight; growth restriction; and fetal, neonatal, and infant mortality than all other racial and ethnic groups.[7] In most instances the rate is two- to threefold higher when compared with the Caucasian population. Hispanics and Asians each have comparable rates

to Caucasians, but when stratified by subpopulations these groups demonstrate significant variation.[6–8,14] For example, Puerto Ricans have rates of preterm birth and infant mortality that parallel African American rates.[45] Likewise, Hawaiians are at increased risk of adverse neonatal outcomes when compared with other subgroups of Asian and Pacific Islanders.

Multiple theories have been espoused to explain these disparities, including decreased access, lower socioeconomic status, increased biologic tendencies toward infection, stress and strain, and lack of social support.[17] The persistent disparity, and the increasing scientific association between antenatal and birth events as contributing factors in an individual's ultimate health have led to a heightened sensitivity of the need to narrow this gap, which constitutes a major national public health priority.[10] Despite improved access and enhanced use of prenatal care, these disparities remain, and, in fact, the rate of preterm birth has actually increased in recent years.[7] Many authorities have suggested that because of the complex, multifactorial etiology of preterm birth and poor growth, a comprehensive, multilevel, multidisciplinary, community-based approach, comparable to the IOM's determinants of population health model, is the only strategy likely to have an impact on these factors. Evidence to support this broad change in policy is gleaned largely from international data, but systematic evaluation of specific multitiered interventions in the United States is promising (see later discussion of Healthy Start and Perinatal Periods of Risk).[46–50]

Postpartum and Interconceptional Health Maintenance

Postpartum and interconceptional health maintenance care is an opportunity for further prevention, screening, and interventions, and the importance of postpartum follow-up visits has been recognized by ACOG and the National Center for Quality Assurance (NCQA).[2,51] Table 3–4 lists key reproductive health conditions that are relevant to this time period. Although the indicators in the table are primarily

▶ **TABLE 3-3.** Reproductive Health Conditions Along the Women's Health Continuum: Newborn Period

Condition	Total	White	Black	Hispanic[b]	Asian[c]	Other[d]	Reference
1. Perinatal mortality[a]	—	1.9	4.7	1.9	—	—	8
2. Fetal deaths (>20 weeks per 1000 live births)[a]	6.6	5.6	12.4	—	—	—	6
3. Neonatal mortality[a] (< 28 days per 1000 live births)	4.6	3.8	9.4	3.7	—	—	8
4. Infant mortality (1 year)[a]	6.9[6]	5.7[8]	14.1[8]	5.6[8] 5.5 MA[6] 8.1 PR[6] 4.3 CU[6] 4.9 CA[6]	5.1[6] 3.8 JA[6] 3.5 CH[6] 5.9 FIL[6] 5.2 OTH[6] 8.7 HA[6]	9.0 NA[6]	6, 8 (as specified in, columns 2–7)
5. Preterm birth (% < 37 weeks)[a]	12.1	11.1	17.5	11.6 11.4 MA 14.0 PR 10.5 CU 12.2 CA	10.4 9.2 JA 7.7 CH 12.7 FIL 10.5 OTH 13.3 HA	13.1 NA	14
6. Low birth weight (< 2500 g)[a]	7.8	6.8	13.3	7.8 6.2 MA 9.7 PR 6.5 CU 6.5 CA	7.8 7.6 JA 5.5 CH 8.6 FIL 8.6 OTH 8.1 HA	7.2	14
7. Very low birth weight (< 1500 g)[a]	1.5	1.2	3.1	1.5 1.1 MA 2.0 PR 1.2 CU 1.2 CA	1.1 1.0 JA 0.7 CH 1.3 FIL 1.2 OTH 1.6 HA	1.3	14
8. Intrauterine growth restriction (% ≥ 37 weeks)	2.9	2.5	5.2	4.0	—	—	14

[a] *Healthy People 2010* indicator.

[b] NA, Native American.

[c] CA, Central American; CU, Cuban; MA, Mexican American; PR, Puerto Rican.

[d] CH, Chinese; FIL, Filipino; HA, Hawaiian; JA, Japanese American; OTH, Other Asian and Pacific Island heritage.

▶ **TABLE 3–4**. Reproductive Health Conditions Along the Women's Health Continuum: Postpartum and Interconceptional Health Maintenance

Condition	Total	White	Black	Hispanic	Asian	Other	Reference
1. Breast feeding[a]	55.2	59.1	25.1	62.2	—	—	39
2. Depression[a]	8.0						10
3. Fibroids (per 1000 women)	9.2	8.2	16.9	—	—	—	56
4. Chronic gynecologic condition (per 1000 women)	97.1						

[a] *Healthy People 2010* indicator.

clinical—related to the prevention, detection, and early treatment of complications such as hemorrhage, eclampsia, infection, and postpartum depression—it should be emphasized that maternal (and neonatal) needs in the immediate postpartum period are commonly related to information, education, and support.[52] Information and education about child care, breast feeding, nutrition, and contraception are critical during this time period. In the United States, this occurs in a brief time period during hospitalization and may be reinforced 2 weeks later for cesarean patients and 6 weeks postpartum for all patients. However, there is a growing consensus that more health-care provider interactions are needed, both more frequently and spread out over a longer period of time.[52,53] The WHO Technical Working Group on Postpartum Care suggested 6 hours, 6 days, 6 weeks, and 6 months as critical times when provider visits might be valuable in identifying maternal or neonatal health needs or complications.[52] Moreover, this is an ideal regimen to support, encourage, and emphasize the maternal and neonatal merits of breast feeding. In addition to the recognized neonatal benefits, maternal benefits include weight loss and reduced risk of breast and ovarian cancer.[9] Further, recent data suggest that women's health after pregnancy influences child outcomes.[54,55]

In a longitudinal study using data from the National Maternal and Infant Health Survey,[55]

women's self-reported poor health had a strong association with the ratings of their children's physical health and poor behavior symptoms. Maternal self-reported depressive symptoms were associated with delayed speech and behavior problems in children 3 years postdelivery. The authors emphasized that the adverse child outcomes spanned multiple maternal conditions and cut across various domains of child health and development, furthering the importance of the need for researchers to understand the complex interactions of biobehavioral, psychosocial, and genetic intergenerational determinants of health. Hence, improving or optimizing a mother's health in the postpartum period could directly influence the well-being of her child and family. Unfortunately, the current model of care in the United States does not support sustained, ongoing interactions between mothers and their caregivers, nor are the political will or resources available to assure these interactions.

The postpartum and interconception period also is a time where gynecologic disorders might be manifested, such as fibroids, endometriosis, menstrual disorders, or chronic pelvic pain. A population-based study using National Health Interview Survey data estimated the annual prevalence of chronic gynecologic conditions at 97.1 per 1000 women aged 18 to 50 years.[56] Menstrual disorders were the most common, followed by adnexal conditions (eg, ovarian cyst) and fibroids. Approximately 20%

of reproductive-age women have fibroids, and their prevalence increases with age. African American women are at increased risk for fibroids and are twice as likely to undergo hysterectomy for this disorder.[57]

Postreproduction and Menopause

The predominant issues related to the postreproduction phase include those symptoms related to menopause—a biologic process that affects each woman differently (Table 3–5). There is evidence to suggest significant racial, ethnic, and sociocultural differences in how menopause is experienced and perceived, some of which are mediated by personal factors.[58–62] The Study of Women's Health Across the Nation (SWAN)—a large, multicenter, multiethnic, community-based survey—found the median age of natural menopause was 51.4 years of age after adjusting for smoking, education, marital status, heart disease, parity, race and ethnicity, employment, and prior use of oral contraceptives. Current smoking, lower SES (education, employment, single marital status) were associated with earlier menopause. Parity, prior oral contraceptive use, and Japanese race and ethnicity were associated with later age of natural menopause.[61] In general, Japanese and Chinese women reported the fewest symptoms, while Hispanic women reported the most, and there was significant variation in the number and type of symptoms by race and ethnicity. For example, African American women were more likely to report hot flashes and vaginal dryness, whereas Caucasian women were more likely to report urine leakage and difficulty sleeping. Reported symptoms were mediated by body mass index, smoking, and SES.[62] These studies suggest that lifestyle, race and ethnicity, SES, and cultural expectations affect symptoms, function, and quality of life during this time period. Recent findings from the Women's Health Initiative have made variations in prescription of and compliance with use of hormonal treatment a nonissue.[63]

Although not exclusive to the postreproductive period, other conditions that are more likely to occur during this time period include pelvic prolapse, incontinence disorders, and reproductive tract cancers. Limited data suggest that Caucasians have higher rates of incontinence and prolapse than African Americans, Hispanics, and Asian and Pacific Islanders, but this may be a reflection of ascertainment bias, because Caucasians are more likely to seek treatment for these disorders.[64–66] Many women find urinary incontinence too embarrassing to report, even to a health-care provider.[64]

Lastly, with regard to reproductive tract cancers, African Americans and Hispanics have lower incidence rates but consistently higher mortality rates when compared with Caucasians.[67,68] This is due in part to the fact that poor and minority women present at later stages, reflecting complex interactions: high-risk behaviors, such as drinking; smoking; denial; health beliefs; and lack of access due to lack of coverage or lack of usual source of care.[69–71] This may be another area in which a comprehensive, multilevel, integrated approach might be associated with significant improvement in screening, diagnosis, and treatment for selected populations.[72,73]

Implications of Health Disparities in Pregnancy and Women's Reproductive Health

What underlies the differential of adverse reproductive health conditions across the childbearing life span? Differences in individual women's behaviors play a part, and adverse behaviors can be demonstrated across all ethnic and socioeconomic groups. For example, recent surveillance data from 19 states showed that black and Hispanic women and women with less education reported lower percentages of adequate preconceptional multivitamin use than white and higher-educated women.[74]

▶ **TABLE 3-5.** Reproductive Health Conditions Along the Women's Health Continuum: Postreproduction and Menopause

Condition	Total	White	Black	Hispanic	Asian[b]	Other	Reference
1. Menopause (median age at onset; adjusted)	51.4	51.4	51.4	51.0	51.8 JA 51.4 CH	—	60
2. Pelvic prolapse (per 1000 women)	2.1	—	—	—	Varies by subgroup; incidence in Chinese and Japanese is decreased relative to whites	—	64
3. Incontinence GUI (%)	59	59	29	8	14	—	65
DI (%)	15	15					
4. Cancer incidence[a]							67
Breast	135.8	140.8	120.8	83.6	102.0	54.4	
Cervix	9.1	8.8	12.3	16.1	8.6	—	
Ovary	16.7	17.6	11.8	12.4	13.1	—	
Uterus	24.3	25.6	17.3	15.3	18.0	—	
Cancer deaths[a]							67
Breast	—	27.2	35.9	17.9	12.5	14.9	
Cervix	—	2.7	5.9	3.7	2.9	2.9	
Ovary	—	—	—	—	—	—	
Uterus	—	—	—	—	—	—	

DI, diabetes insipidus; GUI, genitourinary incontinence.

[a] *Healthy People 2010* indicator.

[b] CH, Chinese; JA, Japanese American.

Although the prevalence of smoking among pregnant women in all racial and ethnic groups is relatively low, non-Hispanic white women are more than twice as likely to smoke during pregnancy than non-Hispanic black women, and the rate of smoking during pregnancy among white women has long exceeded that of black women.[75] Nor are racial disparities fully explained by maternal age or education or income, among other leading demographic risk factors.[76] For example, African American women have a greater likelihood of adverse perinatal outcomes even after controlling for income and education.

As with long-standing disparities in infant mortality, differences in pregnancy and women's health most likely reflect a dynamic interaction between social and medical forces.[77] In addition to racial differences in maternal medical conditions (including bacterial vaginosis and prior preterm delivery), it has been suggested that stress, lack of social support, and maternal health experiences unique to black women might better explain persistent black–white disparities in preterm delivery as well as other adverse health outcomes.[78] Indeed, a convergence of complex barriers to self- and health care conspire to prevent many women of color and of lower socioeconomic means—and their infants—from enjoying the same health status as their white and more affluent counterparts. Accordingly, it will be the strategic combination of prevention and intervention across the life span and at multiple levels that will result in closing the gap in pregnancy and women's health.

▶ SUMMARY AND RECOMMENDATIONS: CLOSING THE GAP

Essential Actions at Multiple Levels

As emphasized by our selected frameworks, disparities in health outcomes are the manifestation of complex and interactive forces that operate at multiple levels, from individual to societal. Therefore, effective actions to eliminate disparities in pregnancy and women's health must take place at all levels to yield comprehensive, integrated, and sustainable change in individual and institutional knowledge, attitudes, behaviors, practices, and policies. We outline below an overview of issues (Table 3–6) and general actions or recommendations (Table 3–7) that can contribute to such meaningful change.

Individual Level Actions

According to the Centers for Disease Control and Prevention (CDC), "prevention measures to reduce maternal and infant mortality and promote the health of all childbearing-aged women and their newborns" should include preconception, screening for preexisting chronic conditions and health risks; counseling about contraception and access to effective family planning to prevent unintended pregnancy and unnecessary abortion; counseling about good nutrition, including consumption of iron and folic acid; and advice about the value of regular physical exercise and the avoidance of alcohol, tobacco, and illicit drugs.[79] Pregnant women should receive early, continuous, and high-quality care throughout pregnancy, labor, delivery, and postpartum. In addition to the monitoring and treatment of preexisting conditions, pregnant women should be screened and treated for group B streptococcus, bacterial vaginosis, and human immunodeficiency virus (HIV). Wide-scale studies have shown that access to and utilization of this broader range of reproductive health care beyond prenatal care—including family planning and abortion—manifests in benefits to both mother and child.[3,46,47] However, not all women conform to these global "shoulds" in their individual behaviors nor are they equal beneficiaries of optimal clinical care. Personal responsibility to conform to healthy behaviors, while laudable and appropriately anticipated for most women, may be especially challenging for isolated, less-educated women with competing personal priorities who are not part of a regular health-care system. Effective health behavior change interventions will need to take into account such factors as a woman's cultural

▶ **TABLE 3–6.** Summary of Major Issues Relating to Pregnancy and Women's Reproductive Health

- Pregnancy is a significant event in a woman's life that has profound impact on her personal and family well-being.
- Women's reproductive health encompasses more than pregnancy alone; it can best be conceptualized as a life span continuum with different health-care issues at the various stages of her life course: puberty and preconception, pregnancy, caring for a newborn, interconception, and postreproduction and menopause.
- Focusing on reproductive health in the broader context of a woman's life course allows for greater opportunities to consider mediating factors and potential interventions for prevention and treatment.
- Measuring maternal health assists population-based assessment of women's reproductive health. There is widespread variation by race and ethnicity in maternal health in the United States as measured by maternal and neonatal mortality and morbidity.
- There are significant racial and ethnic disparities in each major category across a woman's life span. African American women experience significantly higher rates of STDs, teen pregnancy, maternal and perinatal mortality, and deaths due to breast and cervical cancer than their white counterparts. Additional effort is needed to understand why these differences persist.
- Additional data are needed to better understand and improve reproductive health outcomes for women of Hispanic and Asian descent. Although insufficient published population data for Native American women's reproductive health were available for inclusion in this review, attention to their health status and improved monitoring of health disparities also is essential for comprehensive assessment.
- Eliminating health disparities in pregnancy and women's health requires strategic action at multiple levels: individual behaviors; social, family, and community networks; living and working conditions; and broad social, economic, cultural, health, and environmental conditions and policies at the global, national, state, and local levels.

and language preferences, literacy level, and access to basic resources to increase the likelihood of healthier choices. Clinical care must reach all women for guaranteed access to essential services during their childbearing years. Special efforts and additional resources will be needed to assure that those who are at greatest risk for adverse outcomes, who disproportionately are poor and women of color, are the equal beneficiaries of comprehensive, quality prevention, diagnosis, and treatment services.[80]

In addition, international models for safe motherhood call for increased attention to women and children postpartum, with an emphasis on education, support, and promoting maternal wellness. In the United States, this would require modifications within the current system, such as increased emphasis on the content, quality, and the promotion of more postpartum visits, as well as incorporation of other health personnel (eg, doulas, nurse midwives,

and advanced practice nurses).[53] Pediatricians might also be included, because they have periodic interactions with the mother consistent with the child's immunization schedule, and recent studies suggest that awareness of the need for maternal screening and referral is a mechanism for optimizing maternal and child health.[81–83]

Family and Community Level

Social, family, and community networks are essential to support healthy pregnancy and optimal women's health; these networks are not equally present, positive, or sustaining across racial, ethnic, and socioeconomic lines. Among the challenges that call for greater social supports are single parenting, domestic violence, mental illness, and substance abuse; many of these challenges are found disproportionately among women of color. National initiatives—

▶ **TABLE 3-7.** Summary of Recommendations for Action Across the Life Span

- **Advance Preconception Health.** The importance of preconception health, including preconception counseling at every routine gynecologic visit, is central to the prevention of adverse maternal and perinatal outcomes and the promotion of women's health. Given that nearly half of all pregnancies are unintended, preconception health can facilitate access to family planning and reinforcement of dietary supplementation of folate to prevent birth defects. For women of color, preconception health can become the portal for addressing underlying and often unattended chronic health conditions, such as diabetes, hypertension, and obesity. Adoption of emerging national standards for the content and quality of preconception health care should be encouraged, and preconception health-care services must become readily accessible and affordable for all women.
- **Support Research and Interventions to Eliminate Preterm Births.** For reasons not yet fully understood, prematurity continues to manifest at significantly higher rates in African American women, and the adverse sequelae of prematurity have an impact on both mother and child. The nation must rally behind the national March of Dimes Prematurity Campaign and other related efforts to raise national awareness about what must be done to keep infants from being born too small, too soon. Greater support for focused research is needed to clarify the causal pathways of premature birth and identify interventions that work to prevent and reverse preterm labor.
- **Acknowledge and Address Women's Health Issues Following and Between Pregnancies.** Outreach and advocacy for women's well-being after delivery is essential for the prevention of adverse mental and physical health conditions in both mother and child across racial and ethnic groups. Services and financing have not been universally available to support postpartum health care, including for maternal depression and family planning. The traditional intensive focus on well-child care in the first year of life must be coupled with accessible and affordable well-mother care for greater family success. Services and interventions must be tailored to diverse groups of women whose language, traditions, and values demand cultural competence.
- **Improve Data on Women's Health Disparities.** Although attention to the differences in reproductive health risks and outcomes between African American and white women has been the leading focus, equal emphasis must be given to disparities within and among diverse subgroups of women of Hispanic origin, and Native American and Asian American women. Smaller numbers must not become an excuse for not knowing, at least nationally, the magnitude and trend in health disparities. Local, state, and tribal leaders and consumers of women's reproductive health must have the capacity to understand and use data to address health disparities and shape data-driven solutions.
- **Assure Affordable Women's Health Care Through the Life Span.** Among the 45 million Americans currently uninsured are more than 20 million women of reproductive age who are more likely to be immigrants and minorities. Health insecurity threatens the basic well-being of women, their children, and their families. Greater government funding and regulation of the health-care industry is needed to eliminate the gap in access to essential care between women who can afford it and those who cannot.

such as the federal Healthy Start program—that target communities with the greatest maternal and child health disparities, establish or strengthen community support networks for pregnant women and their families as a primary infant mortality prevention strategy to improve women's health.[48] More recently some local Healthy Start sites and other urban com-

munities have reexamined perinatal disparities through the Perinatal Periods of Risk (PPOR) approach, a community planning process for translating newly framed and analyzed data on fetal and infant mortality into prioritized actions. Based on PPOR-based identification of "Maternal Health and Prematurity" (deaths of fetuses, neonates, and postneonates weighing less than

1500 g at birth) as the "period of risk" with the greatest perinatal disparity, these communities have shifted their emphasis to preconception health women's services and comprehensive primary health care for women as a longer-term strategy for prevention.[48–50]

Other examples in which multitiered, systematic approaches have been beneficial include perinatal regionalization and maternal and fetal–infant mortality review boards. The March of Dimes Birth Defect Monitoring Program's Committee on Perinatal Health published two documents addressing the importance of regionalized perinatal services.[84,85] Since the first study was published in 1976, studies have consistently shown that development and implementation of regionalized systems of care have resulted in reduced rates of mortality among low- and very-low-birth-weight infants.[84–91] Considerable networking was required between hospitals and regional health departments to build and sustain an infrastructure that standardized inpatient care into three levels of risk-appropriate care based on facilities' capabilities and providing mechanisms for referral to ensure that specialty and subspecialty care are readily available among and between institutions.[92] Work is ongoing with regard to standardizing clinical care processes at the provider level, such as that promoted by the Vermont Oxford Network, Leapfrog, and the California Perinatal Quality Care Collaborative, but more work is needed at the regulatory, policy, and fiscal levels to support and facilitate these changes.[93–96]

Regulatory, political, and financial support is similarly needed to support the recommendations offered by Fetal and Infant Mortality Review (FIMR) boards. Using maternal mortality reviews as a historic model, FIMR boards have evolved as a national multidisciplinary program that provides a technical advisory panel and a local community panel to look at potential contributing causes of mortality, including medical care, health system issues, and individual patient factors, and then propose geographic-specific interventions to factors identified

locally.[97] The success has been variable, largely due to structural and process barriers related to implementing proposed recommendations.[98–101]

Living and Working Conditions

The health of a woman is intricately interwoven with the conditions in which she lives and works each day. Those conditions are not equal across lines of race and income. The last half-century has witnessed the unprecedented entrance into and sustained presence of women in the workforce in this nation, elevating occupational health and workplace wellness as key components of women's health, particularly during the reproductive years. This movement has been accelerated by recent changes in national social policy, such as the Welfare Reform Act of 1996, which mandated the transition of able-bodied adults from welfare to work, especially among low-income women. The work environment can adversely affect the health of women of reproductive age psychologically and physically through stress and noxious environments. Women with less education are more likely to be working in jobs that pay less, have fewer benefits, and are more physically demanding. Affordable housing of sufficient quality, reliable transportation, adequate food supplies, quality education, and accessible recreation are among the basic needs that can be beyond the reach of many families, especially those of color and new immigrants.

Compromised health can tip the delicate balance; hence the fundamental need for accessible public health services combined with essential health-care services for women at the center of their families' lives. However, primary health care in the United States for women of reproductive age independent of pregnancy has been termed "abysmal."[77] The major barrier is access to affordable health care, as underscored by the nearly 20 million adult women overall—30% of Hispanic women and 20% of black women in the United States—estimated to be without health insurance.[102,103] The 2001 Kaiser

Women's Health Survey documented "unstable health coverage" in half (49%) of Latina women and 30% of African American women surveyed, who lacked continuous insurance coverage during the previous 12 months, compared to 24% of white women surveyed.[103] Among immigrant women older than 18 years who are noncitizens—most of whom are minorities—nearly 20% lack a usual source of health care (a place they usually go to when they are sick), and more than 40% have no health insurance.[104] Higher rates of uninsurance among women of color are related to their lower rates of job-based coverage. Although two thirds (66%) of white women have employer-based insurance, only 52% of their African American and 44% of their Latina counterparts are insured through their work.[103] Access to basic health care for women throughout the life span, and health coverage that assures such access, is a basic strategy for all women that will improve their daily living conditions. Lack of health insurance and a usual source of care have a significant impact on use of preventive services, management of chronic medical conditions, and cancer survival.

Public Policy

Three things must converge to achieve the broad social, economic, cultural, health, and environmental conditions and policies necessary for optimal pregnancy and women's health.[104] First is better and more accessible information and research about women's health and health disparities for health professionals and their partners to use in planning and monitoring change. Greater national awareness and championship of women's health, with special emphasis on the elimination of disparities, has been manifest in the parallel development within the US Department of Health and Human Services (HHS) of coordinating infrastructures to address both women's health and minority health. Offices of Women's Health and Minority Health have been established in each major agency of HHS (eg, the National Institutes

of Health, CDC, Health Resources and Services Administration [HRSA], as well as in each state health department). Centralized and shared data on women and health disparities regularly available in print (eg, Women's Health USA) and through the Internet (*www.4women.gov*) serve to increase health practitioners' knowledge base as a precursor to informed action. Greater government funding is being directed at both women's health and minority health, while private funds are supporting national research on key issues, such as prematurity, a bellwether of racial and ethnic disparities in pregnancy and women's health.[105]

Second is the identification and dissemination of effective, proven, population-based programs designed to reduce disparities in pregnancy and women's health. One such example is HRSA's Bright Futures for Women's Health and Wellness Initiative (BFWHWI).[106] The vision of the BFWHWI, a public–private partnership, is to "achieve physical, mental, social, and spiritual health" by identifying "opportunities for integrating prevention into self-care, culturally competent health care, and community action." The mission of the BFWHWI is to "plan, develop, implement, and evaluate a variety of culturally competent consumer, provider, and community-based products to increase awareness and use of preventive services for all women across their life span."[104] Amidst great effort and a wide array of multiple projects in almost every state and major locality, programs to improve pregnancy outcomes and promote women's health tend to be fragmented and underfunded, rendering less-than-optimal and unsustainable results. Some programs have become entrenched, assumed to be unaccountable. In a time of increasing fiscal constraint, program evaluation must be encouraged to ensure that effort is aligned with measurable and intended outcomes.

Third is the mustering of sufficient political will to tackle the more difficult, underlying forces that keep women in the United States, especially women of color, from experiencing optimal health before, during, and after pregnancy.

In the realm of health disparities in women's health and beyond, the acknowledgment of larger institutional factors that manifest in racism is key to unlocking the greater potential of all.[107] Efforts to understand and eliminate racism in the practices and policies on which health care for women and their children is based can serve to strengthen the very health-care institutions that serve our nation's most vulnerable and vital citizens.

When critical knowledge, effective practice, and sufficient political will come together, there is greater likelihood of optimal pregnancy outcomes and significant improvements in the health and well-being of all women and, ultimately, the goal of a healthier nation.

▶ REFERENCES

1. Barker DJP. *Mothers, Babies and Disease in Later Life*. London, England: Br Med J Publ Group; 1994.
2. American Academy of Pediatrics and the American College of Obstetricians and Gynecologists. *Guidelines for Perinatal Care*, 4th ed. Elk Grove Village, Ill: AAP; 1997.
3. Brown SS, Eisenberg L, eds. *The Best Intentions: Unintended Pregnancy and the Well-being of Children and Families*. Washington, DC: National Academy of Sciences; 1995.
4. *Infant and Under Five Mortality Rates by WHO Region; Year 2000*. Available at http://www.who.org.
5. Chang J, Elam-Evans LD, Berg CJ, et al. Pregnancy-related mortality surveillance—United States, 1991–1999. *MMWR Morb Mortal Wkly Rep* Surveill Summ 2003;52(2):1–8.
6. National Center for Health Statistics. *Health, United States, 2003*. Hyattsville, Md: NCHS; 2003.
7. Arias E, MacDorman F, Strobino DM, et al. Annual summary of vital statistics—2002. *Pediatrics* 2003;112(8):1215–1230.
8. MacDorman MF, Minino AM, Strobino DM, et al. Annual summary of vital statistics—2001. *Pediatrics* 2002;110(6):1037–1052.
9. Henry J Kaiser Family Foundations and Jacobs Institute of Women's Health. *Women's Health Data Book*. Available at: http://www.kff.org.
10. US Dept of Health and Human Services. *Healthy People 2010*, 2nd ed. Washington, DC: USDHHS; 2000. Available at: http://www.healthypeople2010.com.
11. Institute of Medicine, Committee on Using Performance Monitoring to Improve Community Health. *Improving Health in the Community: A Role for Performance Monitoring*. Washington DC: National Academy Press; 1997.
12. Institute of Medicine, Committee on Assuring the Health of the Public in the 21st Century. *The Future of the Public's Health in the 21st Century*. Washington, DC: National Academy Press; 2002.
13. Gregory KD, Hobel CJ, Korst LM, et al. *A Framework for Developing Maternal Quality Care Indicators*. Monograph prepared for the California Dept of Health and Human Services, Maternal and Child Health Branch; 2001.
14. Martin JA, Hamilton BE, Ventura SJ, et al. Births: Final data for 2000. *National Vital Statistics Reports*, Vol 50, issue 5. Hyattsville, Md: National Center for Health Statistics; 2002.
15. Halfon N, Inkelas M, Hochstein. The health development organization: An organizational approach to achieving child health development. *Milbank Q* 2000;78:447–497.
16. Collins K, Schoen C, Duchon L, et al. *Health Concerns Across a Woman's Life Span: The Commonwealth Fund 1988 Survey of Women's Health*. New York, NY: Commonwealth Fund; 1999.
17. Lu MC, Halfon N. Racial and ethnic disparities in birth outcomes: A life-course perspective. *Matern Child Health J* 2003:7(1):13–30.
18. Misra DP, Guyer B, Allston A. Integrated perinatal health framework: A multiple determinants model with a life span approach. *Am J Prev Med* 2003; 25(1):65–75.
19. Expert Panel on the Content of Prenatal Care. *Caring for Our Future: The Content of Prenatal Care*. Washington, DC: Public Health Service; 1989.
20. Barker DJP. Fetal origins of coronary heart disease. *BMJ* 1995;311:171–174.
21. Kuh D, Ben-Shlomo Y, eds. *A Life Course Approach to Chronic Disease Epidemiology*. Oxford, England: Oxford Univ Press; 1997.
22. Bateson P. Design for a life. In: Masnusson D, ed. *The Life Span Development of Individuals: Behavioral, Neurobiological, and Psychological*

Perspectives. New York, NY: Cambridge Univ Press; 1996:1–20.

23. Godfry KM. Maternal regulation of fetal development and health in adult life. *Eur J Obstet Gynecol Reprod Biol* 1998;78:141–150.

24. Garbarin K. The human ecology of early risk. In: Meisels SJ, Shonkoff TP, eds. *Handbook of Early Childhood Intervention*. New York, NY: Cambridge Univ Press; 1990:78–96.

25. Hertzman C, Weins M. Child development and long-term outcomes: A population health perspective and summary of successful interventions. *Soc Sci Med* 1996;43(7):1083–1095.

26. Power CT, Hertzman C. Social and biological pathway linking early life and adult diseases. *Br Med Bull* 1997;53(1):210–297.

27. Rich-Edwards JW, Stampter MJ, Mammson JAE, et al. Birthweight and the risk of cardiovascular disease in a cohort of women followed up since 1976. *BMJ* 1997;315:396–400.

28. Herman-Giddons ME, Slora EJ, Wasserman RC, et al. Secondary sexual characteristics and menses in young girls seen in office practice: A study from the Pediatric Research in Office Settings Network. *Pediatrics* 1997;99(4):505–512.

29. Biro FM, McMahon RP, Striegel-Moore R, et al. Impact of timing of pubertal maturation on growth in black and white female adolescents: The National Heart, Lung, and Blood Institute Growth and Health Study. *J Pediatr* 2001;138(5):636–643.

30. Russell DL, Keil MF, Bonat SH, et al. The relation between skeletal maturation and adiposity in African American and Caucasian children. *J Pediatr* 2001;139(6):844–848.

31. Graham EA, Sugar N. Secondary sexual characteristics and menses in young girls. Letter to the editor. *Pediatrics* 1998;101(5):949.

32. Villareal SF, Martorell R, Mendoza F. Sexual maturation of Mexican American adolescents. *Am J Hum Biol* 1989;1:87–95.

33. Selevan SG, Rice DC, Hogan KA, et al. Blood lead concentration and delayed puberty in girls. *N Engl J Med* 2003;348(16):1527–1536.

34. Eveleth PB, Tanner JM. Sexual development. In: Eveleth PB, ed. *Worldwide Variation in Human Growth*. Cambridge, England: Cambridge Univ Press; 1990:161–175.

35. American College of Obstetricians and Gynecologists. *Preconceptional Care*. ACOG Technical Bulletin No. 205; 1995.

36. Henshaw SK. Unintended pregnancy in the United States. *Fam Plann Perspect* 1998;30(1):24–29,46.

37. World Health Organization. *Family Planning*. Available at: http://www.who.org.

38. Meis PJ, Goldenberg RL, Mercer BM, et al. Preterm prediction study: Is socioeconomic status a risk factor for bacterial vaginosis in black or white women? *Am J Perinatol* 2000;17:41–45.

39. Abma JC, Chandra A, Mosher WD. Fertility, family planning and women's health: New data from the 1995 National Survey of Family Growth. *Vital Health Stat* 1997;23:1–28.

40. Freed GL, Clark SJ, Pathman DE, et al. Influences on the receipt of well-child visits in the first two years of life. *Pediatrics* 1999;103:864–869.

41. Green JA, Robbins JC, Scheiber M, et al. Racial and economic demographics of couples seeking infertility treatment. *Am J Obstet Gynecol* 2001;184:1080–1082.

42. Callahan TL, Hall JE, Ettner SL, et al. The economic impact of multiple gestation pregnancies and the contribution of assisted-reproduction techniques to their incidence. *N Engl J Med* 1994;331:244–249.

43. Rossing MA, Daling JR, Weiss NS, et al. Ovarian tumors in a cohort of infertile women. *N Engl J Med* 1994;331:771–776.

44. Kurinczuk JJ. Safety issues in assisted reproduction technology. From theory to reality—just what are the data telling us about ICSI offspring health and future fertility and should we be concerned? *Hum Reprod* 2003;18(5):925–931.

45. Varela R, Perez R, Sappenfield W, et al. Infant health among Puerto Ricans—Puerto Rico and U.S. Mainland, 1989–2000. *MMWR Morb Mortal Wkly Rep* 2003;52(42):1012–1016.

46. Ehiri JE, Prowse JM. Child health promotion in developing countries: The case for integration of environmental and social interventions. *Health Pol Plann* 1999;14(1):1–10.

47. World Health Organization. *Reduction of Maternal Mortality: A Joint WHO/UNFPA/UNICEF World Bank Statement*. Geneva, Switzerland, WHO; 1999.

48. Health Resources and Services Administration, USDHHS. *Federal Healthy Start*. Available at: https://performance.hrsa.gov/mchb/MCHProjects/

49. Perinatal Periods of Risk. Available at: http://www.citymatch.org/ppor.

50. Peck M, Brady C, et al. Strategies for strengthening state–local collaboration through PPOR implementation. Presentation at the 2003 MCH Epidemiology Workshop, Tempe, Ariz; December 2003.

51. National Committee for Quality Assurance. *State of Managed Care Quality 2000.* Washington, DC: National Committee for Quality Assurance; 2000.

52. Technical Working Group, World Health Organization. Postpartum care of the mother and newborn: A practical guide. *Birth* 1999;226(4):255–258.

53. Bradley P, Bray H. What we can learn from the British maternal child health system. *MCN Am J Matern Child Nurs* 2003;28(3):192–197.

54. Haas JS, McCormick M. Hospital use and health status of women during the 5 years following the birth of a premature, low birthweight infant. *Am J Public Health* 1997;87(7):1151–1155.

55. Kahn RS, Zuckerman B, Bauchner H, et al. Women's health after pregnancy and child outcomes at age 3 years: A prospective cohort study. *Am J Public Health* 2002;92:1312–1318.

56. Kjerulff KH, Erickson BA, Langenberg PW. Chronic gynecologic conditions reported by US women: Findings from the National Health Interview Survey, 1984–1992. *Am J Public Health* 1996;86:195–199.

57. Lepine L, Hillis S, Marchbanks P, et al. *Hysterectomy Surveillance: United States 1980–1993.* Atlanta, Ga: National Center for Chronic Disease Prevention and Health Promotion, Centers for Disease Control and Prevention; 1997: 1–15.

58. Brett KM, Cooper GS. Associations with menopause and menopausal transition in a nationally representative US sample. *Maturitas* 2003;45(2):89–97.

59. Wise LA, Krieger N, Zierler S, et al. Lifetime socioeconomic position in relation to onset of perimenopause. *J Epidemiol Comm Health* 2002;56(11):851–860.

60. Sampselle CM, Harris V, Harlow SD, et al. Midlife development and menopause in African American and Caucasian women. *Health Care Women Int* 2002;23(4):351–363.

61. Gold EB, Bromberger J, Crawford S, et al. Factors associated with age at natural menopause in a multiethnic sample of midlife women. *Am J Epidemiol* 2001;159(9):865–874.

62. Gold EB, Sternfeld B, Kelsey JL, et al. Relationship of demographic and lifestyle factors to symptoms in a multi-racial/ethnic population of women 40–55 years of age. *Am J Epidemiol* 2000;152(5):463–473.

63. Friedman-Koss D, Crespo CJ, Bellantoni MF, et al. The relationship of race/ethnicity and social class to hormone replacement therapy: Results from the Third National Health and Nutrition Examination Survey 1988–1994. *Menopause* 2002;9(4):264–272.

64. Gray Mikel L. Gender, race and culture in research on UI: Sensitivity and screening are integral to adequate patient care. *Am J Nurs* 2003; (103):20–25.

65. Brizzolara S, Grandinetti A, Mor J. Percentage of hysterectomy for pelvic prolapse in five ethnic groups. *Urogyn J* 2002;13(6):372–376.

66. Duong TH, Korn AP. A comparison of urinary incontinence among African American, Asian, Hispanic and white women. *Am J Obstet Gynecol* 2001.

67. Nelson K, Geiger AM, Mangione CM. Effects of health beliefs on delays in care for abnormal cervical cytology in a multi-ethnic population. *J Gen Intern Med* 2002;17(9):709–716.

68. National Cancer Institute. Cancer Health Disparities: Fact Sheet 2002. Available at: http://www.nci.nih.gov/cancertopics/factsheet/cancerhealthdisparities/

69. Selvin E, Brett KM. Breast and cervical cancer screening: Sociodemographic predictors among white, black and Hispanic women. *Am J Public Health* 2003;93(4):618–623.

70. Corbie-Smith G, Flagg EW, Doyle JP, et al. Influence of usual source of care on differences by race/ethnicity in receipt of preventive services. *J Gen Intern Med* 2002;17(6):458–464.

71. Ferrante JM, Gonzalez EC, Roetzheim RG, et al. Clinical and demographic predictors of late-stage cervical cancer. *Arch Fam Med* 2000; 9(5):439–445.

72. Hiatt RA, Pasick RJ, Stewart S. Community-based cancer screening for underserved women: Design and baseline findings from the Breast and Cervical Cancer Intervention Study. *Prev Med* 2001;33(3):190–203.

73. Harlan LC, Clegg LX, Trimble EL. Trends in surgery and chemotherapy for women diagnosed with ovarian cancer in the United States. *J Clin Oncol* 2003;21(18):3488–3494.

74. Centers for Disease Control and Prevention. Surveillance for selected maternal behaviors and experiences before, during, and after pregnancy-PRAMS 2000. *MMWR Morb Mortal Wkly Rep* 2003;52(SS11):1–14.

75. US Dept of Health and Human Services, Health Resources and Services Administration, Maternal and Child Health Bureau. *Women's Health USA 2003*. Rockville, Md: USDHHS; 2003:25.

76. Schoendorf K, Hogue CJ, Kleinman J, et al. Mortality among infants of black as compared to white college graduates. *N Engl J Med* 1992;326:1552–1556.

77. Wise PH. The anatomy of a disparity in infant mortality. *Annu Rev Public Health* 2003;24:341–362.

78. Hogan VK, Richardson JL, Ferre CD, et al. A public health framework for addressing black and white disparities in preterm delivery. *J Am Med Women Assoc* 2000;56:1780.

79. Centers for Disease Control and Prevention. Opportunities to reduce maternal and infant mortality. *MMWR Morb Mortal Wkly Rep* 1999;48(38);856.

80. Institute of Medicine. *2001 Unequal Treatment. Confronting Racial and Ethnic Disparities in Health Care*. Washington, DC: National Academies Press; 2003.

81. Kahn RS, Wise PH, Finkelstein JA, et al. The scope of unmet maternal health needs in pediatric settings. *Pediatrics* 1999;103:576–581.

82. Klerman LV, Reynold DW. Interconception care: A new role for the pediatrician. *Pediatrics* 1994;93(2);327–329.

83. Zuckerman B, Parker S. Preventive pediatrics—New models of providing needed health services. *Pediatrics* 1995;95(5):758–762.

84. Committee on Perinatal Health. *Toward Improving the Outcome of Pregnancy: Recommendations for the Regional Development of Maternal and Perinatal Health Services (TIOP I)*. White Plains, NY: March of Dimes Birth Defects Foundation; 1976.

85. Committee on Perinatal Health. *Toward Improving the Outcome of Pregnancy: The 90s and Beyond (TIO II)*. White Plains, NY: March of Dimes Birth Defects Foundation; 1993.

86. McCormick MC, Shapiro S, Starfield BH. The regionalization of perinatal services. Summary of the evaluation of a national demonstration program. *JAMA* 1985;253(6):799–804.

87. Mayfield JA, Rosenblatt RA, Baldwin LM, et al. The relation of obstetrical volume and nursery level to perinatal mortality. *Am J Public Health* 1990;80(7):819–823.

88. Cifuentes J, Bronstein J, Phibbs CS, et al. Mortality in low birth weight infants according to level of neonatal care at hospital of birth. *Pediatrics* 2002;109(5):745–751.

89. Powell SL, Holt VL, Hickok DE, et al. Recent changes in delivery site of low-birth weight infants in Washington: Impact on birth weight-specific mortality. *Am J Obstet Gynecol* 1995;173(5):1585–1592.

90. Yeast JD, Poskin M, Stockbauer JW, Shaffer S. Changing patterns in regionalization of perinatal care and the impact on neonatal mortality. *Am J Obstet Gynecol* 1998;178(1 Pt 1):131–135.

91. Menard MK, Liu Q, Holgren EA, Sappenfield WM. Neonatal mortality for very low birth weight deliveries in South Carolina by level of hospital perinatal service. *Am J Obstet Gynecol* 1998;179(2):374–381.

92. Strobino DM, Silver GB, Allston AA, Grason HA. Local health department perspectives on linkages among birthing hospitals. *J Perinatol* 2003;23(8):610–619.

93. Horbar JD, Carpenter JH, Buzas J, et al and Vermont Oxford Network. Timing of initial surfactant treatment for infants 23–29 weeks' gestation: Is routine practice evidence based. *Pediatrics* 2004;113(6):1593–1602.

94. Edwards WH, Conner JM, Soll RF, Vermont Oxford Neonatal Skin Care Study Group. The effect of prophylactic ointment therapy on nosocomial sepsis rates and skin integrity in infants with birth weights 501–2000 g. *Pediatrics* 2004;113(5):1195–1203.

95. Jackson JK, Velluci J, Johnson P, Kilbride HW. Evidence-based approach to change in clinical practice: Introduction of expanded nasal continuous positive airway pressure use in an intensive care nursery. *Pediatrics* 2003;1(4 pt 2):e542–547.

96. Stevenson DK, Quaintance CC. The California Perinatal Quality Care Collaborative: A model for national perinatal care. *J Perinatol* 1999;19(4):249–250.

97. Davidson ED Jr. A strategy to reduce infant mortality. *Obstet Gynecol* 1991;77(1):1–5.

98. Klerman LV, Cleckley DC, Sinsky RJ, Sams SH. Infant mortality review as a vehicle for quality

improvement in a local health department. *Jt Comm J Qual Improv* 2000;26(3):147–159.

99. Buckley K, Chapin JL. Fetal and Infant Mortality Review; an evolving process. *Matern Child Health J* 1999;3(3):173–176.

100. Grason H, Misra D. Assessment of Healthy Start Fetal and Infant Mortality Review recommendations. *Matern Child Health J* 1999;(3):151–159.

101. Balatay M, McCormick MC, Wise PH. Implementation of fetal and Infant mortality review (FIMR): Experience from the National Healthy Start program. *Matern Child Health J* 1999;3(3):141–150.

102. National Center for Health Statistics, National Health Interview Survey, 2001. In: *Women's Health USA 2003*; p 64. Available at: http://www.hrsa.gov/womenshealth.

103. Henry J Kaiser Family Foundation. *Racial and Ethnic Disparities in Women's Health Coverage and Access to Care. Findings from the 2001 Kaiser Women's Health Survey.* Menlo Park, Calif: Henry J Kaiser Family Founcation; Pub No. 7018; March 2004.

104. Richmond JB, Kotelchuck M. The effect of the political process on the delivery of health services. In: McGuire C, Foley R, Gorr D, Richards R, eds. *Handbook of Health Professions Education*. San Francisco, Calif: Josey-Bass; 1983:386–404.

105. March of Dimes Birth Defects Foundation, National Prematurity Campaign. White Plains, NY. Available at: http://www.marchofdimes.org.

106. Health Resources and Services Administration, Bright Futures for Women's Health and Wellness Initiative. Available at http://www.hrsa.gov.womenhealth/brightfut.htm.

107. Jones C. Levels of racism: A theoretic framework and a gardener's tale. *Am J Public Health* 2000;90(8):1212–1215.

CHAPTER 4

Health Disparities in Children

FRANCES J. DUNSTON, MD, MPH

▶ INTRODUCTION

Children are particularly vulnerable to factors that adversely influence their health and lead to disparities in health status. During gestation, the developing fetus is subjected to the environmental milieu of the womb, which may be preconditioned by the mother's health or influenced by conditions that arise during pregnancy. These factors determine the health of the infant at birth. At birth, the infant enters a world not of its choosing, the circumstances of which will determine its health and survival.

A child's health is dependent on the family into which it is born and that family's capacity to adequately provide for its care. The capacity to nurture the child may be compromised by the health, socioeconomic status, and emotional well-being of the family. Family variables may be compounded by conditions in the neighborhood or community in which a family lives. The health of children is particularly susceptible to conditions of poverty, social dysfunction, inadequate resources for health care, and the lack of social support systems that plague many neighborhoods. Shared health beliefs and social norms within communities shape the health behaviors and lifestyles of children as they grow and develop. If the family lives in a community that is exposed to environmental health hazards, it is the children who are most likely to be ad-

versely affected. Health and social policy can establish the conditions that define the availability and accessibility of vital health services needed for children to maintain good health. These and other factors that contribute to racial and ethnic health disparities in children are summarized in Table 4–1 and explored in this chapter.

▶ FACTORS ASSOCIATED WITH HEALTH DISPARITIES IN CHILDREN

The health of newborns and infants is predetermined by environmental factors associated with gestation. Whether the mother smokes, drinks alcohol, abuses drugs, has inadequate nutrition, or receives suboptimal prenatal care will determine the health of her newborn infant and, indeed, its chances of life survival. These factors are compounded if the mother is also an unmarried teenager. In 2000, infants died at a rate of 6.9 deaths per 1000 live births prior to the first year of life, largely due to one or more of these factors.[1]

Children are born into sociologic and structural conditions that may place them at high risk for poor health. Being born to a single mother who may also be homeless, jobless, and have poor educational attainment places the infant

▶ **TABLE 4-1**. Factors Contributing to Racial and Ethnic Health Disparities in Children—A Developmental Model

Developmental Stage	Health Limiting Factor	Adverse Health Effect
Adulthood	Differential content of health services	
	Discriminatory provider behavior	Chronic disease in adults
	Racial and ethnic stereotyping	Maladaptive health behaviors
		Distrust of the health system
Adolescence	Lack of health insurance	Dissatisfaction with the health system
	Homicide rates	Underutilization of health services
	Alcohol and drug use	Intentional and unintentional injuries
	Cultural and linguistic barriers	Stress
	Fires	Unhealthy lifestyles
	Inadequate nutrition	Diabetes mellitus, type 2
Childhood	Air pollution	Obesity
	Chronic poverty	Asthma
	Lack of health insurance	Inadequate access to health care
	Substandard housing: indoor	Tuberculosis
	allergies lead poisoning	Neurodevelopmental deficits
	Environmental toxins	
Infancy	Poverty	
	Inadequate nutrition	
	Environmental toxins	
	Lack of customized health education	Iron deficiency anemia
		Nutritional rickets
		Gastroenteritis
Prenatal and birth	Adequacy of prenatal care	Cognitive deficiency
	Exposure to air pollution	Sudden infant death syndrome
	Maternal consumption of fish	Infant mortality
	contaminated with mercury PCBs	Low birth weight
	Maternal drug use	Very low birth weight
	Maternal smoking	
	Bacterial vaginosis	
	Maternal nutritional status	

at similar risk for inadequate health care and poor access to preventive and health education services. Being born into a neighborhood where these socioeconomic conditions prevail increases the risk of poor health for both the mother and infant.

The largest segment of the US population living below the poverty line, or with an income of less than $18,104 for a family of four, is women and children.[1] From the very beginning of life, these children struggle against sometimes overwhelming odds to achieve the optimal health and well-being our society assumes all children should enjoy. Lifestyles and health behaviors are conditioned by the social community in which the child may live. Steady exposure to poverty and deprivation, family violence, alcohol abuse, or sexual bartering sets the stage for children to adopt similar social strategies or coping and survival mechanisms. The longer the exposure is to such conditions, the more likely the child will be to assume the same behaviors.[2]

Children are exposed to varying degrees of environmental hazards and toxins that negatively influence their health. Living in communities with high levels of air pollution is directly associated with an increased incidence of respiratory illness in children.[3] A child living near an unreclaimed landfill, a polluted waterway, certain types of agricultural enterprises, manufacturing industries, nuclear power plants, or toxic waste sites is disproportionately vulnerable to associated environmental health effects. Children are susceptible to these effects because their bodies are still growing and developing. Cellular and molecular mechanisms in children still undergoing dynamic maturation are particularly susceptible to damage with exposure to environmental toxins.

The health of children may also be adversely affected by health policies and inconsistencies within US health-care delivery systems. The same children whose health may be adversely affected by gestational, socioeconomic, or environmental factors may also be prevented from accessing adequate health care due to lack of health insurance. Medicaid, the government-sponsored safety-net health insurance, is an important payer of health services for children. However, health policies, such as changes in eligibility criteria employed to restrain massive state Medicaid budgets, often result in vulnerable segments of the child population being cut off from routine, primary health care. Even when children gain access to basic health care, health delivery system issues may still prevent them from getting adequate care. These issues may include rigid appointment systems, the absence or limited availability of after-work hours, services that are insensitive to the supportive needs of children and families, and exclusionary practices, such as the relative unavailability of health services for adolescent males.

▶ RACIAL AND ETHNIC HEALTH DISPARITIES IN CHILDREN

Disparities in health status among children may be variably explained as biologically determined, rooted in the effects of poverty, or environmentally mediated. Certain health conditions, such as sickle cell disease or Tay Sachs disease, are genetically determined and are prevalent in certain racial and ethnic population groups, such as African Americans and Eastern European Jews.

Figure 4–1 illustrates some of the community factors associated with racial and ethnic health disparities. Living in poverty is highly correlated with suboptimal health status. Poor children are twice as likely to be in fair or poor health, 1.5 times as likely to have spent days in bed during the year, twice as likely to have been hospitalized for short stays, 3.5 times as likely to have blood lead levels greater than the currently recommended safe level, and 1.5 times as likely to die between the ages of 0 and 14 years of age.[3] However, increasingly, population studies have shown that health disparities are heightened on the basis of racial and ethnic background, even when controlling for biologic or socioeconomic factors.[4]

Racial and ethnic health disparities in children are attributed to the lingering effects of historical inequities in health care; current discriminatory practices that have become institutionally ingrained in the delivery of health services; the attitudes of individual health-care providers who respond to patients based on racial or ethnic stereotypes; and lack of cultural awareness resulting in the provision of culturally incompetent health care.[5]

The effects of racial and ethnic health disparities are likely to persist and worsen well into the future. This is because children are the most racially and ethnically diverse segment of the US population, and children from certain racial and ethnic groups represent the fastest growing segments. Currently, 28% of the US population is of African American, Latino or Hispanic, Alaskan Native or Native American, Asian and Native Hawaiian, and other Pacific Islander backgrounds.[6] This represents an increase from 20% in 1980. By 2050, 56% of the adolescent population will be from these groups. Latinos are the most rapidly growing population group;

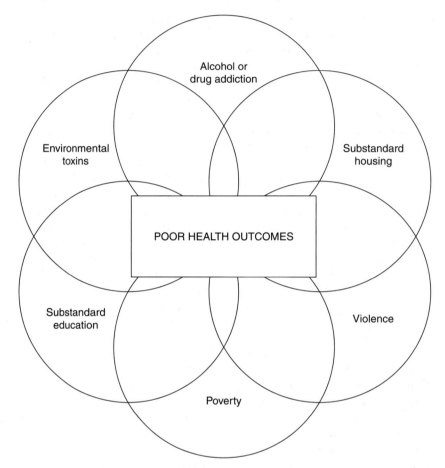

Figure 4–1. Community factors associated with racial and ethnic health disparities.

by 2020 an estimated one in five children living in the United States will be Latino.[7]

The remainder of this chapter examines the factors that contribute to health disparities in children and the effects of race and ethnicity on its expression. In each case, whether it be complications of pregnancy, inadequate family support systems, environmental health effects, lifestyle behaviors shaped by chronic exposure to adverse social influences, health-care system issues, or health policies, the resulting disparities in health status are heightened for children from certain racial and ethnic backgrounds.

Racial and Ethnic Disparities in Pregnancy Outcomes

Although the United States has achieved a significant decline in the rate of low-birth-weight infants and in infant mortality, certain racial and ethnic groups have not enjoyed the same decline. In fact, the infant mortality rate for African Americans has consistently remained twice as high as that of whites since 1945. African American infants are twice as likely to be born low birth weight and three times as likely to be born very low birth weight as white infants. As a consequence, their rate of infant mortality due to very low birth weight and prematurity is five times that of whites. Hispanics as an overall group exhibit low birth weight rates that are comparable to those of whites. However, among Hispanics, infants of mothers from Puerto Rico are 57% more likely to exhibit low birth weight than are infants born to Mexican mothers.[8]

When one examines the causes of these birth outcomes, they are not adequately explained on the basis of socioeconomic status. Although poverty is directly correlated with poor pregnancy outcomes, and the rate of poverty is much higher for African Americans than for whites, the disparity in the rates of low birth weight and infant mortality persist even when controlling for socioeconomic status. The rate of poverty among Hispanics is slightly higher than that of African Americans, yet their rates of low birth weight and infant mortality are similar to those of whites. Therefore, poor pregnancy outcomes among those racial and ethnic groups cannot be explained on the basis of socioeconomic status alone.[8]

Studies have shown that pregnant women living in neighborhoods where they are continuously exposed to air pollution are slightly more likely to experience preterm delivery of a low-birth-weight infant than women who live in areas with acceptable air quality.[9] African Americans, Hispanics, and Native Americans are more likely to live in neighborhoods with chronically polluted air. Other variables that have been shown to be associated with low-birth-weight infants include the content and comprehensiveness of prenatal care. Ten or more prenatal visits starting in the first trimester, along with social support resources offered in a culturally sensitive manner, have been found to be protective against poor pregnancy outcomes. The presence of bacterial vaginosis is another factor that has been associated with poor pregnancy outcomes in African American women. The hypertension of preeclampsia and eclampsia of pregnancy, a frequent cause of prematurity and low birth weight, is found with greater frequency among African Americans.[5]

Sudden infant death syndrome (SIDS) accounts for 10% of all infant deaths in the first year of life. The incidence of SIDS has dropped dramatically as mothers have adopted guidance to place infants to sleep on their backs. The incidence of SIDS is three to four times as high among blacks, Hispanics, and Native Americans as among whites. Behavioral research to explain the failure of these groups to adopt advice regarding SIDS is needed.[7]

Health Disparities and Poverty

Children born into poverty face significant challenges to their health and well-being. These challenges are often made more insurmountable if the child and family are members of certain racial or ethnic groups. For example, in 2001, one million African American children lived in extreme poverty, with income less than 50% of the poverty level, which is defined as $18,104 for a family of four.[1] The percentage of African Americans in extreme poverty increased in 2001, despite what had been a downward trend since 1992.

Mothers living in extreme poverty show diminished capacity for supportive parenting of their children. Poor parenting skills among impoverished mothers is attributed to chronic psychosocial stress and the lack of consistently supportive spousal relationships.[1] These parents generally have diminished capacity to protect their children, to assure their adequate growth and development, or to maintain their health by receiving and benefiting from continuous primary and preventive health care.

Children living is severely impoverished homes are often deprived of basic resources for survival, including adequate nutrition. Twelve million children live in households that are food insecure, and an additional 2.7 million children live in households that skipped or sized back on meals due to lack of food.[10] Nutritional deficiencies in children can translate into iron deficiency anemia, failure to thrive, dampened immunity, delays in cognitive and social development, and increased vulnerability to infectious diseases.[11] Mexican children are six times more likely, and African American children are three times more likely, to have inadequate food resources than whites. Rates of tuberculosis and gastrointestinal infections are also higher among these groups.[12]

The longer a child lives in conditions of poverty, the more likely it is that his or her health will be affected. This is thought to be due to a confluence of factors associated with economic deprivation, including poor housing, lack of transportation, and inadequate social support networks. Other issues, such as maternal substance abuse, single parent, female-headed households, and spousal abuse, also can converge in the domain of extreme poverty. The children whose health is most affected are those who live in a chronically impoverished state, with *chronically* defined as 5 years or more. Twenty-nine percent of African American children are poor for 10 years or more, whereas 6% of white children live in poverty for 5 years.[1]

Impoverished children live in neighborhoods inhabited by others who are similarly socioeconomically situated. As a social group, they are subjected to a wide range of toxic influences that exert adverse health effects. Poor neighborhoods may not have grocery stores where nutritious foods can be purchased. When present, the foods in these stores are more frequently substandard with respect to shelf life, safe food-handling practices, and contamination by pests and hazardous substances. Such neighborhoods are favored sites for fast-food enterprises offering fatty, high-sugar-content foods.[1]

With inadequate recreational resources and the fear of threatened safety, children living in poor neighborhoods may resort to staying inside the home, with little opportunity for physical activity or to play in the sunlight. The health effects of living in these ecologic environments include increased risk for nutritional rickets, obesity, type 2 diabetes, and early signs of adult cardiovascular disease.[8] Studies have shown that the adverse health effects of living in poor neighborhoods over several years are exacerbated

by attendant factors of social deprivation and racism.[13]

Environmental Hazards and Health Disparities

Children from certain racial and ethnic groups, or who are poor, are disproportionately represented in communities burdened with hazardous wastes and environmental pollutants. This is because the communities inhabited by these groups have been selectively chosen as sites for toxic waste disposal and polluting industries because they offer the least political resistance. More than 50% of African Americans and 60% of Hispanics in the United States live near highways and other environmental structures that produce high levels of air pollutants. Half of all Asian and Pacific Islanders live in communities with uncontrolled toxic waste sites.[14]

Examples of exposures to toxic substances associated with residential location are numerous. Pregnant women and children living in proximity to shore lines may have a high consumption of saltwater fish, resulting in chronic exposure to low levels of methyl mercury. Methyl mercury has been found to concentrate in the brains of children and the developing fetus and to exert adverse neurodevelopmental effects. Freshwater fish may be a major dietary source for children living in rural areas and are often obtained from rivers polluted with polychlorinated biphenyls (PCBs) derived from manufacturing runoffs. Native American children are exposed to PCBs through the intake of contaminated fish recovered from polluted streams. In-utero absorption of PCBs has been associated with cognitive deficits in infants, including lower intelligence quotients, short-term memory loss, behavioral problems, and, in children, lower academic achievement.[3]

Inner-city children, mostly racial and ethnic minorities and the poor, are at increased risk of respiratory illness and asthma due to the adverse effects of air pollution, which include aberrations of the ambient ozone layer, acid aerosols, and particulate matter. These children regularly breathe air contaminated with emissions from manufacturing plants and diesel exhaust particles. Definite links exist between geographic proximity to environmental hazards and respiratory illness. Neighborhoods with the greatest number of environmental hazards also have the highest proportion of racial and ethnic minorities.[15]

Asthma morbidity and mortality in children increased dramatically over the period from 1980 through 1998. African American children were three times as likely to be hospitalized for asthma as whites, and more than four times as likely to die of an acute asthmatic episode.[16] African American, Hispanic, and Asian and Pacific Islander children experience higher mean levels of air pollution when compared with whites. This difference in levels of exposure persists even when correcting for the educational attainment of the mothers, a surrogate for economic status.[17] Similarly, African American children are more likely to be sensitized to indoor allergens, such as cockroach droppings and dust mites, that have been linked to asthma.[18]

African American children are five times more likely to suffer from lead poisoning than white children, primarily because they are more likely to live in older, dilapidated housing. Living downstream from manufacturing plants with lead emissions, or on soil contaminated by preexisting lead-burdened enterprises, has been associated with lead poisoning in inner-city children. Twenty-two percent of children living in older housing have lead poisoning.[3] Even low blood lead levels have been associated with neurodevelopmental effects in children later in life. Low blood lead levels in pregnant women have been associated with low-birth-weight babies. Other health effects associated with lead exposure, which may develop as the child matures to adulthood, are hypertension and kidney disease.[3]

Health Services and Health Disparities

Health delivery system factors contributing to racial and ethnic health disparities are summarized in Figure 4–2. The most dramatic health disparity among racial and ethnic minorities is the inability to access health care due to lack of health insurance. Being uninsured is the greatest impediment to acquiring effective health care. Forty-one percent of Hispanic children lack health insurance coverage, as do 28% of Asian and Pacific Islander, 23% of African American, and 17% of white children. When these children have health insurance, it is most likely to be publicly funded rather than private coverage. Thirty-nine percent of Hispanic children rely on publicly funded health insurance, as do 55% of Asian and Pacific Islander, and 46% of African American children, respectively.[19]

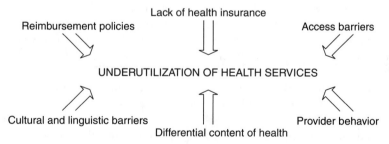

Figure 4–2. Health delivery system factors contributing to racial and ethnic health disparities in children.

The lack of health insurance and, to a lesser extent, coverage with publicly funded insurance, determines the quantity and quality of health care these children receive. It is difficult to find a medical "home" with one customary health-care provider when there is no means to compensate the provider due to lack of or limited health insurance. Only 75% of Hispanic and 81% of Asian and Pacific Islander children have a customary source of primary care, compared with 91% of white children. Without a medical home, these children must rely on public clinics, outpatient departments of hospitals, or hospital emergency departments. Twenty-eight percent of Hispanic, 28% of African American, and 49% of Asian and Pacific Islander children report these facilities as their source of ongoing health care, compared with 17% of white children.[19] Despite these differences, one half to three quarters of racial and ethnic health disparities in access to and use of health care would remain if differences in income and health insurance were eliminated.[20]

Racial and ethnic disparities exist in the provision of health care for children with special health-care needs (ie, children with both static and dynamic chronic health conditions). Like relatively healthy children with episodic illnesses, racial or ethnic minority children with persistent special health care needs experience difficulties with health-care access due to low income and lack of health insurance. As a result, these children are less likely to have used physician office services over a period of 1 year but more likely to have to resorted to emergency care and hospitalization to address their health-care needs. These problems are most striking among Hispanic children, those most likely to be uninsured. However, even when adjustments are made for income, lack of insurance, and health status, racial and ethnic disparities persist in the ability of children with special health-care needs to secure a regular source of physician services, thus limiting their opportunities to benefit from high-quality, continuous, culturally competent health care.[21]

Inner-city children often live in neighborhoods with high access to tertiary care services, because most major medical centers are located in large urban areas. Despite the proximity of a relatively immediate source of tertiary care, child mortality differences are evident among racial and ethnic minorities when compared with whites. Low income is a primary driver, but more is being understood about the relationship of the differential causes of child mortality with socialization to a common set of values, beliefs, and behaviors that are developed and reinforced by living in a community. Differences observed in neonatal and postneonatal infant mortality have been well documented. Beyond the neonatal period, racial and ethnic minority children living in poor inner-city communities have higher mortality rates due to respiratory diseases, fire, and homicide than whites. White children are more likely to die of injuries from motor vehicle collisions, reflecting their having sufficient income to have access to and use of motor vehicles.[22]

Even when children have health insurance coverage, the quality of the patient–provider relationship may reflect racial and ethnic disparities. For children in managed care plans, there is a high degree of dissatisfaction with the relationship between the provider and the patient's family. These parents report a lack of strength of affiliation with providers in networks that are selected by managed care plans. Asian children and families report the least satisfaction with these arrangements and their perceived restrictions. Parental dissatisfaction in interactions with health providers is based on the perceived lack of helpfulness by providers, and language and communication barriers. These findings have led to the conclusion that less-restrictive policies that consider the culture, values, and health beliefs of the patient and family are important considerations directly related to the quality of health care.[23]

There are deviations in other measures of quality in health-care services provided to children from racial and ethnic minority groups compared with white children. Children from racial and ethnic minority backgrounds are less likely to secure an appointment during off-peak hours at times that do not interfere with parental employment. Fifty percent of African American, 52% of Asian and Pacific Islander, 52% of Native American, and 54% of Hispanic children are afforded this option, compared with 64% of white children. At the time of the physician visit, waiting times were more likely to be longer for these groups than for white children. Nineteen percent of African American children wait more than 30 minutes to see their physician compared with 15% of white children. In the emergency department, 33% of African American children waited 1 hour or more as opposed to 25% of white children. Satisfaction with the patient visit was likely to be lower, although this variable improved with the perceived cultural competence of the provider, and with racial and ethnic concordance between the patient and the provider.[19] Dissatisfaction with the health-care encounter may contribute to the finding that racial and ethnic minority parents perceive the health of their children to be less than optimal.[19] Utilization of health-care services is also far less for children of racial and ethnic minorities than for whites, even for families with health insurance.[24]

The content of health care experienced by racial ethnic minorities may vary significantly from that routinely received by whites. The content of care delivered to adolescents in the emergency department setting varies with the race or ethnicity of the patient. Black and Latino adolescents are much less likely to be prescribed opioids than their white counterparts, even where indicated by diagnosis of migraines or acute back pain.[25] Children diagnosed with gastroenteritis are treated differently if they are from certain racial or ethnic backgrounds and are less likely to benefit from proper outpatient management. Hispanic children are hospitalized at a higher rate than white children. Asian and Pacific Islander children are less likely to be hospitalized than whites.[19]

Differences in expressed rates of asthma morbidity and mortality are thought to be mul-

tivariant. Limited access to health care due to lack of health insurance, inadequate quality in one or more domains of health-care services, and failure to adhere to asthma treatment guidelines are factors that have been studied and linked to increased rates of asthma complications. Even when children are insured through enrollment in Medicaid managed care plans, differences in treatment of asthma persist. African American and Latino children were less likely to use inhaled anti-inflammatory medication than were white children. All other modalities recommended in the current asthma treatment guidelines were used equally across all population groups.[26]

▶ SUMMARY AND RECOMMENDATIONS

Specific actions must be taken to eliminate racial and ethnic health disparities among children. Progress has been made in decreasing childhood morbidity in some areas such as alcohol and drug abuse. However, the fact that adverse differences in health status for these children have persisted over decades suggests the need for more aggressive action. Much still needs to be understood regarding which actions are most effective in eliminating health disparities. It will require continued research to understand not only the affected population groups, but also how to optimize the ways in which the health-care system interacts with these children and their families.

There are opportunities for action to eliminate health disparities that have been demonstrated to be effective and to have broad applicability. Health education interventions culturally tailored to Latino families with children with asthma have been found to be effective both in increasing knowledge, and in motivating action to remove asthma triggers from the home environment. The effect of such interventions is that the children experience fewer emergency department visits and hospitalizations due to acute asthma episodes.[27]

Health-care systems must be redesigned to meet the needs of diverse groups. Cultural and linguistic barriers must be removed. Physician performance should be evaluated on ability to acknowledge, understand, and manage sociocultural differences in the patient/family–physician diad.[28] Where these measures have been implemented, there have been measurable improvements in patient satisfaction, adherence to treatment regimens, and improved health outcomes.

Other actions important to the elimination of racial and ethnic health disparities among children include the development of reimbursement policies by third-party payers that specifically address the multiple vulnerable health characteristics of children from certain racial and ethnic groups. Policies that restrict access to culturally competent care, that dampen patient satisfaction, or that discourage appropriate and timely utilization of health care should be eliminated.[22]

Health information materials, signage, consent forms, patient surveys, and other printed materials should be specifically designed to reflect the health literacy, language proficiency, language usage, and cultural norms of families.[29] Health-care providers and staff must be trained to recognize and remediate situations in which negative stereotypes associated with children from different racial and ethnic groups influence the quality and quantity of care patients receive. Racial stereotypes, based on the perception that a patient is lazy, prone to violence, unable to adhere to treatment, or able to endure inordinate pain, negatively influence provider behavior.[5] Children and families who experience racism in the receipt of health services are more likely to suffer psychological stress and poor health outcomes.[30]

Children and their families report the highest degree of satisfaction with their primary care provider when there is the greatest concordance in racial and ethnic background and primary language use between patient and health-care provider. Yet the current diversity of the pediatric workforce is grossly mismatched with that of the child population. The racial and ethnic makeup of the US child population is currently far more diverse than that of pediatricians as a group. With the projected growth in racial and ethnic diversity among children in the foreseeable future, the disproportionate underrepresentation of physicians from certain racial and ethnic backgrounds will increase.[31] To address this problem, concerted efforts must be made to substantially increase the representation of African American, Hispanic, Asian and Pacific Islander, and Native American pediatricians in the United States. The recruitment of racial and ethnic minorities into the health-care workforce must be pursued with vigor by all sectors engaged in the education and training of health-care professionals, and supported by the federal government.[32]

The elimination of health disparities among children also depends on the recognition and remediation of the disproportionate exposure to environmental hazards experienced by some racial and ethnic groups. Certain racial and ethnic groups overrepresented among migrant farm workers and children living in rural areas engaged in agricultural work must be protected. Screening and monitoring programs targeted to the needs of workers and their families should be implemented. Regulatory policies that limit the exposure of these children to environmental hazards must be established.

The built environment of highways, nuclear energy facilities, and manufacturing plants with hazardous effluents should be sited with consideration for their proximity to residential communities, and without regard to racial, ethnic, or economic demographics of residents. Where hazardous or toxic situations exist, cleanup and remediation should be mandated by regulation. Environmental genomics promises to identify genetic variations that increase individual susceptibility to toxic environmental exposures. With this information, preventive measures can be taken.

Socioeconomic inequities experienced by children in certain racial and ethnic groups must be corrected. The lingering effects of poverty, substandard education, and limited economic opportunities directly impair the growth, neurodevelopment, and health outcomes of children. Not until these fundamental societal conditions are adequately addressed can all children enjoy optimal health and well-being, the ability to develop to their fullest capacity, and to contribute to a thriving society.

▶ REFERENCES

1. Federal Interagency Forum on Child and Family Statistics. *America's Children: Key Indicators of Well-Being*. Washington, DC: US Government Printing Office; 2003.

2. Wood D. Effect of child and family poverty on child health in the United States. *Pediatrics* 2003;112–3(Pt 2):707.

3. National Institute of Environmental Health Sciences. *Health Disparities Research—Children's Heath Disparities Fact Sheet*. Washington, DC: NIEHS Clearinghouse; 2001.

4. Elster A, Jarosik J, Van Geest J, et al. Racial and ethnic disparities in healthcare for adolescents: A systematic review of the literature. *Arch Pediatr Adolesc Med* 2003;157(9):850–851.

5. Smedley BD, Stith AY, Nelson AR, eds. *Unequal Treatment: Confronting Racial and Ethnic Disparities in Health Care*. Washington, DC: National Academy Press; 2003.

6. National Center for Health Statistics. *Health, United States, 2000, with Adolescent Health Chartbook*. Hyattsville, Md: NCHS; 2000.

7. Henry J Kaiser Foundation. *Key Facts: Race, Ethnicity, and Medical Care*. Menlo Park, Calif: Henry J Kaiser Foundation; 1999.

8. National Institute of Child Health and Human Development. *Health Disparities: Bridging the Gap*. Washington, DC: NICHD Clearinghouse; 2000.

9. Woodruff TJ, Parker JD, Kyle AD, et al. Disparities in exposure to air pollution during pregnancy. *Environ Health Perspect* 2003;117(7):942–946.

10. Andrews M, Nord M, Bicker G, et al. *Household Food Security in the United States, 1999*. Food Assistance and Nutrition Research Report No. 8. Washington, DC: Food and Rural Economic Division, Economic Research Service, US Dept of Agriculture; 1999.

11. Alaimo K, Olson SM, Frongillo EA, et al. Food insufficiency, family income, and health in US preschool and school-aged children. *Am J Public Health* 2001;88:419–426.

12. Maimo K, Brutel RR, Frongillo EA, et al. Food insufficiency exists in the United States. *Am J Public Health* 1999;88:419–426.

13. McLoyd VC. The impact of economic hardship on black families and children: Psychological distress, parenting, and socioeconomic development. *Child Dev* 1990;61(2):311–346.

14. Hatfield H. *Toxic Communities: Environmental Racism*. Web MD, 2003. Available at: http://www.webmd.com.

15. Wooddruff TJ, Parker SD, Kyle AD, et al. Disparities in exposure to air pollution during pregnancy. *Environ Health Perspect* 2003;111(7):942–946.

16. Akinbami LJ, Schoendorf KC. Trends in childhood asthma: Prevalence, health care utilization and mortality. *Pediatrics* 2002;110:315–332.

17. Sexton K, Gong H Jr, Bailar JC III, et al. Air pollution health risks: Do class and race matter? *Toxicol Ind Health* 1993;9(5):843–878.

18. Stevenson LA, Gergan PJ, Hoover DR, et al. Sociodemographic correlations of indoor allergy sensitivity among United States Children. *J Allergy Clin Immunol* 2001;108(5):747–752.

19. Agency for Healthcare Research and Quality. *National Healthcare Disparities Report*. Rockville, Md: US Dept of Health and Human Services; 2003.

20. Brach C, Fraser I. Can cultural competency reduce racial and ethnic health disparities? A review and conceptual model. *Med Care Res Rev* 2000;57(suppl 1):181–217.

21. Newacheck PW, Hung YY, Wright KK. Racial and ethnic disparities in access to care for children with special health care needs. *Ambul Pediatr* 2002;2(4):247–254.

22. Wise PH, Kotelchuck M, Wilson ML, et al. Racial and socioeconomic disparities in childhood mortality in Boston. *N Engl J Med* 1985;313(6):360–366.

23. Stevens GD, Shi L. Effect of managed care and children's relationships with their primary care physicians: Differences by race. *Arch Pediatr Adolesc Med* 2002;156(4):369–377.

24. Weinick RM, Zuvekas SH, Cohen JW. Racial and ethnic differences in access to and use of health care services, 1977 to 1996. *Med Care Res Rev* 2000;57(suppl 1):36–54.

25. Elster A, Jarosile J, VanGeest J, et al. Racial and ethnic disparities in health care for adolescents: A systemic review of the literature. *Arch Pediatr Adolesc Med* 2003;157(9):867–874.

26. Lieu TA, Lozano P, Finkelstein JA, et al. Racial/ ethnic variation in asthma status and management practices among children in managed Medicaid. *Pediatrics* 2002;109(5):857–865.

27. Jones JA, Wahlgreen DR, Meltzer SB, et al. Increasing asthma knowledge and changing home environments for Latino families with asthmatic children. *Patient Educ Couns* 2001;42(1):67–79.

28. Levine RS, Foster JE, Fullilove RE, et al. Black–white inequalities in mortality and life expectancy, 1933–1999: Implications for Healthy People 2010. *Public Health Rep* 2001;116(5):474–483.

29. Betancourt JR, Green AR, Carrillo JE. Cultural Competence in Health Care: *Emerging Frameworks and Practical Approaches*. New York: Commonwealth Fund, 2002.

30. Williams DR. Race, socioeconomic status, and health. The added effects of racism and discrimination. *Ann N Y Acad Sci* 1999;896:173–188.

31. Stoddard JJ, Back MR, Brotherton SE. The respective racial and ethnic diversity of US pediatricians and American children. *Pediatrics* 2000;105(1 pt 1):27–31.

32. Smedley BD, Stith AY, Colburn L. *The Right Thing to Do; Enhancing Diversity in the Health Professions*. Washington DC: National Academy Press; 2001.

CHAPTER 5

Health-Care Access for Children of Immigrants

Nicole Prudent, MD, MPH

Mathilda B. Ruwe, MD, MPH

Alan Meyers, MD, MPH

John Capitman, PhD

▶ INTRODUCTION

Many view the United States as a nation of immigrants, a welcoming nation, strengthened by offering opportunities to newcomers and their children. Traditional accounts hold out hope to immigrant families that their children can become full participants in civic life and prosperous economic contributors. Another, more ethnocentric perspective on immigration has also remained popular: By offering a range of health-care and social services to immigrant families, our nation has become a magnet for immigration, creating overwhelming obligations that stymie efforts to meet the needs of citizens. Ongoing political and cultural struggles around these contrasting views have created a surprisingly varied mosaic of health policies and programs geared to children of immigrant families across the country. Yet, given continued immigration and the number of children in immigrant families who are US citizens by birth, such children will continue to form a notable segment of the population. How these children are treated will play a major role in shaping the nation's future.

This chapter begins by examining the social context of immigration, and the health risks and barriers to health-care access borne by children in immigrant families. We then explore how health-care policies, practices, and other factors contribute to these outcomes, before offering some possible solutions.

Social Context of Immigration

The political, economic, social, and other contextual issues associated with parents' migration are significant determinants of a child's

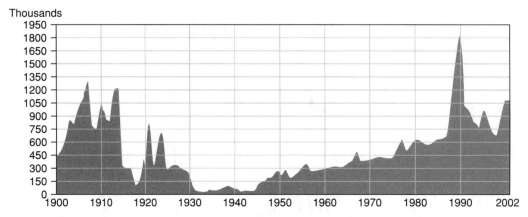

Figure 5–1. Immigrants admitted: Fiscal years 1900–2002. *(Source: US Citizenship and Immigration Services.* Immigrants 2003 Yearbook of Immigration Statistics. *Washington, DC: Office of Immigration Statistics, Dept of Homeland Security; September 2004.)*

physical and psychological adjustment.[1] Except for those in American Indian and Alaskan Native communities, almost all persons in the United States have roots in other parts of the world. Following the waves of settlers from Europe and enslaved persons from Africa, the United States saw a huge spike in immigration around the dawn of the 20th century. The 1950s witnessed a steady increase in immigration, forming a second wave, with the largest surge occurring in the 1990s (Fig. 5–1).

Sociodemographics

Unlike the first wave of immigrants, who were predominately of European descent, contemporary immigrants come from all regions of the world. Although 58% of the foreign-born are from Latin America,[2] the largest share of those accorded legal permanent residence come from North America and Europe.[3] The foreign-born population now constitutes about 33.5 million, accounting for 11.7% of the US population.[2] By 2050, the US population is projected to include 80 million post-1994 immigrants and their descendants, accounting for 25% of the total population.[2] Although technically the federal term *immigrant* refers only to legal permanent residents,[2] in this chapter we focus on children

whose parents would be termed "immigrants" in colloquial usage. This group includes legal permanent residents, refugees and asylees, undocumented immigrants, and persons with non-immigrant visas (Fig. 5–2). Based on parental nativity, children of newcomers can be classified as native-born with native-born parentage (NNP), native-born with mixed status parentage (NMP), native-born with foreign-born parentage (NFP), and foreign-born with foreign-born parentage (FFP). Significantly, there are broad variations between and within families in their socioeconomic characteristics and eligibility for public services based on the legal status of their newcomer parents.

- **Age.** One striking feature of the new immigrant population is its youth. Most immigrants are in the economically active age group (18 to 64 years). One in every five children under the age of 18 years is a child of an immigrant (born either of a mixed status or of a purely immigrant parentage).[4]
- **Race/Ethnicity and Language.** As shown in Table 5–1, the new immigrants are predominantly classified racially as white. About 75% come from regions in which English is not spoken. Hispanic ethnicity of

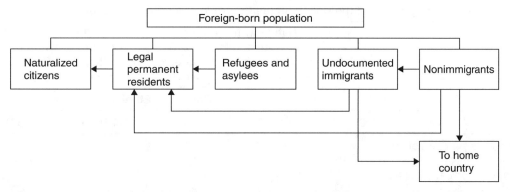

Figure 5–2. Immigrant categories and pathways to legal immigration. *(Source: Based on US Citizenship and Immigration Services.* Immigrants 2003 Yearbook of Immigration Statistics. *Washington, DC: Office of Immigration Statistics, Dept of Homeland Security; September 2004).*

any race also constitutes a substantial proportion (23.5 to 45.2%, of NMP and FFP respectively).

- **Economic Indicators.** NMP (ie, children with one foreign-born parent) show more favorable outcomes on economic measures. FFP children have the worst social indicators; they are disproportionately poor, with limited access to well-paying jobs or health insurance (see Table 5–1).

These data and related studies[5,6] suggest that social integration requires a more complex conceptualization than is offered by traditional acculturation theory. Traditionally, it was assumed that over time immigrants would assimilate into the US cultural and economic mainstream, and their offspring and successive generations would acculturate more fully and experience economic progress. However, the broad variability in the well-being and economic status of children in immigrant families seems more consistent with so-called segmented assimilation. According to this view, children of contemporary immigrants have very different outcomes as a reflection of the conditions of their parents' immigration, the social and economic resources brought by their families, and the opportunity structures of the communities

in which they settle. Based on these factors, the children of immigrants can take different routes within the system of stratification in the United States, from growing acculturation and parallel integration into the white middle-class to declining status relative to their parents, permanent poverty, and assimilation into the underclass.[5,6] Sociologic research suggests that public services are crucial factors in characterizing the reception offered by host communities. Cultural and economic integration is accelerated in communities that are more consistently welcoming.

Policy Significance

Both academic debates and public opinion reflect considerable controversy about whether it is in the best interest of the United States to offer adequate health and social services for immigrants. Economic analyses by Borjas[7] and others show that immigrants provide a net economic benefit to the domestic economy, but others studies report the opposite.[8] Nonetheless, a public health argument for services has been advanced, especially with regard to certain infectious diseases. For example, if denied access to preventive care, immigrants with active tuberculosis can be expected to expose many others in their community.[9] Despite

▶ **TABLE 5–1.** Demographics of the United States Population by Nativity of Parents: 2000

	Total Population	Native with Native Parentage (NNP)	Native with Mixed Parentage (NMP)	Native with Foreign Parentage (NFP)	Foreign-Born with Foreign Parentage (FFP)
Age, Race, and Ethnicity					
	274,087	245,708	12,703	14,808	28,379
Age < 18 years (% of N)	26.4	26.6	34.3	48.0	10.0
18–64 years	61.7	62.4	49.7	28.2	79.0
Race or ethnicity (% of N)					
White	82	83.6	88.7	79.6	67.9
Black	13.0	14.6	4.5	5.4	7.8
American Indian and Alaskan Native	1	1.1	0.8	0.5	0.7
Asian and pacific Islander	4	0.6	6	14.5	23.6
Hispanic (of any race)	12	4.9	23.5	42.9	45.2
White–not Hispanic	71	79	66.5	38.4	24.8
Selected Social Indicators					
High school or higher (% of N)	84.1	86.9	88.4	78.0	67.0
Total median income	$31,607	$32,080	$36,152	$31,597	$25,533
Poverty rate: < 18 years	16.9	15.4	13.8	25.7	29.4
Health insurance					
No health coverage	15.5	13.1	12.5	19.4	33.4
Medicaid	10.2	9.8	9.4	16.8	9.6
Private insurance	71	74.1	73.3	57.5	53.1
Managerial and professional specialty (% of N)	30.1	30.6	36.8	32.2	24.7

Source: US Census Bureau. The Foreign–Born Population in the United States: 2003. *Washington, DC: US Dept of Commerce, Economics and Statistics Administration; 2004.*

deep-seated anti-immigrant attitudes, US public opinion has consistently supported increased government efforts to aid the uninsured,[10] and a Kaiser Family Foundation health poll[11] showed that a large majority agreed that "health should be provided equally to everyone." Such support appears consistent with enlightened self-interest, particularly for the native-born white population, which can expect to rely increasingly on the economic productivity and commitments to social solidarity of immigrants and their children.[12]

▶ HEALTH STATUS AND WELL-BEING OF CHILDREN OF IMMIGRANTS

The World Health Organization (WHO) definition of health as not only the absence of infirmity but also complete physical and social well-being has provided the framework for developing measures of child well-being. These indicators range from measures of economic security and education to measures of health behavior and social environment.[13] This section reviews available health indicators for children in immigrant families (general health, low birth weight, mortality rates, vaccine rates, and vaccine-preventable childhood infectious diseases) and selected chronic health conditions (asthma, diabetes, mental health, nutritional problems, and dental health problems). Highlighted are indicators having (1) well-established primary care standards and subject to management in primary care, and (2) potentially greater risk to immigrant children given their physical and social environments. The section also discusses selected non–vaccine-preventable communicable diseases. Because of limited data on mental health, the section focuses on the extraordinary stress experienced by immigrants. Other important measures for which national data are not available (and which are not discussed here) include child abuse and neglect.[13]

Although national data are available for most of the health indicators discussed in this section, little is known about the health status of all children of immigrants, because the data are not usually aggregated by nativity or parental status. Three types of children of immigrants— (1) native-born of foreign parentage (NFP), (2) native-born of mixed status parentage (NMP), and (3) foreign-born children born of foreign parentage (FFP)—are identified only where data are available.

General Health

Children of immigrants are likely to be in good health, although their health status may vary depending on region of origin. Paradoxically, given the relative wealth of the United States, some children who are initially in good health status may deteriorate due to socioeconomic conditions. Yu et al,[14] using the National Health Interview Surveys for 1997–2000, found that Asian ethnicity and being foreign-born were generally associated with good to excellent health. Kou and Porter[15] found that differences in health status emerge when data on the Asian or Pacific Islander (API) population is analyzed by national origin. Guendelman et al[16] studied 708 infants of Mexican immigrants, finding that health status was eroded for 26% due to adverse socioeconomic conditions.

Birth Weight and Infant Mortality

Several studies suggest that immigrant women have better pregnancy outcomes than native-born women. In a study comparing pregnancy outcome of foreign-born and US-born women among 49,904 deliveries,[17] Forna et al found foreign-born women had a lower risk of preterm delivery, lower perinatal mortality, and new-borns with higher mean birth weight (3315 to 3084 g). Factors such as selectivity of the immigration process, more beneficial health behaviors, and less exposure to environmental toxins might account for these findings, but these possibilities have not been adequately explored.

Infectious Diseases

Children in immigrant families have an elevated risk for childhood vaccine-preventable infectious diseases because of suboptimal rates of immunization.[18] Although rubella now mostly occurs among persons born in countries that do not have routine vaccination programs, 176 cases of rubella were reported by the Centers for Disease Control and Prevention (CDC) in 2000, of which 78% occurred among Hispanics.[19] Lifson et al,[20] in Minnesota, reported a high prevalence of chronic hepatitis B infection (7%). Similarly, rates of non–vaccine-preventable infectious diseases are higher among immigrant children. Tuberculosis is mostly reported in foreign-born persons and is increasing in the United States.[19,21–23] Lifson et al[20] found a high prevalence of intestinal parasites (22%) among immigrant children. Tropical diseases such as malaria and typhoid fever are almost exclusively reported among refugee children.

Chronic Health Conditions

Asthma is the most common chronic childhood illness, affecting 1 in 3 children younger than 18 years of age. Asthma is most common in non-Hispanic black children followed by Hispanic children.[24] A study conducted in the Boston Public School system[25] found that 16% of Asian immigrant children had been diagnosed with asthma, and 3% had possible undiagnosed asthma. Beckett et al[26] reported the prevalence of asthma to be 18.4% among Hispanic children older than 9 months, compared with 7.4% for white children.

Severe iron-deficiency anemia, as well as folate and vitamin B_{12} deficiency, are among common chronic nutritional problems reported in Vietnamese immigrants living in southern California.[27] Strikingly high rates of food insecurity and hunger were documented among legal immigrants in California, Illinois, and Texas.[28] Data from the National Survey of Adolescent Health show that the process of immigrants' assimilation into US culture is accompanied by increasing rates of childhood overweight; second- and third-generation immigrant children had higher rates of overweight than first-generation children.[29] This effect is ultimately attributable to dietary and lifestyle changes, but the complex interplay between genetic susceptibility and culturally specific experiences with food security also play a role.

Dental Health

In 1987, Pollick et al[30] reported that of 1012 recent immigrant elementary school children screened in San Francisco, 77% of children needed dental treatment on first screening compared with 25% in a 1979–1980 survey of the western United States. Nonrefugee immigrants had more serious dental needs but used dental services less often than children with refugee status. Watson et al[31] studied a convenience sample of children aged 2 to 5 years and their parents and found that only 53% of the children were free of dental caries, whereas 18% needed emergency dental care and 26% needed early or nonurgent dental care. The strongest predictors of dental caries after adjusting for child's age and mother's education was the tenure of mother's residence in the United States.

Mental Health

Newly arrived immigrants—children and parents alike—may suffer from post-traumatic stress disorder (PTSD),[32] especially those who have witnessed natural disaster, political unrest, war, and other traumatic events. Even for those who emigrate under less-stressful conditions, arrival in a new country and the intergenerational conflicts associated with cultural and economic assimilation are significant potential sources of mental and behavioral health challenges. Nonetheless, there is a dearth of studies on the prevalence of mental health problems among children of immigrants. The few available studies suggest that despite multiple predisposing factors, immigrants' children are less likely to be diagnosed with mental illness. The reasons for this are not clear and may reflect inadequate measurement or blocked access to care.[33] Cultural bias and insensitivity by providers leading to misdiagnosis has also been suggested.[34] A 3-year follow-up study of 27 Cambodian youth (aged 8 to 12 years) who were traumatized as children found post-traumatic stress disorder and depression to be highly prevalent, at 48% and 41%, respectively. These researchers also found that avoidance behavior was highly prevalent, even among those without PTSD.[35]

▶ HEALTH CARE UTILIZATION BY CHILDREN OF IMMIGRANTS

Ambulatory and Emergency Care

Several studies have demonstrated that children of immigrants are less likely to have regular contact with the health-care system, use preventive care, have a usual source of care, and use ambulatory care. Berk et al,[36] using data from a 1996–1997 survey of undocumented Latino immigrants in four sites, found rates of ambulatory care utilization to be much lower than the average for all Latinos. Clark[37] found that immigrant mothers of Mexican origin described more barriers to children's health-care services than more acculturated mothers. Yu et al[14] examined the health status and health services access and utilization characteristics of children with diverse backgrounds using data from the National Health Interview Survey. They found that Asians had more favorable health status measures but were less likely to have had contact with the health-care system. Citizenship and nativity status, maternal education attainment, and poverty status were all significant independent risk factors for health-care access and utilization. According to the Kaiser Family Foundation Report,[38] immigrants are more likely to use clinics, less likely to use the physician's office, and more likely to report no usual source of care.

Given these access barriers, immigrant children are at greater risk for delayed emergency care. In a cross-sectional analysis of a full-year sample of cases of acute appendicitis in children aged 4 to 18 years from California and New York, Guagliardo et al[39] found that Hispanic and Asian children in California, as well as Asian and African American children in New York, had higher odds of appendix rupture.

Immunization Completion

Access barriers may hinder timely completion of vaccinations for both FFP and NFP children of immigrants. Studies of immunization status have revealed three basic problems: (1) low rates of immunization in some racial and ethnic groups; (2) lack of hepatitis B and *Haemophilus influenzae* coverage in others; and (3) some immigrant children being vaccinated at older ages.[40] Very low immunization rates were found among

Lao (43%) and Cambodian adolescents (35%). Findley et al[41] surveyed 314 Latino children younger than 5 years of age at two immunization clinics in New York City, finding that foreign-born children were underimmunized with regard to *H influenzae* and hepatitis B. Similarly, Jacobson et al,[42] in Rochester, New York, found that Somali children were more likely to receive vaccinations at older ages than were Hispanics. Barnett et al[43] evaluated 669 refugee children aged newborn to 20 years, and found that 82% had antibodies to measles and rubella and 64% had antibody to varicella.

Access to Dental Care

Milgrom et al[44] examined factors related to the utilization of dental care by 895 mothers and their 5- to 11-year-old children from low-income households, randomly selected from public schools for the period 1991 to 1992. The overall utilization rate was 63.2%; the rate for nonemergent (preventive) visits was 59.9%. Race and years the guardian lived in the United States were predictive of receiving care. Preventive medical visits and perceived need were strong predictors of a visit to the dentist, as were beliefs in the efficacy of dental care. Mothers who were satisfied with their own care and oral health and whose children were covered by insurance were more likely to utilize children's dental care.

▶ BARRIERS TO HEALTH-CARE ACCESS BY CHILDREN OF IMMIGRANTS

Gardel, a 7-year-old, is frequently seen in the pediatric neurology clinic for seizures. He also has a speech delay and asthma. Gardel was born in the United States. Both parents were legal immigrants. They came as refugees and did not speak English very well. A few weeks after the husband lost his job and associated health benefits, the mother found out that she was pregnant. Her job did not provide health insurance. She delayed prenatal care to the second trimester. Although the clinic quickly arranged for her to gain Medicaid coverage, it was discontinued on Gardel's second birthday. At 2½, Gardel became ill with severe cough, runny nose, and poor appetite. His parents waited and hoped that he would get better. They were still paying the bill for a Saturday emergency room visit for a similar illness one month earlier. One evening, after an episode of intense coughing, Gardel became limp and could barely breathe. His father called the ambulance and, while waiting, Gardel had his first seizure. He was admitted to the pediatric intensive care unit where he required mechanical ventilation for 3 weeks. After discharge, his parents observed with deep sadness that their son had lost his ability to understand and express words. He now required speech therapy and special education. His mother has never stopped blaming herself.

As this case and preceding sections emphasize, children of immigrants face disparate health-care access and outcomes, which in most cases vary by parental region of origin, nativity status, and residential location. These patterns show that a complex set of barriers to health-care access may be influencing their experiences, including (1) structural factors (ie, policies that systematically exclude immigrants from full participation in health and social services or limit integration into host communities), (2) sociocultural factors, and (3) individual economic factors.

Structural Barriers

The Personal Responsibility and Work Opportunity Reconciliation Act (PRWORA) of 1996, popularly known as "welfare reform," limited public benefits available even to legal immigrant adults and encouraged states to deny all services to undocumented persons. Because many immigrant adults do not have employment that provides health insurance, they are forced to seek pub-

licly covered services. Yet because of PRWORA rules and their varied interpretations around the country, many immigrant families fear that by seeking public services even for children who are US-born, they may limit their potential to become citizens.

Many immigrants feel vulnerable, especially the undocumented. Undocumented (and sometimes documented) immigrants live anonymously, to elude the attention of US immigration authorities. This fear is not totally unfounded, as evidenced by a bill introduced in Congress in 2004 (HR 3722) by Representative Rohrabacher (D-CA) that would have required hospitals to report undocumented patients to the US Citizenship and Immigration Services (CIS) within 2 hours of providing treatment. This bill was not enacted, but even its introduction and discussion in the news could have a chilling effect on immigrants seeking health services for themselves or their children. For medical care, many immigrants turn to private sources whose capacity is limited, or rely on lay healers or folk remedies, or both.[45]

Lack of Health Insurance

The ability to pay (income and insurance status) plays a major role in gaining access to the US health-care system. Several studies have shown that children of immigrants are more likely to lack health insurance. Huang,[46] using data from the 1994 and 1996 Current Population Survey, found that 27.3% of children of immigrants were without health insurance and 34.1% received public insurance. Foreign-born children who had not yet become US citizens were the most likely to lack health insurance. Huang also found that children of Haitian and Korean (45.3%) immigrants were more likely to be uninsured than children of other nationalities. These findings have been replicated in more recent studies.[47]

Insurance Status and Access to Care

Passel[48] found that both children of racial and ethnic minorities and children of immigrants reported being in worse health and were less likely to have health insurance than were white, non-Hispanic children and children of US natives. A number of studies indicate these findings may reflect the impact of insurance status on access to regular care. Guendelman et al[49] reported that 52% of foreign-born children were uninsured and 66% had a regular care source, compared with 20% and 92%, respectively, among native-born children. Ku and Matani[50] found that fewer noncitizen immigrants and their children had Medicaid or job-based insurance and many more were uninsured than were native citizens or children of citizens. Noncitizens and their children also had worse access to both regular ambulatory and emergency care, even when insured. Halfon et al[51] surveyed 817 Latino families in urban California; only 40% of eligible children had continuous Medicaid coverage since birth, 18.6% had never been insured, and 20.7% had received episodic Medicaid coverage. Granados et al[52] found that 64% of Latino children were uninsured when both parents and child were noncitizens, compared with 23% of US-born children of Latino immigrant parents and 10% of US-born children of Latino parents who were US citizens. A similar pattern was seen for access to regular primary care.

Lack of health insurance has also been associated with lower levels of immunization among some children of immigrants. Sun et al[53] found a significant difference in the accessibility to immunization services between non–US-born and US-born children. Vryheid[40] found that barriers to child immunization included transportation, language, lack of knowledge of immunizations, missed opportunities, and cultural barriers.

Sociocultural Barriers

The capacity and willingness of the health-care system to negotiate cultural and linguistic differences also appears as a barrier to appropriate care for children in immigrant families. Cultural barriers include language and communication styles that are different from those in the host country. Approximately 75% of immigrants come from countries where English is not the dominant or official language.[54] A lack of proficiency in Spanish or other languages and a lack of trained interpreters are barriers to health-care system use for non-English speakers.[53,55] Other influential cultural factors include health beliefs as well as values and attitudes that are different from biomedical concepts of disease and treatment approaches.

Most developing countries from which new immigrants to the United States migrate do not have a primary health care system. Some of the children, particularly those from rural areas, have never been to a clinician trained in Western medicine. Family members, especially those with low educational attainment, may have a distorted concept regarding the practice and efficacy of health care. For example, a medical visit without any prescribed medicine may be unacceptable to some; medication delivered by injection is often preferred over oral medication; and failure to provide it may lead to dissatisfaction with care. These attitudes may limit trust in the health-care system and affect adherence. Practitioners also need to understand who typically makes health care decisions in the cultural tradition of the patient's family (eg, grandmother, father, extended family) and adapt interventions to this knowledge.

▶ INTERVENTIONS TO REDUCE BARRIERS TO HEALTH-CARE ACCESS FOR CHILDREN OF IMMIGRANTS

As discussed in the foregoing sections, barriers to health-care access by children of immigrants exist at multiple levels, including policy, structure, program, and individual family levels. Interventions are needed at each.

Interventions to Reduce Economic Barriers

At the policy level, a number of developments have helped to cushion the impact of PRWORA.

The State Children's Health Insurance Program (SCHIP), enacted in 1997, gave states matching funds to provide health-care coverage to children whose families' income was above Medicaid level but below 200% of the federal poverty level. Eleven million children in the United States were uninsured when SCHIP was enacted, and it opened up opportunities for immigrant families who had been excluded under Medicaid. States have the opportunity under SCHIP and other legislation to increase the number of children in immigrant families with regular access to health care. But sustaining and promoting coverage for undocumented immigrants will require continuing subsidies through a mix of private and public funding.[56] The California Endowment funded a 2-year demonstration project to provide subsidized health insurance coverage to more than 7500 children through five nonprofit organizations. Locally based, comprehensive initiatives are in place or emerging in a growing list of California counties. Other states are also exploring how programmatic changes and mixing public with private financing can increase the accessibility of health care for children in immigrant families.

Intervention to Reduce Cultural Barriers

Cultural Competence

Eliminating disparities in the health status of people of diverse backgrounds and improving health-care quality appears to require increasing the cultural and linguistic competence of health-care settings and practitioners. To meet this challenge, changes in policies, structures, practices, and procedures are needed.[57] Checklists have been developed by the National Center for Cultural Competence (NCCC) for use by individual practitioners, programs, and institutions in assessing aspects of cultural competence. Many institutions have established cultural competency training for their medical workforce. The Bureau of Primary Health Care of the US Department of Health and Human Services (DHHS) has recommended National Standards for Culturally and Linguistically Appropriate Health Care Services (NCLAS). The Liaison Committee on Medical Education has led medical schools to develop curricula to teach cultural competency. Similar strategies have been developed for nursing and most other disciplines in medicine and public health. Insurance companies and health plans have developed their own policies and training programs. Private foundations are active in funding health resources, training programs, interpreter services, research, and national conferences to support cultural competency programs and improve access to care and education for immigrant families and culturally diverse communities.

Reducing Intergenerational Conflicts

Improving parent–child communication skills is another method that has been used to provide culturally competent services to immigrant children. In a randomized pre-/post-study, Litrownik et al[58] found that culturally sensitive parent–child communication strategies were effective in promoting healthy youth decision making (eg, not to engage in alcohol or tobacco use).

Reducing Language Barriers

Approximately 40 states have addressed language access in health-care settings. Although some states, such as California and New York, offer specific guidance to providers on what they must do to meet language needs, other states, such as Illinois, leave it to providers to decide on the service they will offer.[59]

Cultural Humility and Use of Cultural Brokers

Practitioners need to understand their limitations in learning and understanding the culture of their patients. The use of cultural brokers is one method that is popular and effective in reducing this limitation. Ikeda et al[60] found that with appropriate training, bilingual, bicultural women effectively delivered culturally relevant nutrition education that resulted in improved diets of low-income Vietnamese women. Castaneda et al[61] found that outreach workers were particularly effective in enrolling and retaining hard-to-reach populations in California, especially immigrant families, into low-income health insurance programs such as MediCal and Healthy Families.

Collaborative research is another method to help practitioners and researchers learn more about the culture of their patients. Stein et al[62] describe an academic-community partnership used in the Mental Health for Immigrants Program (MHIP), a school-based mental health intervention. They provide examples of how a participatory research partnership may work at various stages of the project, including design, implementation, and program evaluation, to meet a specific community's needs and produce generalizable knowledge.

▶ SUMMARY AND RECOMMENDATIONS

Irrespective of citizenship, children of immigrants face multiple barriers to health-care access. Parental legal status has an influence on indicators of social-well being for children of immigrants, reducing the potential for economic and cultural assimilation. Studies of emerging interventions provide some confidence that integrated health insurance and services programs, public–private partnerships, and culturally competent initiatives can increase access for children of immigrants. However, research into the health and well-being of children of immigrants, who are traditionally underrepresented, as well as research into best-practice models and efficacy and cost-effectiveness of interventions aimed at improving their outcomes, are necessary. Summaries of the findings and recommendations discussed in this chapter appear in Tables 5–2 and 5–3.

▶ **TABLE 5–2.** Summary of Major Findings Regarding Health Disparities in Children of Immigrants

- Parental legal status has an influence on indicators of social-well-being for children of immigrants, reducing potential for economic and cultural assimilation for significant numbers of future citizens.
- Data on health status, health-care access, and utilization for children in immigrant families by parental source country, legal status, and region are inadequate.
- Available data suggest that children in immigrant families have less access to health care; they are likely to lack a usual source of care, have fewer routine ambulatory visits, and delay emergency care; and their health status tends to deteriorate over time in the United States.
- Inadequate health-care access for children in immigrant families increases risk for communicable disease in the general population.
- Children in immigrant families, irrespective of citizenship, face multiple barriers to health-care access, including lack of health insurance, parental fear of using public programs, linguistic and cultural barriers.
- Current public policies that limit insurance for immigrant families and low parental access further complicate children's access.
- Lack of cultural competence limits capacity of health-care organizations and practitioners to provide quality care for children in immigrant families.
- Studies of emerging interventions provide some confidence that integrated health insurance and services programs, public–private partnerships, and culturally competent initiatives can increase access for children of immigrants.
- There are no systematic efficacy or cost-effectiveness evaluations of best-practice models for increasing access and preventing deterioration in health status for children in immigrant families.

▶ **TABLE 5–3**. Summary of Recommendations

- Reduce health-care access disparities by increasing insurance coverage for immigrant families and their children
- Improve health-care access for immigrant families and their children through programs of linguistic and cultural navigation by trained paraprofessionals
- Hold providers accountable for delivery of culturally competent care by tracking adherence to practice standards and linking reimbursement to demonstrated cultural competence
- Increase immigrant family awareness and proficiency in using health care by including health literacy training in settlement programs
- Encourage research into the health and well-being of children of immigrants who are traditionally underrepresented, such as immigrants from the Caribbean, Southeast Asia, and Africa
- Encourage research into best-practice models and efficacy and cost-effectiveness of interventions in improving outcomes for children in immigrant families
- Accelerate research on children of immigrants by requiring collection of health and health-care data by parental status, region of origin, and source country

▶ REFERENCES

1. Guarnaccia PJ, Lopez S. The mental health and adjustment of immigrant and refugee children. *Child Adolesc Psychiatr Clin N Am* 1998;7(3):537–53, viii–ix.
2. US Census Bureau. *The Foreign-Born Population in the United States: 2003.* Washington, DC: US Dept of Commerce, Economics and Statistics Administration; 2004.
3. USCIS. *United States Citizenship and Immigration Services.* 2004. Available at: http://www.USCIS.gov.
4. Fix ME, Zimmerman W, Passel JS. *The Integration of Immigrants Families in the United States.* Washington, DC: The Urban Institute; 2001.
5. Zhou M. Segmented assimilation: Issues, controversies and recent research on the new second generation. In: Hirschman C, Kasinitz P, Dewind J, eds. *Handbook of International Migration: The American Experience.* New York, NY: Sage Foundation; 1997:196–211.
6. Portes A, Rumbaut R. *Legacies: The Story of the Immigrant Second Generation.* Berkeley, Calif: Univ of Calif Press; 2001.
7. Borjas GJ. The economic benefits of immigration. *J Econ Perspec* 1995;9(2):3–22.
8. Camarota SA. *The High Cost of Cheap Labor: Illegal Immigration and the Federal Budget.* Washington, DC: Center for Immigration Studies; 2004. Available at: http://www.cis.org/articles/2004/fiscal.pdf.

9. Asch S, Leake B, Gelberg L. Does fear of immigration authorities deter tuberculosis patients from seeking care? *West J Med* 1994;161:373–376.
10. Blendon RJ, Young JT, DesRoches CM. The uninsured, the working uninsured, and the public. *Health Aff* 1999;18(6):203–211.
11. *Kaiser Health Poll Report, 2003.* Available at: http://headlines.kff.org/healthpollreport/templates/printfriendly.php?p=6&d=detail&feature=feature3.
12. Capitman J. Defining diversity: A primer and review. *Generations* 2002;Fall:8–15.
13. National Institute for Child Health and Human Development: *America's Children: Key National Indicators of Well-Being, 2003.* Available at: http://www.nichd.nih.gov/publications/pubs/childstats/americas03.htm.
14. Yu SM, Huang ZJ, Singh GK. Health status and health services utilization among U.S. Chinese, Asian Indian, Filipino, and other Asian/Pacific Islander Children. *Pediatrics* 2004;113(1):101–107.
15. Kuo J, Porter K. Health status of Asian Americans: United States, 1992–1994. *Adv Data* 1998;(298):1–16.
16. Guendelman S, English P, Chavez G. Infants of Mexican immigrants: Health status of an emerging population. *Med Care* 1995;33(1):41–52.
17. Forna F, Jamieson DJ, Sanders D, et al. Pregnancy outcomes in foreign-born and US-born women. *Int J Gynaecol Obstet* 2003;83(3):257–265.
18. World Health Organization. *State of the World's Vaccines and Immunizations.* Geneva,

Switzerland: WHO Dept of Vaccines and Biologicals; 2002. Available at: http://www.unicef.org/publications/pub_sowvi_en.pdf.

19. Centers for Disease Control and Prevention. Rubella among Hispanic adults in Kansas 1998 and Nebraska, 1999. *MMWR Morb Mortal Wkly Rep* 2000;49:225–228.

20. Lifson AR, Thai D, O'Fallon A, et al. Prevalence of tuberculosis: Hepatitis B and intestinal parasitic infections among refugees to Minnesota. *Public Health Rep* 2002;117(1):69–77.

21. Recommendations for prevention and control of tuberculosis among foreign-born persons. Report of the Working Group on Tuberculosis among Foreign-Born Persons. Centers for Disease Control and Prevention. *MMWR Recomm Rep* 1998;47(RR-16):1–29.

22. Preventing and controlling tuberculosis along the U.S.–Mexico border. *MMWR Recomm Rep* 2001;50(RR-1):1–27.

23. Centers for Disease Control and Prevention. *Reported tuberculosis in the United States, 2000.* Atlanta, Ga: US Dept of Health and Human Services; 2001b. Available at: http://www.cdc.gov/nchstp/tb/.

24. Childtrends Databank: 2004. Available at: http://www.childtrendsdatabank.org/pdf/43_PDF.pdf.

25. Lee T, Brugge D, Francis C, et al. Asthma prevalence among inner-city Asian American School children. *Public Health Rep* 2003;118(3):215–220.

26. Beckett WS, Belanger K, Gent JF, et al. Asthma among Puerto Rican Hispanics: A multi-ethnic comparison study of risk factors. *Am J Respir Crit Care Med* 1996;154(4):894–899.

27. Luong KV, Nguyen LT. Folate and vitamin B_{12}-deficiency anemias in Vietnamese immigrants living in Southern California. *South Med J* 2002; 93(1):53–57.

28. Kasper J, Gupta SK, Tran P, et al. Hunger in legal immigrants in California, Texas, and Illinois. *Am J Public Health* 2000;90:1629–1633.

29. Popkin BM, Udry JR. Adolescent obesity increases significantly in second and third generation US immigrants: The national longitudinal study of adolescent health. *Am Soc Nutr Sci* 1997;128:1–706.

30. Pollick HF, Rice AJ, Echenberg D, et al. Dental health of recent immigrant children in the Newcomer Schools, San Francisco. *Am J Public Health* 1987;77(6):731–732.

31. Watson MR, Horowitz AM, Garcia I, et al. Caries conditions among 2–5-year-old immigrant Latino children related to parents' oral health knowledge, opinions and practices. *Community Dent Oral Epidemiol* 1999;27(1):8–15.

32. Locke CJ, Southwick K, McCloskey LA, et al. The psychological and medical sequelae of war in Central American refugee mothers and children. *Arch Pediatr Adolesc Med* 1996;150(8):822–828.

33. Escobar JI, Hoyos NC, Gara MA. Immigration and mental health: Mexican Americans in the United States. *Harv Rev Psychiatry* 2000;8(2):64–72.

34. Choi H. Understanding adolescent depression in ethnocultural context. *ANS Adv Nurs Sci* 2002; 25(2):71–85.

35. Kinzie JD, Sack W, Angell R, et al. A three-year follow-up of Cambodian young people traumatized as children. *J Am Acad Child Adolesc Psychiatry* 1989;28(4):501–504.

36. Berk ML, Schur CL, Chavez LR, et al. Health care use among undocumented Latino immigrants. *Health Aff* 2000;19(4):51–64.

37. Clark L. Mexican-origin mothers' experiences using children's health care services. *West J Nurs Res* 2002;24(2):159–179.

38. Kaiser Family Foundation Report. *Immigrants' Health Care Coverage and Access.* Menlo Park, Calif: Kaiser Commission on Medicaid and Uninsured; 2004. Available at: http://www.kkf.org/Medicaid/2241-index.cfm.

39. Guagliardo MF, Teach SJ, Huang ZJ, et al. Racial and ethnic disparities in pediatric appendicitis rupture rate. *Acad Emerg Med* 2003;10(11):1218–1227.

40. Vryheid RE. A survey of vaccinations of immigrants and refugees in San Diego County, California. *Asian Am Pac Island J Health* 2001;9(2):221–230.

41. Findley SE, Irigoyen M, Schulman A. Children on the move and vaccination coverage in a low-income, urban Latino population. *Am J Public Health* 1999;89(11):1728–1731.

42. Jacobson RM, Vierkant RA, Jacobsen SJ, et al. Association of parental vaccination reports with measles, mumps, and rubella protective antibody levels: Comparison of Somali immigrant, Hispanic migrant, and US children in Rochester, MN. *Mayo Clin Proc* 2002;77(3):241–245.

43. Barnett ED, Christiansen D, Figueira M. Seroprevalence of measles, rubella, and varicella in refugees. *Clin Infect Dis* 2002;35(4):403–408.

44. Milgrom P, Mancl L, King B, et al. An explanatory model of the dental care utilization of low-income children. *Med Care* 1998;36(4):554–566.

45. Colucciello ML, Woelfel V. Child care beliefs and practices of Hispanic mothers. *Nursingconnections* 1998;11(3):33–40.

46. Huang FY. Health insurance coverage of the children of immigrants in the United States. *Matern Child Health J* 1997;1(2):69–80.

47. Carrasquillo O, Carrasquillo AI, Shea S. Health insurance coverage of immigrants living in the United States: Differences by citizenship status and country of origin. *Am J Public Health* 2000;90(6):917–923.

48. Passel JS. Demographic and social trends affecting the health of children in the United States. *Ambul Pediatr* 2002;2(2 suppl):169–179.

49. Guendelman S, Schauffler HH, Pearl M. Unfriendly shores: How immigrant children fare in the U.S. health system. *Health Aff* 2001;20(1):257–266.

50. Ku L, Matani S. Left out: Immigrants' access to health care and insurance. *Health Aff* 2001;20(1):247–256.

51. Halfon N, Wood DL, Valdez RB, et al. Medicaid enrollment and health services access by Latino children in inner-city Los Angeles. *JAMA* 1997;277(8):636–641.

52. Granados G, Puvvula J, Berman N, et al. Health care for Latino children: Impact of child and parental birthplace on insurance status and access to health services. *Am J Public Health* 2001;91(11):1806–1807.

53. Sun WY, Sangweni B, Butts G, et al. Assessment of an outreach program that links children who use New York City immunization clinics to primary care. *Health Mark Quart* 1999;17(1):9–22.

54. National Forum of Immigration. *1999 National Immigration Forum.* Washington, DC: 2001. Available at: http://www.immigrationforum.org.

55. Garrett CR, Treichel CJ, Ohmans P. Barriers to health care for immigrants and non-immigrants: A comparative study. *Minn Med* 1998;81(4):52–55.

56. Frates J, Diringer J, Hogan L. Models and momentum for insuring low-income, undocumented immigrant children in California. *Health Aff* 2003;22(1):259–263.

57. Developing cultural competence in health care settings. National Center for Cultural Competence. *Pediatr Nurs* 2002;28(2):133–137.

58. Litrownik AJ, Elder JP, Campbell NR, et al. Evaluation of a tobacco and alcohol use prevention program for Hispanic migrant adolescents: Promoting the protective factor of parent-child communication. *Prev Med* 2000;31(2 pt 1):124–133.

59. Perkins J. *Ensuring Linguistic Access in Health Care Settings: An Overview of Current Legal Rights and Responsibilities.* Menlo Park, Calif: Kaiser Commission on Medicaid and the Uninsured, Henry J Kaiser Family Foundation. Available at: http://www.kkf.org/medicaid/2241-index.cfm.

60. Ikeda JP, Pham L, Nguyen KP, et al. Culturally relevant nutrition education improves dietary quality among WIC-eligible Vietnamese immigrants. *J Nutr Educ Behav* 2002;34(3):151–158.

61. Castaneda X, Clayson ZC, Rundall T, et al. Promising outreach practices: Enrolling low-income children in health insurance programs in California. *Health Promotion Pract* 2003;4(4):430–438.

62. Stein BD, Kataoka S, Jaycox LH, et al. Basis and program design of a school-based mental health intervention for traumatized immigrant children: A collaborative research partnership. *J Behav Health Serv Res* 2002;29(3):318–326.

CHAPTER 6

Geriatrics and End-of-Life Care

JAMEHL L. DEMONS, MD

RAMON VELEZ, MD, MSC

► INTRODUCTION

The US population is growing older. This population includes increasing numbers of people of color. The over-85 age group is the fastest-growing segment of the population. Over the past 100 years, the total population has increased by five times, while the number of those older than 65 years has multiplied 18 times. One in eight people is over 65—35.6 million in 2002.[1] It is imperative that our health-care systems become sensitive to the specific concerns unique to this population.

The health needs of minority elders are the same as those for any other group: affordable, accessible, and competent care. However, this is not available for all minority patients. Racial biases seen in health care are magnified for the elderly because of their high prevalence of chronic disease and increased use of the health-care system. When minorities have equal access to physicians, they are less often advised to have screening tests such as mammograms or preventive measures such as flu shots. Minorities are hospitalized more often for complications of advanced disease, such as limb amputations in diabetes and orchiectomy in prostate cancer, suggesting they do not receive early interventions.[2]

Advances in technology have led to increased survival from acute illness, resulting in more people living with and dying of chronic diseases than ever before. The top five chronic illnesses that lead to death are congestive heart failure, chronic obstructive pulmonary disease, dementia, stroke, and cancer. These conditions are frequently accompanied by prolonged disability, characterized by exacerbations of illness prior to death. Optimal care of chronic disease requires close monitoring, often by an interdisciplinary health-care team. Minorities are less likely to receive this comprehensive care. Trust in the health-care provider and buy-in of the patient to the concept of control of disease is required to allow adequate management of chronic diseases. These aspects may also assist in preparing the patient and his or her family for the ultimate patient outcome—death.

End-of-life care is largely an elderly issue. Eighty-six percent of the 2.3 million people who died in 1997 were Medicare recipients. Twenty-seven percent of the yearly Medicare budget is spent on care in the last year of life.[3] Consequently, laws governing Medicare often influence end-of-life care, including hospice.

This chapter examines end-of-life care in elderly minorities, particularly African Americans and Hispanics, from a racial and cultural perspective. It provides examples of how quality end-of-life care that is provided for some is not provided for all. The chapter concludes by discussing what has been done and what should be done to narrow this racial and cultural divide.

▶ IN SEARCH OF A GOOD DEATH

If I'm lucky, I'll be wired every which way in a hospital bed. Tubes running into my nose. But try not to be scared of me, friends! I'm telling you right now that this is okay. It's little enough to ask for at the end. Someone, I hope, will have phoned everyone to say, "Come quick, he's failing!" And they will come. And there will be time for me to bid goodbye to each of my loved ones... be glad for me if I can die in the presence of friends and family. If this happens, believe me, I came out ahead. I didn't lose this one.[4]

This excerpt points out two stark contrasts. Initially it is as if the writer is counting it a good thing to be in the hospital at the end of life with "tubes running into my nose." However, as the writer goes on, you realize that he or she wants to be able to know when death is imminent, to have someone gather his family and friends to say that final goodbye. The poem indicates that the person perceives medical treatment or hospitalization as the vehicle to prolong his life momentarily, not as a healing entity or a long-term solution, but just long enough to give him the opportunity to end on his own terms and say goodbye, to have a good death.

The Institute of Medicine Committee on End of Life Care defined high-quality dying as a death free from avoidable distress and suffering for patients, families, and their caregivers.[5] Steinhauser et al convened a focus group to identify domains integral to a good death. The 75 participants were from different disciplines and included physicians, nurses, social workers, chaplains, hospice volunteers, patients, and recently bereaved family members who all could give insight into different perspectives on end-of-life care. From the qualitative analysis, six domains—pain and symptom management, clear decision making, preparation for death, completion, contributing to others, and affirma-

tion of the whole person—were identified as the most important to gauge a good death.[6] Family members have defined higher quality dying as better symptom management, good clinician–patient communication, and good clinician–family communication.[5] Dying patients want to receive adequate pain and symptom management, avoid inappropriate prolongation of dying, achieve a sense of control, relieve burden, and strengthen relationships with loved ones.[7]

These domains concur with the World Health Organization definition of palliative care. Palliative care is the total active care of patients who have received a diagnosis of a serious, life-threatening illness. The goal of palliative care is achievement of the best possible quality of life for patients and their families.[8]

Hospice

The word *hospice* stems from the root "hospitality" and is a form of medical care that began in London, England, around 1967. It was not until 1978 that the US Department of Health, Education, and Welfare suggested providing federal funds to support the hospice movement in the United States. The Medicare Hospice Benefit was established in 1986. Hospice care involves a team-oriented approach to medical treatment, pain management, and emotional and spiritual support for patients who are terminally ill as well as their families. Hospice focuses on caring, not curing. Hospice care may be provided in freestanding hospice centers, or as an integrated part of hospitals and nursing homes. Hospice care is covered under Medicare, Medicaid, most private insurance plans, health maintenance organizations (HMOs), and other managed care organizations.[9]

Baer and Hanson surveyed family members of recently deceased individuals from nursing homes who had received hospice care. They were asked to evaluate hospice services based on quality of care for symptoms before and after hospice, the monetary value of hospice, the effect of hospice on hospitalization, and special services provided. Sixty-four percent of respondents felt their loved one was receiving good or excellent care before the initiation of hospice. However, after hospice services began, 93% reported good to excellent care. The family members' comments included the statement that "Hospice offers nurturing for both the emotional and spiritual sides plus solid medical information" to both patient and family.[10]

Patients and families express desire for pain and symptom management, preparation for death, and affirmation of the whole person, which hospice typically provides. Yet hospice care is not provided equitably to the entire population. There is very little ethnic and racial diversity in the more than 3000 hospice programs in the United States. Most recent statistics indicate that 84% of hospice patients are white, whereas 8% are African American, and 1% of other origins.[11,12] No matter what the geography, these numbers remain the same. In some rural areas these demographics accurately represent the surrounding population, but this is not representative of most metropolitan areas, where minorities equal 30% or more of the population.[13]

Many surmise that minorities do not use hospice more because patients and physicians do not know of its services or how to gain access. However, even after they learn of a terminal illness and are informed about hospice, nearly 40% of African Americans still do not use the service.[14] African Americans are less likely than whites to have completed a living will or durable power of attorney for health care, and this is not always associated with education or income. One reason cited in a study of patients with advanced cancers was the belief that formal documentation was not needed because family would know of the patient's treatment preferences.[15] The same holds true for Hispanic patients. The New Mexico Elder Health Study surveyed elderly Hispanics and whites. Hispanics were less likely to correctly define a living will or durable power of attorney. Of the 70% of Hispanic men and women who even thought they knew what advance directives were, less than one-half had signed one compared with 60% of whites who had similar knowledge.[14]

Cultural and Spiritual Views

There are barriers to palliative end-of-life care, particularly in the African American community. The reasons are multifactorial. For one, a good death may not be defined the same by all. Some traditional Christian religions view death as involving pain and suffering that should not be avoided but rather endured ("Jesus suffered at his death, should I expect any less?"). Many African American Muslims hold the Islamic teaching that pain is sent by God as a test of one's faith.[12] In these instances, a health professional offering palliation, particularly pain medicine, may be considered outside the will of God. Among many African Americans, the family, usually a female member, is expected to care for terminally ill family members and outside help from hospice team members is viewed as a sign of weakness.

Systematic Barriers

Other barriers are built on institutional injustices. Lack of insurance leads to poor access to the health-care system. African Americans are twice as likely as whites to be uninsured. A further indication of institutional barriers related more closely to end-of-life issues is the use of less analgesia for Hispanics and African Americans, even in the face of equal pain assessments.[2] Morrison et al found that pharmacies in neighborhoods with mostly nonwhite residents carried lower or no stock of medicines to treat severe pain. In a survey of New York City pharmacies, many reported fear of robbery as the reason for low supplies. After controlling for the crime rate in those areas, pharmacies in communities with higher nonwhite population still had statistically fewer supplies.[16,17] Underrepresentation of minorities in medicine creates yet another barrier. Cultural differences between provider and patient can be a nidus for poor communication. This is particularly true when one participant, either clinician or patient, is insensitive to the differences. The stress of a terminal illness has been proven to worsen these barriers.

Racial Preference

There are ethnic differences in preferences for end-of-life care. Blackhall et al surveyed African American, Mexican American, and Korean American elders.[18] The African American elders, as a group, pointed out some situations where withholding or withdrawing medical care is acceptable. However, the elders surveyed had a personal desire to use life support at least "for a little while." Some wanted to continue life support because they did not trust physicians' motives for suggesting withdrawal or withholding lifesaving measures. They indicated a perception that the motives might be based on economic reasons—"Do they need this bed and want to get rid of me? Did they find out I have no insurance?"—rather than true concern for the patient. Many also felt it was not the responsibility of a health-care provider to determine that a patient's condition is terminal, because the provider is not God and a miracle might occur.

Mexican Americans in the same study generally wanted to continue life support even when presented with situations that were described as hopeless. They also had more of a desire for life support for themselves in all medical situations presented. In-depth conversation with a subset of participants revealed the feeling that the physician would not even discuss life support if it were truly a hopeless situation. This finding reveals a conflict with the principle of patient autonomy in Western medicine.[18] The emphasis in end-of-life care planning is based on patient autonomy, the right of the patient with sound mind to make decisions regarding medical treatment. The Patient Self-Determination Act enacted in 1991 requires all states to recognize

advance directives such as living wills. It also requires that all persons admitted to a medical facility be given the opportunity to complete such documents.[15] In the Hispanic culture, the matriarch makes the medical decisions for her family. Korean Americans feel it is the responsibility of the family to do all possible for the patient within the family out of *nyodo* (family devotion) despite the wishes of the patient and without the help of those outside the family.[18] In fact, many Mexican-Americans and Korean-Americans feel that only the family should know the truth abut a patient's diagnosis and prognosis.[19]

The difference in individuals' preference for aggressive care to the end-of-life is truly ethnic and not based on economic considerations, as evidenced by a survey of African American and white physicians. In a self report of physician attitudes toward end-of-life care for themselves and their patients, six times as many black physicians as whites wanted aggressive treatment for themselves, even if in a persistent vegetative state.[20]

▶ PHYSICIANS AS BARRIERS

There is a professional culture of denying death as a natural part of life. Many physicians feel it is their role to heal, not to tell someone they or a loved one is dying. Death is viewed as a failure of medicine or the medical provider. That provider then fails to have any role in palliation and the ultimate death of their terminally ill patient.[21] Many hospital and medical school cultures do not support educating students in end-of-life care. Some 50% of medical school faculty and residents do not feel there is much to be learned from a dying patient and often "protect" students from these "poor teaching cases."[22]

Medical Student Education

Physicians are often the primary source of education for their patients. When a physician or other primary care provider lacks knowledge of the range of issues related to palliative care, the educational possibilities for the patient are lost. Minority physicians care disproportionately for minority patients; thus, their knowledge deficit has more impact on end-of-life care in a minority community.

Medical students and other trainees have the most open minds regarding personal differences. They learn through lectures from school faculty but also rely heavily on textbooks. Carron et al reviewed several textbooks in 1999 to determine their coverage of 12 illnesses that often led to death.[23] Each book was scored on the presence of helpful advice regarding end of life. *Harrison's Principles of Internal Medicine,* 13th edition, the *Merck Manual,* 16th edition, *Scientific American on CD-ROM,* 1994 edition, and *The Washington Manual,* 28th edition were used. With a rating scale that gave a score of 0 for the lack of discussion, 1 point for information that was present but not particularly helpful, and 2 points for information that was helpful, the researchers determined how well these texts prepared students for end-of-life care. The nine domains were epidemiology, prognostic factors, disease progression, medical interventions that can change the course of a disease, advance care planning, mode of death, decision making, effect of death and dying on the patient's family, and symptom management.

In the scoring system, *Harrison's,* the most widely used text, failed, scoring 38%. The *Merck Manual* scored 36%, *Scientific American,* 42% and the *Washington Manual,* 11%. The researchers reported their findings to the textbook editors. Some recognized their shortfall and at least one, *Merck Manual,* immediately began asking chapter authors to include care of the dying patient. *Scientific American* also assigned it as a task for one of its associate editors.[23]

This study revealed that most textbooks do not provide the needed guidance to students for palliative care and its complexities. The foundation for change in the US health-care system is education. The lack of information in some of the most popular texts begs the question, where will the education come from? How can physicians and other health-care providers be considered comprehensively educated if they are not adequately trained to help break down these barriers and offer complete care to the individual regardless of culture or ethnicity?

Mistrust

Mistrust is a large barrier to optimal care for minority patients. Racism and injustice date back to the history of slavery. The reason for distrust was augmented by more recent experimentation, including the US Public Health Department–funded Tuskegee Study.[24] Older Hispanics report even less trust in physicians than African Americans.[2] Recruitment of minority participants into research projects is still hindered by the mistrust garnered many decades ago. African Americans often report feeling their physician has given them experimental treatment without their consent or would not tell them all the risks of participating in protocols known to be experimental. The frequently seen "do everything" mentality may stem from an inherent fear that refusal of the most aggressive care will result in no care at all. This situation is exacerbated by the fact that the majority of physicians are white.

The wariness may not be completely based on historical occurrences. Each encounter with the health-care system can weaken or strengthen the wall built by years of injustices. Racial bias exists among many clinicians. According to one survey of physicians, there were significant negative stereotypes about African American patients, including perceived higher rates of patients not adhering to physician recommendations and substance abuse as well as lower intelligence than whites.[25]

Communication

Good patient–clinician communication is essential for improved end-of-life care. Survivors associate communication with a better experience during the illness and death of a loved one. Open dialogue regarding patient desires for their own end-of-life care is the best way to ensure they receive the services they really want.

This can be difficult when the clinician and patient are from different ethnic and cultural backgrounds.[5] A patient's health is an intensely personal matter. It is imperative that patient and physician develop a personal relationship, and the development of this relationship is often lost in a hospital setting in the midst of treatment of one or more diseases. Failure to establish this relationship may lead to ineffective patient care and patients becoming "stuck" in the medical model. Physicians may neglect the patient's feelings about his or her disease or the treatment plan. In addition, patients may be depersonalized in the clinical setting, with reference being made to "that lady with the widely metastatic breast cancer" rather than the 65-year-old mother of four who is expecting her second grandchild in five months. This woman may want "everything done" to allow her the joy of seeing that grandchild. However, unless there is a therapeutic bond between patient and health-care provider, the patient is unlikely to state the reasons behind her request.

It is most important to treat the patient as well as the disease. Communication is the key to beginning that bond. However, many minorities do not feel comfortable allowing persons who are unlike them to know their inner thoughts and a barrier is set up, as illustrated by a recent case in an academic hospital in North Carolina.

> CS was a 52-year old African American woman who lived in an assisted living facility with her sister. She had end-stage renal disease, congestive heart failure, a seizure disorder, and an above-the-knee amputation. She was able to move independently through her facility in a wheelchair. She fell out of her wheelchair without losing consciousness or having a seizure but hit her neck. X-rays in the emergency department found a cervical stenosis with acute central cord compression. She was alert, conversant and only had complaint of upper extremity weakness. She was hospitalized and treated with steroids and close monitoring. Two days later she had an unwitnessed cardiac arrest. She was intubated, resuscitated, and placed in the intensive care unit, now unresponsive. She was never again able to communicate or follow commands, although after 2 months in the hospital she was able to open her eyes spontaneously. Her son, her closest relative, refused to discuss anything except the most aggressive care, including ventilator, hemodialysis, gastrostomy tube placement, and full resuscitation should she have another cardiac arrest. Although capable clinicians, the previous physicians had all been white. It was not until a minority physician talked with the son that he felt his concerns were understood. He, like many African Americans, felt that palliative care meant no care and that the health-care system was against him and his mother because of their background and ethnicity. After that conversation, he agreed to have her code status changed to DNR but refused withdrawal of care. With aggressive pulmonary toilet she was weaned off the ventilator and discharged to a nursing home after a 4-month hospitalization. However, 2 days later, on her way to dialysis, she had cardiopulmonary arrest and died. Her son had been unwilling or unable to see the need for aggressive palliation. She died without peace, and he did not have the opportunity to receive prolonged grief counseling, which hospice could have provided.

▶ ACCESS TO END-OF-LIFE CARE

Although hospice provides the palliation that many people want at the end of life, it is not available to all. In the British medical system, all terminally ill patients have access to hospice services. There is an acceptance of palliation throughout the course of a terminal disease. In the United States, the hospice benefit through Medicare limits access by requiring a primary care physician to certify the patient has

6 months or less to live. Establishing a prognosis is an imperfect science. Many physicians, even those who can recognize the transition from treat to palliate, have difficulty certifying the time frame. This becomes even more difficult when dealing with chronic illnesses, which invariably have frequent exacerbations and recoveries. Many are hesitant to refer patients to hospice in the face of this uncertainty. Access to hospice is limited because it is intimately tied to an insurance program. Hospice is covered by Medicare, Medicaid in some 43 states, or private insurance. Uninsured patients are often not able to benefit.

> EC was a 47-year-old Hispanic woman who moved from Mexico 2 years ago to be with her daughter. She worked hard as a domestic but had no health insurance. She developed progressive weakness in her lower extremities that led her to be wheelchair bound. An MRI of her cervical spine revealed demyelinating disease. Additional testing and history confirmed multiple sclerosis. Without insurance she could not afford the medicines recommended by the consulting neurologist. She presented again to an academic institution with infected pressure ulcers. These were treated aggressively with IV antibiotics and debridement of wounds. She was discharged to a nursing home to complete antibiotics and obtain wound care. Because of lack of personal finances, the hospital paid her bills while on IV antibiotics but once those were completed there were no funds available to continue care in the nursing home for wound care. She was discharged home to the care of her family, also without the assistance of home health care. She again returned to the hospital with multiple infected pressure ulcers, which were once more treated fully in the hospital. She was discharge home again with family but without services. She returned 1 month later with pneumonia and sepsis and died in the intensive care unit.

In this case, the patient was deprived of access to high-quality end-of-life care. In addition, she had no access to any type of in-home care, a problem that would be solved by a national health insurance program.

▶ CURRENT EFFORTS TO REMOVE BARRIERS

National Programs

Foundations have begun to support initiatives to improve end-of-life care in the United States. In 1998, the Robert Wood Johnson Foundation began a $12 million national program entitled "Promoting Excellence in End-of-Life Care." The goal is to help health-care institutions improve care provided to seriously ill and dying patients.[26] With this funding, hospitals and hospices have been able to determine the largest barriers to hospice referrals. These include the discomfort of many physicians and families in confronting end-of-life issues. Physicians often know very little about the services hospice can provide and, as noted earlier, the limit on Medicare hospice benefit has narrowed the use of hospice to the last 6 months of life, which is difficult to predict. The investigations undertaken also led to the recognition of enablers to effective hospice referrals. One such enabler is providing early outreach to patients with terminal diagnoses to allow for smoother transitions. Educating physicians about hospice services through continuing medical education (CME) programs and educating the community through local mass marketing can be enormous enablers.[27]

Last Acts is a national organization dedicated to improving end-of-life care. It is sponsored by a coalition of professional and consumer groups that believe in palliative care. Last Acts is focused on managing pain and making life better for individuals and families facing death. Coalitions developed across the country to address end-of-life issues often focus on minorities because of their low numbers in palliative care programs. Last Acts publishes *Diversity Notes* which focuses on differences in African American and Hispanic views regarding end of life to help community coalitions develop more culturally sensitive programs.[28]

Another nonprofit organization, Aging with Dignity, with the help of physicians, nurses, attorneys, and other end-of-life experts, has created Five Wishes, a tool to help patients address their personal, emotional, and spiritual needs regarding medical requests. It allows the person, through a checklist, to specify the following preferences:

1. The person I want to make care decisions for me when I cannot.
2. The kind of medical treatment I want or do not want.
3. How comfortable I want to be.
4. How I want people to treat me.
5. What I want my loved ones to know.

Five Wishes meets requirements for a living will in 35 states and helps patients communicate their desires to family and facilitate needed discussion with physicians.[29]

The Initiative to Improve Palliative and End of Life care in the African American community was formed to help create a society in which African American patients, their families, the physicians who treat them, and the community at large have knowledge and access to state-of-the-art palliative and hospice care through the elimination of racial and socioeconomic disparities.[30,31]

Community Initiatives

In addition to the national efforts, there are many local groups working to focus attention on disparities related to minorities and end-of-life care. The Duke Institute on Care at the End of Life began in 2000 with a grant from a former graduate of the Duke Divinity School. Its seven main goals are to (1) promote interdisciplinary scholarship and collaborative research, (2) advance education on end-of-life care, (3) provide practical training in palliative and bereavement care, (4) nurture traditional practices of compas-

sionate presence, (5) enhance public awareness of the opportunities and challenges at the end of life, (6) guide public policy toward improving services for the dying and their families, and (7) create partnerships with other universities and institutions, particularly those representing minority communities.[32]

The Harlem Palliative Care Network is a community initiative centered in the North General Hospital of New York that serves to improve care offered to dying patients. The consortium of community providers set as their objectives to (1) increase access to palliative care services for patients and their families, (2) overcome cultural and environmental barriers among minority populations, (3) enhance continuity and coordination of care, (4) improve quality of life through better pain and symptom management, and (5) provide support services to meet the spiritual and emotional needs of patients at the end of life and their families.[33]

Medical Education

Many medical students, residents, and practicing physicians recognize their paucity of knowledge regarding the foundations of quality end-of-life care. These areas include but are not limited to delivering bad news, recognizing emotional stress, discussing prognoses, and addressing advance care planning.[34–36] Medical schools are beginning to see the need to develop curricula specific to these issues. Senior medical students who have formal education in end-of-life care are more likely to feel prepared to address treatment of symptoms, psychosocial issues, and cultural and spiritual issues surrounding the dying process. Students without a dedicated curriculum but with some clinical experiences in palliative care are also more likely to feel prepared to discuss these issues.[37]

Practicing physicians may gain education on the essential clinical competencies required to provide quality end-of-life care through the EPEC Project (Education for Physicians on End-of-life Care). EPEC was developed by the

American Medical Association, funded by a grant from The Robert Wood Johnson Foundation.[38] The American Association of Colleges of Nursing has developed ELNEC (End-of-Life Nursing Education Consortium), with a primary goal of coordinating national nursing education efforts in end-of-life care.[39] The module on cultural considerations delivers the three key messages that (1) culturally sensitive care encompasses recognition of multiple factors including ethnicity, gender, sexual orientation, and social class; (2) cultural factors significantly influence communication with patients and families; and (3) culturally appropriate care is best provided through an interdisciplinary approach. The objective is for each participant to be able to identify the influence culture has on end-of-life care and conduct a cultural assessment of patients facing the end of life.[40]

▶ FURTHER ACTION

Spiritual Assessment

Spirituality, or those things affecting the soul, is a strong determinant of decision making for many minority cultures. Spirituality may or may not involve a particular religion but can be a very vital component of a comprehensive approach to end-of-life issues. Religious practices or rituals may need to be performed for the patient and family to feel at peace, placing the chaplain or minister in a position of extreme importance in the health-care team. To assess a patient's spiritual beliefs, one expert has devised a helpful mnemonic, FICA, which stands for faith, influence, community, address.

- **Faith**. What is your faith or belief? Do you consider yourself a spiritual or a religious person? Does religious faith or spirituality play an important part in your life? What do you feel gives your life meaning?
- **Influence.** How does your religious faith or spirituality influence your thoughts about

health? How does it affect the way that you take care of yourself?
- **Community.** Do you consider yourself part of a spiritual or a religious community or congregation? How is that community or congregation a source of support for you?
- **Address.** Do you have any religious or spiritual issues or concerns that you would like me to address with you? Is there someone else you would like to speak with about these matters?[41]

Cultural Competency

Only by knowing a patient's cultural background and accompanying spiritual needs can clinicians hope to understand the patient's specific expectations regarding care in general and at end of life. Health-care providers must first be aware of their own perspective, and self-assessment can be of use. One example is the Cultural Self-Assessment Tool, which asks the clinician to examine questions such as, "Where were your grandparents born," "What are the gender issues in your culture and in your family structure," and "What are your customs and beliefs around such transitions as birth, illness, and death?"[41] The Cultural Knowledge Beliefs preassessment developed by the Oncology Nursing Society asks respondents to rank the most common resources they use to learn about people from other cultural groups, including television, radio, movies, or ongoing personal relationships. It also asks why the participant is reluctant to or does not interact with people from other cultural groups. Responses include fear of rejection, lack of interest, nothing in common, or not knowing where to meet them.[40] Once cultural sensitivity, which requires awareness of how culture shapes patients' values, beliefs, and world views, is developed, the clinician must acknowledge that differences exist and respect them. Clinicians must then develop cultural competency, which requires skills of communication, including use of an interpreter if necessary, and attention to nonverbal communication.

Cultural competence is not only a moral obligation, it is a legal mandate. In December 2000, the Office of Minority Health of the Department of Health and Human Services created national standards for culturally appropriate health services.[42] These standards include knowledge that mainstream Western ideas of patient autonomy are often not relevant in the Hispanic community (because the matriarch of the family is responsible for the health-care decisions of her family and decisions are often made by the extended family), and that African Americans are often unwilling to speak of advance directives (because they feel that planning for something will make it happen). Understanding these concepts will help the health-care provider communicate better with patients.[43]

Research

Without question, more research is needed to describe and analyze demographics, prevalence of symptoms, and morbidity of minority elders at the end of life. There must be research into patient–provider relationships and how to encourage better communication. Decreasing patient distrust of the medical system is one way to open communication, but this will require improving access and decreasing institutional racism.

▶ CONCLUSION

Care for aged patients at the end of life (see Fig. 6-1) should be taught as thoroughly as care for patients at the beginning of life. Health-care

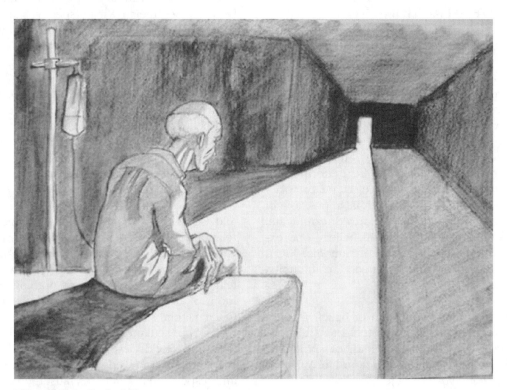

Figure 6–1. End of life.

providers and patient advocates must be taught cultural sensitivity during the introduction to patient–client care, always keeping in mind that each person should be treated as an individual. Only through these measures can the barriers hindering good-quality end-of-life care be eliminated.

► ACKNOWLEDGMENTS

The authors wish to thank Richard Stephenson, MD, medical director of Forsyth County Hospice and Palliative Care, for his encouragement and advice.

► REFERENCES

1. Dept of Health and Human Services, Administration on Aging. *A Profile of Older Americans.* Available at: http://www.aoa.gov.
2. Krakauer EL, Crenner C, Fox K. Barriers to optimum end-of-life care for minority patients. *J Am Geriatr Soc* 2002;50(1):182–190.
3. Bird CE, Shugarman LR, Lynn J. Age and gender differences in health care utilization and spending for Medicare beneficiaries in their last years of life. *J Palliat Med* 2002;5(5):705–712.
4. Carver R. My Death. In: Reynolds R, Stone J, eds. *On Doctoring.* New York, NY: Simon and Schuster; 1991:368.
5. Patrick DL, Curtis JR, Engelberg RA, et al. Measuring and improving the quality of dying and death. *Ann Intern Med* 2003;139(5Pt2):410–415.
6. Steinhauser KE, Clipp EC, McNeilly M, et al. In Search of a good death: Observations of patients, families, and providers. *Ann Intern Med* 2000; 132(10):825–832.
7. Singer PA, Martin DM, Kelner M. Quality end-of-life care: Patients' perspectives. *JAMA* 1999; 281(2):163–168.
8. World Health Organization. Cancer pain relief and palliative care. *WHO Technical Report Series* 1990;804:1–75.
9. National Hospital and Palliative Care Organization. *History of Hospice Care.* 2004. Available at: http://www.nho.org.
10. Baer WM, Hanson LC. Families' perception of the added value of hospice in the nursing home. *J Am Geriatr Soc* 2000;48(8):879–882.
11. Kaplan KO. Women of color and end-of-life care. *Am J Public Health* 2002;92(9):1386–1387.
12. Crawley L, Payne R, Bolden J, et al. Palliative and end-of-life care in the African American Community. *JAMA* 2000;284(19):2518–2521.
13. O'Mara AM, Arenella C. Minority representation, prevalence of symptoms, and utilization of services in a large metropolitan hospice. *J Pain Symptom Manage* 2001;21(4):290–297.
14. Romero LJ, Linderman RD, Koehler KM, et al. Influence of ethnicity on advance directives and end-of-life decisions. *JAMA* 1997;277(4):298–299.
15. Phipps E, True G, Harris D, et al. Approaching the end of life: Attitudes, preference, and behaviors of African-American and white patients and family caregivers. *J Clin Oncol* 2003;21(3):549–554.
16. Morrison RS, Wallenstein S, Natale DK, et al. We don't carry that—Failure of pharmacies in predominantly nonwhite neighborhoods to stock opioid analgesics. *N Engl J Med* 2000;342(14): 1023–1026.
17. Freeman HP, Payne R. Racial injustice in health care. *N Engl J Med* 2000;342(14):1045–1047.
18. Blackhall LJ, Frank G, Murphy ST, et al. Ethnicity and attitudes towards life sustaining technology. *Soc Sci Med* 1999;48(12):1779–1789.
19. Blackhall LJ, Murphy ST, Gelya F, et al. Ethnicity and attitudes toward patient autonomy. *JAMA* 1995;274(10):820–825.
20. Mebane EW, Oman RF, Kroonen LT, et al. The influence of physician race, age, and gender on physician attitudes toward advance care directives and preferences for end-of-life decision-making. *J Am Geriatr Soc* 1999;47(5):579–591.
21. Weissman DE. Talking about dying: A clash of cultures. *J Palliat Med* 2000;3(2):145–147.
22. Sullivan AM, Lakoma MD, Block SD. The status of medical education in end-of-life care. *J Gen Intern Med* 2003;18(9):685–695.
23. Carron AT, Lynn J, Keaney P. End-of-life care in medical textbooks. *Ann Intern Med* 1999;130(1): 82–86.
24. Corbie-Smith G, Thomas SB, St George DM. Distrust, race, and research. *Arch Intern Med* 2002;162(21):2458–2463.
25. Crawley LM. Palliative care in African American communities. *J Palliat Med* 2002;5(5):775–779.

26. *Promoting Excellence in End-of-Life Care.* 2004. Available at: http://www.promotingexcellence. org.

27. Friedman BT, Harwood MK, Shields M. Barriers and enablers to hospice referrals: An expert overview. *J Palliat Med* 2002;5(1):73–84.

28. *Rallying Points. Improving Community End-of-Life Care through Coalitions.* 2004. Available at: http://www.lastacts.org.

29. Aging with Dignity. *Five Wishes Tool.* 2004. Available at: http//www.agingwithdignity.org.

30. *Initiative to Improve Palliative Care for African-Americans.* 2004. Available at: http://www.iipca. org.

31. Crawley LM, Marshall PA, Lo B, et al. Strategies for culturally effective end-of-life care. *Ann Intern Med* 2002;136(9):673–677.

32. Duke Institute on Care at the End of Life. 2004. Available at: http://www.iceol.duke.edu.

33. Payne R, Payne TR. The Harlem palliative care network. *J Palliat Med* 2002;5(5):781–792.

34. Haq C, Steele DJ, Marchand L, et al. Integrating the art and science of medical practice: Innovations in teaching medical communication skills. *Fam Med* 2004;36 Suppl:S43–S50.

35. Ury WA, Berkman CS, Weber CM, et al. Assessing medical students' training in end-of-life communication: A survey of interns at one urban teaching hospital. *Acad Med* 2003;78(5):530–537.

36. Bradley EH, Cramer LD, Bogardus ST, et al. Physicians' ratings of their knowledge, attitudes, and end-of-life-care practices. *Acad Med* 2002;77(4):305–311.

37. Fraser HC, Kutner JS, Pfeifer MP. Senior medical students' perceptions of the adequacy of education on end-of-life issues. *J Palliat Med* 2001;4(3): 337–343.

38. American Medical Association. *The EPEC Project.* 2004. Available at: http//www.ama-assn.org.

39. American Association of Colleges of Nursing. *ELNEC Project.* 2004. Available at: http//www.aacn. nche.edu.

40. Matzo ML, Sherman DW, Mazanec P, et al. Teaching cultural consideration at the end of life: End of Life Nursing Education Consortium program recommendations. *J Contin Educ Nurs* 2002;33(6):270–278.

41. Mazanec P, Tyler MK. Cultural considerations in end-of-life care: How ethnicity, age and spirituality affect decisions when death is imminent. *Am J Nurs* 2003;103(3):50–58.

42. Office of Minority Health. Standards for Culturally and Linguistically Appropriate Health Care Services. Available at: www.omhrc.gov/clas/

43. Kagawa-Singer M, Blackhall LJ. Negotiating cross-cultural issues at the end of life: "You got to go where he lives." *JAMA* 2001;286(23):2993–3001.

SECTION II

---

*The Disparate Burden
of Disease*

CHAPTER 7

Cardiovascular Disease and Hypertension

CHARLOTTE JONES-BURTON, MD
ELIJAH SAUNDERS, MD, FACC, FACP

▶ INTRODUCTION

African Americans and other ethnic minorities are disproportionately represented among persons with lower education, lower socioeconomic status (SES), and medical diseases. In 1996, approximately 20% of African Americans and 40% of Hispanics had fewer than 12 years of schooling, compared with less than 10% of Caucasians. In addition, approximately 40% of African American and Hispanic children younger than 18 years of age live below the poverty line.[1] Income level is closely associated with educational attainment, and these statistics reflect the inequalities in SES and education. These inequalities are undoubtedly related to the health disparities that exist in the United States. Higher education and income status afford opportunities for individuals to live in safe neighborhoods, access medical care on a regular basis, and engage in eating and lifestyle behaviors that promote wellness. More importantly, SES has been linked to cardiovascular risk factors[2] and has been found to be a predictor of coronary disease mortality.[3]

▶ RACIAL DISPARITIES IN HEALTH

There are significant racial disparities in the incidence of most diseases, including hypertension, renal disease, and cardiovascular diseases. Even when the incidence of disease is lower in African Americans (eg, breast cancer), the morbidity and mortality is higher in African Americans. Since 1932, it has been evident in medical literature that there is a difference in blood pressure among blacks and whites in the United States.[4] Today, hypertension is a common disease worldwide. The prevalence of hypertension in the United States in people 18 years old or older is approximately 29%, affecting more than 58 million individuals.[5] African Americans are disproportionately represented in this number. Even though African Americans constitute approximately 12% of the US population, 33.5% have hypertension compared with 28.9% of non-Hispanic whites.[5] This disparity in hypertension begins after puberty and persists into adult life. The greatest racial difference is seen among those aged 40 through 59 years: 50% of blacks in this age group are hypertensive compared with 30% of whites.[6]

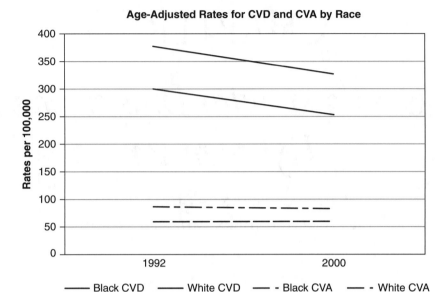

Figure 7–1. Age-adjusted rates in African Americans and Caucasians for cardiovascular and cerebrovascular diseases. (CVA, cerebrovascular accident; CVD, cardiovascular disease.) (*Based on information in Saunders E, ed. Racial Differences in Cardiovascular Health. Pfizer Facts; 2003.*)

By age 65, as many as 75% of African American women are hypertensive, compared with approximately 50% of Caucasian women in the same age group.

Not only is hypertension precocious in African Americans, the disease is more severe and results in more target organ damage.[7] More importantly, the morbidity and mortality associated with hypertension from stroke, kidney disease, and heart disease affect African Americans disproportionately. In the 1990s, heart disease and stroke death rates declined in both Caucasians and African Americans, but age-adjusted rates for African Americans remained higher (Fig. 7–1). Specifically, age-adjusted heart disease and stroke death rates are 29% and 40% higher in African Americans, respectively.[6] Hypertension in African Americans leads to an 80% higher stroke mortality rate, a 50% higher heart disease mortality rate, and a 32% higher rate of hypertension-related end-stage renal dis-

ease (ESRD) than the general population.[8] In 1950, the cardiovascular disease mortality rate was 1.6 times higher for African Americans than Caucasians.[9] Even when the general population has exhibited a decline in mortality, the rate of decline in African Americans is consistently lower than the decline in Caucasians.[10] Therefore, it is not surprising that in 1995, the cardiovascular disease mortality rate for African Americans remained the same as it was in 1950.

Medical literature has documented the existence of racial disparities in health care for cardiovascular diseases (ie, ischemic heart disease and congestive heart failure). Superficially, this is thought to be a result of limitations in access to medical care for African Americans. However, even when access to care is not an issue, such as in Department of Veterans Affairs hospitals, physicians are less likely to refer African American patients for cardiac catheterization,[11] and African Americans are less likely to undergo

invasive cardiac procedures.[12] Additionally, it has been shown that among Medicare patients enrolled in managed health care plans, blacks were less likely than whites to receive β-blockers after myocardial infarction, a known standard of care.[13]

It has been well documented that African Americans are less likely to receive invasive cardiovascular procedures, even after controlling for health insurance.[14] Even though the rate of percutaneous transluminal coronary angioplasty in US blacks has doubled since 1992, African Americans are still less likely to receive this procedure (248 procedures per 1000 circulatory system discharges compared with 396 per 1000 discharges for Caucasians).[6] Similarly, blacks are half as likely to undergo coronary artery bypass graft than whites, 40 and 81 per 1000 hospital discharges, respectively.[6] Among those with inducible arrhythmias, blacks are less likely to receive implantable cardioverter-defibrillators than whites.[15]

The inequalities in access to health care suggest that racial discrimination influences the type of health care received by African Americans. The impact of racism—defined as "an organized system, rooted in an ideology of inferiority, that categorizes, ranks, and differentially allocates societal resources to human population groups"[10]—on African Americans in the United States is difficult to assess in clinical studies. To date, the Jackson Heart Study is the only study designed to focus on racial disparity in cardiovascular disease. This prospective study, currently ongoing, includes approximately 6000 African Americans, aged 35 to 84 years, from Jackson, Mississippi. It is the largest study of its type of African Americans in the United States[16] and has been called by some the "Black Framingham Heart Study."

Genetics and Pathophysiology

For at least the past half century, the observation that blacks in the United States experience higher levels of blood pressure than whites[17] spawned the doctrine that blacks and whites are fundamentally distinct, biologically and physiologically. Research has attempted to characterize blacks as biologically inferior, and thus more prone to illness.[18] Titles of articles in peer-reviewed literature perpetuate this notion of innate distinction and inferiority; for example, "The pathogenesis of hypertension: Black–white differences,"[19] and "Hypertension in African-Americans: A paradigm of metabolic disarray."[20] Likewise, statements have been made without factual basis, equating racial disparity with increased virulence. Even though several hypotheses have been generated regarding the racial differences that exist between African Americans and Caucasian Americans, there remains a paucity of evidence supporting a unique pathophysiology for the occurrence of hypertension in African Americans.

One frequently cited explanation for the increased rate of hypertension in African Americans is based on the voyage from Africa to America on slave ships (the so-called Middle Passage). Grim and others have speculated that during these arduous trips, the slaves were placed in a Darwinian situation of "survival of the fittest," in which survival depended on "high-sodium-retaining" genes.[19] Once an individual with these genes assumed a lifestyle in an environment in which sodium was plentiful (acculturation), the hypothesis suggests, the risk of hypertension escalated. This theory is problematic and controversial.[21]

Another explanation espouses the significant differences in sodium handling between blacks and whites. Studies demonstrate that African Americans have increased sodium sensitivity, retaining more sodium than whites and exhibiting a greater rise in blood pressure.[19] Although many hypertensive African Americans have normal to high circulating renin activity, as a group, they are more likely to manifest suppressed circulating renin activity than hypertensive Caucasians. However, this does not prove a genetic basis. In fact, this could be the result of a secondary effect on the kidneys, caused by prolonged exposure to elevated blood pressure that has been unrecognized, untreated, or undertreated. If this is the norm in African American families, then certainly this pattern could be passed on through generations.

The pursuit for a specific genetic mutation to explain the racial differences in hypertension is ongoing. Various genes, including renin, angiotensinogen, angiotensin-converting enzyme (ACE), and kallikrein, have been studied,[22] but this area of study has been plagued by small study samples. One exciting area of genetic interest involves the epithelial sodium channel (ENaC) located in the cortical collecting duct of the kidney. This channel is involved in sodium reabsorption, and a gain of function mutation in this channel leads to increased sodium reabsorption, increased effective circulating blood volume, and salt-sensitive, low-renin hypertension. Polymorphisms of this channel have been identified, and one allele has been found to be present in approximately 6% of individuals of African origin, but not in white populations.[23] Changes in the sympathetic nervous system, the adrenocorticotropic hormone–cortisol axis, and vascular reactivity, particularly endothelial function, have also been examined.[23]

Despite the various hypotheses, hypertension is likely the result of a complex interplay of genetics and pathophysiology, such as differences in excretion of sodium and potassium, environment (particularly diet and stress), and demographic factors, especially, age, race or ethnicity, and geographic location.

Target Organ Damage

There is a strong and independent relationship between elevated blood pressure and congestive heart failure (CHF),[24] coronary heart disease (CHD), stroke, and kidney disease.[25] Pooled information from nearly 400,000 adults in nine observational studies reveals a five times higher risk of CHD and 10 times higher risk of stroke

in individuals with a diastolic blood pressure of 105 mm Hg versus those with a diastolic blood pressure of 74 mm Hg.[26] Numerous studies have clarified the role of hypertension in the racial disparity of prevalence and death rates for cardiovascular disease, CHF, stroke, and ESRD.[27]

Congestive Heart Failure and Hypertension in African Americans

CHF is twice as common in hypertensive as in normotensive individuals.[28] The development of left ventricular hypertrophy is proportional to the elevation in blood pressure. A 20 mm Hg increase in systolic blood pressure increases the relative risk of left ventricular hypertrophy by 43% in men and 25% in women.[29] It is not surprising that hypertension in African Americans contributes to the increased incidence of left ventricular hypertrophy and CHF in this racial group. Even though the overall prevalence of CHF is similar for African Americans and Caucasians,[6] African Americans with left ventricular hypertrophy have a greater risk, 30% to 50% higher, for hospitalization[14] and mortality that is 2.5 times higher than Caucasians.[14] In a cohort of African Americans with essential hypertension and the absence of angiographic coronary artery disease, left ventricular hypertrophy was found to be a powerful, independent predictor of cardiovascular morbidity and mortality. Furthermore, cardiovascular mortality from left ventricular hypertrophy was twice as likely in women as in men.[30] In 1999, the age-adjusted death rates for cardiomyopathy were approximately twice as high in African Americans as in Caucasians.[31] Hypertension is the most common cause of cardiomyopathy in African Americans. It is often associated with left ventricular diastolic dysfunction, which can lead to heart failure with normal systolic function.

Not only is left ventricular hypertrophy a risk factor for CHD and cardiovascular mortality, it is also an independent risk factor for ischemic stroke in all age, sex, and racial or ethnic groups.[32,33] Specifically, concentric hypertrophy has been found to be associated with a 2.5-fold increase in ischemic stroke after adjustment of other risk factors for stroke.[34] Additionally, left ventricular hypertrophy appears to predispose individuals to arrhythmias, and it is known that sudden death is more prevalent in African Americans than in Caucasians.[15,35]

Coronary Heart Disease and Hypertension in African Americans

Thirteen million Americans have coronary artery disease (CAD).[31] More than 1 million people experience a myocardial infarction (MI) each year. In NHANES 1999–2000, the prevalence of MI among Caucasians was greater than in African Americans, approximately 4% and 2.25%, respectively.[6] MI is the leading cause of all deaths in both African Americans and Caucasians.[31] Even though the age-adjusted death rate for CHD decreased by 20% for the total population from 1987 to 1995, the decrease was only 13% for African Americans.[36] Thus, African Americans still experience the highest death rates from heart disease of any racial or ethnic group in industrialized countries.[37] Compared with Caucasians, who had an age-adjusted death rate from heart disease of 253.6 per 100,000, African Americans die from heart disease at an alarming 326.5 per 100,000.[6]

Aside from the contribution that differences in risk factors, time to presentation and access to medical care prior to MI, and SES contribute to this obvious racial disparity, the pathogenesis of CAD in African Americans remains unclear. It is unknown whether significant biologic differences exist. One hypothesis focuses on abnormalities in coronary endothelial function and vasoactivity on the basis of race.[38,39] It has been shown that African Americans with left ventricular hypertrophy experience a blunted response to acetyl-choline, a nitric oxide–dependent vasodilator, compared with Caucasians with similar left-ventricular hypertrophy. Furthermore, augmentation of coronary blood flow was shown to be significantly depressed in African Americans as compared with Caucasians with left ventricular hypertrophy.[38]

Psychosocial stress increases the development of atherosclerosis.[40] Anger has been linked to cardiovascular disease, including hypertension and CAD.[41] The experience of anger is particularly relevant to blacks in the United States, a society built on institutionalized racism. In 1995, a study published by the Federal Glass Ceiling Commission found that African Americans earn 21% less than Caucasians in the same jobs.[42] This suggests that skin color continues to be the vehicle used to allocate African Americans to lower SES, an unjust appointment that predicates health disparities.

Cerebrovascular Accidents and Hypertension in African Americans

Stroke is the third leading cause of death in the US population, accounting for approximately 7% of all deaths in the United States in 2000.[43] The age-adjusted prevalence of stroke for Americans is higher in both African American men and women than in white American men and women (Fig. 7–2). African Americans possess a disproportionate burden of the risk factors for stroke and stroke mortality. This racial disparity is multifactorial, but strongly correlated to the increased prevalence of other cardiovascular disease risk factors—diabetes and hypertension in African Americans. Another factor that may contribute to this epidemic in blacks in addition to greater severity of risk factors is lack of access to care.[34]

There are racial differences in the subtypes of stroke. In particular, African Americans have a higher incidence of cerebral infarction, subarachnoid hemorrhage, and intracerebral hemorrhage.[34] Similarly, different subtypes of

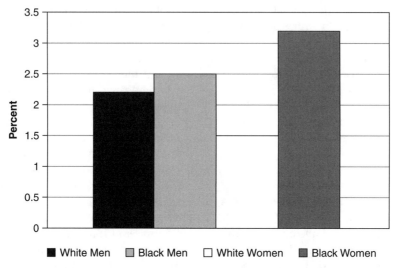

Figure 7–2. Age-adjusted prevalence of stroke by race and gender in the United States. (*Based on information in Saunders E, ed. Racial Differences in Cardiovascular Health. Pfizer Facts; 2003*).

ischemic stroke may occur in African Americans, namely, lacunar infarcts and large artery intracranial occlusive disease.[34] These racial disparities in subtypes of stroke are greatest at younger ages. Young African Americans have a two- to threefold greater risk of ischemic stroke than their white counterparts and are more likely to die as a result of stroke.[44] In fact, in 2000, stroke mortality was higher in blacks than in whites at all ages.[31]

Kidney Disease and Hypertension in African Americans

African Americans suffer from kidney disease in disproportionate numbers to Caucasians. Previous studies have suggested that the higher prevalence of kidney disease is linked to the higher prevalence of hypertension in this population.[45] Indeed, African Americans have the highest rate of hypertension-related ESRD of any other racial or ethnic group (five times higher than in Caucasians).[46] In addition, African Americans have a higher rate of diabetes-related ESRD, second only to Native

Americans. Over the past decade, the overall incidence of ESRD has steadily increased, and the racial disparity related to this disease has persisted.[47] Although African Americans comprise approximately 12% of the US population, they represent 31% of patients with ESRD.[48] African American males aged 25 to 44 years of age are 20 times more likely to develop ESRD as a result of elevated blood pressure than are white males in the same age group.[49] Additionally, African Americans with ESRD on the average are younger than Caucasians, with the median ages for each group 59.4 and 67.1, respectively.[50]

A recent data analysis of the National Health and Nutrition Examination Surveys III (NHANES III) and the United States Renal Data System (USRDS) did not find a higher prevalence of chronic renal insufficiency (defined as a glomerular filtration rate from 15 to 59 mL/min per 1.73 m^2) in African Americans as compared with Caucasians.[51] This leads to speculation that African Americans have an increased susceptibility to ESRD compared with Caucasians. In fact, even when similar levels of blood pressure control occur, renal function in African Americans has been shown to decline five times faster than in non-African Americans.[52] The cause of this rapid progression to ESRD is likely multifactorial, including the higher prevalence of renovascular disease, decreased use of "renoprotective" agents, and higher prevalence of obesity in African Americans. Other factors that contribute to this rapid demise include lower SES and education, leading to suboptimal medical care, cultural aspects (delaying presentation to the health system, health care beliefs), and environmental exposures, such as illicit drug use.[53,54]

Although causation is difficult to identify, it is clear that risk factors for and incidence of cardiovascular disease are higher in patients with kidney disease. The Heart Outcomes Prevention Evaluation (HOPE) study revealed that patients with microalbuminuria, a marker of kidney disease, had a 61% increased risk of MI, stroke, and death from cardiovascular causes.[55] In fact, patients with kidney disease are more likely to die of cardiovascular disease than of kidney failure.[56] In a group of dialysis patients, mortality related to cardiovascular disease was 10 to 30 times higher than in the general population.[57] This increased burden of cardiovascular disease in patients with kidney disease is a result of multiple factors, including anemia,[58] impaired vasculature,[59] increased inflammation,[60] and increased oxidative stresses[61] in this population. Although many patients with kidney disease have multiple cardiovascular risk factors, it is important to note that the presence of chronic kidney disease is an independent risk factor for cardiovascular disease.[63]

Treatment of Hypertension in African Americans

The rates of cardiovascular mortality have declined over the past decade.[6] Undoubtedly, better hypertension control has contributed to this decline in mortality. Awareness of hypertension remains high, as well. Specifically, among African Americans aged 40 years and over, 71% to 83% reported awareness of hypertension. In this group, a majority reported that their hypertension was being treated (83% to 97%). Despite the high awareness and treatment of this disease, it is astounding that a minority of African Americans receiving treatment achieve blood pressures below 140/90 mm Hg, only 31% of all hypertensive patients meet this criteria[63] and 25% of African American hypertensive patients.[64] In other words, despite increased knowledge regarding hypertension and therapeutic agents to treat hypertension, adequate blood pressure control remains the exception, not the rule.

The seventh report of the Joint National Committee on Prevention, Detection, Evaluation, and Treatment of High Blood Pressure (JNC 7) revised the classification of hypertension[65] (Table 7–1). Because African Americans develop a more severe hypertension, and do so earlier, the identification of "prehypertensive" should identify a larger group of patients to enable more aggressive targeting prior to the onset of hypertension. JNC 7 recommends a goal of blood pressure lower than 140/90 mm Hg and lower than 130/80 mm Hg in patients with diabetes and chronic kidney disease.

Until recently, clinical trials have not included large numbers of African American patients to test hypotheses regarding therapeutic regimens for hypertension. Two landmark

► **TABLE 7–1.** JNC 7 Classification of Blood Pressure[65]

Classification	Systolic BP (mm Hg)	Diastolic BP (mm Hg)
Normal	< 120	< 80
Prehypertension	120–139	80–89
Stage 1 hypertension	140–159	90–99
Stage 2 hypertension	> 160	> 100

BP, blood pressure; JNC 7, seventh report of the Joint National Committee on Prevention, Detection, Evaluation, and Treatment of High Blood Pressure.

trials, African American Study of Kidney Disease and Hypertension (AASK)[66] and Antihypertensive and Lipid-Lowering Treatment to Prevent Heart Attack Trial (ALLHAT)[67] have provided insight into the management of African Americans with hypertension.

AASK, a randomized, double-blind trial, was designed to evaluate two different blood pressure goals (strict, 125/75 mm Hg, and usual, 140/90 mm Hg) and three different antihypertensives as first-step agents (a dihydropyridine calcium channel blocker, amlodipine; an ACE inhibitor, ramipril; and a β-blocker, metoprolol) on the progression of hypertensive kidney disease in African Americans.[66] This trial enrolled 1094 African Americans and is the first trial with significant power to evaluate the effects of inhibition of the renin-angiotensin-aldosterone system in African Americans. For patients with proteinuria, data revealed that the decline in glomerular filtration rate, the primary outcome, was 36% slower in the ramipril group compared with the amlodipine group over 3 years. There was a similar decline in glomerular filtration rate in the metoprolol group. However, unique to the ramipril group was a statistically significant risk reduction in secondary outcomes (a decline in glomerular filtration rate, ESRD, or death) and less proteinuria. Blood pressure was considerably lower during the follow-up period than at baseline in a large percentage of participants (78.9%), but there was no statistically significant difference in blood pressure between the treatment groups (of note, additional agents were added in a stepwise approach to achieve blood pressure goals with furosemide, used in the majority of participants).

Additionally, the observed benefits occurred at similar blood pressure levels. These data support the initial use of an ACE inhibitor in African Americans with hypertensive kidney disease, despite the degree of albuminuria. This represents a paradigm shift from limited use of ACE inhibitors in African Americans (because of the lower potency in blood pressure reduction when used as monotherapy) to an essential use of ACE inhibitors in these patients be-

▶ **TABLE 7–2.** Lessons Learned From AASK

- African American hypertensive patients with mild renal insufficiency can attain the usual BP goal (< 140/90 mm Hg)
- Multidrug therapy is often need to achieve usual BP goal (including a diuretic)
- In African American hypertensive patients with mild renal insufficiency, an ACE-inhibitor-based regimen was as effective in achieving BP targets as a dihydropyridine calcium-channel-blocker–based regimen
- In African American hypertensive patients with mild renal insufficiency and proteinuria > 300 mg/d, an ACE-inhibitor based regimen provided more renal protection than a dihydropyridine patients based regimen

AASK, African American Study of Kidney Disease and Hypertension; ACE, angiotension-converting enzyme; BP, blood pressure.

cause of additional benefits other than blood pressure reduction. Perhaps the most important lesson learned from the AASK trial is that African Americans can achieve target blood pressure goals through persistent and intense treatment Table 7–2).

ALLHAT, the largest antihypertensive treatment trial to date, enrolled approximately 15,000 African Americans (35% of the total study group).[67] Patients were randomly assigned to initial therapy with four antihypertensive medications: a diuretic, chlorthalidone; an ACE inhibitor, lisinopril; an α-blocker, doxazosin; and a dihydropyridine calcium channel blocker, amlodipine. The doxazosin arm of the trial was terminated early after patients in this arm developed CHF at a greater rate than did the patients treated with chlorthalidone. There was no significant difference observed in the remaining three drugs in preventing the primary outcome of the trial, major coronary events, or in their effect on overall survival. However, chlorthalidone was superior to lisinopril in lowering blood pressure and in preventing aggregate cardiovascular disease, including stroke and CHF.

▶ **TABLE 7–3.** Average Number of Antihypertensive Agents Used to Achieve Target Blood Pressure in Four Randomized, Controlled Trials

	MDRD	ABCD	HOT	UKPDS
Goal BP (mm Hg)	MAP < 92	DBP < 75	DBP < 80	DBP < 85
Average number of drugs per patient	3.6	2.7	3.3	2.8

ABCD, Appropriate Blood Pressure Control in Diabetes trial; DBP, diastolic blood pressure; HOT, Hypertension Optimal Treatment; MAP, mean arterial pressure; MDRD, Modification of Diet in Renal Disease Study; UKPDS, UK Prospective Diabetes Study Group.

Note: The goal MAP of < 92 mm Hg specified in the MDRD trial corresponds to a systolic/diastolic blood pressure of approximately 125/75 mm Hg.

Adapted from Lea JP, Brown DT, Lipkowitz M, et al. Preventing renal dysfunction in patients with hypertension: Clinical implications for the early AASK trial results. Am J Cardiovasc Drugs 2003; 3(3):193–200.

As well, chlorthalidone was superior to amlodipine in preventing CHF. In African American patients, the data revealed a greater reduction in systolic blood pressure (4 mm Hg) that was more favorable for chlorthalidone than for lisinopril. As well, this greater reduction in systolic blood pressure appears to account for the decrease in stroke risk observed only in African American patients (RR 1.40, 95% CI 1.17–1.68).[68] Based on these results, the authors concluded that thiazide diuretics are superior in preventing one or more major forms of cardiovascular disease and should be the preferred agent for first-step antihypertensive therapy. However, it should not be overlooked that a majority of patients in ALLHAT, and other major clinical trials[69] (Table 7–3), require multiple agents to lower blood pressure. In other words, monotherapy is usually insufficient to treat hypertension, particularly in African Americans (Table 7–4).

In light of these clinical data and other trials, the Hypertension in African Americans Working (HAAW) Group of the International Society on Hypertension in Blacks (ISHIB) published an evidence-based consensus statement regarding the management of high blood pressure in African Americans[70] (Fig. 7–3). This evidence-based approach is a marked departure from the traditional "stepwise" approach of starting with a drug and titrating up. For the first time, dual therapy was recommended as initial treatment for patients with markedly elevated blood pressure (systolic blood pressure ≥15 mm Hg or diastolic blood pressure ≥10 mm Hg above their target). JNC 7,[65] published shortly afterward, supports a similar approach for all patients with hypertension. It is also of note that in the HAAW/ISHIB document, it was suggested that among the highest risk patients (diabetes, kidney disease) with blood pressures above 145/90 mm Hg, combination therapy should be instituted with a drug that blocks the renin-angiotensin-aldosterone system.

▶ **TABLE 7–4.** Lessons Learned From ALLHAT

- African Americans have a greater benefit in systolic blood pressure reduction (4 mm Hg) with the use of a thiazide-like diuretic than an ACE inhibitor.
- African Americans have a greater reduction in stroke with the use of a thiazide-like diuretic.
- African Americans have a greater reduction in heart failure with the use of a thiazide-like diuretic.
- Thiazide-like diuretics should be a part of every therapeutic regimen to control BP in African Americans, unless contraindicated.
- Multidrug therapy is often needed to achieve usual BP goal (< 140/90 mm Hg).

ALLHAT, Antihypertensive and Lipid-Lowering Treatment to Prevent Heart Attack Trial; ACE, angiotension-converting enzyme; BP, blood pressure.

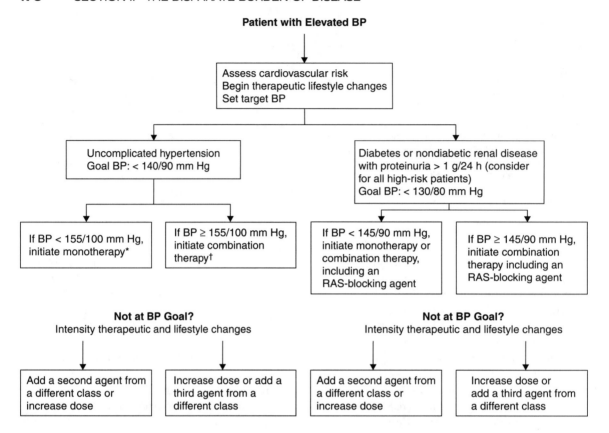

Figure 7–3. Clinical algorithm for achieving target BP in African American patients with high blood pressure (BP). (*) Indicates to initiate monotherapy at the recommended starting dose with an agent from any of the following classes: diuretics, β-blockers, calcium channel blockers, angiotensin-converting enzyme (ACE) inhibitors, or angiotensin receptor blockers (ARBs). (†) Indicates to initiate low-dose combination therapy with any of the following combinations: β-blocker and diuretic, ACE inhibitor and diuretic, ACE inhibitor and calcium channel blocker, or ARB and diuretic. (RAS, renin-angiotensin-aldosterone system.) (*Reprinted with permission from Douglas JG, Bakris GL, Murray-Epstein M, et al. Management of high blood pressure in African Americans: Consensus statement of the hypertension in African Americans working group of the International Society on hypertension in Blacks. Arch Intern Med 2003;163(5):525–541*).

► CLOSING THE RACIAL GAP IN HYPERTENSION AND CARDIOVASCULAR DISEASE

With cardiovascular disease being the leading cause of death in the industrialized world, it is appropriate to examine whether this applies consistently to all racial and ethnic groups, especially in a country as diverse as the United States. It is clear from the numerous data cited in this chapter that this is not true. It seems that ethnic minorities, particularly African Americans, in a multicultural society experience considerable health disparities, as discussed in various chapters of this book. Considerable racial disparities have been reported in the incidence and prevalence of cardiovascular and renal diseases and hypertension. Although genetics have been examined as a possible source of these differences, they account for little of the observed difference between populations.

There is an inverse correlation between poor health and socioeconomic, educational, and psychosocial factors. This has been demonstrated conclusively with cardiovascular and related diseases in African Americans, who have higher morbidity and mortality compared with their white counterparts. Disparity in cardiovascular health is not limited to the diseases themselves, but also to the health care given for these diseases. Therefore, it is not a surprise that health outcomes are considerably worse in minority groups, such as African Americans, than in the majority population.

In this chapter, we presented data to support the disparities in health and health care, along with studies in African Americans indicating that the risk of cardiovascular disease can be reduced by offering the same care and access that is routinely given to the white population. Barriers to such care include stereotyping, bias in diagnosis and treatment, and lack of cultural competence. There was a time in the near past when prominent cardiologists and academicians believed that African Americans had CAD infrequently, if at all. It took the effort of a number of minority medical groups [National Medical Association, ISHIB, Association of Black Cardiologists (ABC)] as well as unbiased researchers and social activists to refute these misconceptions. Thus, we need to supplement the education, and in some cases, retrain certain cardiovascular specialists. Medical students need to learn, early in their careers, to diagnose and to treat cardiovascular, renal, and hypertensive diseases in minorities in a culturally sensitive manner. Finally, health-care providers rendering care to minority patients with cardiovascular risk factors and diseases need to understand the differences in the presentation and clinical course of the disease that may be unique to these patients.

▶ REFERENCES

1. US Department of Health and Human Services. *Healthy People 2010: Understanding and Improving Health,* 2nd ed. Washington, DC: US Government Printing Office; November 2000.
2. Kaplan GA, Keil JE. Socioeconomic factors and cardiovascular disease: A review of the literature. *Circulation* 1993;88:1973–1998.
3. Keil JE, Sutherland SE, Knapp RG, Tyroler HA. Does equal socioeconomic status in black and white men equal risk of mortality? *Am J Public Healt* 1992;82:1133–1136.
4. Adams JM. Some racial differences in blood pressures and morbidity in a group of white and colored workmen. *Am J Med Sci* 1932;184:342–350.
5. Hajjar I, Kotchen TA. Trends in prevalence, awareness, treatment, and control of hypertension in the United States, 1988–2000. *JAMA* 2003;290(2):199–206.
6. Saunders E, ed. *Racial Differences in Cardiovascular Health*. Pfizer Facts; 2003.
7. Hildreth C, Saunders E. Hypertension in blacks: Clinical overview. In: Saunders E, ed. *Cardiovascular Diseases in Blacks*. Philadelphia, PA: FA Davis; 1991:85–96.
8. Ayala C, Mensah GA, Croft JB. Trends in hypertension-related mortality in the United States. ACC 2003: American College of Cardiology 62nd Annual Scientific Sessions, March 30–April 2, 2003, Chicago, Illinois. *J Am Coll Cardiol* 2003; 41:277A:1133–1150.
9. Williams DR. Race, socioeconomic status, and health: The added effects of racism and discrimination. *Ann N Y Acad Sci* 1999;896:173–188.
10. Wyatt SB, Williams DR, et al. Racism and cardiovascular disease in African Americans. *Am J Med Sci* 2003;325(6):315–331.
11. Ibrahim SA, Whittle J, et al. Racial/ethnic variations in physician recommendations for cardiac revascularization. *Am J Public Health* 2003; 93(10):1689–1693.
12. Whittle J, Conigliaro J, Good CB, Lofgren RP. Racial differences in the use of invasive cardiovascular procedures in the Department Of Veterans Affairs Medical System. *N Engl J Med* 1993; 329(9):621–627.

13. Schneider EC, Zaslavsky AM, Epstein AM. Racial disparities in the quality of care for enrollees in medicare managed care. *JAMA* 2002; 287(10):1288–1294.

14. Alexander M, Grumbach K, Selby J, et al. Hospitalization for congestive heart failure: Explaining racial differences. *JAMA* 1995;274(13):1037–1042.

15. Russo AM, Hafley GE, et al. Racial differences in outcome in the multicenter unsustained tachycardia trial (MUSTT): A comparison of whites versus blacks. *Circulation* 2003;108(1):67–72.

16. Sempos CT, Bild DE, Manolio TA. Overview of the Jackson heart study: A study of cardiovascular diseases in African American men and women. *Am J Med Sci* 1999;317(3):142–146.

17. Lackland DT, Keil JE. Epidemiology of hypertension in African Americans. *Semin Nephrol* 1996;16(2):63–70.

18. Krieger N. Shades of difference: Theoretical underpinnings of the medical controversy on black/white differences in the United States, 1830–1870. *Int J Health Serv* 1987;17:250–278.

19. Blaustein MP, Grim CE. The pathogenesis of hypertension: Black–white differences. In: Saunders E, ed. *Cardiovascular Diseases in Blacks*. Philadelphia, PA: FA Davis; 1991:97–114.

20. Weir MR, Hanes DS. Hypertension in African-Americans: A paradigm of metabolic disarray. *Semin Nephrol* 1996;16(2):102–109.

21. Kaufman JS, Hall SA. The slavery hypertension hypothesis: Dissemination and appeal of a modern race theory. *Epidemiology* 2003;14(1):111–118.

22. Grim CE, Robinson M. Blood pressure variation in blacks: Genetic factors. *Semin Nephrol* 1996;16(2):83–93.

23. Nesbitt S, Victor RG. Pathogenesis of hypertension in African Americans. *CHF* 2004;10(1):24–29.

24. Kannel WB, Belanger AJ. Epidemiology of heart failure. *Am Heart J* 1991;121:951–957.

25. Flack JM, Neaton JD, Daniels B, Esunge P. Ethnicity and renal disease: Lessons from the Multiple Risk Factor Intervention Trial and the Treatment of Mild Hypertension Study. *Am J Kidney Dis* 1993;21(suppl 1):31–40.

26. MacMahon S, Peto R, Cutler J, et al. Blood pressure, stroke, and coronary heart disease. Part 1, prolonged differences in blood pressure: Prospective observational studies corrected for the regression dilution bias. *Lancet* 1990;335:765–774.

27. Sowers JR, Ferdinand KC, Bakris GL, Douglas JC. Hypertension-related disease in African Americans: Factors underlying disparities in illness and its outcome. *Postgrad Med* 2002; 112(4):24–48.

28. National Institutes of Health, National Heart, Lung, and Blood Institute. Congestive heart failure in the United States: A new epidemic. Data Fact Sheet. Available at: http://www.nhlbi.nih.gov/health/public/heart/other/CHF.htm.

29. Levy D, Larson MG, Vason RS, et al. The progression from hypertension to congestive heart failure. *JAMA* 1996;275(20):1557–1562.

30. Liao Y, Cooper RS, Mensah GA, McGee DL. Left ventricular hypertrophy has a greater impact on survival in women than in men. *Circulation* 1995;92(4):805–810.

31. *NHLBI Morbidity and Mortality Chartbook, 2002.* Bethesda, MD: National Heart, Lung, and Blood Institute; May 2002. Accessed March 15, 2004. Available at: http://www.nhlbi.nih.gov/resources/docs/cht-book.htm.

32. Gardin JM, McClelland R, Kitzman D, et al. M-mode echocardiographic predictors of six- to seven-year incidence of coronary heart disease, stroke, congestive heart failure, and mortality in an elderly cohort (the Cardiovascular Health Study). *Am J Cardiol* 2001;87(9): 1051–1057.

33. Di Tullio MR, Zwas, DR, Sacco RL, et al. Left ventricular mass and geometry and the risk of ischemic stroke. *Stroke* 2003;34(10):2380–2384.

34. Gorelick PB. Cerebrovascular disease in African Americans. *Stroke* 1998;29:2656–2664.

35. Nabel EG. Genomic medicine: Cardiovascular disease. *N Engl J Med* 2003;349(1):60–72.

36. Available at: http://www.raceandhealth.omhrc.gov/3rdpgBlue/Cardio/3pgGoalsCardio.htm.

37. Gillum RF. Cardiovascular disease in the United States: An epidemiologic overview. In: Saunders E, ed. *Cardiovascular Diseases in Blacks*. Philadelphia, PA: FA Davis; 1991:3–16.

38. Houghton JL, Strogatz DS, Torosoff MT, et al. African Americans with LVH demonstrate depressed sensitivity of the coronary microcirculation to stimulated relaxation. *Hypertension* 2003;42(3):269–276.

39. Treiber FA, Kamarck T, Schneiderman N, et al. Cardiovascular reactivity and development of preclinical and clinical disease states. *Pyschosom Med* 2003;65(1):46–62.

40. Castillo-Richmond A, Schneider RH, Alexander CN, et al. Effects of stress reduction on carotid atherosclerosis in hypertensive African Americans. *Stroke* 2000;31(3):568–573.

41. Smith TW. Hostility and health: Current status of a psychosomatic hypothesis. *Health Psychol* 1992;11:139–150.

42. Available at: http://www.ethnicmajority.com/glass_ceiling.htm.

43. Mokdad AH, Marks JS, Stroup DF, Gerberding JL. Actual causes of death in the United States, 2000. *JAMA* 2004;291(10):1238–1245.

44. Available at: http://www.strokecenter.org/pat/stats.htm.

45. Whittle JC, Whelton PK, Seidler AJ, Klag MJ. Does race variation in risk factors explain black–white differences in the incidence of hypertensive end-stage renal disease? *Arch Intern Med* 1991;151:1359–1364.

46. Martins D, Tareen N, Norris KC. The epidemiology of end-stage renal disease among African Americans. *Am J Med Sci* 2002;323:65–71.

47. Jones CA, McQuillan GM, Kusek JW, et al. Serum creatinine levels in the US population: Third National Health and Nutrition Examination Survey. *Am J Kidney Dis* 1998;32:992–999.

48. Prevalence of chronic kidney disease and decreased kidney function in the adult U.S. population: Third National Health and Nutrition Examination Survey. *Am J Kidney Dis* 2003;41(suppl 2):S29–40.

49. National Kidney Disease Education Program. (NIH Publication No. 03-53490). Bethesda, MD: National Institutes of Health; 2003.

50. US Renal Data System. *USRDS 2003 Annual Data Report: Atlas of End-Stage Renal Disease in the United States*. Bethesda, MD: National Institutes of Health, National Institute of Diabetes and Digestive and Kidney Diseases; 2003.

51. Hsu CY, Lin F, Vittinghoff E, Shlipak MG. Racial differences in the progression from chronic renal insufficiency to end-stage renal disease in the United States. *J Am Soc Nephrol* 2003;14(11):2902–2907.

52. Klag MJ, Whelton PK, Randall BL, et al. End-stage renal disease in African-American and white men. 16-year MRFIT findings. *JAMA* 1997;277(16):1293–1298.

53. Tarver-Carr ME, Powe NR, Eberhardt MS, et al. Excess risk of chronic kidney disease among African-American versus white subjects in the United States. A population-based study of potential explanatory factors. *J Am Soc Nephrol* 2002;13:2363–2370.

54. Perneger TV, Whelton PK, Klag MJ. Race and end-stage renal disease. Socioeconomic status and access to health care as mediating factors. *Arch Intern Med* 1995;155:1201–1208.

55. The Heart Outcomes Prevention Evaluation Study Investigators. Effects of an angiotensin-converting-enzyme inhibitor, ramipril, on cardiovascular events in high-risk patients. *N Engl J Med* 2000;342(3):145–153.

56. Shulman NB, Ford CE, Hall WD, et al. Prognostic value of serum creatinine and effect of treatment of hypertension on renal function: Results from the hypertension detection and follow-up program. The Hypertension Detection and Follow-up Program Cooperative Group. *Hypertension* 1989;13(5 suppl):180–193.

57. Levey AS, Beto JA, Coronado BE, et al. Controlling the epidemic of cardiovascular disease in chronic renal disease: What do we know? What do we need to learn? Where do we go from here? National Kidney Foundation Task Force on Cardiovascular Disease. *Am J Kidney Dis* 1998;32:853–906.

58. Ma JZ, Ebben J, Xia H, et al. Hematocrit level and associated mortality in hemodialysis patients. *J Am Soc Nephrol* 1999;10:610–619.

59. Guerin AP, London GM, Marchais SJ, et al. Arterial stiffening and vascular calcifications in end-stage renal disease. *Nephrol Dial Transplant* 2000;15:1014–1021.

60. Arici M, Walls J. End-stage renal disease, atherosclerosis, and cardiovascular mortality: Is C-reactive protein the missing link? *Kidney Int* 2001;59:407–414.

61. Himmelfarb J, Stenvinkel P, Ikizler TA, et al. The elephant in uremia: Oxidant stress as a unifying concept of cardiovascular disease in uremia. *Kidney Int* 2002;62:1524–1538.

62. Sarnak MJ, Levey AS, Schoolwerth AC, et al. Kidney disease as a risk factor for development of cardiovascular disease: A statement from the American Heart Association Councils on kidney in cardiovascular disease, high blood pressure research, clinical cardiology, and epidemiology and prevention. *Circulation* 2003;108:2154–2169.

63. *NHLBI Fact Book, Fiscal Year 2002*. Bethesda, MD: National Heart, Lung, and Blood Institute;

February 2003. Accessed March 15, 2004. Available at: http://www.nhlbi.nih.gov/about/factpdf.htm.

64. Price EG, Cooper LA. Hypertension in African Americans: Strategies to help achieve blood pressure goals. *Consultant* 2003;1330–1336.

65. Chobanian AV, Bakris GL, Black HR, et al. The seventh report of the Joint National Committee on prevention, detection, evaluation, and treatment of high blood pressure: The JNC 7 report. *JAMA* 2003;289(19):2560–2572.

66. Wright JT Jr, Bakris G, Greene T, et al. Effect of blood pressure lowering and antihypertensive drug class on progression of hypertensive kidney disease: Results from the AASK trial. *JAMA* 2002;288:2421–2431.

67. ALLHAT Officers and Coordinators for the ALLHAT Collaborative Research Group. Major outcomes in high-risk hypertensive patients randomized to angiotensin-converting enzyme inhibitor or calcium channel blocker vs diuretic: The anthihypertensive and lipid-lowering treatment to prevent heart attack trial (ALLHAT). *JAMA* 2002;288:2981–2997.

68. Ferdinand KC. Recommendations for the management of special populations: Racial and ethnic populations. *Am J Hypertens* 2003;16:50S–54S.

69. Lea JP, Brown DT, Lipkowitz M, et al. Preventing renal dysfunction in patients with hypertension: Clinical implications for the early AASK trial results. *Am J Cardiovasc Drugs* 2003;3(3):193–200.

70. Douglas JG, Bakris GL, Murray-Epstein M, et al. Management of high blood pressure in African Americans: Consensus statement of the hypertension in African Americans working group of the International Society on hypertension in Blacks. *Arch Intern Med* 2003;163(5):525–541.

CHAPTER 8

Diabetes

SAMUEL DAGOGO-JACK, MD, FRCP
JAMES R. GAVIN III, MD, PhD

▶ INTRODUCTION

The US Census Bureau's 2000 data indicate that ethnic minorities constitute approximately 29% of the total US population, with African Americans accounting for 13%. The population of minority groups has been increasing at a faster rate than the national average, and there are several reasons why attention should be paid to special populations in relation to diabetes. First, minority groups have a disproportionately higher prevalence of type 2 diabetes than the majority population. Second, the ethnic disparity in diabetes prevalence is associated with increased risk for diabetes complications in minority groups. Third, hospitalization rates and disability due to diabetes for African Americans and other minority populations are nearly double those for Caucasians. Fourth, diabetes-related mortality is increasing among African Americans and other minority populations whereas it is stable or decreasing among Caucasians.

Disparities in diabetes are likely to become worse in the future: Projected rates for diagnosed diabetes by the year 2020 indicate a 107% increase for Latinos and a 50% increase for African Americans, compared with a 27% increase for Caucasians. Genetic and lifestyle factors drive the ethnic disparities in diabetes

prevalence, but the increased morbidity from diabetes is due to suboptimal control of blood glucose levels. Data from the Third National Health and Nutrition Examination Survey (NHANES III) showed that diabetic control, as indicated by hemoglobin A $_{1c}$ (HbA)$_{1c}$ levels, was poorer among African Americans than among Caucasians. Socioeconomic factors contribute to the disparities in morbidity and mortality from diabetes: Disparities in access to care, quality of metabolic control, and health insurance coverage create conditions that favor increased risk for complications. Increased insulin resistance has been demonstrated in minority groups, even after correction for obesity and lifestyle factors. Thus, interventions that reduce insulin resistance (notably, caloric restriction, weight reduction, physical activity, and medications that increase insulin sensitivity) are desirable in these populations and have been shown to be particularly effective in controlling or preventing diabetes. Ethnic disparities exist at several levels in the prevalence and complications of diabetes, but not in the efficacy of interventions used for the prevention and control of diabetes. Much of the ethnic difference in morbidity from diabetes complications is eliminated when Caucasians and non-Caucasians are treated to identical degrees of glycemic control.

Diabetes Mellitus and Prediabetic States

Diabetes mellitus is a group of metabolic disorders that results in hyperglycemia. These disorders have different etiologies but a common manifestation, hyperglycemia, which is associated with acute and long-term complications regardless of underlying etiology. The occurrence of diabetes complications can be prevented or markedly reduced by a treatment approach that results in normalization or near-normalization of blood glucose levels. Most cases of diabetes fall into one of two categories, although overlap may occur and the distinction may not always be clear.[1]

Type 1 diabetes accounts for less than 10% of all cases of diabetes, tends to occur in younger subjects, and is caused by severe insulin deficiency. The latter results from autoimmune destruction of the insulin-secreting β cells of the pancreas. The risk factors for autoimmune β-cell destruction include inheritance of disease susceptibility genes (HLA haplotypes) in the major histocompatibility locus and possible exposure to environmental triggers. Type 1 diabetes is predominantly a disease of persons of European ancestry and is much less prevalent among persons of African, Asian, and other non-European descent. The highest prevalence of type 1 diabetes is found in Finland.

Type 2 diabetes accounts for more than 90% of all cases of diabetes. It is usually a disease of older adults, but is being diagnosed with increasing frequency in younger age groups, including children and adolescents.[2] Obesity and physical inactivity are major risk factors for type 2 diabetes in adults, adolescents, and children. Other hallmarks of type 2 diabetes in childhood include increased risk among ethnic minority groups, female preponderance, acanthosis nigricans (dark, velvety skin discoloration in the neck, axilla, and other flexural areas), and absence of ketoacidosis. Insulin resistance and relative insulin deficiency are characteristic pathophysiologic findings in persons with type 2 diabetes. Obesity, physical inactivity, and genetic predisposition increase the risk for insulin resistance; the etiology of the insulin secretory defect in type 2 diabetes is not well understood. Endogenous insulin production may be sufficient to prevent ketogenesis under basal conditions, but diabetic ketoacidosis can develop during stress. Unlike type 1 diabetes, type 2 diabetes is disproportionately more prevalent in non-European than European populations.

Prediabetic States

The term *prediabetes* refers to impaired glucose tolerance (IGT) and impaired fasting glucose (IFG), two intermediate metabolic states between normal glucose tolerance and diabetes. IGT is defined by a plasma glucose level of 140 to 199 mg/dL, 2 hours following ingestion of a 75-g oral solution. IFG is defined by a fasting plasma glucose level of 100 to 125 mg/dL.[1] IFG and IGT are risk factors for type 2 diabetes, and persons with these conditions progress to type 2 diabetes at variable rates. In addition, epidemiologic studies indicate that IGT is associated with increased risk for macrovascular disease (coronary artery disease, stroke, and peripheral vascular disease). The insulin resistance (metabolic) syndrome appears to be the link between prediabetes and macrovascular disease. Most patients with prediabetes have features of the metabolic syndrome, including upper body obesity, hypertriglyceridemia, decreased high-density lipoprotein cholesterol levels, and hypertension, among others. Major criteria for recognition of the metabolic syndrome have been developed by the American Association of Clinical Endocrinologists[3] (Table 8–1), and the National Cholesterol Education Program[4] has put forth a simplified diagnostic tool (Table 8–2). The case for routine drug treatment for persons with IGT or IFG has not been established, but clinical trials have demonstrated the efficacy of lifestyle intervention (exercise, dietary modification) and certain medications in preventing progression from prediabetes to type 2 diabetes.

▶ **TABLE 8–1.** Major Criteria for Dysmetabolic Syndrome X^a (ICD-9 277.7)

- Insulin resistance (hyperinsulinemia relative to glucose levels), or
- Acanthosis nigricans
- Central obesity (waist circumference > 102 cm in men or > 88 cm in women)
- Dyslipidemia: HDL cholesterol < 45 mg/dL in women or < 35 mg/dL in men or triglyceride levels > 150 mg/dL
- Hypertension (blood pressure 130/85 mm Hg)
- Impaired fasting glucose (> 110 mg/dL) or type 2 diabetes
- Hyperuricemia

HDL, high-density lipoprotein.

^{a}Diagnostic criteria and operational definition developed by American Association of Clinical Endocrinologists.

Reproduced with permission from American Association of Clinical Endocrinologists. New ICD-9-CM Code for Dysmetabolic Syndrome X. 2002.

▶ ETHNIC DISPARITIES IN THE PREVALENCE OF DIABETES AND PREDIABETES

The prevalence of type 2 diabetes has been increasing at alarming rates in all populations around the world[5] and has reached epidemic proportions in the United States.[6,7] The Be-

▶ **TABLE 8–2.** Adult Treatment Panel III (ATP III): Criteria for Diagnosis of the Metabolic Syndrome^a (ICD-9 277.7)[4]

Abdominal obesity (waist circumference)	
Men	> 102 cm (> 40 in)
Women	> 88 cm (> 35 in)
Triglycerides	≥150 mg/dL
HDL cholesterol	
Men	< 40 mg/dL
Women	< 50 mg/dL
Blood pressure	≥ 130/ ≥ 85 mm Hg
Fasting glucose	≥110 mg/dL

HDL, high-density lipoprotein.

^{a}Diagnosis is established when more than 3 of these risk factors are present.

havioral Risk Factor Surveillance Study (BRFSS) found that the prevalence of diagnosed diabetes increased by approximately 60% between 1990 and 2001.[8] The increase was particularly striking among minority groups and in persons aged 30 to 39 years.[8] As previously noted, 2000 census data indicate that ethnic minorities constitute approximately 29% of the overall US population, with African-Americans accounting for approximately 13%. The population of minority groups has been increasing at a faster rate than the national average. Compared with white Americans, the relative increase in the prevalence of type 2 diabetes is approximately 1.5-fold in African Americans, 2.5-fold in Hispanic Americans, 3- to 4-fold in Asian Americans and Pacific Islanders, and 10-fold or greater in certain Native American ethnic groups.[9]

The disparities in the prevalence of diabetes are likely to escalate in the future because the projected rates for the prevalence of diagnosed diabetes by the year 2020 indicate a 107% increase among Hispanic Americans and 50% increase for African Americans, as compared with 27% increase for Caucasians.[10] Of even greater concern, 47 million Americans have prediabetes or the metabolic syndrome based on the NHANES III data.[11] Data on disparities in prediabetes are less clear: the prevalence of IGT was 16% in NHANES III in the United States,[12] 13% in DECODE in Europe,[13] 15% in the DECODA study of 11 Asian populations,[14] and 20% in young African Americans.[15] Because the definition of IGT employs the more sensitive postchallenge glucose measurements, the prevalence of IGT is two to four times higher than IFG in the general population.[16]

Although the prevalence of type 1 diabetes has increased, the current diabetes epidemic is accounted for by increases in the rates of type 2 diabetes. Ethnic minority populations in the United States carry a disproportionately heavier diabetes disease burden than whites. This chapter discusses several aspects of disparities in diabetes, including susceptibility factors, complications, health-care delivery, and prevention. The role of nature and nurture is evaluated in the context of socioeconomic mediators and modifiers of the disparities in the prevalence and ferocity of diabetes.

▶ GENETIC AND ENVIRONMENTAL FACTORS

The exact reasons for the ethnic and racial differences in the incidence and prevalence of type 2 diabetes are not known precisely. A collusion of genetic predisposition and environmental triggers likely accounts for the development of type 2 diabetes in any population. The nature and identity of the diabetogenes are still being actively investigated.[17]

Genetic Factors

The thrifty gene hypothesis[18] posits that ancestors of modern humans that lived millions of years ago might have been selected for survival based on certain genetically transmitted metabolic traits. In those primeval times, when food availability was insecure and natural disasters (floods, fires, famine, etc) were rampant, people who were metabolically efficient or "thrifty" survived better than others. Metabolic thriftiness ensured efficient storage of energy as fat when food was available for utilization during famine. Ancient humans were also hunter-gatherers for whom daily physical activity was mandatory. Over time, these "thrifty" genes have been transmitted to progeny down to the present era, when famine is no longer rampant and use of modern exercise-sparing devices (automobile, elevator, escalator, remote control, the Internet, etc) is a universal addiction. The result of guaranteed food surplus and markedly reduced physical activity, superimposed on a background of ancestral genetic thriftiness, is the epidemic of obesity in affluent countries and among the elite in developing countries.[19,20] Genes that once ensured survival in an era of starvation have become a handicap in a time of plenty (Fig. 8–1).

The thrifty gene hypothesis is generally accepted as a plausible explanation for obesity, but its extension to explain type 2 diabetes has been challenged.[20] Indeed, as argued by Lev-Ran,[20] the evolutionary advantages of genes that lead to diabetes are unclear, whereas the connection between thrifty genes and obesity is much clearer. Obesity ensured survival by making available stored energy during starvation;

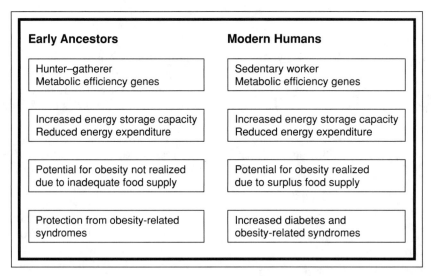

Figure 8–1. Schema for thrifty gene hypothesis. *(Based on reference 18).*

diabetes, on the other hand, is teleologically maladaptive in that it reduces survival by a full decade and compromises quality of life through its numerous complications. Thus, the application of the thrifty gene hypothesis to type 2 diabetes appears not to be as convincing as its link to obesity.

Another problem with the thrifty gene hypothesis is that it does not quite explain the lower prevalence of type 2 diabetes in persons of European ancestry as compared with other ethnic and racial groups (the "European paradox"); especially since obesity rates are comparable across major regions of the world. By definition, every modern human is a beneficiary of ancestral thrifty genes. Throughout history, intermittent starvation had been rife in all parts of the world until the very recent era, and the historically "better-fed European is a myth."[20] As Lev-Ran[20] argued, "the explanation of the European paradox by (invoking) early development of successful agriculture or by high degree of urbanization is unacceptable; hunger was a permanent reality of life in Europe no less than elsewhere." Furthermore, the contention that better nutrition promoted "nonthrifty" genotype among Europeans, which led to reduced risk for type 2 diabetes, is not supported by the higher prevalence of type 2 diabetes among Chinese (despite exposure to centuries of successful agricultural developments that preceded European agronomic awakening).

Other Hypotheses

Based on the foregoing premise, alternative hypotheses have been proposed. One of these is called *antagonistic pleiotropy*.[21] This concept suggests that there might be a trade-off between fitness components during earlier and later stages of life. As proposed under this scheme, thriftiness at a younger age ensured survival and reproductive viability, but, after middle age, these thrifty genes predispose to diabetes. The major weakness of antagonistic pleiotropy is that it lacks empirical examples in nature. The second alternative is the so-called genetic trash can hypothesis: The conservation of multiple, individually neutral gene mutations

that confer aggregate risks for type 2 diabetes when accumulated and concentrated in a given population.[20,22] Because diabetogenes are generally transmitted as recessive traits, such a hypothesis would be consistent with the increased prevalence of type 2 diabetes in ethnic populations that have been less exogamous than European populations.[20] Exogamy, migrations, conquests, invasions, interbreeding, and admixtures exert a dilutional effect on mutant genes, and many aboriginal societies have experienced less of these diluting events than have Caucasians.[20]

Environmental Triggers

The role of the environment in uncovering latent genetic predisposition is well known. This was clearly demonstrated in the studies that showed a threefold increase in the rate of type 2 diabetes in Japanese immigrants to the United States compared with native Japanese.[23] Such a dramatic increase in disease prevalence in humans cannot be attributed to sudden new genetic mutations. Environmental triggers, including change in diet and lifestyle, most probably account for the expression of the innate genetic predisposition to type 2 diabetes in the Japanese immigrants. The exact mechanisms whereby environmental triggers induce diabetes in genetically predisposed persons are not known with certainty. However, the traditional environmental factors associated with increased occurrence of type 2 diabetes, often referred to as risk factors, include obesity, physical inactivity, history of gestational diabetes, hypertension, and dyslipidemia, among others (Table 8–3).

The distribution of these individual risk factors varies across the different ethnic groups, but the aggregate risk factor burden in various populations must overlap considerably. Therefore, ethnic differences in conventional risk factors alone cannot account for the marked disparities in diabetes prevalence. For example, although obesity is the single most compelling (and most predictable) of the traditional risk factors for type 2 diabetes in the general population, the incidence of diabetes among even massively

▶ **TABLE 8–3**. Risk Factors for Type 2 Diabetes

Family history of type 2 diabetes in first-degree relatives
Overweight or obesity
Physical inactivity
Ethnicity
Gestational diabetes
Delivery of infant weighing ≥ 9 lb
Hypertension
Dyslipidemia
Major psychiatric disorder (schizophrenia, depression, bipolar disease, etc.)

obese persons is far from being 100%. Indeed, obesity triggers diabetes only in a susceptible minority, the majority of obese persons being capable of escaping diabetes as a metabolic consequence of their obesity. Nonetheless, because the prevalence of obesity (especially among women) is higher in African Americans, Latinos, and Native Americans compared with Caucasians, it is possible that individual risk factors may exert differential effects on diabetes risk across ethnic groups. Also, national surveys indicate that the accrual of habitual physical activity minutes is at endemically low levels across all ethnic groups. In a recent report, the decline in voluntary physical activity was striking among young African American women, who had virtually no such activity after age 16 years.[24] Thus, physical inactivity is an obvious target of opportunity for reduction of the ethnic disparities in obesity and diabetes.

Insulin Resistance and Pancreatic β-Cell Function

The key metabolic defects that lead to type 2 diabetes include insulin resistance and impaired insulin secretion by the pancreatic β cells.[25] The concurrent roles of insulin resistance and β-cell dysfunction in predicting the development of type 2 diabetes was confirmed in a longitudinal study of Pima Indians[26] and may represent a general model in other ethnic groups. Studies that compared various populations of West

African descendants (including African Americans and native Ghanaians) and Caucasians have reported higher degrees of insulin resistance among the West African descendants.[27] The Insulin Resistance Atherosclerosis Study (IRAS) also showed higher degrees of insulin resistance among African American and Latinos than Caucasians, even after adjusting for age, gender, body mass index, and other pertinent variables.[28] These studies suggest a role for genetically driven insulin resistance in the pathophysiology of ethnic disparities in the prevalence of type 2 diabetes.

However, as demonstrated in the study of Pima Indians,[26] progression from normal glucose tolerance to impaired glucose tolerance or diabetes is not inevitable among susceptible individuals. Among Pima Indians, impaired first-phase insulin secretion proved to be the major predictor for progression to higher glycemic states. However, data on β-cell function in relation to risk of diabetes remain unsettled. European relatives of type 2 diabetes patients have been reported to have intact[29] or decreased[30] insulin secretion. A high concordance rate for subnormal insulin secretion has been reported among European identical twins discordant for type 2 diabetes,[31] consistent with an inherited component of β-cell dysfunction. Insulin secretion was maintained and insulin clearance decreased in nondiabetic subjects of West African heritage as compared with Caucasians.[27] One cross-sectional study of West African offspring of diabetic parents indicated low insulin secretory responses,[32] but there is a dearth of longitudinal studies in African Americans and other ethnic minorities.

▶ DISPARITIES IN THE COMPLICATIONS OF DIABETES

Acute Complications

Acute diabetic complications (such as ketoacidosis, nonketotic hyperosmolar syndrome, and hypoglycemia) occur with varying frequencies in the different ethnic groups, but there are suggestions that the rate of hospitalization for diabetic ketoacidosis and nonketotic coma may be higher among certain minority groups, such as African Americans.[33] In the general diabetes population, diabetic ketoacidosis often is triggered by intercurrent infections, but cessation of insulin therapy appears to be a major precipitating factor among African American patients.[34] In many instances, the cessation of insulin was involuntary and was due to lack of resources for replenishment of insulin stock in economically disadvantaged patients.[34]

Long-term Complications

In the United States, diabetes now accounts for approximately 50% of all cases of end-stage renal disease, adult blindness, and lower extremity amputation. Patients with diabetes have a 25-fold increase in risk of renal failure, a 20-fold increase in risk of blindness, and a 40-fold increased risk of lower extremity amputation.[35] Diabetes also confers a two- to fivefold increase in risk of heart disease.[36] Moreover, the economic costs of diabetes are staggering— diabetes accounted for approximately 8% of total U.S. health care expenditures in 1997 ($78 billion).[37] Sadly, the long-term complications of diabetes are disproportionately higher among ethnic minority patients than Caucasians. During the 1980s, diabetes-related mortality for Caucasian men and women decreased 1.6% and 4.5%, respectively; in contrast, mortality increased among African-American men (11%) and women (5.5%).[38] Thus the ethnic disparity in the prevalence of type 2 diabetes translates to increased burden from diabetes complications in minority populations. It must be emphasized that improved metabolic control has been demonstrated to reduce diabetes complications and the related health care costs.[39]

Microvascular Complications

The diabetes-specific microvascular complications include retinopathy, nephropathy, and neuropathy. These complications do not occur in persons with impaired glucose tolerance, but require hyperglycemia as an initiating factor. The development of microvascular complications is a function of both the duration of diabetes and the state of metabolic control; nearly 25% of patients with type 2 diabetes already have developed one or more microvascular complications by the time of diagnosis. The single most modifiable factor underlying microvascular complications is hyperglycemia, and intensive control of blood glucose levels is the only strategy known to prevent the development and slow progression of microvascular complications.

In NHANES III, a fundus photograph of a single eye was taken with a nonmydriatic camera, and a standardized protocol was used to grade diabetic retinopathy in subjects from a cross section of the US population. The prevalence of any lesions of diabetic retinopathy in people with diagnosed diabetes was 46% higher in African Americans and 84% higher in Mexican Americans, compared with non-Hispanic whites. African Americans and Mexican Americans also had higher rates of moderate and severe retinopathy and higher levels of many putative risk factors for retinopathy.[40] Similarly, the rates of end-stage renal disease (ESRD) are approximately threefold higher in African Americans, Latinos, and Native Americans compared with Caucasians.[41] Diabetic nephropathy now accounts for 50% of ESRD cases requiring dialysis treatment. Microalbuminuria (defined as 30 to 300 mg of albumin per 24 hours), a potentially reversible stage of incipient nephropathy, precedes overt proteinuria (more than 500 mg of protein per liter, or more than 300 mg of albumin per day) by several years in patients with diabetes. After gross proteinuria has developed, progression to nephrotic syndrome and ESRD occurs over a shorter time frame. The mean duration from diagnosis of diabetes to development of overt proteinuria is approximately 17 years, and the time from the occurrence of gross proteinuria to ESRD averages 5 years.[25] Thus, a wide window of opportunity exists for preventing progressive renal failure in patients with diabetes. The proven methods for doing so include aggressive control of blood glucose and blood pressure levels; use of medications that inhibit angiotensin-converting enzyme or angiotensin II receptors in patients with microalbuminuria; and modification of other risk factors, such as smoking and hyperlipidemia.[42]

The third microvascular complication, diabetic neuropathy, encompasses a wide variety of focal as well as diffuse neurologic syndromes, the best recognized example of which is peripheral neuropathy. The loss of protective pain sensation predisposes the diabetic limb to injuries, infections, gangrene formation, and lower extremity amputation. The rates of hospitalization for lower extremity ulcers are similar across all ethnic groups, but lower extremity amputation rates are two to three times higher in Mexican American and African American patients compared with Caucasians.[43] Diabetic neuropathy can be prevented by a policy of tight glycemic control (HbA_{1c} less than 7%).[44] Furthermore, the consequences of established diabetic neuropathy (especially gangrene and amputation) are not inevitable. Screening for foot sensation using the 5.07 monofilament identifies patients at high risk, who can then be triaged to intensive limb preservation practices.[42]

Macrovascular Complications

There is a two- to fivefold increase in the prevalence of coronary artery disease (CAD), stroke, and peripheral vascular diseases (collectively referred to as macrovascular complications) in patients with diabetes compared with nondiabetic subjects. The risk of first myocardial infarction (MI) in diabetes patients is similar to that of recurrent MI in nondiabetic persons who have had a previous heart attack.[45] Thus, diabetes is not merely a risk factor but a CAD risk-equivalent. Moreover, a strong correlation between hyperglycemia and cardiovascular disease has been observed in several studies, including the Paris Prospective study, the Whitehall Study, the Chicago Heart Study, the Tecumseh Study, and the Honolulu Heart Study, among others. Patients with diabetes present with atypical man-ifestations of CAD (including painless MI) that could delay timely diagnosis and intervention. Sadly, myocardial infarction carries a worse prognosis, and percutaneous coronary angioplasty gives less satisfactory results in diabetic patients compared with nondiabetic individuals. These tragic features of macrovascular disease in diabetes operate across all ethnic lines.

Unlike microvascular complications, the relative risks for macrovascular complications have not been shown consistently to be higher among ethnic minorities. In fact, the collective data indicate similar or lower rates of MI and stroke in African American, Asian, and Hispanic populations compared with white Americans.[46,47] Given the higher prevalence of hypertension and diabetes in African Americans compared with whites, the findings of reduced relative risks for MI and stroke suggest the presence of possible mitigating factors, among which may be a less atherogenic lipoprotein profile.[48] In contrast to the similar or reduced rates of macrovascular disease, mortality from CAD is disproportionately higher in minority populations (especially African American women) than Caucasians.[49] This suggests that the conventional markers used for predicting macrovascular risk in the general populace may be less informative in minority populations. The mortality data are also consistent with possible ethnic disparities in the biologic expression of macrovascular disease or quality of care following myocardial infarction, or both. Further studies are needed to determine whether ethnic minority subjects exhibit greater atheroinflammatory markers, and how this may relate to increased mortality despite their similar or lower incidence of macrovascular disease compared with Caucasians.

▶ ETIOLOGY OF THE DISPARITIES IN DIABETES COMPLICATIONS

Theoretically, the greater rates of complications of diabetes among ethnic minorities may be due to primary (ie, genetic) susceptibility or secondary (ie, acquired) factors.

▶ **TABLE 8–4**. Diabetes Management: Patient Compliance and Practices by Ethnicity[a]

	Hispanic (%)	African American (%)	Caucasian (%)
Missed clinic	1.4	1.9	1.5
Noncompliance	34.0	27.0	26.0
Alcoholism	3.4	2.2	2.5
Missed foot clinic	0.0	2.7	5.6
Missed weight visit	17.0	15.0	9.0
Missed eye clinic	0.0	2.0	7.0

[a]There were no significant racial or ethnic differences in compliance behavior.

Adapted with permission from Martin TL, Selby JV, Zhang D. Physician and patient prevention practices in NIDDM in a large urban managed-care organization. Diabetes Care 1995;18(8):1124–1132.

Primary or Genetic Susceptibility

There is some evidence for familial clustering of microvascular complications, especially diabetic nephropathy, in certain ethnic minority populations, which would suggest a role for hereditary factors in the pathogenesis of diabetes complications. However, data from landmark studies argue strongly against a primary and major role for genetics in driving diabetes complications. In the Diabetes Control and Complications Trial,[50] intensive glycemic control resulted in a 50% to 70% reduction in the risk of development of retinopathy, neuropathy, or nephropathy. In the UK Prospective Diabetes Study, intensive glucose control reduced the risk of doubling of serum creatinine by 74%, among other benefits.[44] These rather large effects of glycemic control in preventing target organ complications indicate that genetic factors are permissive rather than obligate determinants of risk. In the NHANES III retinopathy data, the black–white disparity no longer was significant after adjusting for known risk factors for retinopathy, such as chronicity of diabetes, HbA$_{1c}$ level, and blood pressure.[51]

Secondary or Acquired Factors

Nongenetic factors that could promote the development of complications from a chronic disease include patient practices, suboptimal care, and socioeconomic factors. What follows is a discussion of the role of these factors in de-termining increased morbidity from diabetes in ethnic minorities.

Patient Compliance

Physicians and other health-care providers often explain away suboptimal outcome on the basis of possible noncompliance with therapeutic recommendations. Such sentiments are frequently expressed in clinical settings around the world. Yet careful studies have revealed no evidence of significant ethnic or racial differences in global compliance with diabetes-related tasks[52] (Table 8–4). A notable exception is self-monitoring of blood glucose, where approximately 18% of African American patients were testing at the minimal recommended frequency compared with approximately 30% of Latino and Caucasian patients.[33] It must be noted, however, that the frequency of self-monitoring is suboptimal even among Latinos and Caucasians.

An unsubstantiated impression of general noncompliance tends to undermine further aggressive therapeutic action by the physician. This could be tragic for the effective management of diabetes, an undertaking that draws sustenance from positive iterative interactions between patient and physician. It is therefore imperative that the label of noncompliance be avoided, unless admitted to by patients or proven by objective criteria. Even after a patient has been found to be noncompliant, it behooves the caring physician to understand and attempt to correct the barriers or misguided premise that led to such behavior.

Physician Practices

Another plausible explanation for the increased morbidity from diabetes in ethnic minorities is systematic delivery of suboptimal care. Indeed, reduced HbA$_{1c}$ testing frequency and poorer results have been reported in African Americans compared with Caucasians, even in the setting of presumed equal access to care.[53] Such reports indicate that there are disparities in the quality of care rendered to persons with diabetes. However, national surveys do not indicate a widespread practice of systematic undertreatment of minority patients as an explanation for the increased morbidity from diabetes[54] (Table 8–5). What is evident is a poor overall state of diabetes control in the nation at large.[55] Because persons from ethnic minority groups suffer disproportionately from diabetes complications, it is imperative for diabetes caregivers to use all available resources to achieve excellent diabetes control in these subjects.

Socioeconomic Factors

There is abundant literature on the contributions of low socioeconomic status, limitations

▶ **TABLE 8–5**. Medical Care for Black Adults and White Adults with Type 2 Diabetes[a]

	Black (%)	White (%)
≥ 4 Physician visits/year	62.4	58.9
Insulin	51.9	35.9
Oral agents	50.1	39.9
Following diet	88.9	88.2
SMBG	18	35
Visit dietitian	28	19
Diabetes education	43	32
Eye examination	64	60
Visit podiatrist	19	16

SMBG, self-monitoring blood glucose.

[a]National Diabetes Data Group. Analysis based on 1989 clinical data.

Adapted with permission from Cowie CC, Harris MI. Ambulatory medical care for non-Hispanic whites, African-Americans, and Mexican-Americans with NIDDM in the U.S. Diabetes Care 1997;20(2): 142–147.

in access of care, lack of health insurance or underinsurance, and other socioeconomic barriers to increased burden of diabetes and its complications.[53,56] One striking example is the life-threatening acute diabetes complication, diabetic ketoacidosis (DKA): In a study of economically disadvantaged African Americans seen at an urban clinic, cessation of insulin was the major precipitating cause of DKA.[34] Further analysis indicated that 43% of patients had stopped taking insulin because they had run out of supplies and had no means of replenishing their spent stock of insulin; 25% stopped taking insulin because of a fundamental misunderstanding of the role of insulin therapy during sick days[34] (Fig. 8–2). Thus, two thirds of the cases of DKA among African Americans in that study were preventable, either through renewal of insulin supplies or education to improve self-management skills. Indeed, much of what passes for ethnic disparities in clinical outcomes may be mediated to a large extent by socioeconomic factors. For example, the marked ethnic disparity in lower extremity amputation rates observed in the general diabetic population is not evident in an ethnically diverse population with uniform health-care coverage.[47] Even the low frequency of self-monitoring of blood glucose has socioeconomic underpinnings: with identical health insurance coverage, the frequency of self-monitoring of blood glucose among African Americans increased to match or exceed that of Asian, Latino, or Caucasian patients.[47]

Overriding Mechanism

Studies have shown that controlling blood glucose levels to comparable degrees eliminates or dampens the ethnic disparities in diabetes complications; also, lifestyle and pharmacologic interventions for prevention of type 2 diabetes were equally efficacious in persons of African, Asian, European, Hispanic, and Native American ancestry.[57] The targets for glycemic control for persons with diabetes, as recommended

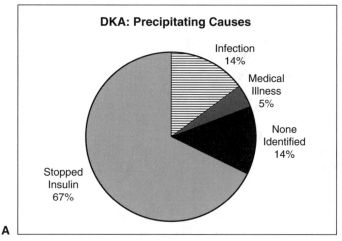

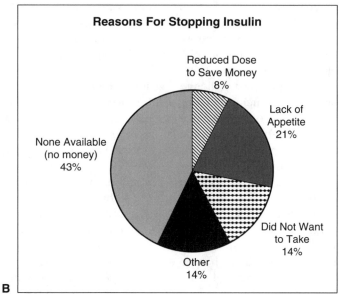

Figure 8–2. A. Cessation of insulin as the major precipitating cause of diabetic ketoacidosis among African American patients at an urban clinic **B.** Reasons for cessation of insulin among African American patients presenting with diabetic ketoacidosis. *(Based on reference 34).*

by the American Diabetes Association (ADA) are: average preprandial blood glucose values of 80 to 120 mg/dL; bedtime blood glucose level of 100 to 140 mg/dL; and HbA$_{1c}$ of less than 7% or lower. The American College of Endocrinology Diabetes Mellitus Consensus Conference recommends a fasting glucose target of less than

110 mg/dL and an HbA$_{1c}$ of less than 6.5%. All recommendations are in general agreement that the goals of diabetes management are normalization or near-normalization of fasting and postprandial blood glucose levels and prevention of acute and long-term complications. The vigorous pursuit of these standards in all

patients with diabetes, particularly those from ethnic minority populations, is the dominant strategy for prevention of diabetes complications. Such a strategy also has the greatest prospect of eliminating ethnic disparities in diabetes-related morbidity and mortality.

► STRATEGIES FOR DIABETES PREVENTION AND MANAGEMENT

Prevention of Diabetes

Persons identified as having prediabetes or IGT progress to type 2 diabetes over several years at a rate that ranges from 1% to more than 10% per year, depending on the specific population. Risk factors that influence progression from IGT to diabetes include family history of type 2 diabetes, higher levels of fasting or postchallenge hyperglycemia, obesity, and ethnicity. Persons with prediabetes often have insulin resistance and components of the metabolic syndrome (see Table 8–1) that predict increased risk for macrovascular disease. Data from several large studies, including NHANES II, the prospective Rancho Bernardo study, the Lipid Research Clinic program, and the San Antonio Heart Study, consistently indicate that individuals with IGT have a cardiovascular risk profile that is between that of individuals with type 2 diabetes and those with normal glucose tolerance.

The long prodrome from prediabetes to diabetes presents great opportunity for primary prevention of type 2 diabetes. Because obesity and physical inactivity are major risk factors for prediabetes (and type 2 diabetes) in virtually all populations, several studies have addressed whether the risk associated with these factors is reversible through intervention. The results have been overwhelmingly positive, demonstrating the efficacy of caloric restriction and physical activity in preventing progression from IGT to type 2 diabetes.[57] On average, walking briskly for 30 minutes five times weekly together with modest caloric restriction that results in modest weight loss (5% to 7%) can be expected to reduce the risk of diabetes by more than 50%. Medications such as metformin and acarbose have also been shown to prevent progression to type 2 diabetes, but the effect is only about one half or less compared with that observed with diet and exercise. Clinical trials are in progress to determine whether other agents (eg, thiazolidinediones) can also prevent diabetes.

The findings from the Diabetes Prevention Program (DPP) offer interesting new perspectives with regard to ethnic disparities. In the DPP, the rate of progression from prediabetes (IGT) to type 2 diabetes was similar (approximately 11%) among African Americans, Asian Americans and Pacific Islanders, Caucasian Americans, Hispanic Americans, and Native Americans.[57] In other words, the well-known ethnic disparity in type 2 diabetes was surprisingly not evident among the DPP cohort (approximately 3000 subjects) with impaired glucose tolerance, who were followed for 2 to 4 years. By definition, persons with IGT have normal fasting plasma glucose levels and 2-hour levels of 140 to 199 mg/dL during a 75-g oral glucose tolerance test. The finding of similar transethnic diabetes rates in the DPP suggests that once individuals have progressed from normal glucose tolerance to IGT, the risk of further progression to diabetes is largely independent of ethnic and racial influences. Thus, the ethnic or genetic factors that predispose to diabetes must have exerted their maximal effects during the transition from normal metabolism to prediabetes. This intriguing and novel notion has obvious implications for the design and translation of primary prevention strategies.

► PRINCIPLES OF MANAGEMENT

Nonpharmacologic Interventions

The mnemonic *MEDEM* (*M*onitoring, *E*ducation, *D*iet, *E*xercise, *M*edications) can be used to recall the key modalities of diabetes management. Self-monitored blood glucose (SMBG) is an important (but underutilized) tool of diabetes management and education. The recommended frequency of SMBG is two to four times or more daily for insulin-treated patients. The optimal frequency has not been established for patients with type 2 diabetes treated with oral agents, but regular SMBG (at least once daily) is recommended. Diabetes education and dietary and exercise counseling are effective in minority populations; these approaches should be promoted as important adjuncts to drug therapy of type 2 diabetes. Regular physical activity enhances insulin sensitivity, decreases abdominal obesity, and improves blood pressure and lipid levels. Exercise programs should be tailored to individual patients' physical condition and should always include warm-up and cool-down periods. To be effective, programs should utilize aerobic exercise (eg, walking, cycling, swimming) at about 60% of maximum oxygen utilization (VO_2 max) for about 30 minutes, three or more times per week. Cardiac screening with stress electrocardiogram is recommended for patients aged 35 years or older, especially those who have been sedentary.

Medications

The ideal treatment for type 2 diabetes should reverse insulin resistance (and the associated metabolic syndrome), normalize hepatic glucose production, improve pancreatic β-cell function, and prevent the development of long-term complications. The medications used for treating diabetes include insulin and oral agents. Most patients with type 2 diabetes respond initially to oral antidiabetic agents but may require insulin as the disease progresses. The currently available oral agents include insulin secretagogues (sulfonylureas, repaglinide, and nateglinide); metformin, which is a biguanide; α-glucosidase inhibitors (acarbose and miglitol); and insulin sensitizers or thiazolidinediones (rosiglitazone and pioglitazone). Pharmacotherapy for diabetes is most effective if initiated as part of a comprehensive management plan that includes self-monitoring of blood glucose, pa-

tient education, and dietary and exercise counseling. The maintenance of long-term glycemic control (necessary for prevention of complications) in persons with type 2 diabetes often requires the use of multiple agents in combination. Medications for combination therapy should be selected from drug classes that lower blood glucose by different mechanisms, to ensure additive or synergistic effects and to maximize nonglycemic benefits related to alterations in cardiovascular risk markers.

▶ SUMMARY AND RECOMMENDATIONS

There are many reasons why attention should be focused on minority issues in relation to diabetes. First, minorities suffer disproportionately from type 2 diabetes, the subtype that accounts for 95% of all cases of diabetes. Second, several of the long-term complications of diabetes, including premature death, occur more frequently among minorities compared with non-Hispanic whites, thus compromising quality and quantity of life. Third, there are indications of disparities in access to care and socioeconomic factors that aggravate the unequal burden of diabetes among minority populations.

Pathophysiologically, several studies have documented alterations in glucoregulatory physiology (especially insulin action) across demographic groups. Some studies, notably the Insulin Resistance Atherosclerosis Study, have shown a higher prevalence of insulin resistance in minority groups, even after correction for obesity and lifestyle factors. These findings underscore the need for a more aggressive approach to diabetes management in high-risk populations. Biobehavioral interventions that reduce insulin resistance have profound effects on glycemic control and reduce the requirement for medications in African American patients and diabetic subjects from other ethnic groups. These measures also are effective in primary prevention of diabetes. Thus, weight reduction and physical activity need to be vigorously promoted as potent and safe remedies for the amelioration of insulin resistance. In addition to lifestyle modification, endemic insulin resistance in minority populations compels judicious use of pharmacologic agents that act primarily by increasing tissue sensitivity to insulin. Thus, although there are wide ethnic disparities in the prevalence of type 2 diabetes, probably related to genetically driven insulin resistance, there is no ethnic resistance to the prophylactic effects of lifestyle interventions for prevention of diabetes. Similarly, there is no ethnic disparity in the responsiveness to lifestyle or pharmacologic interventions for the treatment of established diabetes.

The ethnic disparities in many of the complications of diabetes are largely erased by equalization of glycemic control. Indeed, all interventions tested to date (lifestyle and pharmacologic) have been equally effective in controlling diabetes and preventing complications in all populations. This realization ought to trigger a policy of aggressive diabetes management in patients from ethnic minority backgrounds in an effort to minimize the ravages of diabetes in these populations. Early detection through screening is the answer to the high burden of undiagnosed diabetes among ethnic minority populations. For the general US population, screening is recommended for all persons at age 45 years or older; normal tests should be repeated at 3-year intervals. Screening should be performed at a younger age and more frequently in individuals from high-risk populations (Native American, Asian American and Pacific Islander, Hispanic American, African American), and those with other risk factors for diabetes (eg, obesity, family history of diabetes mellitus, physical inactivity, hypertension, dyslipidemia, etc). The oral glucose tolerance test and fasting plasma glucose are both suitable screening tests, but the fasting plasma glucose is more convenient and less expensive. Ultimately, a well-articulated public health policy[58] focusing on primary prevention would be an even more compelling approach to elimination of ethnic disparities in diabetes.

▶ REFERENCES

1. American Diabetes Association. Diagnosis and classification of diabetes mellitus. *Diabetes Care* 2004;27(suppl 1):S5–S10.
2. Rosenbloom AL, Joe JR, Young RS, Winter WE. Emerging epidemic of type 2 diabetes in youth. *Diabetes Care* 1999;22:345–54.
3. American Association of Clinical Endocrinologists. *New ICD-9-CM Code for Dysmetabolic Syndrome X.* 2002. Available at: http://www.aace.com/members/socio/syndromex.php.
4. Executive Summary of The Third Report of The National Cholesterol Education Program (NCEP) Expert Panel on Detection, Evaluation, And Treatment of High Blood Cholesterol in Adults (Adult Treatment Panel III). *JAMA* 2001;285(19): 2486–2497.
5. King H, Aubert RE, Herman WH. Global burden of diabetes, 1995–2025: Prevalence, numerical estimates, and projections. *Diabetes Care* 1998;21(9):1414–1431.
6. Mokdad AH, Ford ES, Bowman BA, et al. Diabetes trends in the U.S.: 1990–1998. *Diabetes Care* 2000;23(9):1278–1283.
7. Mokdad AH, Ford ES, Bowman BA, et al. The continuing increase of diabetes in the US. *Diabetes Care* 2001;24(2):412.
8. Mokdad AH, Bowman BA, Ford ES, et al. The continuing epidemics of obesity and diabetes in the United States. *JAMA* 2001;286(10):1195–1200.
9. Dagogo-Jack S. Ethnic disparities in type 2 diabetes: Pathophysiology and implications for prevention and management. *J Natl Med Assoc* 2003; 95(9):774, 779–789.
10. Hogan P, Dall T, Nikolov P. Economic costs of diabetes in the US in 2002. *Diabetes Care* 2003; 26(3):917–932.
11. Ford ES, Giles WH, Dietz WH. Prevalence of the metabolic syndrome among US adults: Findings from the third National Health and Nutrition Examination Survey. *JAMA* 2002;287(3):356–359.
12. Harris MI, Flegal KM, Cowie CC, et al. Prevalence of diabetes, impaired fasting glucose, and impaired glucose tolerance in U.S. adults. The Third National Health and Nutrition Examination Survey, 1988–1994. *Diabetes Care* 1998;21(4):518–524.
13. Will new diagnostic criteria for diabetes mellitus change phenotype of patients with

diabetes? Reanalysis of European epidemiological data. DECODE Study Group on behalf of the European Diabetes Epidemiology Study Group. *BMJ* 1998;317(7155):371–375.

14. Qiao Q, Nakagami T, Tuomilehto J, et al. Comparison of the fasting and the 2-h glucose criteria for diabetes in different Asian cohorts. *Diabetologia* 2000;43(12):1470–1475.

15. Falkner B, Sherif K, Sumner AE, et al. Blood pressure increase with impaired glucose tolerance in young adult American blacks. *Hypertension* 1999;34(5):1086–1090.

16. Lindahl B, Weinehall L, Asplund K, et al. Screening for impaired glucose tolerance. Results from a population-based study in 21,057 individuals. *Diabetes Care* 1999;22(12):1988–1992.

17. Silver K, Shuldiner A. Candidate genes for type 2 diabetes mellitus. In LeRoith D, Taylor S, Olefsky J, eds. *Diabetes Mellitus—A Fundamental and Clinical Text,* 2nd ed. Philadelphia, Pa: Lippincott; 2000:705–719.

18. Neel JV, Weder AB, Julius S. Type II diabetes, essential hypertension, and obesity as "syndromes of impaired genetic homeostasis": The "thrifty genotype" hypothesis enters the 21st century. *Perspect Biol Med* 1998;42(1):44–74.

19. Sobal J, Stunkard AJ. Socioeconomic status and obesity: A review of the literature. *Psychol Bull* 1989;105(2):260–275.

20. Lev-Ran A. Thrifty genotype: How applicable is it to obesity and type 2 diabetes? *Diabetes Rev* 1999; 7:1–22.

21. Curtsinger JW, Service P, Prout T. Antagonistic pleiotropy, reversal of dominance, and genetic polymorphism. *Amer Naturalist* 1994;144:210–228.

22. Turner RC, Levy JC, Clark A. Complex genetics of type 2 diabetes: Thrifty genes and previously neutral polymorphisms. *Q J Med* 1993;86(7):413–417.

23. Fujimoto WY, Leonetti DL, Kinyoun JL, et al. Prevalence of diabetes mellitus and impaired glucose tolerance among second-generation Japanese-American men. *Diabetes* 1987;36(6):721–729.

24. Kimm SY, Glynn NW, Kriska AM, et al. Decline in physical activity in black girls and white girls during adolescence. *N Engl J Med* 2002;347(10):709–715.

25. Dagogo-Jack S, Santiago JV. Pathophysiology of type 2 diabetes and modes of action of therapeutic interventions. *Arch Intern Med* 1997;157(16):1802–1817.

26. Weyer C, Tataranni PA, Bogardus C, et al. Insulin resistance and insulin secretory dysfunction are independent predictors of worsening of glucose tolerance during each stage of type 2 diabetes development. *Diabetes Care* 2001;24(1):89–94.

27. Osei K, Schuster DP, Owusu SK, et al. Race and ethnicity determine serum insulin and C-peptide concentrations and hepatic insulin extraction and insulin clearance: Comparative studies of three populations of West African ancestry and white Americans. *Metabolism* 1997;46(1):53–58.

28. Haffner SM, D'Agostino R, Saad MF, et al. Increased insulin resistance and insulin secretion in nondiabetic African-Americans and Hispanics compared with non-Hispanic whites. The Insulin Resistance Atherosclerosis Study. *Diabetes* 1996;45(6):742–748.

29. Eriksson J, Franssila-Kallunki A, Ekstrand A, et al. Early metabolic defects in persons at increased risk for non-insulin-dependent diabetes mellitus. *N Engl J Med* 1989;321(6):337–343.

30. Skarfors ET, Selinus KI, Lithell HO. Risk factors for developing non-insulin dependent diabetes: A 10 year follow up of men in Uppsala. *BMJ* 1991; 303(6805):755–760.

31. Vaag A, Henriksen JE, Madsbad S, et al. Insulin secretion, insulin action, and hepatic glucose production in identical twins discordant for non-insulin-dependent diabetes mellitus. *J Clin Invest* 1995;95(2):690–698.

32. Mbanya JC, Pani LN, Mbanya DN, et al. Reduced insulin secretion in offspring of African type 2 diabetic parents. *Diabetes Care* 2000;23(12):1761–1765.

33. Tull E, Roseman J. Diabetes in African Americans. In: *Diabetes in America,* 2nd ed. Bethesda, Md: National Diabetes Data Group, National Institutes of Health; 1995:613–629. Available at: http://diabetes.niddk.nih.gov/dm/pubs/america/pdf/chapter31.pdf

34. Musey VC, Lee JK, Crawford R, et al. Diabetes in urban African-Americans. I. Cessation of insulin therapy is the major precipitating cause of diabetic ketoacidosis. *Diabetes Care* 1995;18(4):483–489.

35. Nathan DM. Long-term complications of diabetes mellitus. *N Engl J Med* 1993;328(23):1676–1685.

36. Laditka SB, Mastanduno MP, Laditka JN. Health care use of individuals with diabetes in an

employer-based insurance population. *Arch Intern Med* 2001;161(10):1301–1308.

37. Economic consequences of diabetes mellitus in the U.S. in 1997. American Diabetes Association. *Diabetes Care* 1998;21(2):296–309.

38. Centers for Disease Control, Division of Diabetes Translation. Diabetes Surveillance, 1980–1987 Policy Program Research, Annual Report. *DHHS9-12,* 1990.

39. Wagner EH, Sandhu N, Newton KM, et al. Effect of improved glycemic control on health care costs and utilization. *JAMA* 2001;285(2):182–189.

40. Harris MI, Klein R, Cowie CC, et al. Is the risk of diabetic retinopathy greater in non-Hispanic blacks and Mexican Americans than in non-Hispanic whites with type 2 diabetes? A U.S. population study. *Diabetes Care* 1998;21(8):1230–1235.

41. Rostand SG, Kirk KA, Rutsky EA, et al. Racial differences in the incidence of treatment for end-stage renal disease. *N Engl J Med* 1982;306(21):1276–1279.

42. Dagogo-Jack S. Preventing diabetes-related morbidity and mortality in the primary care setting. *J Natl Med Assoc* 2002;94(7):549–560.

43. Lavery LA, Ashry HR, van Houtum W, et al. Variation in the incidence and proportion of diabetes-related amputations in minorities. *Diabetes Care* 1996;19(1):48–52.

44. Intensive blood-glucose control with sulphonylureas or insulin compared with conventional treatment and risk of complications in patients with type 2 diabetes (UKPDS 33). UK Prospective Diabetes Study (UKPDS) Group. *Lancet* 1998;352(9131):837–853.

45. Haffner SM, Lehto S, Ronnemaa T, et al. Mortality from coronary heart disease in subjects with type 2 diabetes and in nondiabetic subjects with and without prior myocardial infarction. *N Engl J Med* 1998;339(4):229–234.

46. Lowe LP, Liu K, Greenland P, et al. Diabetes, asymptomatic hyperglycemia, and 22-year mortality in black and white men. The Chicago Heart Association Detection Project in Industry Study. *Diabetes Care* 1997;20(2):163–169.

47. Karter AJ, Ferrara A, Liu JY, et al. Ethnic disparities in diabetic complications in an insured population. *JAMA* 2002;287(19):2519–2527.

48. Cowie C, Harris M. Physical and metabolic characteristics of persons with diabetes. In: *Diabetes in America,* 2nd ed. Bethesda, Md: National Diabetes Data Group, National Institutes of Health; 1995:117–164. Available at: http://diabetes.niddk.nih.gov/dm/pubs/america/pdf/chapter31.pdf

49. Tofler GH, Stone PH, Muller JE, et al. Effects of gender and race on prognosis after myocardial infarction: Adverse prognosis for women, particularly black women. *J Am Coll Cardiol* 1987;9(3):473–482.

50. The Diabetes Control and Complications Trial Research Group: The effect of intensive treatment of diabetes on the development and progression of long-term complications in insulin-dependent diabetes mellitus. *N Engl J Med* 1993;329:978–986.

51. Harris MI, Klein R, Cowie CC, et al. Is the risk of diabetic retinopathy greater in non-Hispanic blacks and Mexican Americans than in non-Hispanic whites with type 2 diabetes? A U.S. population study. *Diabetes Care* 1998;21(8):1230–1235.

52. Martin TL, Selby JV, Zhang D. Physician and patient prevention practices in NIDDM in a large urban managed-care organization. *Diabetes Care* 1995;18(8):1124–1132.

53. Wisdom K, Fryzek JP, Havstad SL, et al. Comparison of laboratory test frequency and test results between African-Americans and Caucasians with diabetes: Opportunity for improvement. Findings from a large urban health maintenance organization. *Diabetes Care* 1997;20(6):971–977.

54. Cowie CC, Harris MI. Ambulatory medical care for non-Hispanic whites, African-Americans, and Mexican-Americans with NIDDM in the U.S. *Diabetes Care* 1997;20(2):142–147.

55. Jencks SF, Cuerdon T, Burwen DR, et al. Quality of medical care delivered to Medicare beneficiaries: A profile at state and national levels. *JAMA* 2000;284(13):1670–1676.

56. Harris MI. Racial and ethnic differences in health care access and health outcomes for adults with type 2 diabetes. *Diabetes Care* 2001;24(3):454–459.

57. Diabetes Prevention Program Research Group. Reduction in the incidence of type 2 diabetes with lifestyle intervention or metformin. *N Engl J Med* 2002;346:393–403.

58. Steinbrook R. Disparities in health care—from politics to policy. *N Engl J Med* 2004;350(15):1486–1488.

CHAPTER 9

Oncology

OTIS W. BRAWLEY, MD
SUSAN G. MOORE, MD, MPH

▶ INTRODUCTION

Population studies demonstrate tremendous disparities among populations in cancer incidence, mortality, and survival. Narrowing and eliminating these disparities is a significant challenge in cancer prevention and control. Study of the variation in cancer rates among populations provides clues to the causes, risk factors, and forces that influence the development and progression of cancer as well as the interventions necessary to control the disease and decrease the disparities.

Cancer Rates in Populations

Cancer incidence and mortality rates in the United States are published annually by the National Cancer Institute's Surveillance Epidemiology and End Results (SEER) Program and the Center for Disease Control and Prevention's National Center for Health Statistics.[1] US incidence and mortality rates for selected cancers are shown in Table 9–1.

The accuracy of incidence and mortality rates for some smaller racial and ethnic groups must be interpreted with extreme caution. These rates are less precise than rates in larger populations such as blacks and whites. For smaller populations, rates are frequently averaged over

5 years to provide more reliable data. As a result, rates for Hispanic and Native American populations are especially nebulous.

Overall cancer incidence and mortality rates are higher in men than in women. Among Americans, black men have the highest overall cancer rates and non-Hispanic white men the second highest. The major causes of cancer death among American men are from cancers of the lung, prostate, colon, and rectum. Among women, racial and ethnic disparities are not as extreme as among men. Among US women, cancers of the lung, breast, colon, and rectum are major causes of cancer death. Worldwide, cancer of the liver, stomach, lung, and cervix are leading causes of death among many populations.

▶ POPULATION CATEGORIES

In health statistics, populations are frequently described by race or ethnicity, although both terms are not well understood and frequently misused. Race and ethnicity is not a scientific categorization, but a categorization of population based on sociopolitical considerations. This must be taken into account when interpreting cancer data. Another interesting way to assess cancer statistics is by socioeconomic status (SES).

▶ **TABLE 9–1.** Annualized Cancer Incidence and Mortality Rates Obtained by Averaging 1997–2001 Data[a]

Disease	All	NH White	Black	API	AI/AN	Hisp
US Female Cancer Incidence Rates						
Brain and nervous system	5.3	6.2	3.4	2.7	2.3	4.6
Breast	135.2	149.9	119.9	96.8	54.2	89.6
Cervix	9.3	7.3	11.8	9.5	6.0	16.2
Colon and rectum	46.4	47.2	56.5	38.6	32.7	32.5
Corpus and uterus, NOS	24.5	27.1	18.2	17.2	10.2	16.8
Esophagus	2.0	2.0	3.8	1.1	0.0	1.2
Hodgkin lymphoma	2.4	2.9	2.0	1.0	0.0	2.0
Kidney and renal pelvis	7.8	7.8	9.4	4.3	7.0	8.2
Larynx	1.4	1.5	2.4	0.5	0.0	0.9
Leukemia	9.4	9.7	7.9	5.9	4.5	7.6
Liver and intrahepatic bile duct	3.5	2.4	3.9	7.7	4.8	5.8
Lung and bronchus	49.1	53.4	54.5	28.5	23.4	23.9
Melanoma of the skin	13.8	19.5	0.7	1.5	0.0	4.5
Myeloma	4.6	4.1	9.8	3.0	3.4	4.4
Non-Hodgkin lymphoma	15.7	16.9	11.7	11.4	7.7	13.5
Oral cavity and pharynx	6.4	6.7	6.2	5.8	3.8	3.9
Ovary	13.9	15.3	10.1	10.3	9.0	11.4
Pancreas	9.7	9.2	13.9	8.6	8.4	9.4
Stomach	6.1	4.1	9.9	12.4	8.9	10.0
Thyroid	10.4	11.2	5.7	11.8	6.3	9.9
Urinary bladder	9.1	10.2	7.7	4.5	0.0	5.0
US Female Cancer Mortality Rates						
Brain and nervous system	3.8	4.2	2.3	1.5	1.8	2.5
Breast	27.0	26.7	35.4	12.6	13.6	17.3
Cervix	2.9	2.5	5.6	2.8	2.8	3.6
Colon and rectum	17.7	17.2	24.5	10.8	11.7	11.6
Corpus and uterus, NOS	4.1	3.8	6.9	2.1	2.3	3.2
Esophagus	1.8	1.7	3.2	1.0	1.4	1.0
Hodgkin lymphoma	0.4	0.4	0.3	0.2	0.0	0.4
Kidney and renal pelvis	2.8	2.9	2.7	1.3	3.2	2.4
Larynx	0.5	0.5	0.9	0.1	0.0	0.2
Leukemia	5.9	6.1	5.4	3.3	3.1	4.3
Liver and intrahepatic bile duct	2.9	2.6	3.8	6.6	4.3	5.1
Lung and bronchus	40.8	43.3	39.9	19.2	26.6	14.9
Melanoma of the skin	1.8	2.1	0.5	0.3	0.0	0.6
Myeloma	3.2	2.9	6.6	1.6	2.7	2.8
Non-Hodgkin lymphoma	6.9	7.2	4.6	4.1	4.4	5.3
Oral cavity and pharynx	1.6	1.7	2.0	1.3	1.1	0.9
Ovary	8.9	9.3	7.5	4.6	4.9	6.1
Pancreas	9.2	8.9	12.8	6.6	5.9	7.5
Stomach	3.3	2.6	6.3	7.0	4.1	5.3
Thyroid	0.5	0.4	0.5	0.8	0.0	0.7
Urinary bladder	2.3	2.3	2.9	1.0	1.0	1.3

► **TABLE 9–1.** (*Continued*)

Disease	All	NH White	Black	API	AI/AN	Hisp
US Male Cancer Incidence Rates						
Brain and nervous system	7.6	9.0	4.6	4.0	3.0	5.8
Colon and rectum	63.4	63.8	72.9	56.3	38.3	49.6
Esophagus	7.7	7.9	10.6	5.1	4.9	6.0
Hodgkin lymphoma	3.0	3.4	2.9	1.2	0.0	3.1
Kidney and renal pelvis	15.7	16.0	18.8	8.9	13.9	15.1
Larynx	6.7	6.5	12.1	3.4	0.0	5.4
Leukemia	15.9	17.0	12.8	9.6	5.6	11.4
Liver and intrahepatic bile duct	9.1	6.2	11.8	21.1	8.3	13.5
Lung and bronchus	79.1	79.1	117.2	60.5	46.0	45.2
Melanoma of the skin	21.4	28.4	1.5	1.7	0.0	4.4
Myeloma	6.9	6.7	12.9	4.1	0.0	6.0
Non-Hodgkin lymphoma	23.3	25.1	18.3	16.7	9.7	18.5
Oral cavity and pharynx	15.7	16.3	19.5	12.2	10.7	9.6
Pancreas	12.6	12.5	17.1	10.2	8.3	10.4
Prostate	172.3	166.7	271.3	100.7	51.2	140.0
Stomach	12.6	9.7	18.8	21.9	15.7	17.8
Testis	5.2	7.0	1.5	2.1	2.3	3.6
Thyroid	3.8	4.2	2.2	3.9	0.0	2.9
Urinary bladder	36.1	41.3	20.4	16.3	9.5	18.6
US Male Cancer Mortality Rates						
Brain and nervous system	5.6	6.3	3.3	2.3	2.7	3.6
Colon and rectum	25.3	24.8	34.3	15.8	17.1	18.0
Esophagus	7.7	7.6	11.7	3.5	4.8	4.4
Hodgkin lymphoma	0.6	0.6	0.6	0.2	0.0	0.7
Kidney and renal pelvis	6.1	6.3	6.3	2.8	6.8	5.5
Larynx	2.6	2.3	5.4	1.0	2.4	2.2
Leukemia	10.2	10.6	9.0	5.3	4.8	6.8
Liver and intrahepatic bile duct	6.7	5.8	9.3	15.6	8.3	10.6
Lung and bronchus	77.9	79.5	104.1	40.2	49.8	39.6
Melanoma of the skin	3.9	4.7	0.5	0.4	0.8	1.1
Myeloma	4.7	4.5	9.0	2.2	3.4	3.8
Non-Hodgkin lymphoma	10.5	11.0	7.4	6.7	5.9	8.1
Oral cavity and pharynx	4.3	4.0	7.5	3.6	3.8	2.9
Pancreas	12.2	12.0	16.0	8.1	6.5	9.4
Prostate	31.5	29.1	70.4	13.0	20.2	23.5
Stomach	6.6	5.4	13.3	11.9	7.3	9.7
Testis	0.3	0.3	0.2	0.0	0.0	0.2
Thyroid	0.4	0.5	0.4	0.5	0.0	0.5
Urinary bladder	7.6	8.0	5.6	2.9	2.4	4.1

AI/AN, American Indian/Alaska Native; API, Asian or Pacific Islander; NH, non-Hispanic; NOS, not otherwise specified.

[a]Incidence rates are from the 12 surveillance epidemiology and end results registries, and mortality rates are from the United States as a whole and are provided by the National Center for Health Statistics. All rates are per 100,000, age-adjusted to the year 2000 US standard.

Race and ethnicity in the numerator of cancer data is based on information abstracted from medical records or death certificates. The US Bureau of the Census provides population counts used in the denominator such that rates can be presented per 100,000 persons. The US Office of Management and Budget (OMB), an arm of the executive branch of government, defines race and ethnicity as used in the census.[2] The OMB clearly states that its categories are social constructs and are not based on taxonomic efforts of physicians, anthropologists, or biologists. Race, as used in the OMB scheme, has no biologic basis.[3] It is important to note that science has found no genetic basis for race or racial classification. Although race is a classification scheme that is of value for social science research, inferences about cancer cause and genetics require extreme caution. Race should not be used as a scientific categorization in cancer health statistics, although it may be viewed as a surrogate to identify social and cultural subgroups whose environmental exposures may be similar.

The OMB directive recognizes "Hispanic" as an ethnicity. These are "Spanish speaking people from North, South, and Central America." In the most recent OMB directive, Hispanics can also classify themselves as "Black," "White," or "Native American." Most data is still published using the categories "Hispanic," "White Hispanic," "non-Hispanic White," and "non-Hispanic Black." The anthropology and medical sociology literature heavily link ethnicity to culture. Common threads that may tie one to an ethnic group include skin color, religion, language, customs, ancestry, and occupational or regional features.[4]

Members of an ethnic group may also be associated with common behavioral, environmental, and other extrinsic factors, which may increase or decrease the likelihood of an illness. It is useful in cancer epidemiologic research to distinguish ethnic groups from one another, provided that researchers are clear as to the nature and source of human variation (eg, cultural and behavioral patterns, lifestyle, and other environmental influences) and their relationship to disease and health outcomes. Such research,

however, can be accomplished only by clearly identifying population groups and understanding that human identity is not static or mutually exclusive.

A substantial body of literature suggests that cancer incidence and mortality are higher among persons in the lower socioeconomic strata.[5] Common socioeconomic indicators include education, household income, and occupation.[6] There is controversy over which indices most appropriately assess SES to characterize social determinants of health. The European literature uses the term *deprivation*, taking into account numerous markers of wealth and education. Variables of increased deprivation have been correlated with increased cancer mortality and worse cancer pathologies.[7,8] In Europe, health-care disparities between strata have been found to persist in an equal-access health-care system.

US SEER data have been published showing cancer mortality rates in American census tracts in which less than 10% of residents live in households with incomes below the US poverty level (wealthier areas),[10] 10% to 19.9% of persons live in households below the poverty level (intermediate), and 20% of residents or more live below the poverty level.[9,10] Cancer mortality rates are consistently higher in counties in which more than 20% of residents live below the poverty level (poor areas). When using SES indices, the disparity in cancer incidence and mortality is greater among men than women. These effects are true for almost all cancers in almost all races or ethnicities (Fig. 9–1).

▶ ETIOLOGY OF CANCER

The causes of cancer are genetic (intrinsic to the individual), environmental (extrinsic forces on the individual), or both.[11] Indeed, most cancers are due to both factors, or so-called gene-environment interaction. Although there has been tremendous interest in US society concerning genetics and race, the relationship among race, ethnicity, socioeconomic status, and environment leading to cancer is less well

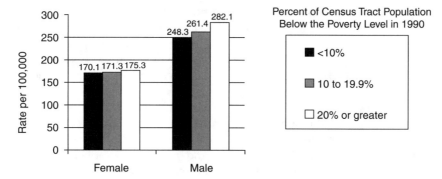

Figure 9–1. Cancer incidence by census tract poverty rate, 1996–1999. (*Data from Singh GK, Miller BA, et al.* Area Socioeconomic Variations in U.S. Cancer Incidence, Mortality, Stage Treatment, and Survival, 1975–1999. *NCI Cancer Surveillance Monograph Series No. 4. Bethesda, Md: National Cancer Institute; 2003. NIH Publication No. 03-5417.*)

appreciated, but truly more important. Race, ethnicity, and socioeconomics are correlated with a number of environmental influences that cause cancer, cause a delay in diagnosis of cancer, or cause a patient to receive less than optimal treatment.

Race, Genetics, and Cancer

Biologic and especially phenotypic differences clearly exist among the racial groups as commonly defined in the United States; however, these differences usually track poorly with genetics. Indeed, genetic variation within a race is greater than that between races.[12]

Several genetic mutations have been linked to cancer. The prevalence of a specific genetic mutation can be higher in a specific population or specific racial group, but that population is unlikely to monopolize the mutation.[13] A specific gene or series of genes can be conserved among families. Most genetic differences that have been correlated or associated with race should be considered familial and not racial. A closed society will conserve genetic traits within that society. Segregation on the basis of race, ethnicity, economics, or other factors can lead to increased prevalence of a specific gene or series of genes in the segregated population. This phenomenon has been demonstrated in non-

malignant diseases such as Tay-Sachs disease, cystic fibrosis, and sickle cell disease.[14,15] Each of these diseases has a higher prevalence in, but is not exclusive to, a specific racial or ethnic group. As the United States becomes more interracial, these genetic differences will lessen.[16]

Certain mutations of the *BRCA1* and *BRCA2* genes have been associated with an increased risk of breast cancer.[17–20] Although these mutations of *BRCA1* and *BRCA2* have been found in women of all races, several distinct mutations are common, but not exclusive, to people who identify themselves as Ashkenazi Jews. These mutations are likely common among Jewish families due to ethnic segregation among families. Indeed, genetic epidemiologists link one specific *BRCA* mutation found in Ashkenazi Jews (185delAG) to one woman who is believed to have lived about AD 800.

There are genetic differences in how a specific individual metabolizes drugs (pharmacogenetics).[21] The prevalence or activity of a specific enzyme will differ in defined groups or populations versus others, however the group is defined. These prevalences are familial and sometimes track with ethnicity or race as a result of genetic segregation. Genetic differences in drug metabolism also correlate with differences in metabolism of environmental toxins, rendering them more or less carcinogenic. There is a growing body of literature, for example, on genetic differences in cytochrome enzyme phenotypes that may correlate with an increased or decreased risk for development of cancer.[22–24]

Environment and Cancer

There are nutritional, social, cultural, and behavioral factors that lead to environmental stimuli of cancer. Important knowledge about the environmental influences on the etiology of cancers has been gained through studies of similar populations with differing environmental stimuli. Culture and ethnicity may influence cancer risk through diet, which is an environmental stimulus.

Prentice et al[25] studied the incidence of breast cancer in 21 countries and found a 5.5-fold increase in breast cancer incidence in countries with the highest fat intake (45% of daily caloric intake) compared with those with the lowest fat intake (15% of daily caloric intake). When Italian immigrants to Australia were studied, it was found that those who adopted the regional high-fat diet doubled their age-adjusted breast cancer mortality rates over a nearly 20-year period, nearly equaling the Australian rates.[26] In immigration studies done before the prostate-specific antigen (PSA) screening era, Japanese immigrants to the United States were shown to have a marked increase in prostate cancer, although the rates of Japanese Americans are still less than those of whites.[27] Similarly, although prostate cancer incidence rates are very low in Eastern Europe and Russia, Polish immigrants to the United States acquire significantly higher rates upon migration. Population studies also suggest that there may be a genetic component to prostate cancer.

The United States is currently battling an epidemic of obesity. For sociologic reasons, this has afflicted some populations more than others. A disproportionate number of black and Native American women are obese. It has also been noted that a disproportionate number of poor women are obese. Calle et al, in a 16-year prospective study of a cohort of nearly 1 million people, found that those with a very high body mass index (BMI greater than 40 kg/m^2) had a 50% to 60% percent increased risk of cancer.[28] Gordon et al have associated increased BMI with increased stage of breast cancer and even increased histologic grade of breast cancer.[29]

Tobacco use is an environmental stimulant of several cancers. Alcohol in combination with tobacco has been linked to cancer of the head and neck and esophagus. Patterns in alcohol and tobacco use vary by economic status, social situation, and culture. The prevalence and manner of smoking varies considerably by race and ethnicity. There are also SES differences in smoking patterns. Those with lower education and lower household incomes have higher smoking rates. These SES differences can manifest as different lung cancer incidence and death rates.[30]

Some cancer differences among populations are associated with environmental factors unique to a particular geography. Indeed, some cancers once hypothesized to be due to a genetic predisposition on the part of the population in that area are now known to be due to the environment. Inhabitants of Linxian, a county in the Henan province of north-central China, have one of the highest rates of esophageal squamous cell carcinoma in the world.[31,32] Most squamous cell cancer in low-risk groups is due to alcohol and tobacco consumption. The rates in Linxian were not fully explained by the prevalence of smoking and drinking. The cause of esophageal cancer in the high-risk Linxian population is now believed to be due to high-level exposure to polycyclic aromatic hydrocarbons in the diet.[33] Similarly, the African form of Burkitt lymphoma has been correlated with the Epstein-Barr virus and is of increased prevalence in areas where malaria is endemic.[34,35]

► CONTROL OF CANCER

Cancer is best controlled by prevention through avoidance of exposures to cancer-causing agents and early detection of disease.

Early detection of disease is accomplished through encouraging subjects to recognize symptoms early and to present for medical attention. Cancer screening is often encouraged, but the reader should be aware that few screening modalities have been assessed and found to save lives. Detailed structured systematic reviews of the screening literature with recommendations are published by the US Preventive Services Task Force (*http://www.ahcpr.gov/clinic/uspstfix.htm*) and the Canadian Task Force on Preventive Health Care (*http://www.ctfphc.org*). The American Cancer Society (ACS) publishes cancer screening guidelines that are the most widely quoted in the lay literature (*http://www.cancer.org*). The recommendations of these groups are shown in Table 9–2.

The US National Cancer Institute (NCI) publishes extensive reviews of the screening literature with frequent updates (*http://cancernet.nci.nih.gov*). The NCI generally does not make screening recommendations but explicitly examines and attempts to quantify benefits and harms that can be used in an informed, shared, decision process between patient and health professional.

▶ DISPARITIES IN TREATMENT

Numerous patterns of care studies in virtually every cancer assessed have demonstrated that there are black–white differences in patterns of care.[36] That is to say that white Americans with cancer are more likely to receive optimal screening and diagnosis and, once diagnosed, optimal cancer treatment. There are some data to suggest that a proportion of these disparities in cancer care are more of a socioeconomic phenomenon than a racial phenomenon. Poor people, be they white, black, or others, are less likely to receive optimal care.[37] Discrimination based on race and on socioeconomic status are both problems within the US health-care system.[5]

There is significant evidence in most cancers to show that "equal treatment yields equal outcome and race need not be a factor in outcome," even though there are significant data to show that race is a factor in amount and quality of care received.[38,39] Even in diseases such as breast cancer, in which this mantra has been questioned, there is evidence of the influence of unequal care on the disparate outcomes.[40] It is noteworthy that the availability of adequate treatment combined with a culture that seeks that treatment eliminates the majority of the black–white disparity.

▶ DISEASE-SPECIFIC REVIEW

Breast Cancer

Racial disparities are better studied in breast cancer than in any other cancer. In this section, correlations between race, socioeconomic status, and outcomes in breast cancer are discussed. Lessons in breast cancer are likely applicable to other diseases. It is well appreciated that black Americans have poorer cancer outcomes when compared with whites.[41] Unfortunately, there are limited data for Hispanics, Asians, and Native Americans as to whether their outcomes are better or worse than those for whites.

Compared with white Americans, black Americans have a lower incidence of breast cancer, but greater mortality from it. It is accepted that as a group, a larger proportion of black women present with higher stage tumors and with more aggressive pathologies compared with whites.[42,43] These poor prognostic factors suggest differences in biology. Many observers use these facts to argue that there are racial differences in the biology of breast cancer. Some assume there are differences in the genetics predisposing to the tumors that black women develop versus those occurring in white women. Indeed, when the genetics of black and white women with breast cancer are very carefully studied, overexpression of *HER2 NEU* is

▶ **TABLE 9–2.** Screening Recommendations for Asymptomatic Normal-Risk Subjects[a]

Test or Procedure	USPSTF	CTFPHC	ACS
Sigmoidoscopy	> 50: Periodically < 50: Not recommended	Insufficient evidence	Age 50 and over: Every 3–5 years
Fecal occult blood testing	Age 50 and over: Every year	Insufficient evidence	≥ 50 Every year
Digital rectal examination	No recommendation	Poor evidence to include or exclude in men over 50	≥ 40: Every year
Prostate-specific antigen	Insufficient evidence to recommend	Recommendation against	Men ≥ 50: Every year
Pap test	Women 18–65: Every 1–3 years	Fair evidence to include in examination of sexually active women	Women with uterine cervix: Beginning 3 years after start of intercourse or by age 21; yearly for standard Pap; every 2 years with liquid test
Pelvic examination	Do not recommend; advise adnexal palpation during exam for other reasons	Not considered	Women 18–40: Every 1–3 years with Pap test Women > 40: Every year
Endometrial tissue sampling	Not considered	Not considered	At menopause if obese or a history of unopposed estrogen use
Breast self-examination	No recommendation	Insufficient evidence to make a recommendation	≥ 20: Monthly
Breast clinical examination	Women > 50: Every year	Women > 50: Every year	Women 20–40: Every 3 years Women > 40: Yearly
Mammography	Women 40–75: Every 1–2 years (labeled as fair evidence)	Women 50–69: Every year	Women ≥ 40: Every year Women ≥ 50: Every 1–2 years
Complete skin examination	Not recommended	Poor evidence to include or exclude in men > 50	Age 20–39: Every 3 years

[a] The following table is a summary of the screening procedures recommended for the general population by the US Preventive Services Task Force (USPSTF), the Candian Task Force on Preventive Health Care (CTFPHC), and the American Cancer Society (ACS). These recommendations refer to asymptomatic persons who have no risk factors, other than age or gender for the targeted condition.

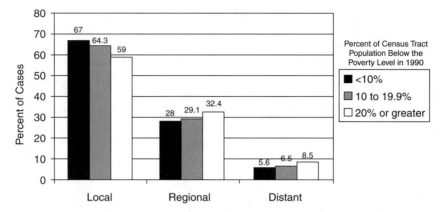

Figure 9–2. SEER female breast cancer stage by census tract poverty rate, 1995–1999. (*Data from Singh GK, Miller BA, et al.* Area Socioeconomic Variations in U.S. Cancer Incidence, Mortality, Stage Treatment, and Survival, 1975–1999. *NCI Cancer Surveillance Monograph Series No. 4. Bethesda, Md: National Cancer Institute; 2003. NIH Publication No. 03-5417.*)

comparable in blacks and whites, as are aberrations in p53 status.[44,45]

The assumption of inherent racial differences in genetics fails to take into account numerous extrinsic differences that influence breast cancer. First, black women had essentially the same breast cancer mortality rate as whites prior to 1981. The disparity in mortality has increased every year since. Race is far less important when stage and socioeconomic factors are considered.[46,47]

More is known about the risk factors for breast cancer than about risk factors for any other malignancy except lung cancer. Breast cancer risk factors are early age at onset of menarche, late age at onset of menopause, first full-term pregnancy after age 30, and history of breast cancer in a first-degree relative.[48] These are risk factors for women of all races, but they are influenced by culture and SES. For example, early-onset menarche is more common among some racial and ethnic populations and has been linked to increased caloric intake in childhood, which is influenced by culture and socioeconomics.[49] Birthing patterns are also a cultural and SES phenomena. Much of the increased breast cancer incidence found among white women compared with other popula-

tions is a "professional woman" effect. Delaying childbirth past age 30, due to career, increases risk of breast cancer. Obesity, which is again influenced by culture and SES, has also been linked to increased stage at diagnosis and worse outcome.[50] It has also been suggested that racial differences in survival may be partly explained by differences in nutritional status.[51]

SES correlates with stage of disease at diagnosis (Fig. 9–2) and may have some effect on grade of tumor at diagnosis.[29] Data suggest that both black and white American cancer patients living in census tracts with lower median education and income are diagnosed in later stages of disease than are patients in census tracts with higher median education and income values.[52] African Americans and Hispanics as a group are disproportionately poorer. Despite the consistent and strong association of social class with health status, the extent to which racial and ethnic disparities in cancer screening reflect social class is rarely addressed.[53]

In a case-control study comparing black and white women with breast cancer, Coates et al[54] demonstrated that the median time from recognition of symptoms to medical consultation was longer for black women than white women. The authors were unable to directly relate the delay in seeking treatment to increased mortality, but it is a possible contributor. Other studies suggest that delay in reporting symptoms was a significant factor in stage of disease at diagnosis and survival.[55,56]

Population-based data demonstrate that black American women have an increased risk of cancer at a younger age and an increased number of cancers with high pathologic grade. In a case-control study, adjusting for age and stage at diagnosis, Chen et al[43] found black–white differences, but also found that white women of high SES had more favorable tumor pathologies than white women of lower SES. This is highly suggestive that an extrinsic influence, perhaps diet, is causing the increasing disparity.

Others have similar findings and have shown that the question "why do poor women have a higher risk of cancer at a younger age and a higher risk of high pathologic grade disease?" is a more appropriate scientific question than "why do black women have a higher risk of cancer at a young age and a higher risk of high pathologic grade disease?"[57,58] Another important question is why do wealthier women have increased rates in older age and more low-grade disease.

Screening and Diagnosis of Breast Cancer

A number of studies demonstrate that high-quality mammography combined with high-quality assessment and treatment lowers mortality rates by 20% to 35% among women aged 50 to 70 years. Many organizations recommend a screening mammogram and breast examination performed by a health professional every 1 to 2 years for women aged 40 and older. Although it is difficult to assess disparities in quality, it is known that there are differences in mammography utilization rates by race or ethnicity and SES. In the 2000 National Health Interview survey, 71.4% of white, 67.8% of black, 47.3% of Native American, 53.3% of Asian, and 53.3% of Hispanic women surveyed said they had received a mammogram in the past 2 years. In a similar survey in 1990, 45% to 50% of women of all races said they had received a mammogram in the previous 2 years.[59] In the 2000 survey, 55.2% of women who were considered poor had a mammogram in the previous 2 years, whereas 72.2% of women categorized as near poor or nonpoor had had a mammogram. Unfortunately the accuracy of this type of survey data has not been confirmed through assessment of medical records.

Substantial scientific literature has developed concerning methods to increase minority participation in screening programs in special populations.[60] Much of the work focuses on tailoring messages such that they are culturally acceptable and educating the health educator and health care giver to be culturally competent.[61]

When assessing outcomes in breast cancer clinical trials, equal treatment yields equal outcomes regardless of race.[62,63] After adjusting for all other prognostic factors, race appears to have no independent prognostic significance in survival.

Three clinical trials[62–64] and eight case control studies[40,46,57,65–69] have focused on outcomes by race. Most of these studies look at black–white differences, and the cumulative result suggests that race is a not a biologic factor in outcomes. This is not to say that blacks as a group do not have worse outcomes than whites as a group, but rather that disproportionate stage, grade, and comorbid disease account for most of the disparities in outcomes. Black women, diagnosed at a disease stage comparable to white women and treated appropriately, tend to experience similar breast cancer prognoses and survival. In most studies reported in the literature, the primary explanatory factor alone, such as stage of disease at diagnosis, did not fully account for differences in outcome between groups; when additional factors were taken into account, however, prognoses became more similar. Results from the National Surgical Adjuvant Breast and Bowel Project clinical trials similarly indicated that when stage of disease and treatment were comparable, outcomes for blacks did not differ markedly from those for whites.

Some case series have reported black–white differences in outcome. Many of these studies have not normalized for disparities in risk factors.[62] In a retrospective review of Department of Defense (DoD) medical beneficiaries with breast cancer, black women were found to have a decrease in survival compared with whites. The 5-year mortality rate for African American women was 24.8% compared with 18.1% for white women.[40] In the US SEER registry, the 5-year mortality rate was 34.2% for black women and 18.4% for white women. These observations suggest that ready access to medical facilities and the full complement of treatment options that are standard for all DoD patients dramatically improves survival rates for African American women. The improved prognosis among women treated in the military system, while not an equalization of risk, is still clear solid evidence of the positive impact of equal access to and increased utilization of health care. Importantly, the Wojcik study did not adjust for differences in the population, such as BMI or treatment received. These types of adjustments as well as an assessment of cultural differences might have equalized risk.

At a minimum, the Wojcik results represent what can occur in the real world, suggesting that logistical issues, such as getting early detection and appropriate therapy to African American patients could result in a substantial reduction in the current disparity in breast carcinoma mortality between African Americans and whites.

Patterns of cancer care received often differ among populations categorized by race or ethnicity. For example, it has been demonstrated that black women with breast cancer are less likely to receive aggressive therapy compared with white women.[70–72] Breen et al[71] demonstrated that 21% of black women with breast cancer received less than minimum expected therapy compared with 15% of white women drawn from the same geographic area.

In a study of patients in the Detroit SEER registry, Bradley et al found that race was not statistically significantly associated with unfavorable breast cancer outcomes. However, low socioeconomic status was associated with late-stage breast cancer at diagnosis, type of treatment received, and death.[73] Similar studies have not been done on other racial and ethnic groups, but there is evidence that the message translates to all groups. A substantial effort to get appropriate high-quality care to all Americans can result in substantial saving of lives.

Melanoma

Melanoma is a disease that is caused by sun exposure, an environmental stimulus. It disproportionately affects individuals with a light complexion. Persons of African and Asian heritage are known to get melanoma. The risk factor for melanoma is not race or ethnicity, but complexion.

Lung Cancer

Lung cancer is the leading cause of cancer death among Americans. Incidence and mortality rates vary by race and ethnicity, primarily because of the cultural differences in how people smoke. There are even cultural differences in how smoke is inhaled.[74] In 2002, approximately 22.5% of all Americans were cigarette smokers: 22.4% of black Americans smoked, 23.6% of whites, 19.1% of Hispanics, and 13.7% of Asian Americans. During the period from 1983 to 2002, adults with household incomes below the poverty level and those with less than some college education consistently had higher smoking prevalence.

Black Americans tend to start smoking in their late teens and early twenties, whereas whites generally become addicted in the early to mid-teen years.[75,76] Even a relatively new smoker is at risk for lung cancer and cancers of the head and neck. A smoker's disease risk increases dramatically after more than 20 pack-years (eg, one pack per day for 20 years or two packs per day for 10 years). As the number of pack-years increases, risk of tobacco-related cancers, heart disease, and pulmonary disease also increases. The peak incidence of lung cancer is between the ages of 65 and 79 years.

Screening for lung cancer has not been proven to save lives. Currently, screening of asymptomatic individuals for lung cancer should only be done within the context of a clinical trial to prove that it is of benefit.[77] The use of spiral computerized tomography and positron emission tomography in lung cancer screening are actively being studied. A proportion of those who are diagnosed when disease is localized (usually due to symptoms) can be cured through surgical removal of the tumor.[78] In a landmark article, Bach et al[79] noted that eligible blacks are less likely to receive this therapy compared with whites. In an analysis of outcomes, equal treatment yields equal outcome.

Cancer of the Colon and Rectal Cancer

This is the second most common cause of cancer death among Americans as a whole. It is highly linked to diets low in fiber and high in fat. Diet, culture, and SES are highly correlated to the incidence of disease.

When diagnosed early, a substantial proportion of colon cancers is curable. Screening to detect blood or hemoglobin in stool has been found to save lives in randomized trials,[80,81] and screening with sigmoidoscopy has been found to save lives in case-control studies.[82] The efficacy of colonoscopy screening is the subject of a large, ongoing, randomized National Cancer Institute study begun in 1992 and expected to end around 2006.[83]

Black Americans are less likely than whites to undergo surgical resection.[84] Black and white patients who receive less-than-optimal care generally have poverty and access to poor-quality health care in common. Very little data on patterns of care are available in other racial and ethnic groups.

Prostate Cancer

The incidence of prostate cancer increased dramatically in the United States in the early 1990s

due to the availability of the serum PSA for screening.[85]

Black Americans have prostate cancer mortality rates far higher than those of whites, who have rates higher than other American populations. The reasons are largely unknown. This may be due to shared genetic or environmental influences, which includes diet. There is the suggestion that the Asian diet, which is high in soy content and low in animal fat, may prevent prostate cancer and that the American diet, high in animal fat, may encourage prostate carcinogenesis.[86] Asians migrating to the United States are at higher risk than those who remain in their native countries. Second- and third-generation Asian Americans who acculturate to the American culture have prostate cancer incidence rates near those of white Americans.

Men with a family history of the disease are clearly at higher risk.[87] Certain genetic polymorphisms (minor changes in DNA sequences) that are thought to increase prostate cancer risk have been found to predominate in some populations.[88] These populations can be defined by race or more scientifically by area of geographic origin. In a study of primarily white physicians, the number of CAG nucleotide repeats at the beginning of the gene coding for the androgen receptor was correlated with risk of prostate cancer risk.[89] Men with prostate cancer had an average of 16 repeats, whereas the average number for men who had not developed prostate cancer was 17 to 18.[89] Variation in polymorphic alleles of genes such as CAG repeats could explain a large proportion of the difference in population risk for prostate cancer. This influence of family genetics is far stronger than that of racial classification.

In a study of military beneficiaries, obese patients with prostate cancer presented for radical prostatectomy at a younger age with higher grade and more pathologically advanced cancers. Blacks have higher grade cancers than other ethnic groups and, at the same time, have significantly higher BMIs. These findings suggest that obesity is associated with progression of latent to clinically significant prostate cancer, and that BMI may account, in part, for the racial variability in prostate cancer risk.[90,91] Military medical center studies also show that socioeconomic status is associated with pathologic grade of disease. Poorer men tend to have a disproportionate share of higher grade cancers.[92] In the equal-access health-care system of the DoD, African American race is not associated with a consistently negative prognosis in patients treated with surgery or definitive radiation therapy for prostate cancer.[93,94]

Although there are legitimate questions about the effectiveness of prostate cancer screening and treatment, both screening and aggressive treatment of localized disease have become a common therapy in the United States.[95,96] Both are not proven to save lives and are the subject of great debate among prostate cancer specialists. Screening, however, clearly identifies a large proportion of men who have prostate cancer but do not need treatment.[97,98] Unfortunately, there is no reliable test to differentiate between the individual who is in need of therapy and the individual who needs to be observed. There are patterns of care studies to show that black men and uninsured men are less likely to receive aggressive therapy for the same stage of disease compared with white and middle-class patients.[96,99]

Cancer of the Head and Neck

Cancer of the nasopharynx occurs with greater frequency among Asians. Americans who have immigrated from China, Vietnam, Laos, Cambodia, and the Philippine Islands have higher rates of nasopharyngeal cancer compared with white Americans.[100,101] The cause is thought to be related to consumption of fermented foods and salted fish. Exposure to the Epstein-Barr virus and certain dust and smoke particles may also increase risk. Squamous cell carcinomas of the mouth and throat are also heavily linked to tobacco and alcohol use. The human papillomavirus has also been linked to squamous cell cancer of the head and neck.[102]

Shavers et al[103] studied head and neck cancers in the SEER populations and found racial differences in early detection and the receipt of cancer treatment. They concluded that more equitable receipt of cancer treatment combined with preventive measures and earlier detection would reduce racial and ethnic disparities in survival and mortality from cancers of the oral cavity, pharynx, and larynx.

Cancer of the Liver

Hepatocellular cancer is one of the leading causes of death in the world. This is primarily due to the very high incidences in Asia. Primary cancer of the liver accounts for only 1.5% of all cancers in the United States.[104] Nearly 70% of hepatocellular cancers are associated with hepatitis B or hepatitis C.[105] Certain types of mold and aflatoxins in stored food are risk factors for liver cancer among Africans and Asians. Individuals at risk are often screened with serum liver function tests and hepatic ultrasound. The effectiveness of screening is unproven in this disease.

Gastric Cancer

In the 1930s, gastric cancer was one of the leading causes of cancer death in the United States. Today, it is one of the five leading causes of cancer death among many Asian and Hispanic American populations. US rates have dropped due to the declining use of salted, smoked, and pickled meats and the increased use of refrigeration. These are all influences that are mediated by culture and socioeconomic status. *Helicobacter pylori* infection of the gastrium has been linked to gastric ulcers and gastric cancer.[106] *H pylori* can be treated with standard antibiotics.

Gastric reflux and scarring of the lower esophagus at the level of gastroesophageal junction has been associated with increased rates of an adenocarcinoma, which some consider gastric cancer. Screening of persons at high risk for this and classic gastric cancer is common, even though these methods have not yet been proven effective.

Cervical Cancer

Cervical cancer was once the leading cause of cancer death in American women and is still a leading cause of death in the third world.[107] Screening for cervical dysplasia with the Pap smear and treatment of abnormalities has had significant impact in the prevention of this disease. The major cause of cervical cancer is the human papillomavirus (HPV). Exposure to HPV is in some ways influenced by socioeconomic status. Cervical cancer rates are currently very high among Vietnamese American women. This is due to a lack of screening over a 10- to 20-year period. Cervical cancer rates are also higher in black and Hispanic Americans, apparently due to barriers to high-quality early detection and treatment services.[108,109]

▶ SUMMARY AND RECOMMENDATIONS

Much can be learned through the study of cancer rates among special populations. This knowledge benefits all who are at risk for the disease. These populations have been defined in political, not in scientific, terms, but it is apparent that their cancer rates are influenced by numerous extrinsic factors. The full effect of these disparities in treatment on mortality is unknown.

Although much of the data on health disparities focuses on black–white differences, there is evidence that SES plays a key role in cancer risk and in quality of health-care received. In terms of race, there are studies showing that equal treatment yields equal outcome in prostate, colon, and lung cancer. There are studies suggesting that much of the breast cancer disparity would not exist if there was equal treat-

▶ **TABLE 9–3.** Summary of Major Findings Regarding Health Disparities in Cancer Rates

- US cancer demographic data for black and white populations is of good quality
- Data for Native Americans, Asian, and Hispanic populations is less reliable
- Major cancers in all racial and ethnic groups are cancers of the lung, breast, and colon

ment. There are also studies that show racially defined differences in patterns of care for breast cancer, colon cancer,[110] prostate cancer,[99] lung cancer,[79,111] and cancer of the cervix, with blacks disproportionately receiving less-aggressive or less-preferred therapies than whites.

The reasons for these disparities in cancer care are active areas for research. Some studies suggest that among patients, cultural differences in the acceptance of a disease and its resultant

▶ **TABLE 9–4.** Summary of Recommendations

- Race or ethnicity need not be a factor in cancer treatment outcome
- Equal cancer treatment yields equal outcome
- There is not equal treatment among the races
- Studies demonstrate that the poor and ethnic minorities are more likely to receive less-than-optimal care because of:
  - Cultural differences in acceptance of therapy
  - Disparities in comorbid diseases among population groups, making aggressive therapy inappropriate
  - Lack of access to therapy
  - Racism and SES discrimination
- Patient compliance can be increased by staff attention to:
  - Patient education regarding the disease and treatment
  - Patient financial needs
  - Logistical considerations such as transportation
  - And, most of all, demonstrating care and respect for the patient

treatment are important.[56] In other cases, treatment disparities may be due to disparities in comorbid diseases that make aggressive therapy inappropriate.[112,113] Socioeconomic barriers such as lack of insurance, lack of access to treatment, and discrimination can also be contributing factors to these health disparities.[114] Unfortunately, few studies of practice patterns have been done in populations other than blacks and whites. There is, however, evidence to show that many of these disparities are due to socioeconomic barriers that are also prevalent elsewhere, especially among Hispanic, Native American, and some Asian populations. Very solid case-control studies demonstrate an association between lower SES and worse pathologic grade in breast and prostate cancers, and several studies demonstrate a correlation with increasing BMI and worse histologic grade.[29,91,92] Important work still needs to be done to discern the full influence of socioeconomic status on tumor behavior (stage and pathology). Table 9–3 summarizes key findings from this chapter. Recommendations for the future are outlined in Table 9–4.

► REFERENCES

1. SEER Cancer Statistics Review, 1973–1999; 2002. Available at: http://seer.cancer.gov/csr/1973_1999/.

2. Recommendations from the Interagency Committee for the Review of the Racial and Ethnic Standards to the Office of Management and Budget Concerning Changes to the Standards for the Classification of Federal Data on Race and Ethnicity (Directive 15). 1997;62(131): 36873–36946. 131-369466.

3. Witzig R. The medicalization of race: Scientific legitimization of a flawed social construct. *Ann Intern Med* 1996;125(8):675–679.

4. American Anthropological Association. *AAA Response to OMB Directive 15; Race and Ethnic Standards for Federal Statistics and Administrative Reporting.* AAA; 1997.

5. Freeman H. Race, poverty, and cancer. *J Natl Cancer Inst* 1991;83(8):526–527.

6. Adler NE, Boyce T, Chesney MA, et al. Socioeconomic status and health. The challenge of the gradient. *Am Psychol* 1994;49(1):15–24.

7. Taylor A, Cheng KK. Social deprivation and breast cancer. *J Public Health Med* 2003;25(3): 228–233.

8. Whynes DK, Frew EJ, Manghan CM, et al. Colorectal cancer, screening and survival: The influence of socio-economic deprivation. *Public Health* 2003;117(6):389–395.

9. Ward E, Jemal A, Cokkinides V, et al. Cancer disparities by race/ethnicity and socioeconomic status. *CA Cancer J Clin* 2004;54(2):78–93.

10. Singh GK. Area deprivation and widening inequalities in US mortality, 1969–1998. *Am J Public Health* 2003;93(7):1137–1143.

11. Doll R, Peto R. The causes of cancer: Quantitative estimates of avoidable risks of cancer in the United States today. *J Natl Cancer Inst* 1981; 66(6):1191–1308.

12. Freeman HP. The meaning of race in science—considerations for cancer research: Concerns of special populations in the National Cancer Program. *Cancer* 1998;82(1):219–225.

13. Liu ET. The uncoupling of race and cancer genetics. *Cancer* 1998;83:1765–1769.

14. Kelly TE, Chase GA, Kaback MM, et al. Tay-Sachs disease: High gene frequency in a non-Jewish population. *Am J Hum Genet* 1975;27(3): 287–291.

15. Trabuchet G, Elion J, Baudot G, et al. Origin and spread of beta-globin gene mutations in India, Africa, and Mediterranea: Analysis of the 5′ flanking and intragenic sequences of beta S and beta C genes. *Hum Biol* 1991;63(3): 241–252.

16. Parra EJ, Marcini A, Akey J, et al. Estimating African American admixture proportions by use of population-specific alleles. *Am J Hum Genet* 1998;63(6):1839–1851.

17. Newman B, Mu H, Butler LM, et al. Frequency of breast cancer attributable to *BRCA1* in a population-based series of American women. *JAMA* 1998;279(12):915–921.

18. Offit K, Gilewski T, McGuire P, et al. Germline BRCA1 185delAG mutations in Jewish women with breast cancer. *Lancet* 1996; 347(9016):1643–1645.

19. Robson M, Gilewski T, Haas B, et al. BRCA-associated breast cancer in young women. *J Clin Oncol* 1998;16(5):1642–1649.

20. Struewing JP, Hartge P, Wacholder S, et al. The risk of cancer associated with specific mutations of BRCA1 and BRCA2 among Ashkenazi Jews. *N Engl J Med* 1997;336(20):1401–1408.

21. Flaws JA, Bush TL. Racial differences in drug metabolism: An explanation for higher breast cancer mortality in blacks? *Med Hypotheses* 1998; 50(4):327–329.

22. Bouchardy C, Mitrunen K, Wikman H, et al. *N*-acetyltransferase NAT1 and NAT2 genotypes and lung cancer risk. *Pharmacogenetics* 1998; 8(4):291–298.

23. Ishibe N, Wiencke JK, Zuo ZF, et al. Susceptibility to lung cancer in light smokers associated with CYP1A1 polymorphisms in Mexican- and African-Americans. *Cancer Epidemiol Biomarkers Prev* 1997;6(12):1075–1080.

24. Wu X, Amos CI, Kemp BL, et al. Cytochrome P450 2E1 DraI polymorphisms in lung cancer in minority populations. *Cancer Epidemiol Biomarkers Prev* 1998;7(1):13–18.

25. Prentice RL, Sheppard L. Validity of international, time trend, and migrant studies of dietary factors and disease risk. *Prev Med* 1989;18(2): 167–179.

26. Margetts BM, Hopkins SM, Binns CW. Nutrient intakes in Italian migrants and Australians in Perth. *Food Nutrition* 1981;38:7–10.

27. Haenszel W, Kurihara M. Studies of Japanese migrants. I. Mortality from cancer and other diseases among Japanese in the United States. *J Natl Cancer Inst* 1968;40(1):43–68.

28. Calle EE, Rodriguez C, Walker-Thurmond K, et al. Overweight, obesity, and mortality from cancer in a prospectively studied cohort of U.S. adults. *N Engl J Med* 2003;348:1625–1638.

29. Gordon NH. Association of education and income with estrogen receptor status in primary breast cancer. *Am J Epidemiol* 1995;142:796–803.

30. Cigarette smoking among adults—United States, 2002. *MMWR Morb Mortal Wkly Rep* 2004;53: 427–431.

31. Blot WJ, Li JY, Taylor PR, et al. The Linxian trials: Mortality rates by vitamin–mineral intervention group. *Am J Clin Nutr* 1995;62:1424S–1426S.

32. Taylor PR, Wang GQ, Dawsey SM, et al. Effect of nutrition intervention on intermediate endpoints in esophageal and gastric carcinogenesis. *Am J Clin Nutr* 1995;62:1420S–1423S.

33. Roth MJ, Strickland KL, Wang GQ, et al. High levels of carcinogenic polycyclic aromatic hydrocarbons present within food from Linxian, China may contribute to that region's high incidence of oesophageal cancer [letter]. *Eur J Cancer* 1998;34:757–758.

34. Araujo I, Foss HD, Bittencourt A, et al. Expression of Epstein-Barr virus-gene products in Burkitt's lymphoma in Northeast Brazil [see comments]. *Blood* 1996;87:5279–5286.

35. Morrow RH. Epidemiological evidence for the role of falciparum malaria in the pathogenesis of Burkitt's lymphoma. *IARC Sci Publ* 1985;177–186.

36. Shavers VL, Brown ML. Racial and ethnic disparities in the receipt of cancer treatment. *J Natl Cancer Inst* 2002;94:334–357.

37. Ball JK, Elixhauser A. Treatment differences between blacks and whites with colorectal cancer. *Med Care* 1996;34:970–984.

38. Brawley OW, Freeman HP. Race and outcomes: Is this the end of the beginning for minority health research? *J Natl Cancer Inst* 1999; 91:1908–1909.

39. Bach PB, Schrag D, Brawley OW, et al. Survival of blacks and whites after a cancer diagnosis. *JAMA* 2002;287:2106–2113.

40. Wojcik BE, Spinks MK, Optenberg SA. Breast carcinoma survival analysis for African American and white women in an equal-access health care system. *Cancer* 1998;82:1310–1318.

41. Wingo PA, Ries LA, Parker SL, et al. Long-term cancer patient survival in the United States [see comments]. *Cancer Epidemiol Biomarkers Prev* 1998;7:271–282.

42. Lyman GH, Kuderer NM, Lyman SL, et al. Importance of race on breast cancer survival. *Ann Surg Oncol* 1997;4:80–87.

43. Chen VW, Correa P, Kurman RJ, et al. Histological characteristics of breast carcinoma in blacks and whites. *Cancer Epidemiol Biomarkers Prev* 1994;3:127–135.

44. Elledge RM, Clark GM, Chamness GC, et al. Tumor biologic factors and breast cancer prognosis among white, Hispanic, and black women in the United States [see comments]. *J Natl Cancer Inst* 1994;86:705–712.

45. Krieger N, Van Den Eeden SK, Zava D, et al. Race/ethnicity, social class, and prevalence of breast cancer prognostic biomarkers: A study of white, black, and Asian women in the

San Francisco bay area. *Ethn Dis* 1997;7:137–149.

46. Perkins P, Cooksley CD, Cox JD. Breast cancer. Is ethnicity an independent prognostic factor for survival? *Cancer* 1996;78:1241–1247.

47. Eley JW, Hill HA, Chen VW, et al. Racial differences in survival from breast cancer. Results of the National Cancer Institute Black/White Cancer Survival Study [see comments]. *JAMA* 1994;272:947–954.

48. Gail MH, Brinton LA, Byar DP, et al. Projecting individualized probabilities of developing breast cancer for white females who are being examined annually [see comments]. *J Natl Cancer Inst* 1989;81:1879–1886.

49. Britton JA, Wolff MS, Lapinski R, et al. Characteristics of pubertal development in a multi-ethnic population of nine-year-old girls. *Ann Epidemiol* 2004;14:179–187.

50. Jones BA, Kasi SV, Curnen MG, et al. Severe obesity as an explanatory factor for the black/white difference in stage at diagnosis of breast cancer. *Am J Epidemiol* 1997;146:394–404.

51. Coates RJ, Clark WS, Eley JW, et al. Race, nutritional status, and survival from breast cancer. *J Natl Cancer Inst* 1990;82:1684–1692.

52. Wells BL, Horm JW. Stage at diagnosis in breast cancer: Race and socioeconomic factors. *Am J Public Health* 1992;82:1383–1385.

53. Hoffman-Goetz L, Breen NL, Meissner H. The impact of social class on the use of cancer screening within three racial/ethnic groups in the United States. *Ethn Dis* 1998;8:43–51.

54. Coates RJ, Bransfield DD, Wesley M, et al. Differences between black and white women with breast cancer in time from symptom recognition to medical consultation. Black/White Cancer Survival Study Group. *J Natl Cancer Inst* 1992;84:938–950.

55. Howard DL, Penchansky R, Brown MB. Disaggregating the effects of race on breast cancer survival. *Fam Med* 1998;30:228–235.

56. Lannin DR, Mathews HF, Mitchell J, et al. Influence of socioeconomic and cultural factors on racial differences in late-stage presentation of breast cancer. *JAMA* 1998;279:1801–1807.

57. Gordon NH, Crowe JP, Brumberg DJ, et al. Socioeconomic factors and race in breast cancer recurrence and survival. *Am J Epidemiol* 1992;135:609–618.

58. Taylor A, Cheng KK. Social deprivation and breast cancer. *J Public Health Med* 2003;25:228–233.

59. Swan J, Breen N, Coates RJ, et al. Progress in cancer screening practices in the United States: Results from the 2000 National Health Interview Survey. *Cancer* 2003;97:1528–1540.

60. Meissner HI, Breen N, Coyne C, et al. Breast and cervical cancer screening interventions: An assessment of the literature. *Cancer Epidemiol Biomarkers Prev* 1998;7:951–961.

61. Rimer BK, Glassman B. Tailoring communications for primary care settings. *Methods Inf Med* 1998;37:171–177.

62. Roach M, Cirrincione C, Budman D, et al. Race and survival from breast cancer: Based on Cancer and Leukemia Group B trial 8541 [see comments]. *Cancer J Sci Am* 1997;3:107–112.

63. Dignam JJ. Differences in breast cancer prognosis among African-American and Caucasian women. *CA Cancer J Clin* 2000;50:50–64.

64. Dignam JJ, Redmond CK, Fisher B, et al. Prognosis among African-American women and white women with lymph node negative breast carcinoma: Findings from two randomized clinical trials of the National Surgical Adjuvant Breast and Bowel Project (NSABP). *Cancer* 1997;80:80–90.

65. Heimann R, Ferguson D, Powers C, et al. Race and clinical outcome in breast cancer in a series with long-term follow-up evaluation. *J Clin Oncol* 1997;15:2329–2337.

66. Franzini L, Williams AF, Franklin J, et al. Effects of race and socioeconomic status on survival of 1,332 black, Hispanic, and white women with breast cancer [see comments]. *Ann Surg Oncol* 1997;4:111–118.

67. Nomura AM, Marchand LL, Kolonel LN, et al. The effect of dietary fat on breast cancer survival among Caucasian and Japanese women in Hawaii. *Breast Cancer Res Treat* 1991;18(suppl 1):S135–S141.

68. Yood MU, Johnson CC, Blount A, et al. Race and differences in breast cancer survival in a managed care population. *J Natl Cancer Inst* 1999;91:1487–1491.

69. McWhorter WP, Mayer WJ. Black/white differences in type of initial breast cancer treatment and implications for survival. *Am J Public Health* 1987;77:1515–1517.

70. Diehr P, Yergan J, Chu J, et al. Treatment modality and quality differences for black and white breast-cancer patients treated in community hospitals. *Med Care* 1989;27:942–958.

71. Breen N, Wesley MN, Merrill RM, et al. The relationship of socio-economic status and access to minimum expected therapy among female breast cancer patients in the National Cancer Institute Black-White Cancer Survival Study. *Ethn Dis* 1999;9:111–125.

72. Brawley OW, Freeman HP. Race and outcomes: Is this the end of the beginning for minority health research? *J Natl Cancer Inst* 1999; 91:1908–1909.

73. Bradley CJ, Given CW, Roberts C. Race, socioeconomic status, and breast cancer treatment and survival. *J Natl Cancer Inst* 2002;94:490–496.

74. Vineis P, Alavanja M, Buffler P, et al. Tobacco and cancer: Recent epidemiological evidence. *J Natl Cancer Inst* 2004;96:99–106.

75. Flint AJ, Yamada EG, Novotny TE. Black-white differences in cigarette smoking uptake: Progression from adolescent experimentation to regular use. *Prev Med* 1998;27:358–364.

76. Griesler PC, Kandel DB. Ethnic differences in correlates of adolescent cigarette smoking. *J Adolesc Health* 1998;23:167–180.

77. Preventive Services. *Guide to Clinical Preventive Services: Report of the U.S. Preventive Services Task Force;* 1996.

78. Eddy DM. Screening for lung cancer [see comments]. *Ann Intern Med* 1989;111:232–237.

79. Bach PB, Cramer LD, Warren JL, et al. Racial differences in the treatment of early-stage lung cancer [see comments]. *N Engl J Med* 1999;341: 1198–1205.

80. Ransohoff DF, Lang CA. Screening for colorectal cancer with the fecal occult blood test: A background paper. American College of Physicians [see comments]. *Ann Intern Med* 1997;126: 811–822.

81. Mandel JS, Bond JH, Church TR, et al. Reducing mortality from colorectal cancer by screening for fecal occult blood. Minnesota Colon Cancer Control Study [published erratum appears in N Engl J Med 1993;329(9):672] [see comments]. *N Engl J Med* 1993;328:1365–1371.

82. Newcomb PA, Norfleet RG, Storer BE, et al. Screening sigmoidoscopy and colorectal cancer mortality [see comments]. *J Natl Cancer Inst* 1992;84:1572–1575.

83. Kramer BS, Gohagan J, Prorok PC, et al. A National Cancer Institute sponsored screening trial for prostatic, lung, colorectal, and ovarian cancers. *Cancer* 1993;71:589–593.

84. Cooper GS, Yuan Z, Rimm AA. Racial disparity in the incidence and case-fatality of colorectal cancer: Analysis of 329 United States counties. *Cancer Epidemiol Biomarkers Prev* 1997;6:283–285.

85. Potosky AL, Miller BA, Albertsen PC, et al. The role of increasing detection in the rising incidence of prostate cancer. *JAMA* 1995;273: 548–552.

86. Kolonel LN, Nomura AM, Cooney RV. Dietary fat and prostate cancer: Current status. *J Natl Cancer Inst* 1999;91:414–428.

87. Whittemore AS, Wu AH, Kolonel LN, et al. Family history and prostate cancer risk in black, white, and Asian men in the United States and Canada. *Am J Epidemiol* 1995;141:732–740.

88. Shibata A, Whittemore AS. Genetic predisposition to prostate cancer: Possible explanations for ethnic differences in risk. *Prostate* 1997;32:65–72.

89. Kantoff P, Giovannucci E, Brown M. The androgen receptor CAG repeat polymorphism and its relationship to prostate cancer. *Biochim Biophys Acta* 1998;1378:C1–C5.

90. Amling CL, Riffenburgh RH, Sun L, et al. Pathologic variables and recurrence rates as related to obesity and race in men with prostate cancer undergoing radical prostatectomy. *J Clin Oncol* 2004;22:439–445.

91. Amling CL, Kane CJ, Riffenburgh RH, et al. Relationship between obesity and race in predicting adverse pathologic variables in patients undergoing radical prostatectomy. *Urology* 2001; 58:723–728.

92. Tarman GJ, Kane CJ, Moul JW, et al. Impact of socioeconomic status and race on clinical parameters of patients undergoing radical prostatectomy in an equal access health care system. *Urology* 2000;56:1016–1020.

93. Optenberg SA, Thompson IM, Friedrichs P, et al. Race, treatment, and long-term survival from prostate cancer in an equal-access medical care delivery system. *JAMA* 1995;274:1599–1605.

94. Johnstone PA, Kane CJ, Sun L, et al. Effect of race on biochemical disease-free outcome in patients with prostate cancer treated with definitive radiation therapy in an equal-access health care system: Radiation oncology

report of the Department of Defense Center for Prostate Disease Research. *Radiology* 2002; 225:420–426.

95. Middleton RG, Thompson IM, Austenfeld MS, et al. Prostate Cancer Clinical Guidelines Panel summary report on the management of clinically localized prostate cancer. *J Urol* 1995;154: 2144–2148.

96. Harlan LC, Potosky A, Gilliland FD, et al. Factors associated with initial therapy for clinically localized prostate cancer: Prostate cancer outcomes study. *J Natl Cancer Inst* 2001;93:1864–1871.

97. Thompson IM. Counseling patients with newly diagnosed prostate cancer. *Oncology (Huntingt)* 2000;14:119–126,131.

98. Thompson IM, Pauler DK, Goodman PJ, et al. Prevalence of prostate cancer among men with a prostate-specific antigen level < or = 4.0 ng per milliliter. *N Engl J Med* 2004;350:2239–2246.

99. Klabunde CN, Potosky AL, Harlan LC, et al. Trends and black/white differences in treatment for nonmetastatic prostate cancer. *Med Care* 1998;36:1337–1348.

100. Tsai ST, Jin YT, Mann RB, et al. Epstein-Barr virus detection in nasopharyngeal tissues of patients with suspected nasopharyngeal carcinoma. *Cancer* 1998;82:1449–1453.

101. Bouzid M, Buisson M, Morand P, et al. Different distribution of H1-H2 Epstein-Barr virus variant in oropharyngeal virus and in biopsies of Hodgkin's disease and in nasopharyngeal carcinoma from Algeria. *Int J Cancer* 1998;77: 205–210.

102. Atula S, Auvinen E, Grenman R, et al. Human papillomavirus and Epstein-Barr virus in epithelial carcinomas of the head and neck region. *Anticancer Res* 1997;17:4427–4433.

103. Shavers VL, Harlan LC, Winn D, et al. Racial/ethnic patterns of care for cancers of the oral cavity, pharynx, larynx, sinuses, and salivary glands. *Cancer Metastasis Rev* 2003;22:25–38.

104. El Serag HB, Mason AC. Rising incidence of hepatocellular carcinoma in the United States [see comments]. *N Engl J Med* 1999;340:745–750.

105. Evans AA, O'Connell AP, Pugh JC, et al. Geographic variation in viral load among hepatitis B carriers with differing risks of hepatocellular carcinoma. *Cancer Epidemiol Biomarkers Prev* 1998;7:559–565.

106. Alexander GA, Brawley OW: Association of Helicobacter pylori infection with gastric cancer. *Mil Med* 2000;165:21–27.

107. Liu T, Wang X, Waterbor JW, et al. Relationships between socioeconomic status and race-specific cervical cancer incidence in the United States, 1973–1992 [in process citation]. *J Health Care Poor Underserved* 1998;9:420–432.

108. Kjellberg L, Wang Z, Wiklund F, et al. Sexual behaviour and papillomavirus exposure in cervical intraepithelial neoplasia: A population-based case-control study. *J Gen Virol* 1999;80:391–398.

109. Solomon D, Frable WJ, Vooijs GP, et al. ASCUS and AGUS criteria. International Academy of Cytology Task Force summary. Diagnostic Cytology Towards the 21st Century: An International Expert Conference and Tutorial. *Acta Cytol* 1998;42:16–24.

110. Cooper GS, Yuan Z, Landefeld CS, et al. Surgery for colorectal cancer: Race-related differences in rates and survival among Medicare beneficiaries. *Am J Public Health* 1996;86:582–586.

111. Greenwald HP, Polissar NL, Borgatta EF, et al. Social factors, treatment, and survival in early-stage non-small cell lung cancer. *Am J Public Health* 1998;88:1681–1684.

112. Havlik RJ, Yancik R, Long S, et al. The National Institute on Aging and the National Cancer Institute SEER collaborative study on comorbidity and early diagnosis of cancer in the elderly. *Cancer* 1994;74:2101–2106.

113. Ballard-Barbash R, Potosky AL, Harlan LC, et al. Factors associated with surgical and radiation therapy for early stage breast cancer in older women. *J Natl Cancer Inst* 1996;88:716–726.

114. Andrulis DP. Access to care is the centerpiece in the elimination of socioeconomic disparities in health [see comments]. *Ann Intern Med* 1998;129:412–416.

CHAPTER 10

Transplantation and Organ Donation

Clive O. Callender, MD*
Gwendolyn D. Maddox, MSM
Patrice Miles

▶ INTRODUCTION

More than half a century has now elapsed since the first successful kidney transplantation was performed. From 1954 to the present, transplantation has evolved from novel and experimental into the primary treatment modality for end-stage renal disease (ESRD). The consequences of this transformation have been profound. In the 1950s, a diagnosis of ESRD was associated with a greater mortality rate than many cancers and survival for more than 1 year was unusual. Today, through the use of markedly improved methods of dialysis and transplantation as renal replacement therapy, 20-year survival rates are the rule rather than the exception. Likewise, 1- to 2-year patient and graft survival rates, formerly less than 50% in the 1960s and 1970s, now exceed 90%.[1]

Several factors contribute to these outcomes. The first immunosuppressants—azathioprine, prednisone, and antilymphocyte globulin (poly-

clonal antibodies)—have been replaced by newer polyclonals (Thymoglobulin) and monoclonal antibodies (OKT3, Zenapax, Simulect, Campath). These newer therapeutics are less diffuse and more specific. When used along with calcineurin inhibitors such as Neoral, tacrolimus (Prograf), sirolimus (rapamycin) or their derivatives, these agents make the concept of "transplant tolerance" a near-reality, leading to the introduction of the term *propé tolerance*.[2] Such advances, along with the steroid avoidance therapies that now seem possible, have led transplantation specialists to hypothesize that with improved knowledge of microchimerism,[3] the previously unreachable goal of transplant tolerance may be soon attainable. The extraordinary success associated with extrarenal transplants (liver, kidney–pancreas, heart–lung, pancreas, small intestine, and pancreas islet cell transplantation), all of which are associated with 1- to 2-year patient and graft survival rates of better than 60%, has been no less exciting.

A growing body of research suggests that patient and graft survival rates will be even higher in the future. Induction immunosuppression

*The McGraw-Hill Companies acknowledge the substantial editorial contributions of Donna M. Frassetto and Nancy N. Woelfl in preparation of this chapter.

strategies for kidney transplantation are being carefully assessed so that long-term adverse outcomes can be carefully weighed against the risk of rejection. Obese or overweight patients are being more carefully monitored for microalbuminuria or proteinuria so that the progression to renal insufficiency can be halted. The notion that the more expensive mycophenolate mofetil is superior to azathioprine with recipients of cadaver kidney transplants has been challenged.[4] Other evidence-based approaches are also being used to support further refinements in the area of transplantation.

All Americans, however, have not been the equal beneficiaries of this progress. Although patient and graft survival rates have generally soared, patient and graft survival rates for African Americans have consistently lagged behind rates recorded for all other ethnic subgroups.[5] For the past five decades, graft survival rates for African Americans have been 10% to 20% lower than for their majority counterparts.[6]

This unique disparity separates African Americans from all other ethnic groups. Closer analysis reveals this disparity is nonsingular in nature. As the literature in this area is more closely examined, it becomes clear that many other transplantation and donation disparities exist for this unique subpopulation.[7] This chapter explores these disparities and recommends strategies for their elimination.

▶ THE NATURE AND MAGNITUDE OF ETHNIC DISPARITIES IN KIDNEY TRANSPLANTATION

Organ and tissue transplantation is characterized by some of the most severe disparities in outcomes and processes in the field of medicine. The origins of these disparities are systemically, behaviorally, and biomedically based. Because these factors operate in an interactive rather than a linear fashion, their impact on the African American population is most severe. Not only does the literature of transplantation confirm and document prevailing disparities, the evidence is expanded when combined

with observations acquired during more than 30 years as a transplantation surgeon. These combined information sources suggest that disparities are operative in several different areas, which are outlined in Table 10–1.

▶ TRANSPLANTATION AND ORGAN DONATION: AN ANALYSIS OF ETHNIC DISPARITIES

As Table 10–1 indicates, current disparities in organ and tissue transplantation as well as donor levels are associated with a number of factors. Remediation of the identified problems requires systematic approaches that are directly linked with the causal variables. In the sections below, each of the factors associated with organ and tissue disparities is discussed and strategies for their resolution are recommended.

Organ Donor Shortage

Equity in the market for organs and tissues requires that the supply of organs and tissues be increased and that strategies to reduce demand for these biologic commodities be implemented. The primary tool that has been used to address the organ donor shortage is health communication and education, and this intervention must be increased.

Growing Shortage of Organs and Tissues

The increasing shortage of donors has been astounding. In 1984, approximately 1000 persons were on the waiting list.[8] By 1996, this number had increased exponentially to approximately 20,000 persons.[9] In the 8-year period from 1996 to 2004, the number of persons on the waiting list increased to 83,000. Although approximately 25,000 persons did receive transplants, more than 58,000 persons remained on the waiting list. As noted, organ and tissue transplantation has, because of the nature of the therapy, one of the largest disparity rates in the field of medicine. The disparities are even larger for African Americans who are in need of kidneys.

▶ **TABLE 10–1.** Ethnic Disparities in the Area of Organ Transplantation

Disparities Regarding the Magnitude of Need for Organ and Tissue Transplantation
- The organ donor–recipient disparity
  — For all Americans, disparities are observable between persons on the waiting list and the pool of patients who receive a transplant for all Americans; however, the disparities are even greater for African Americans, a group that disproportionately requires kidney transplants
  — Currently, there are 86,178 people waiting for organs. Approximately 89.9% of all African Americans on the waiting list are waiting for a kidney
  — As of August 27, 2004, there were 59,375 persons on the waiting list for a kidney. Approximately 35.4% of these persons were African American
  — In the year 2003, there were only 1605 African American kidney donors of all donor types
  — African Americans constitute 13.1% of all donors
  — Thus, a tremendous disparity exists between African American kidney donors and African Americans who are in need of a kidney

Systemic Disparities That Occur Within the Organ Transplantation Infrastructure
- Delayed African American and other minority patient referral rates for kidney transplants: African Americans are referred later for kidney transplants, are wait-listed later, and are transplanted later than the majority population regardless of financial status
- Longer waiting times for African Americans and other minorities: African Americans and other minorities wait twice as long as Caucasians for kidney transplants
- Inequitable allocation schema: From 1988 to 2002, HLA-A and HLA-B matching led to ethnic discrimination in the allocation of organs
- Institutional racism: A race-based oncology prevails within US society that operates consciously or unconsciously within providers, causing them to be subjective in their transplantation referral processes
- Race and science: The subjective intrusion of race into medicine and science lends itself to the perpetuation of asymmetries in providers' decision making
- The "green screen": The absence of proven financial resources to pay for health care or the medications needed to sustain health after transplantation lends itself to disparities

Biomedical Disparities
- The prevalence and incidence rates for kidney failure in African Americans and other minorities: The incidence and prevalence rates of end-stage renal disease is higher among African Americans and other minorities because of their increased susceptibility to diabetes and hypertension. African Americans and other minorities are hypertensive or diabetic 200 to 400 times as often as Caucasians
- Nephropathy occurs disproportionately in African Americans with HIV relative to their majority counterparts: For reasons that have not yet been identified, the disproportionately large African American population with HIV or AIDS has a higher incidence of renal disease than their majority counterparts
- Dialysis survival rates: Longer patient survival rates for African Americans on dialysis and a higher reported quality of life delays kidney transplantation among African Americans
- Post-transplantation drug responses in African Americans: African Americans, after transplantation, metabolize transplant medications differently than Caucasians or other groups; this tendency alters their responsiveness to immunosuppression and other agents.
- The differential outcomes of donated African American kidneys and other organs: When African American organs are transplanted into other African Americans or Caucasians, the probability of graft survival is significantly lower
- Poor transplantation outcomes: As a collective, African Americans, after the transplantation of kidneys or other organs, have graft survival rates that are 10–20% lower than all other ethnic groups (at 2–5 years after transplantation). These trends prevail whether the kidney is received from a living related donor, living unrelated donor, or cadaver donor

Behavioral Disparities: Issues of Noncompliance
- The purported lower compliance rates of African American and Latinos after transplantation has been used as a rationale for the lower patient and graft survival rates; however, recent data suggest that allegations of noncompliance are incorrect

Approximately 35.4% of all persons on the waiting list for a kidney are African American.

Addressing Transplantation Disparities Related to the Donor Shortage

The primary strategy for addressing the organ donor shortage is through health education. Specifically, a two-pronged health promotion and education campaign is needed. First, this campaign must encourage more Americans in general and minorities in particular to sign donor cards and hold family discussions. Second, the campaign must urge at-risk populations to adopt health practices that can prevent organ damage. Toward this goal, policy makers and the health-care community must assign top priority to this area of health disparity. Concomitantly, policy makers must reflect the priority assigned to the donor shortage by increasing funding streams to provide both supply- and demand-related health education.

In the past, the United States has spent wisely and allotted significant resources for basic science and clinical research in transplantation. This investment has paid off handsomely, and the 90% 1-year patient and graft survival rate for most organ transplants has been a direct outcome of this effort. However, a paradox exists. Medical successes in the area of transplantation have intensified the need for donors. Stated another way, as transplantation has become more successful, it has also been recognized as the treatment of choice for end-stage organ failure.

As a result, transplantation has attracted more transplant candidates and created a burgeoning need for more organ donors. The present circumstances require dollars to be allocated on the same scale used for the improvement of clinical transplant survival rates. The allocation of appropriate funding for community, hospital, and professional education is now mandatory. The magnitude of need for an intervention of this type suggests that the strategies used must be national in scope and the strategies for narrowing the donor recipient disparity must have education as the core of a multi-pronged initiative. Educational campaigns must be simultaneously community-based, local, and national.[10] Professional, public, hospital, majority, and minority efforts must be integrated with grassroots efforts and multimedia campaigns to deliver targeted messages using transplant candidates, donors, and their families. The power of messages delivered in this fashion will allow the health-care community to overcome its primary enemies—ignorance and distrust.

The efficacy of education as a strategy has been tested and proven effective. In 1990, the number of organ donors per million population (ODM) for Caucasians, African Americans, Latinos, and Asians was 28.1, 22.4, 22.9, and 10.3, respectively. By the year 2000, health education campaigns had caused the ODMs to rise to 42.8 for Caucasians, 40.8 for African Americans, 40.2 for Latinos, and 26.2 for Asians. Minorities, a group that represents 25% of the US population, made up 15% of donors in 1990. Through education, these groups comprised 28.5% of donors in the year 2000,[10] confirming the efficacy of the education and outreach approach.

MOTTEP, the National Minority Organ Tissue Transplant Education Program, received a $5.8 million grant to establish a community education program for minorities at 15 sites across the United States. As shown in Table 10–2, a recent analysis comparing minority and majority donor rates at MOTTEP versus non-MOTTEP sites revealed significantly higher donorship rates at MOTTEP sites for Caucasians ($P < .02$), African Americans ($P < .01$), Latinos ($P < .02$), and Asians ($P < .02$). The analysis was performed by the Scientific Registry of Transplant Recipients in March 2003, and reviewed organ donor rates from 1995 through 1998.

These data provide compelling evidence of the efficacy of community-based educational programs in combination with the use of mass media. National MOTTEP's experience also confirms the value associated with the use of customized messages that are delivered by members of the community who are culturally and ethnically similar.

▶ **TABLE 10–2.** Cadaveric Donors per 1000 Evaluable Deaths and Number of Donors by Ethnicity and MOTTEP OPOs, 1995–1998

| | MOTTEP | | Non-MOTTEP | | Adjusted Donation Rate | |
| | | | | | Ratio of (MOTTEP to | |
Ethnicity	Donation Rate	Donors	Donation Rate	Donors	Non-MOTTEP)	P valve
White, non-hispanic (Caucasian)	59.3	4938	59.2	11,279	1.07	.02
Hispanic/Latino	106.9	1055	47.4	886	2.29	< .01
African American	43.4	1263	32.9	1286	1.40	< .01
Other	50.7	228	43.4	272	1.59	< .01

MOTTEP = Minority Organ Tissue Transplant Education Program; OPO = Organ Procurement Organizations; OPTN = Organ Procurement Transplant Network.
*Adjusted for age, sex and OPTN region.
Prepared by the Scientific Registry of Transplant Recipients.

MOTTEP's experience suggests that the most effective messengers are community members who are transplant candidates, recipients, donors, their family members, or all of these groups. Despite the recent emphasis on what researchers call community-based translational research, the power of the community as a change agent remains a relatively underutilized resource, the full power of which has not yet been appreciated. The need for public, professional, and hospital-based education programs as part of a nationally coordinated effort to ameliorate the donor shortage will benefit all. When appropriate funding levels are provided by the public and private sectors, a reduction in the enormous donor—recipient disparity of nearly 60,000 persons will occur. This strategy could effectively eliminate the 16 preventable deaths per day that presently occur. However, distribution of resources commensurate with this priority has not yet occurred.

Infrastructural Disparities in Organ and Tissue Transplantation

The organ transplantation infrastructure also produces disparities through its operations. The sections that follow describe some of these factors and discuss strategies for their correction.

Delayed African American and Minority Patient Referrals for Kidney Transplants

The work of Alexander and Seghal in 1998[11] confirmed for the first time a hypothesis that had been previously formulated: There are systemic barriers that reduce transplantations to African Americans, women, and the poor. These findings, along with the work of Schulman and others,[12] demonstrated unequivocally that ethnicity and gender were the primary reasons African Americans and women with heart disease were not referred for cardiac catheterization. In each of these studies, financial status and other factors were controlled across gender and ethnic groups. These findings are consistent with the 2000 Institute of Medicine report *Unequal Treatment: Confronting Racial and Ethnic Disparities in Health Care,* which challenges the US health-care system to address its adverse systemic practices.[13] This report dispelled the illusion that lack of financial resources is the sole reason for unequal health care. It confirmed that in each area of health care, even when fiscal resources and health insurance are comparable, African Americans receive inequitable treatment.

These trends are also observable in the area of transplantation. Current data reveal that African American ESRD patients are referred later for transplantation, and receive transplants later than Caucasians solely because of ethnicity.[12,13] It is also clear that physician ethnic bias is operative. This variable determines the direction and speed of referrals for transplantation. What is clearer now than ever before, due to the reports of Kasiske et al in 1998[14] and Epstein et al in 2000,[15] is that the delay in referrals increases post-transplant mortality and lowers transplant graft survival rates. Danovitch et al[16] argued that the negative impact of physician bias and racism could be overcome by simply following the European (Eurotransplant) model, which is based on the concept that waiting time begins when the patient's dialysis is initiated in an uninterrupted fashion. Because African Americans are discriminated against in this way, this simple change would do much to correct the delayed referral times that African American transplant candidates experience.

Addressing Longer Transplant Waiting Times for African Americans and Other Minorities

Waiting times for all minorities are longer than for their majority counterparts.[8,9,16] In 1998, the median waiting time for Caucasians was 888 days, or nearly 30 months. However, the median waiting time for African Americans was 1468 days, or nearly 49 months. Latinos were waitlisted for 1309 days (44 months) and Asians for 1476 days (49 months). Similar patterns persist today. These highly disparate waiting times, for majority and minority Americans, are disturbing and perplexing.[8,9,17] The Hawthorne effect from the field of management science suggests that behavioral improvements occur when individuals are aware that their behavior is being observed. Despite continual monitoring of health disparities in the area of transplantation, no Hawthorne effect has yet been documented. Inspector General Reports published in 1989 and 1996 [17,18] document an increase in African American waiting times from 21 months in 1989 to 43 months in 1991. Caucasian wait-time for transplants increased from 12 months

to 22 months. Despite monitoring, no improvements have occurred, suggesting that the mechanisms that support this area of disparity are deep seated and systemic.

The evidence that argues for unequal access to transplants for all minorities and especially African Americans is abundant and these barriers require special attention. Educational programs are needed to change the behavior of physicians who serve both majority and minority populations. Additionally, policy changes are needed in the systems used to assign organs.

Inequitable Allocation Schema

In an article published in the *New England Journal of Medicine,*[8] Roberts et al discussed changing the priority for human leukocyte antigen (HLA) matching based on the rates and outcomes of kidney transplantation in minority groups, a change that is long overdue. The USA End Stage Renal Disease Program announced plans to begin sharing organs based on a system that was ethnically discriminatory to African Americans beginning in 1989. Starzl, MOTTEP, and other providers protested this system in 1988; subsequently, the United Network for Organ Sharing (UNOS) abolished HLA-A matching in 1994 and HLA-B matching in the year 2002.

The elimination of this source of inequitable allocation is important for two reasons. First, HLA-A and HLA-B matching destroyed any illusion that a system existed that had the equitable allocation of organs and tissues as a priority. The elimination of these highly discriminatory practices created a foundation for the restoration of trust. Second, this alteration in policy demonstrated an effort to make organ allocation more accessible to all. The greatest concern of opponents was that concern for equity was outweighed by disadvantages associated with increased graft loss. No firm evidence exists to support this hypothesis. HLA matching was ethnically discriminatory and a violation of the Civil Rights Act of 1964. Given this change, if the Danovitch et al plan[16] to make time on dialysis equivalent to transplant waiting time is also implemented, tremendous progress can be made toward the goal of reducing disparities.

Institutionalized Racism

Institutionalized racism is a term that is foreign to the fields of ESRD and transplantation. Yet, as one examines the disparities outlined earlier, a discussion of health disparities in the area of transplantation must necessarily be framed within the context of institutional racism. Institutional racism denotes a set of attitudes, beliefs, and behaviors that are operationally grounded within social norms and social systems that reinforce notions associated with racial inferiority. Although the Human Genome Project has made it clear humans comprise one species, racism persists as a sociopolitical construct that assigns groups of humans to unequal strata. These assignments are insidious and comprise one of the greatest threats to health. The pathophysiologic consequences of institutional racism have been demonstrated by Harrell and others since 1982.[19–26] Their research demonstrates the negative correlates and pathophysiologic outcomes that result from institutional racism and discrimination.

Institutionalized racism is a primary source of the majority–minority health disparities that exist in ESRD and transplantation. First, it is responsible for the fact that African Americans experience longer waiting times. Second, delayed African American patient referral rates for kidney transplants are a direct outcome of the race-based ontology used by physicians who make referrals. Third, African Americans, because they are referred later, receive kidney transplants later than Caucasians and, as a result, have poorer graft survival rates and higher rates of mortality. Fourth, African Americans are referred later, if at all, for extrarenal transplantation (transplants for organs other than kidneys). Again, this trend results in African Americans dying without ever being placed on the waiting lists. Fifth, the aptly named "Green Screen" also disproportionately affects African Americans who are more likely to be uninsured. Because dialysis survival rates for African Americans are higher, healthier African American patients who should be transplanted remain on dialysis while corresponding Caucasians are transplanted. These forces each represent institutional racism in action.

Institutional racism was also observable in the inequitable allocation schema that was in place from 1988 to 2002. The plan was racially discriminatory to African Americans because of the emphasis on HLA, a problem that was not resolved until 2002. Prior to that time, added weight was given to HLA matching, with all HLA types known for Caucasians but not for African Americans. This placed African Americans at a distinct disadvantage until the practice was stopped in 2002. Both of these factors contribute to the fact that African American recipients of kidney, liver, and heart transplants fare 10% to 20% worse than all other groups of recipients regardless of their ethnicity. Finally, institutional racism operates to delay the conduct of new research that could serve as the basis to reverse these trends.

Race and Science

The Human Genome Mapping Project, completed in 2000, demonstrated conclusively that mankind, *Homo sapiens,* is one species and that scientific efforts to define race should be abandoned. Despite the subjectivity that has always accompanied race as a theoretical construct, the concept continues to be deeply embedded in the scientific lexicon. The use of the term *race* is divisive and sustains a sociopolitical construct that denies the positive aspects of each ethnic group while reinforcing stereotypes of superiority and inferiority used in tandem with it. Those interested in any area of health disparities research negate their goal if the premise is not adjusted to reflect that humans are one species socioculturally represented by different ethnicities. This transition must occur within the scientific community, among those who design the US Census, and within the Office of Management and Budget (OMB) until the term *race* is replaced by *ethnicity* in all scientific publications and federally disseminated documents.

The "Green Screen"

In the film *John Q,* Denzel Washington assumed the role of a father whose son has a potentially fatal heart disease. Only a donated heart can save the boy's life. Unfortunately, the father's employment status had changed and consequently, his health insurance benefits had been reduced. His son could not be placed on the heart transplant waiting list because Washington's character fell into the large group of people in the United States who are underinsured.

Although the film is fictional, it reflects a reality that is quite common. Updated census data reveal a national population that now exceeds 300 million Americans. Of these 300 million persons, one third are uninsured or underinsured. By virtue of their insurance status, they do not have access to full health care in general or transplantation in particular. Thus, more than 100 million Americans are health care victims of the "green screen."

In the area of organ transplantation, this dilemma is applicable to all organ transplants, but it is especially noteworthy with respect to organs other than kidneys, where lack of access to transplant waiting lists constitutes a death sentence. Not only will uninsured or underinsured patients die because of lack of an organ, they will never be recorded in a database as needing an organ because they will never be wait-listed. "Green screening" obscures the level of need by allowing patients to fall below the radar screen.

These practices also characterize renal transplantation. Because of lack of insurance coverage, many transplant candidates are denied access to kidney transplant waiting lists either because they do not have the needed insurance coverage or because their insurance will not pay for the medications needed during the post-transplant period. Medicare will pay for transplant medicines for virtually all persons who are eligible for Medicare, but the benefit is available for only 3 years. Ironically, this period is not congruent with the time span after which kidney transplants clearly become cost effective. When compared with hemodialysis, the break-even point is 2.5 years.

Currently, inadequate data exist regarding how many candidates are turned down for transplants because of lack of insurance coverage for the medications associated with the post-transplant period. Discussions between the producer of *John Q* and National MOTTEP strongly support the reality of a "green screen" that prevents access to transplantation for those who do not have the "green." Research is urgently needed to identify the magnitude of this barrier to transplantation and to develop a process for its elimination.

Biomedical Disparities

Several disparities in the field of kidney transplantation appear to be biomedically based; this section reviews some of these factors.

Incidence of Kidney Failure in African Americans and Other Minorities

The elevated incidence of hypertension and type 2 diabetes among African Americans, Latinos and Hispanics, and Native Americans results in an incidence of ESRD that is 200 to 400 times higher than the rate among Caucasians. Although this fact is well known, the etiologic chain involved in these morbidities in ethnic subpopulations has not been fully identified. The causes for higher prevalence and incidence of kidney failure among African Americans and other minorities remain an enigma; however, obesity, lack of exercise, environmental factors, high levels of sugar and salt consumption, and malnutrition are correlates of hypertension, diabetes, and renal disease. The often-quoted cliché, "an ounce of prevention is worth a pound of cure," is highly applicable.

A national strategy to change lifestyles in minority populations to prevent the need for transplantation was developed by MOTTEP and funded by the National Institutes of Health in 1995. The community-based education program designed by MOTTEP was implemented at 15 sites across the United States. It was designed to increase minority organ donation rates

▶ **TABLE 10–3**. Percentage of African American Cases by Nephropathy Type, 1995–1999

Type of Nephropathy	Total No. of Reported Cases	Total No. of Reported Cases in African Americans	Percentage of African American Cases
AIDs nephropathy	4029	3774	93
Heroin nephropathy	285	200	70
Sickle cell nephropathy	458	445	97
SLE nephropathy	4068	2263	55

SLE, systemic lupus erythematosus.

Source: *USRDS 2001 annual data report.*

while simultaneously promoting and changing lifestyles to healthier ones that, in the long run, would decrease the high incidence of hypertension and diabetes.[9,17] This campaign helped not only to increase minority donation rates, but also, MOTTEP's research suggests, to change attitudes and behaviors associated with unhealthy lifestyles.[9,17,27] A sustained national effort to continue to promote prevention among ethnic groups using public and community-based efforts is an absolute necessity.[10,27]

Impact of HIV Nephropathy on African Americans

The disproportionate impact of human immunodeficiency virus (HIV) on the African American and Latino populations in the United States is well known.[28] For the year 2002, 42,745 new cases of acquired immunodeficiency syndrome (AIDS) were reported to the Centers for Disease Control and Prevention (CDC).[29] Approximately 70% of these new cases were among minorities, and 50.8% occurred in African Americans. The CDC estimates that 1 in 160 African American women and 1 in 50 African American men are infected with HIV. African Americans are 10 times more likely to be diagnosed with AIDS and 10 times more likely to die from this disease.[29,30] However, little evidence exists to explain why the nephropathy of HIV is so predominately an African American problem.

The data have been cited repeatedly. African Americans with HIV have AIDS nephropathy 1000% more often than other ethnic groups.[31] A staggering 93% of all AIDS nephropathy cases reported are among African Americans[31] (Table 10–3).

The data in Table 10–3 raise the question, if providers perform transplants for many of the long surviving African American HIV-positive patients, what impact will these cases have on transplant outcomes in the future? Transplantation involving selected HIV-positive patients is now associated with greater than 90% 1-year patient and graft survival rates.[32] Will African American HIV transplant survival rates approach Caucasian transplant survival rates? Research is needed to answer these questions.

Dialysis Survival Rates for African Americans

Data analyzed for end-stage renal disease patients on hemodialysis between 1989 and 1997[32] (Table 10–4) reveal that 1-year death rates for Caucasians, African Americans, Native Americans, and Asians, were 13%, 4.9%, 17.8% and 14.3% respectively. The same pattern was observed when longer intervals were studied. Two-year mortality rates were 16.5% for Caucasians, 9.7% for African Americans, 32.4% for Native Americans, and 30.3% for Asian and Pacific Islanders. African American dialysis patients have, by far, the best dialysis survival rates.[32]

Other recent research indicates African Americans who receive dialysis report a higher quality of life. Based on a survey of 1392

► **TABLE 10–4**. Death Rates on Dialysis by Ethnic Status, 1989–1977

Ethnicity	1-Year Death Rate (%)	2-Year Death Rate (%)
Caucasians	13	16.5
African Americans	4.9	9.7
Native Americans	17.8	32.4
Asian and Pacific Islanders	14.3	30.3

Source: *USRDS 2001 annnual data report.*

patients nationwide, Hicks et al[33] found that African American men and women receiving dialysis self-reported an overall better quality of life whether measured by overall health, energy levels, or fewer negative side effects.

This paradox has not yet been investigated sufficiently to identify the factors associated with these trends. Although longer survival while receiving dialysis and a greater ability to tolerate treatment reduces the number of transplants among African American renal patients, transplantation is the superior treatment modality. Strategies must be implemented to educate African American renal patients about the importance of transplantation. The goal must be to have no more than 80% of the African American patients on hemodialysis and 20% of ESRD African American patients on transplant waiting lists—proportions that reflect the ratios that now exist for majority patients.

Post-Transplantation Drug Responses in African Americans

The experience of transplant specialists in the management of African American patients after transplantation reveals that immunosuppressive therapy is more necessary than for other ethnic groups. African Americans, for reasons that are yet unclear, are more immunoresponsive than other ethnicities. When pretransplant immune responsiveness was studied, 90% of African Americans were hyperimmune compared with 66% of Caucasians. This observation suggests the need for more powerful immunotherapy for African Americans. Cyclosporine was so poorly

absorbed by African American patients in the 1990s that Neoral, a microemulsion form, was required to overcome malabsorption of this drug, one of several problems associated with its use in this target audience.[34] Other complications were associated with use of these drugs in an ethnic group in which hypertension and nephrotoxicity were so high that no new toxicities could be tolerated.

Prednisone, with its many side effects, was particularly problematic in African Americans given that hypertension, Type 2 diabetes, and obesity were already present. Mycophenolate mofetil (CellCept) produced a reduction in acute rejection episodes but the price African Americans paid was high. The effective dose was 3 g for African Americans compared with 2 g for Caucasians. In many of these patients, gastrointestinal and bone marrow intolerance ranged from 60% to 80%; at Howard University Hospital Transplantation Center, the rate for both types of intolerance was 80%. Although reduced dosages were tolerated, these patients experienced an increased likelihood of an acute rejection episode.

Tacrolimus (Prograf) is the most potent immunosuppressant used by the Howard University Hospital Transplantation Center. However, its use in African Americans and Latinos is associated with twice the incidence of post-transplant diabetes seen in Caucasians.[34] In addition, most of the African American transplant patients who become diabetic remain insulin dependent. This differs from Latino and Caucasian patients who become diabetic from tacrolimus because their insulin dependency reverses itself. These unique post-transplant drug responses are not completely understood.

African American cytochrome P450 oxidase systems suggest that genetic differences may be one part of the answer. The presence of a heightened African American immune system is another explanatory hypothesis. It is clear that elucidation of this enigma will help eliminate one of the transplant disparities associated with poorer graft survival in African Americans.

Outcomes for Kidneys and Other Transplanted Organs in African Americans

In 1977, Opelz et al[35] were the first to note that kidney donor and graft survival rates in African Americans were the poorest among all ethnic groups. Since that time, a number of studies have further substantiated this additional area of disparity. Other studies have not revealed such a disparity in patient or graft survival for other organ transplant or ethnic groupings.

In an effort to better understand the lower kidney graft survival rates, data were reviewed on patient and graft survival rates for all ethnic groups for single-organ transplants: kidney, heart, and liver. Data from April 1994 through December 2000, provided by the Organ Procurement Transplant Network/United Network for Organ Sharing (OPTN/UNOS), were analyzed. The 118,769 donor–recipient transplants reviewed included 77,689 living and cadaveric kidneys, 26,124 cadaveric livers, and 14,956 cadaveric hearts. Univariate and multivariate techniques were used to examine the effect of donor–recipient ethnic pairing on post-transplant and patient survival rates. A multivariate regression model was used to analyze the effect of donor–recipient combinations on graft survival in kidney and liver recipients and patient survival in heart recipients. Caucasians, African Americans, Latinos, Asians, and other minority groups were included in the study, which examined other donor, recipient, and transplant characteristics as well. Caucasian-to-Caucasian pairs were used as the baseline for comparison. Findings were presented as ratios indicative of the relative risk (RR) of graft loss and mortality.

The data indicate that African American recipients of cadaveric or living donor kidneys had significantly poorer graft survival regardless of donor ethnicity. African American recipients of cadaveric livers and hearts had significantly lower graft survival rates when receiving organs from Caucasians, other African Americans, or Latinos. African American recipients of kidneys, hearts, and livers have significantly poorer graft survival than all other ethnic groups, and the factors that lead to these outcomes are unknown.

Because the reasons for ethnic differences in the success of kidney transplantation remain unknown, additional analysis is needed. Data on half-lives for kidney transplantation for all ethnic groups reveal the following 1-year and 5-year kidney transplant half-lives: Asians, 12.2 years; Caucasians, 10.2 years; Hispanics and Latinos, 9.0 years; and African Americans, 5.3 years.[35,36] Despite the use of Caucasians as the baseline for the analysis, Asians were the ethnic group with the most favorable half-lives while African Americans had the shortest. For African Americans, this difference is significantly poorer than other ethnic groups and persists whether living or deceased donor organs are used. African American recipients of cadaveric or living donor kidneys have significantly poorer graft survival regardless of donor ethnicity.

Data accumulated over time reveal that African Americans are the ethnic group that, despite improvements in immunosuppressive therapy, continues to have significantly poorer 3-year kidney transplant graft survival rates than all other ethnic groups.[37] The kidney transplant graft survival disparity has continued for nearly 30 years since it was first identified.[5] Many hypotheses have been proposed, tested, and abandoned regarding this phenomenon: too few African American donors, HLA mismatches, inequitable allocation, noncompliance, and the "green screen."[6]

The negative correlation between hypertension, hyperimmune responsiveness, and transplant graft survival is quite clear. However, it is less clear why hypertension is a negative correlate of patient or graft survival, or both. Investigation of this relationship should be a focal point of future research. The same processes that allow hypertension to destroy kidneys initially may be replicated in the transplanted kidney, thereby inducing nephrosclerosis.[38]

Current data also demonstrate that the African American recipients who had poorer kidney graft survival rates were overwhelmingly hyperimmune. However, when this group was controlled for, African American graft survival rates were the same as those of Caucasian patients included in the analysis. Evidence indicates that African Americans have higher immune responsiveness to transplanted organs than do Caucasians.

The effect of ethnicity on pretransplant immune response status was also studied in 124 African American and 241 Caucasian first cadaveric renal allograft recipients. Pretransplant tests of immunity found that 90% of African American patients were strong immune responders compared with 66% of Caucasians. Although 3-year graft survival rates were significantly different ($P < .01$) between Caucasians (75%) and African Americans (55%), when low responders of both ethnicities were analyzed, the differences between African American and Caucasian responders were not significant. These data suggest that African American ESRD patients are stronger immune responders than Caucasians and therefore are at an immunologic disadvantage.[35] If this is the case, the newest immunosuppressive regimens, such as the newer polyclonals (Thymoglobulin), monoclonals, calcineurin inhibitors (rapamycin), and other new immunosuppressants, may provide the answer.

African American recipients of cadaveric livers and hearts also had significantly lower graft survival regardless of donor ethnicity. This trend may reflect the overall poorer health status of African Americans, and educational interventions to change their lifestyles to prevent the need for transplantation may be the best approach. Such an approach requires the use of community education and empowerment, a methodology that MOTTEP has already employed.[38] Among all donor ethnic combinations, African American–to–African American pairs had the highest relative risk of graft loss for kidney or liver and mortality for heart. It appears African American recipients of organs fare the poorest of all ethnic groups regardless of the ethnicity of the donor source. Beginning in 1982, MOTTEP sought to recruit African American donors with the hope that an increase in African American donors would improve the graft survival rates for cadaver and live donor African American transplant recipients. Data from two decades of intervention with 15,000 African American donors now confirm that Opelz's[35] observation was no statistical accident but revealed an enigmatic trend that increases in African American donations cannot overcome.[17,37]

Outcomes for Transplanted Organs Donated by African Americans

African American kidneys and other organs, when transplanted into African Americans or Caucasians, or both, have significantly inferior graft survival. Opelz's observation in 1977 that kidneys donated to African Americans survived for shorter periods than in all other ethnic groups led MOTTEP to examine the survival of kidneys, livers, and hearts. As noted, data from April 1994 through December 2000 provided by UNOS/OPTN were used for analysis. Included were 118,769 donor recipient pairs, including 77,689 living and cadaveric kidney-alone and 14,956 cadaveric heart-alone recipient pairs. The results of the analysis revealed that organs donated by African Americans and transplanted into African Americans or Caucasians were associated with significantly poorer graft survival rates for kidneys and livers ($P < .001$). Kidneys, livers, and hearts donated by African Americans and given to African Americans or Caucasians (kidneys, livers) are associated with highly significant relative risks. However, these organs were not associated with significantly higher relative risks among Asians or Latinos and Hispanics.

This finding contradicts the conclusion that all African American donated organs are inferior and should not be used for transplantation. It would also be inappropriate to conclude that all organs donated by African Americans are high risk and require the special consent form used for the expanded donor category. Without further study, such a policy would be injudicious and could be considered overtly discriminatory.

Among all donor ethnic combinations, African American–to–African American transplants were associated with the highest relative risk of graft loss for kidney or liver, or mortality for heart, or both. It was mentioned earlier that African American recipients of organs fare the worst of all ethnic groups regardless of the ethnicity of the donor source.

In 1982, Howard University Hospital Transplantation Center began to recruit African American donors in the hopes that increasing this donor pool would improve the graft survival rates for African American recipients of both cadaveric and living African American organs. However, the opposite occurred. The data continue to reveal that African American donors have the highest negative correlation to the African American recipient. It appears that factors that cause the graft survival rate to be lower in the African American recipient are intensified by receiving an African American organ. Although other minority recipients may overcome this obstacle, the African American recipient cannot and, in fact, has the highest negative correlate upon receiving an African American organ. This does not mean that African American recipients should not receive African American organs; rather, it reveals the need for more research regarding the reasons for the graft survival disparity. Once these causes are better understood, strategies to overcome the disparity can be implemented.

Behavioral Disparities: The Question of Compliance

In recent years, noncompliance has been used, unfairly, to explain why minorities, especially African Americans and Latinos, do less well after transplants.[39] Jarzembowski et al,[40] using a sample of 50 pediatric kidney transplant patients, argued that 71% of late graft loss among African American pediatric patients was due to noncompliance. This research is consistent with other studies that offer noncompliance as a primary explanation of why African Americans and other minorities have much poorer outcomes after transplantation. However, research by Greenstein and Siegel,[41] using a much larger database, makes clear that rates of noncompliance do not differ among ethnic groups and are not responsible for poorer African American graft survival rates. Poorer graft survival is likely related to other factors. However, consistent with the research, adolescents, regardless of ethnicity, are the group that is the least compliant and whose poorer graft survival may be related to noncompliance.

▶ SUMMARY AND RECOMMENDATIONS

A continual theme pervades this review of the nature and magnitude of disparities in the field of organ transplantation, in general, and kidney transplantation, in particular. Specifically, it suggests a national strategy is required to allocate the level of resources needed for an intensive program of remediation. This program encompasses two subcomponents: additional research, and funding for community-based and media-based education. Table 10–5 describes some of the elements of the proposed initiative.

The theme of this chapter—health care disparities in transplantation—is quite complex. This chapter describes the evidence-based data associated with prevailing disparities. Even more critically, it provides recommendations

▶ **TABLE 10–5.** Summary of Recommendations to Eliminate Disparities in Organ and Tissue Transplantation

---

The Research Agenda

Conduct new research that:

- Identifies why graft survival rates are lower for African Americans than for all other groups
- Analyzes current databases to identify the correlates of poorer graft survival of African American recipients of all organs
- Uncovers why 70–90% of the cases of AIDS and of heroin nephropathy occur in African Americans
- Tracks and validates the operation of the "green screen"
- Analyzes the policy implications of the trends
- Uncovers why there is a higher prevalence of renal failure among minorities
- Discovers why African Americans survive longer than other ethnic groups on dialysis
- Tracks the processes associated with longer transplant waiting times and delayed referrals
- Uncovers why African Americans respond differently to transplant medication
- Critically, identifies the factors that reduce the survival rates and increase graft loss when organs from African American donors are used

The Action Agenda

Launch an education campaign to:

- Increase donorship
- Protect healthy organs
- Educate physicians regarding institutional racism
- Educate communities to trigger greater involvement
- Educate the majority community and enlist its support in addressing disparities
- Educate policy makers to stop using the term *race*
- Educate minorities to better monitor the physician management practices used with their family member

---

that will lead to measurable improvements in observed outcomes if implemented.

▶ REFERENCES

1. US Organ Procurement and Transplantation Network and Scientific Registry of Transplant Recipients. *Transplant Data 1993–2002*. Available at: http://www.ustransplant.org.

2. Calne R, Friend P, Moffatt S, et al. Prope tolerance, perioperative Campath 1H, and low-dose cyclosporin monotherapy in renal allograft recipients. *Lancet* 1998;351(9117):1701–1702.

3. Starzl TE, Demetris AJ, Trucco M, et al. Cell migration and chimerism after whole-organ transplantation: The basis of graft acceptance. *Hepatology* 1993;17(6):1127–1152.

4. Remuzzi G, Lesti M, Gotti E, et al. Mycophenolate mofetil versus azathioprine for prevention of acute rejection in renal transplantation (MYSS): A randomised trial. *Lancet* 2004;364(9433):503–512.

5. Katznelson S, Gjertson DW, Cecka JM. The effect of race and ethnicity on kidney allograft outcome. *Clin Transplant* 1995;379–394.

6. Koyama H, Cecka JM, Terasaki PI. Kidney transplants in black recipients. HLA matching and other factors affecting long-term graft survival. *Transplantation* 1994;57(7):1064–1068.

7. Callender CO, Miles PV, Hall MB. National MOTTEP: Educating to prevent the need for transplantation. Minority Organ Tissue Transplant Education Program. *Ethn Dis* 2002;12(1):S1-34-7.

8. Roberts JP, Wolfe RA, Bragg-Gresham JL, et al. Effect of changing the priority for HLA matching on the rates and outcomes of kidney transplantation in minority groups. *N Engl J Med* 2004;350(6):545–551.

9. Callender CO, Washington AW. Organ/tissue donation the problem! Education the solution: A review. *J Natl Med Assoc* 1997;89(10):689–693.

10. Callender CO, Miles PV, Hall MB. Experience with National Minority Organ Tissue Transplant Education Program in the United States. *Transplant Proc* 2003;35(3):1151–1152.

11. Alexander GC, Sehgal AR. Barriers to cadaveric renal transplantation among blacks, women, and the poor. *JAMA*1998;280(13):1148–1152.

12. Schulman KA, Berlin JA, Harless W, et al. The effect of race and sex on physicians' recommendations for cardiac catheterization. *N Engl J Med* 1999;340(8):618–626.

13. Smedley BD, Stith AY, Nelson AR. *Unequal Treatment: Confronting Racial and Ethnic Disparities in Health Care*. Washington, DC: National Academy Press; 2003. Available at: http://books.nap.edu/openbook/030908265X/html/index.html

14. Kasiske BL, London W, Ellison MD. Race and socioeconomic factors influencing early placement on the kidney transplant waiting list. *J Am Soc Nephrol* 1998;9(11):2142–2147.

15. Epstein AM, Ayanian JZ, Keogh JH, et al. Racial disparities in access to renal transplantation—clinically appropriate or due to underuse or overuse? *N Engl J Med* 2000;343(21):1537–1544, 2 p preceding 1537.

16. Danovitch GM, Cohen B, Smits JM. Waiting time or wasted time? The case for using time on dialysis to determine waiting time in the allocation of cadaveric kidneys. *Am J Transplant* 2002;2(10):891–893.

17. Callender CO, Miles PV, Hall MB, et al. Ethnic disparities in transplantation: A strategic plan for their elimination. In: Livingston IL, ed. *Handbook of Black American Health; Policies and Issues Behind Disparities in Health,* 2nd ed, vol 2.Westport Conn: Praeger; 2004:776–791.

18. Ayanian JZ, Cleary PD, Weissman JS, et al. The effect of patients' preferences on racial differences in access to renal transplantation. *N Engl J Med* 1999;341(22):1661–1669.

19. Harrell JP, Merritt N, Kau J. Racism, stress, and disease. *Afr Am Ment Health* 1998:247–280.

20. Harrell JP. *Manichean Psychology: Racism and the Minds of People of African Descent*. Washington, DC: Howard University Press; 1999.

21. Harrell JP. Psychological factors and hypertension: A status report. *Psychol Bull* 1980;87(3):482–501.

22. Harrell JP, Hall S, Taliaferro J. Physiological responses to racism and discrimination: An assessment of the evidence. Am *J Public Health* 2003; 93(2):243–248.

23. Williams DR. Race, socioeconomic status, and health. The added effects of racism and discrimination. *Ann N Y Acad Sci* 1999;896:173–188.

24. Kreger N. Does racism harm health? Did child abuse exist before 1912? On explicit questions, critical science, and current controversies: An ecosocial perspective. *Am J Public Health* 2003; 93(2):194–199.

25. Williams DR, Neighbors HW, Jackson JS. Racial/ethnic discrimination and health: Findings from community studies. *Am J Public Health* 2003;93(2):200–208.

26. King G. Institutional racism and the medical/health complex: A conceptual analysis. *Ethn Dis* 1996;6(1–2):30–46.

27. Callender CO. Organ and tissue donation in African Americans: A national stratagem. In: *Proceedings of the Surgeon General's Workshop on Increasing Organ Donation*. Background papers. Washington DC: US Dept of Health and Human Services, Public Health Services, Office of the Surgeon General,1991:145–162.

28. Callender CO. The results of transplantation in blacks: Just the tip of the iceberg. *Transplant Proc* 1989;21(3):3407–3410; discussion 13–18.

29. McNeil JI. Aspects of HIV/AIDS management in the African American patient. *J Natl Med Assoc* 2003;95(2 suppl 2):1S.

30. Centers for Disease Control and Prevention, National Center for Health Statistics. *FASTATS AIDS-HIV*. Table 53: AIDS cases, according to age at diagnosis, sex, detailed race, and Hispanic origin: United States, selected years 1985–2002. Available at: http://cdc.gov/nchs/fastats/aids-hiv.htm.

31. Norris KC, Agodoa LY. Race and kidney disease: The scope of the problem. *J Natl Med Assoc* 2002; 94(8 suppl):1S–6S.

32. US Renal Data System. *Annual Data Report*. Bethesda, Md: National Institutes of Health, National Institute of Diabetes and Digestive and Kidney Diseases, Division of Kidney, Urologic, and Hematologic Diseases. Available at: http://purl.access.gpo.gov/GPO/LPS2144.

33. Hicks LS, Cleary PD, Epstein AM, et al. Differences in health-related quality of life and treatment preferences among black and white patients with end-stage renal disease. *Qual Life Res* 2004;13(6):1129–1137.

34. Kerman RH, Kimball PM, Van Buren CT, et al. Possible contribution of pretransplant immune responder status to renal allograft survival differences of black versus white recipients. *Transplantation* 1991;51(2):338–342.

35. Opelz G, Mickey MR, Terasaki PI. Influence of race on kidney transplant survival. *Transplant Proc* 1977;9(1):137–142.

36. Neylan JF. Immunosuppressive therapy in high-risk transplant patients: Dose-dependent efficacy of mycophenolate mofetil in African-American renal allograft recipients. U.S. Renal Transplant Mycophenolate Mofetil Study Group. *Transplantation* 1997;64(9):1277–1282.

37. Young CJ, Gaston RS. Renal transplantation in black Americans. *N Engl J Med* 2000;343(21):1545–1552.

38. Callender CO, Miles PV, Hall MB, et al. Blacks and Caucasians and kidney transplantation: A disparity! But why and why won't it go away? *Transplant Rev* 2002;16:163–176.

39. Schweizer RT, Rovelli M, Palmeri D, et al. Noncompliance in organ transplant recipients. *Transplantation* 1990;49(2):374–377.

40. Jarzembowski T, John E, Panaro F, et al. Impact of non-compliance on outcome after pediatric kidney transplantation: An analysis in racial subgroups. *Pediatr Transplant* 2004;8(4):367–371.

41. Greenstein S, Siegal B. Compliance and noncompliance in patients with a functioning renal transplant: A multicenter study. *Transplantation* 1998;66(12):1718–1726.

CHAPTER 11

Immunization and Preventive Care

WALTER W. WILLIAMS, MD, MPH
SONJA S. HUTCHINS, MD, MPH, DrPH
WALTER A. ORENSTEIN, MD
LANCE RODEWALD, MD

▶ INTRODUCTION

Routine vaccination of children is a major public health success story.[1] As a result of vaccines administered throughout the 20th century, many serious childhood infectious diseases have been eliminated or are under control. Record low incidence of vaccine-preventable diseases is the result of record high vaccination coverage levels. For example, US national average coverage levels among children aged 19 to 35 months exceed or are within one percentage point of the *Healthy People 2010* objective of 90% coverage for all vaccines introduced more than 10 years ago: measles, mumps, and rubella (MMR); diphtheria, tetanus, and activated pertussis (DTaP), inactivated polio vaccine (IPV), hepatitis B, and *Haemophilus influenzae* type b (Hib) vaccines. Vaccination coverage levels among people 65 years of age and older against influenza and pneumococcal disease also are at record high levels but remain substantially below *Healthy People 2010* objectives.

Immunization not only saves lives, it saves society from the direct and indirect costs of illness. As such, immunization is considered one of the most cost-effective clinical preventive services. A recent analysis by the Partnership for Prevention ranked routine childhood immunization first out of 30 clinical preventive services, based on the preventable burden of disease and the cost-effectiveness of the intervention.[2] Ranked highly important for persons over age 65 were immunization with influenza vaccine (ranked 4, tied with six other interventions) and pneumococcal vaccine (ranked 11, tied with three other interventions).

This chapter discusses vaccines recommended for children and older adults, disparities in vaccination levels, and strategies for assuring enhanced use of these vaccines.

▶ CHILDHOOD IMMUNIZATIONS

The routine current immunization schedule in the United States reflects the remarkable progress made in vaccine development during the past several decades. The routine schedule now protects against 12 vaccine-preventable diseases (diphtheria, tetanus, pertussis, po-liomyelitis, measles, mumps, rubella, *H influenzae* type b, hepatitis B, varicella, pneumococcal disease, and influenza). Current recommendations call for administration of up to two doses of vaccines by 18 months of age and up to 25 doses by 12 years of age, depending on the combination of vaccines used.[3,4] In addition, for selected high-risk populations, two doses of hepatitis A vaccine are added to the routine schedule. The current schedule can be found at the CDC website: *http://www.cdc.gov/nip*. To achieve childhood immunization at the recommended ages, continuous access is needed to immunization services. Typically, five to six visits to a primary health-care provider are needed in the first 2 years of life.

In the early days of national efforts to control vaccine-preventable diseases, vaccination of school-aged children had a major impact on diseases such as measles and polio. States enacted laws requiring school entrants to be fully vaccinated. As enactment and full enforcement of school laws in all 50 states became a reality through national childhood immunization initiatives, 95% or more of all school entrants since 1981 have had documentation of immunization, virtually eliminating any disparity in immunization between school-aged children who are white and those of racial and ethnic minorities.[4] Although school laws have had a major impact in early control of vaccine-preventable diseases, the goal of immunization is to protect at the earliest possible age at which the vaccine is reliably effective. This approach best minimizes the morbidity and mortality caused by a vaccine-preventable disease and ultimately can lead to elimination of the disease. Among preschool-aged children, differences in vaccination coverage have been observed for children from racial and ethnic minority groups compared with non-minority children.

This section describes the vaccination levels of preschool-aged children in the United States over several decades, documents initial differences in vaccination coverage of children from racial and ethnic minorities compared with non-minority children, highlights interventions that were effective in improving immunization of all racial and ethnic children, and describes the remaining challenges in childhood immunization.

Vaccination Coverage Levels

From the 1970s through the mid-1980s, data on vaccination coverage by race and ethnicity was first routinely collected by the US Immunization Survey (USIS). USIS vaccination coverage levels with three or more doses of a diphtheria, tetanus, and pertussis vaccine (DTP 3+), three or more doses of polio vaccine (polio 3+), or a measles-containing vaccine (MCV) was approximately 60% for children aged 1 to 4 years. Vaccination coverage was similar for children at the second birthday (24 months of age), the midpoint of the age group. Vaccination levels for nonwhite children (mostly black children) were lower than levels for white children (40% to 50% versus 60% to 70%, respectively) (Centers for Disease Control and Prevention [CDC], unpublished data). The gap in vaccination coverage for DTP 3+, polio 3+, or MCV ranged from 12% to 26% and averaged 20% during this multiyear period.

Routine measurement of vaccination coverage of children nationally was temporarily halted in 1985 just before a large measles epidemic that occurred in 1989 to 1991, producing more than 55,000 cases.[5,6] Routine measurement was reinstituted in 1991, at the end of the epidemic. Therefore, the average disparity of 20% lower vaccine coverage for nonwhite children for DTP 3+, polio 3+, or MCV in 1985[7] (CDC, unpublished data) is taken to be the best baseline estimate of the difference in vaccination coverage between nonwhite and white populations before the changes in immunization activities began during the measles epidemic.

After the epidemic, overall vaccination coverage of children improved. According to the National Health Interview Survey (NHIS), in 1992 vaccination coverage of 2-year-old children (aged 24 to 35 months) was 83% for DTP 3+, 72% for polio 3+, and 83% for MCV (see Appendix A, Fig. A–10).* Although overall coverage levels improved, vaccination levels remained lower for nonwhite children than for white children (14% lower for DTP 3+, 18% lower for polio 3+, and 7% for MCV).[8] From 1992 onward, overall vaccination of children continued to increase, reaching, in 1996, the national goal of at least 90% for DTP 3+, polio 3+, or MCV among children aged 19 to 35 months based on estimates from the National Immunization Survey (NIS), regardless of income level at, above, or below the poverty line.[9]

As overall vaccination levels approached 90%, the immunization gap in vaccination coverage between nonwhite children and white children, which averaged 20% during the 1970s and 1980s, virtually disappeared by the late 1990s. By 1996, the immunization gap narrowed to 3% to 5% (see Fig. A–10).[9] By 1997, 89% to 94% of black children aged 19 to 35 months, 88% to 93% of Hispanic children, and 90% to 92% of American Indian and Alaska Native children received DTP 3+, polio 3+, or MCV, while approximately 91% to 96% of white children and 89% to 96% of Asian and Pacific Islander children received these vaccines and doses, regardless of income level at above or below the poverty line.[9] Since 1997, vaccination coverage levels have remained high.[9]

Although vaccination levels in the population for the oldest individual vaccines in the recommended schedule were very high, lower vaccination levels existed among children for all recommended vaccines in the routine childhood schedule, reflecting lower coverage levels for newer vaccines and receipt of multiple vaccines by an individual. For instance, in 2001 and 2002, vaccination coverage was approximately 10% to 15% lower for all children aged 19 to 35 months who had received multiple vaccines. The vaccination level among children who had received multiple vaccines including four or more doses of DTP (DTP 4+), polio 3+, and MCV (4:3:1) was 79%, and the level for those receiving multiple vaccines that

included DTP 4+, polio 3+, MCV, three doses of Hib vaccine, and three doses of hepatitis b vaccine (4:3:1:3:3) was approximately 75%. The immunization gap between white children and children from racial and ethnic minority groups who had received multiple vaccines varied from 5% to 10%[9] (see Fig. A–11). From 1996 to 2002, an increasing immunization gap observed between African American children and white children was explained by increasing vaccination coverage among white children and no change in coverage among African American children during this period.[9–11] However, the disparity was not as large as the 20% gap observed before interventions began during the 1989–1991 measles epidemic.

To estimate the impact of the success in eliminating disparities in vaccination coverage for the oldest individual vaccines, we assumed that at least a 15% immunization gap has been reduced for individual vaccinations with DTP 3+, polio 3+, or MCV, and that minority children are now being immunized with these vaccines and doses at essentially the same level as in the delivery systems serving the majority population. This translates into an estimated 400,000 minority children 2 years of age or younger being protected earlier or on schedule in the United States each year.[7]

Effective Interventions

Recent narrowing of the immunization gap between white children and children from racial and ethnic minority groups was due to universal and targeted interventions, a dual strategy implemented to improve childhood immunizations[7] (Table 11–1). These interventions were initiated during the 1989–1991 measles epidemic and continued after the epidemic. The epidemic created widespread and unprecedented concern that the nation's immunization system was deficient, and resulted in the launching of a national initiative to improve the immunization delivery system.[12,13] Simultaneously, the initiative declared specific disease reduction and vaccination coverage goals to be

---

* Figures illustrating statistical information presented in this chapter are included in Appendix A at the end of the book.

▶ **TABLE 11-1.** Summary and Impact During 1989–2001 of Dual Strategy Approach (Universal and Targeted) Initiated in Response to 1989–1991 Measles Epidemic[7]

Intervention	Impact
Universal	
1. Second dose of measles vaccine	1. Reduced vaccine failures
2. Presidential priority	2. Increased attention and funding for childhood vaccinations
3. Increased funding for health departments	3. Strengthened immunization activities
4. Immunization Action Plans	4. Guided state immunization programs
5. Annual state survey of vaccine coverage	5. Measured state coverage of children aged 19–35 months
6. Extra funds for state immunization programs	6. Provided financial incentives for above-average performance
7. New standards for pediatric immunization practices	7. Improved vaccination services at the point of delivery
8. Quality improvement activities (AFIX) in clinics	8. Raised immunization coverage
9. Assessments of vaccine coverage (HEDIS) in MCOs	9. Stimulated improvements in coverage through measurement
10. State-based immunization registries of children	10. Tracked and measured vaccination status
11. State-based coalitions of organizations	11. Strengthened and extended existing immunization programs
12. Partnerships with national health organizations	12. Promoted and maintained immunizations as a priority
13. Research	13. Tested interventions and found reasons for low vaccine coverage
14. National public information campaigns	14. Improved knowledge of the benefits of vaccination
15. Enforcement of laws and regulations for child-care centers	15. Achieved high vaccine coverage in child-care centers
Targeted	
16. Vaccines for Children Program	16. Entitled uninsured or underinsured children to free vaccine
17. Extra funding for urban-area health departments[a]	17. Improved vaccine coverage of children in 28 urban areas
18. Annual assessment of vaccine coverage	18. Measured vaccine coverage in the same 28 urban areas
19. Local Immunization Action Plans	19. Guided immunization programs in the 28 urban areas
20. Linkage of WIC and immunization activities	20. Screened 40% of all US births for immunization[b]
21. Discounted vaccine prices for Medicaid programs	21. Enabled Medicaid programs to vaccinate
22. Higher reimbursement rates for Medicaid providers	22. Increased the number of Medicaid providers
23. Quality improvement (AFIX) in public clinics	23. Raised immunization coverage for low-income children
24. More user-friendly hours for public clinics	24. Enabled access to vaccination services of low-income children
25. Partnerships with Minority Health Organizations	25. Promoted and maintained immunizations as a priority
26. Special information campaigns	26. Improved knowledge of Spanish-speaking populations

AFIX, Assessment, Feedback, Incentives, and Exchange; HEDIS, Health Care Employer Data and Information Set; IAPs, Immunization Action Plans; MCOs, managed care organizations; WIC, Special Supplemental Nutrition Program for Women, Infants, and Children.

[a]With at least 50% minority populations.

[b]Screens US births enrolled in WIC and refers eligible children for vaccination.

reached before 2000 for a variety of vaccine-preventable diseases, including renewal of efforts started in the 1960s to eliminate indigenous transmission of measles from the United States.[13,14] This dual strategy was responsible for the recent elimination of endemic measles from the United States and the elimination of the up to four- to seven-fold higher risk of measles incidence among children from racial and ethnic minority groups compared with white children that existed during the epidemic.[6,7]

The dual strategy was a multicomponent set of interventions to improve vaccination coverage against measles and other vaccine-preventable diseases[7] (see Table 11–1). Some of these interventions were applied as temporary measures during the measles epidemic of 1989 to 1991. Others were developed later, in an ongoing manner from 1989 to 1992 as part of the Infant Immunization Initiative, and subsequently as part of the 1993 Childhood Immunization Initiative.[13,15,16–27]

The dual childhood immunization strategy was developed with interventions likely to have an impact on the majority of children (eg, new National Standards for Pediatric Immunization Practices distributed to all providers and others), and because of the long-standing disparity in vaccination, additional interventions more likely to reach subgroups of the population with higher proportions of children from racial and ethnic minority groups (eg, the Vaccines for Children [VFC] program, entitling uninsured or underinsured children to free vaccine).[28] At the same time, outbreak control and enhanced surveillance activities were initiated to respond more effectively to disease occurrence.[29] A major focus for childhood immunization efforts has been on the provider. This includes the new standards for pediatric immunization practice, the VFC program, reminder and recall systems to reduce missed opportunities to vaccinate, and continuous quality improvement activities to assess vaccination coverage and feed this information back to providers with performance incentives for targeted action (see Table 11–1). The

strength of evidence for many of the universal and population-specific interventions is published in the *Guide to Community Preventive Services, Vaccine-Preventable Diseases: Improving Vaccination Coverage of Children, Adolescents and Adults.*[15]

Because the dual strategy contained a number of interventions, it is not possible to determine whether a single intervention or combination of interventions was most responsible for its success. What seems plausible is that the gap in coverage would not have been closed without interventions that sought specifically to have greater impact on, or remediate, racial and ethnic minority populations. The contrary may also be correct; namely, that a strategy targeted only at remediating minority populations without emphasis on raising overall vaccination levels among all children may not have succeeded. Equity was achieved at the higher vaccination coverage levels due to an excellent-performing delivery system characteristic of the 1990s.

Although it is not possible to single out any interventions for their role in the success achieved, the overall program implemented a conceptual model that was effective and was based on core components of the PRECEDE model.[30] This model assumed that predisposing, enabling, and reinforcing factors were needed to achieve desired goals, and several of the interventions noted in Table 11–1 fell into these categories. For example, predisposing factors included the 1989–1991 measles resurgence, which led to childhood immunization becoming a priority of the President and, subsequently, to the availability of national funding to improve childhood immunization and control the measles epidemic.[20] Enabling factors included an effective strategy for eliminating measles based on scientific evidence that recommended a second measles vaccine dose and introduction of the VFC program. A reinforcing factor was setting biennial national vaccine coverage and disease targets and close monitoring of these goals through annual assessments of vaccine coverage at national, state, and local levels through surveys and immunization registries.

A separate evaluation of the VFC program, introduced in 1994 to entitle uninsured and underinsured children to free vaccine, indicates that the program has been instrumental in improving the vaccination coverage of low-income children and closing immunization gaps between white children and children from racial and ethnic minority groups. Newly licensed vaccines introduced after the VFC program began have not shown major differences in vaccination levels between minority and nonminority children. For example, with the introduction of the varicella vaccine in 1995, varicella vaccination levels in 1998 and more recently have not shown an immunization gap between white children and children from racial and ethnic minority groups aged 19 to 35 months.[9] Similarly, introduction of the pneumococcal conjugate vaccine has been associated with essentially no immunization gap between white and black children, aged 19–35 months, who were born in 2000 and 2001. Moreover, this pneumococcal vaccination level has also been associated with a significant reduction in the overall incidence of invasive pneumococcal disease in children younger than 5 years of age, and in a narrower gap in the incidence of disease between white and black children[31] (CDC, unpublished data).

Remaining Challenges

The dual strategy, including the introduction of the VFC program, was successful in essentially eliminating disparities in vaccination coverage levels for individual vaccines recommended for routine use during childhood for the past three or more decades (DTP, polio, and measles) and narrowing the immunization gap for the childhood immunization schedule of 4:3:1 or 4:3:1:3:3. To sustain this success, national immunization efforts must be vigilant: nearly 4 million children are born in the United States each year, each requiring multiple vaccine doses to protect against 12 diseases by school entry. As more vaccines are added to the childhood immunization schedule and problems with vaccine supply and vaccine financing occur, maintaining high vaccination coverage levels and further closing of the immunization gap may become more of a challenge.[32,33]

▶ ADULT IMMUNIZATION

Immunization programs have been viewed primarily as a preventive tool for use in children and have markedly reduced the occurrence of vaccine-preventable diseases in children. A substantial proportion of the remaining morbidity and mortality from vaccine-preventable diseases, however, occurs in older adolescents, adults, and the elderly. Persons who were not infected with these diseases or were not immunized during childhood may be at increased risk for these diseases and their complications as adults. Other adults enter special high-risk groups as a result of disease, occupation, behavior, or increasing age and may require immunizations or booster doses not routinely provided in childhood.

The Advisory Committee on Immunization Practices (ACIP) has recommended an adult immunization schedule by age group and medical condition, or based on behavioral, occupational, or other indications.[34] The recommended immunizing agents include influenza vaccine; pneumococcal polysaccharide vaccine; hepatitis B vaccine; hepatitis A vaccine; varicella vaccine; measles, mumps, and rubella vaccines; and tetanus and diphtheria toxoids. Other vaccines may be indicated for travelers to areas or countries where other diseases may be hyperendemic or epidemic.

The ACIP recommends annual influenza vaccination for certain groups and at least one lifetime dose of pneumococcal polysaccharide vaccine. Influenza vaccine is recommended annually for adults 50 years of age and older and those with chronic medical conditions requiring regular medical follow-up, such as chronic conditions of the cardiovascular or pulmonary systems, or chronic metabolic diseases. Influenza vaccine is also recommended annually for residents of nursing homes and other long-term care facilities, women who will be in the second or third trimester of pregnancy during the influenza season, health-care workers, and persons likely to transmit influenza to individuals at high risk.

Pneumococcal vaccination is indicated for adults 65 years of age and older, and those with medical indications, such as chronic disorders of the cardiovascular or pulmonary systems, diabetes mellitus, chronic liver diseases, chronic renal failure or nephrotic syndrome, functional or anatomic asplenia, and immunosuppressive conditions.[34] Routine revaccination of immunocompetent persons previously vaccinated with pneumococcal polysaccharide vaccine is not recommended. However, revaccination is recommended after 5 years for persons who are at highest risk for serious pneumococcal infection and those who are likely to have a rapid decline in pneumococcal antibody levels. Persons at highest risk and those most likely to have rapid declines in antibody levels include persons with functional or anatomic asplenia (eg, sickle cell disease or splenectomy), human immunodeficiency virus (HIV) infection, or chronic renal failure.

Hepatitis B and hepatitis A vaccines are recommended for those with certain medical, occupational, or behavioral indications. Measles, mumps, rubella, and varicella vaccines are recommended for susceptible adults. All adults should maintain immunity to tetanus and diphtheria by receiving a booster dose every 10 years after completing a primary vaccination series.[34]

Although there is growing awareness and numerous strategies have been developed to address underimmunization of adults, there has been no concerted national effort to promote immunization as a preventive health measure among adults, particularly among African Americans, Latinos, and other minority groups.

Influenza and Pneumococcal Infections

The burden of vaccine-preventable diseases in adults in the United States is staggering—approximately 46,000 to 48,000 adults die each year from these diseases. Special focus has been placed on influenza and pneumococcal infections, however, because these two vaccine-preventable diseases contribute annually to thousands of deaths of older persons in the United States. Epidemics of influenza typically occur during the winter months, and each year, approximately 114,000 people in the United States are hospitalized because of influenza with as many as 57% of these hospitalizations occurring among persons younger than 65 years of age. An average of 36,000 people die annually from influenza and its complications; most are people 65 years of age and older. Influenza viruses can also cause pandemics, during which rates of illness and death can increase dramatically worldwide. The risks for complications, hospitalizations, and deaths from influenza are higher among persons 65 years and older, young children, and persons of any age with certain underlying health conditions. Influenza-related deaths can result from pneumonia as well as from exacerbations of cardiopulmonary conditions and other chronic diseases.

Annually, there are approximately 60,000 cases of invasive pneumococcal disease in the United States (ie, bacteremia, meningitis, or infection of other normally sterile sites) and one third (20,000) of these cases occur in people 65 years of age and older. Approximately half of the 6000 to 7000 annual deaths from invasive pneumococcal disease occur in the elderly. In addition, pneumococcal infections are the most common cause of bacterial pneumonia requiring hospitalization. Pneumococcal infections account for an estimated 40,000 deaths annually in the United States—more deaths than any other vaccine-preventable bacterial disease.[35] Approximately half of these deaths could be prevented through the use of pneumococcal polysaccharide vaccine.

Severe pneumococcal infections result from dissemination of bacteria to the bloodstream and the central nervous system. In the United States, the risk for acquiring bacteremia is lower among white persons than among persons in other racial and ethnic groups (blacks, Alaska Natives, and American Indians).[35–37] The incidence of invasive pneumococcal disease among blacks is two to five times higher than that in whites.[35,36] Black adults have a three- to fivefold higher overall incidence of bacteremia than whites, and incidence rates for meningitis are twice as high for blacks as for whites and Hispanics. Rates of invasive pneumococcal disease are exceptionally high among Alaska Natives and American Indians. Incidence rates for meningitis and bacteremic pneumonia are eightfold to tenfold higher for Alaska Natives of all ages than for other US population groups. The highest incidence rates for any US population have been reported among specific American Indian groups (eg, Apache).[37]

Racial and Ethnic Disparities in Influenza and Pneumococcal Vaccination Levels

Substantial racial and ethnic disparities in adult vaccination have been documented in national surveys and have persisted over time[38–44] (Table 11–2). Although national health objectives for 2010 include increasing influenza and pneumococcal vaccination levels to 90% or greater among persons aged 65 years and older (objective numbers 14.29a and 14.29b, respectively),[45] estimated prevalences of influenza and pneumococcal vaccinations were less than 80% among all racial and ethnic groups, and substantial gaps persist by race and ethnicity.

To characterize racial and ethnic disparities in adult vaccination levels, data have been analyzed from the National Health Interview Survey (NHIS)[38,41] and the Behavioral Risk Factor Surveillance System (BRFSS).[39–42] In both the NHIS and BRFSS, respondents 65 years and older were asked the same questions regarding influenza ("During the past 12 months, have you had a flu shot?") and pneumococcal vaccination ("Have you ever had a pneumonia vaccination [sometimes called a pneumonia shot]?").

In general, influenza vaccination coverage has been highest for non-Hispanic whites, followed by Hispanics and then non-Hispanic blacks (see Table 11–2). For pneumococcal vaccination, coverage has been similar for non-Hispanic blacks and Hispanics. Vaccination coverage was less than 60% for all subgroups of non-Hispanic blacks and the majority of subgroups of Hispanics. Differences in influenza coverage between non-Hispanic whites and Hispanics and between non-Hispanic whites and blacks were as high as 13 and 16 percentage points, respectively. Differences in pneumococcal vaccination coverage between non-Hispanic whites and Hispanics and between non-Hispanic whites and blacks were as high as 25 and 23 percentage points, respectively.[38] In addition, there was wide variability in influenza and pneumococcal vaccination coverage across states and other reporting areas.[39–43] Although a higher proportion of Hispanics than non-Hispanic blacks or whites had fewer than two physician visits during the preceding 12 months, a similar proportion in each of the three racial and ethnic populations reported 10 or more physician visits during the preceding 12 months. The substantial racial and ethnic disparities in vaccination coverage were observed among persons with zero to one, two to nine, as well as 10 or more health-care provider contacts during the preceding 12 months, suggesting that access to care might not be a key factor. Differences in vaccination coverage are observed among persons with similar education levels, similar numbers of health-care encounters, and similar insurance status. Large disparities are also evident for influenza and pneumococcal vaccination between non-Hispanic whites and non-Hispanic blacks at or above poverty level, with more than a high school education, and reporting five or more physician contacts during the previous year.[41] In these studies,

▶ **TABLE 11–2.** Percentage of Non-Hispanic White, Non-Hispanic Black, and Hispanic Persons Aged ≥ 65 Years Who Reported receiving Influenza Vaccination During the Proceeding 12 Months or Over Receiving Pneumococcal Vaccination, by Selected Characteristics—National Health Interview Survey, United States, 2000 and 2001 Combined

Characteristic	Influenza			Pneumococcal		
	White, Non-Hispanic % (95% CI[a])	Black, Non-Hispanic % (95% CI)	Hispanic % (95% CI)	White, Non-Hispanic % (95% CI)	Black, Non-Hispanic % (95% CI)	Hispanic % (95% CI)
Sex						
Men	68.0 (±1.8)	47.6 (±5.5)	54.0 (±5.8)	57.1 (±1.9)	30.3 (±4.9)	32.4 (±6.1)
Women	64.5 (±1.4)	48.7 (±3.8)	53.8 (±4.5)	57.5 (±1.4)	34.4 (±3.6)	31.1 (±4.6)
Age group (yr)						
65–74	62.9 (±1.5)	48.4 (±4.0)	53.4 (±4.1)	62.8 (±1.7)	32.5 (±3.9)	31.4 (±4.1)
≥75	69.5 (±1.8)	48.2 (±4.7)	54.4 (±5.4)	62.5 (±1.8)	33.2 (±4.7)	32.3 (±5.7)
Region[b]						
Northeast	65.9 (±2.6)	40.4 (±7.8)	56.6 (±8.8)	54.3 (±3.1)	30.1 (±8.1)	34.1 (±11.7)
Midwest	68.4 (±2.8)	50.2 (±7.7)	49.4 (±18.2)	58.5 (±2.5)	33.9 (±8.1)	27.8 (±4.1)
South	64.3 (±1.8)	50.4 (±8.0)	42.8 (±6.6)	57.4 (±2.1)	32.2 (±3.8)	22.0 (±1.8)
West	69.0 (±2.8)	44.8 (±7.8)	83.8 (±5.7)	62.4 (±2.7)	40.1 (±10.8)	40.9 (±8.5)
Education level						
High school	61.6 (±1.9)	46.2 (±4.3)	51.4 (±4.8)	52.8 (±2.3)	27.7 (±4.0)	28.2 (±4.7)
High school graduate	65.5 (±2.0)	50.7 (±6.1)	53.0 (±8.5)	58.8 (±2.1)	34.4 (±8.8)	35.5 (±7.5)
>High school	70.0 (±1.8)	49.4 (±6.7)	63.9 (±8.0)	61.8 (±1.9)	38.8 (±8.4)	40.8 (±9.1)
Poverty level[c]						
Below	57.2 (±4.8)	48.8 (±6.4)	48.2 (±7.0)	50.5 (±4.4)	30.6 (±5.9)	23.9 (±5.8)
At poverty	62.5 (±2.4)	50.0 (±5.9)	50.9 (±6.4)	56.7 (±2.6)	29.4 (±5.5)	33.3 (±7.9)
Above	69.0 (±1.7)	49.1 (±7.3)	81.8 (±7.6)	59.8 (±2.0)	32.6 (±7.8)	38.1 (±8.0)
Language[d]						
English	66.1 (±1.1)	48.3 (±3.1)	58.9 (±5.2)	57.5 (±1.2)	32.8 (±2.7)	38.1 (±4.4)
Spanish	—[e]	—[e]	47.9 (±4.3)			24.4 (±6.0)

(*continued*)

▶ **TABLE 11-2.** (*Continued*)

Characteristic	Influenza						Pneumococcal					
	White, Non-Hispanic % (95% CI)[a]		Black, Non-Hispanic % (95% CI)		Hispanic % (95% CI)		White, Non-Hispanic % (95% CI)		Black, Non-Hispanic % (95% CI)		Hispanic % (95% CI)	
Insurance												
Medicare/Medicaid	58.6	(±5.4)	47.2	(±7.3)	51.6	(±6.4)	60.6	(±5.8)	33.8	(±6.9)	27.6	(±7.9)
Medicare only	60.3	(±2.3)	48.8	(±6.1)	50.7	(±5.4)	60.0	(±1.8)	31.3	(±4.9)	29.6	(±5.3)
Medicare/Supplemental[f]	68.7	(±1.4)	54.0	(±5.5)	62.6	(±7.5)	60.8	(±1.5)	38.5	(±4.9)	44.0	(±7.9)
High risk[g]												
Yes	71.5	(±1.6)	54.8	(±4.5)	60.4	(±5.4)	86.8	(±1.6)	39.9	(±4.6)	37.3	(±5.5)
No	60.9	(±1.6)	42.3	(±4.6)	47.9	(±6.0)	90.0	(±1.7)	26.2	(±3.6)	28.4	(±4.8)
No. doctor visits												
0–1	49.7	(±2.7)	29.2	(±6.4)	38.5	(±6.9)	39.5	(±2.8)	21.4	(±6.0)	22.8	(±6.1)
2–9	87.7	(±1.4)	52.6	(±4.1)	56.2	(±4.6)	58.7	(±1.5)	34.9	(±3.5)	32.0	(±4.9)
≥ 10	74.2	(±2.1)	63.1	(±7.1)	83.2	(±6.9)	67.7	(±2.5)	36.9	(±6.2)	39.6	(±7.3)
Total	66.0	(±1.1)	48.3	(±3.0)	53.7	(±3.4)	57.3	(±1.2)	32.8	(±2.7)	31.7	(±3.7)

[a]Confidence interval.

[b]*Northern* – Connecticut, Maine, Massachusetts, New Hampshire, New Jersey, New York, Pennsylvania, Rhode Island and Vermont; *Midwest* – Illinois, Indiana, Iowa, Kansas, Michigan, Minnesota, Missouri, Nebraska, North Dakota, Ohio, South Dakota, and Wisconsin; *South* – Alabama, Arkansas, Delaware, District of Columbia, Florida, Georgia, Kentucky, Louisiana, Maryland, Mississippi, North Carolina, Oklahoma, South Carolina, Tennessee, Texas, Virginia, and West Virginia; *West* – Alaska, Arizona, California, Colorado, Hawaii, Idaho, Montana, Nevada, New Mexico, Oregon, Utah, Washington, and Wyoming.

[c]Calculated on the basis of US Census Bureau 2000 poverty thresholds.

[d]Language in which the interview was conducted.

[e]Quantity was insufficient for analysis: < 30 sampled respondents or relative standard error > 0.3.

[f]Any insurance in addition to Medicare, except Medicaid.

[g]Persons were classified as being at high risk for influenza if they reported diabetes during the preceding 12 months; asthma, emphysema, chronic bronchitis, or tuberculosis during the preceding 12 months; chronic kidney disease during the preceding 12 months; or ever being told by a physician that they had a heart attack, heart failure, chronic heart condition, or rheumatic heart disease. Persons who were classified as being at high risk for pneumococcal related complications either had illness consistent with the criteria for being at high risk for influenza-related complications, with the exception of asthma or reported liver disease or cirrhosis during the preceding 12 months.

non-Hispanic whites were more likely to report influenza and pneumococcal vaccination than non-Hispanic blacks at all poverty levels, education levels, and levels of frequency of care with health-care providers.

Factors Influencing Vaccination of African Americans and Hispanics

Qualitative data have been collected from consumer groups and physicians about factors that contribute to low influenza and pneumococcal vaccination rates among older African American and Hispanic populations. The research has focused on identifying beliefs and behaviors in these populations that are directly related to vaccination against influenza and pneumococcal infections, increasing understanding of physicians' attitudes and behaviors related to these vaccines, and assessing the impact and appeal of messages intended to increase vaccination in these target populations. African American and Hispanic respondents participating in formative research on influenza vaccination have generally expressed concerns that vaccination would make them sick or have stated they did not know they needed it. Some also expressed a strong distrust of the government, physicians, and drug companies.[46] Factors that motivated acceptance of vaccination included past experience with influenza infection, the influence of physicians who convinced them to be vaccinated, and a desire to protect family members, particularly grandchildren. Although physicians reported supporting influenza and pneumococcal vaccination, they did not consider influenza vaccination to be a revenue generator. Short, focused, scientific messages appear to work best to motivate physicians to use vaccines, with hospitals and medical journals serving as prime communication channels. Further studies need to more intensively examine the contribution of factors, such as racial and ethnic differences in the administration of vaccines by health-care providers, and racial and ethnic differences in the acceptance of vaccines by patients.

Missed vaccination opportunities also contribute to less-than-optimal vaccination coverage.[41,47–51] Opportunities to offer influenza and pneumococcal vaccination services during patient–provider encounters are being missed, particularly for African Americans.[50] Missed opportunities to vaccinate occur even among persons who have frequent and multiple contacts with health-care providers during the year. Other barriers to vaccination have also been identified, including limited English proficiency, family size, perceived health status, and age distribution.[52,53] Lower vaccination of blacks, however, cannot be attributed to increased health risk, poverty category, or fewer visits to a health-care provider.[52]

Strategies to Improve Vaccination Levels

National goals for improving prevention of vaccine-preventable diseases among adults include: (1) increasing the demand for adult vaccination by improving provider and public awareness; (2) increasing the capacity of the health-care delivery system to effectively deliver vaccines to adults; (3) expanding financing mechanisms to support the increased delivery of vaccines to adults; (4) monitoring and improving the performance of the nation's immunization program; and (5) enhancing the capability and capacity to conduct research regarding vaccine-preventable diseases in adults, vaccination practices, new and improved vaccines, and international programs for adult vaccination.[41,54,55]

Reasons for differences in coverage are poorly understood. Strategies to improve influenza and pneumococcal vaccination of all those at risk should include continued assessment of factors accounting for differential race- and ethnicity-specific vaccination rates, particularly physician practice patterns and patient attitudes; collaboration between public and private organizations to improve awareness about the need for these vaccines; changes in clinical practice to improve vaccine delivery; expansion of pneumococcal and influenza vaccination services by working with private, medical, and community groups to limit cost and remove accessibility constraints; collaboration of public and private medical providers with Center for Medicare and Medicaid Services Quality Improvement Organizations to increase vaccination levels among Medicare beneficiaries; and encouraging local health departments to enroll as Medicare providers to implement pneumococcal and influenza vaccination programs, and to file claims for these vaccination services which are reimbursable by Medicare.

In addition, every contact with the healthcare system should be used to review and update vaccination status as needed. A physician's recommendation for vaccination services can have a strong influence on a patient's decision to be vaccinated.[56–58] Interventions such as standing orders for vaccination,[59] provider reminders and feedback, and patient recalls and reminders have been effective in increasing adult vaccination levels.[60,61] Although use of reminder-recall systems, standing orders, and provider prompts are effective, operational conditions such as improving staffing ratios, information flow, and adequate time to complete all the clinical tasks necessary for vaccination could assure even higher vaccination rates.[62] Opportunities for vaccination at nontraditional health-care settings, such as pharmacies, churches, and grocery stores, could be increased to reach persons who do not routinely access traditional healthcare settings.[59] Opportunities for vaccination of adults with chronic diseases, such as diabetes and heart disease, could also be increased by incorporating vaccination recommendations in guidelines for clinical care of these patients and conducting special campaigns to educate them and reach their providers. Demonstration and evaluation projects, such as the CDC's Racial and Ethnic Adult Disparities Immunization Initiative (READII), may identify additional strategies for addressing vaccination disparities among older non-Hispanic blacks and Hispanics. In READII, local and state health departments are collaborating with community partners and federal agencies at multiple sites to examine the impact of using culturally specific messages, working with health-care providers who care for elderly non-Hispanic black and Hispanics patients to implement effective interventions, and conducting vaccination clinics in underserved neighborhoods.[38,39] Studies have shown that vaccinating persons with high-risk conditions against influenza and invasive pneumococcal disease saves medical costs and improves health.[63,64]

▶ SUMMARY AND RECOMMENDATIONS

To achieve the full health benefits of immunization, high vaccination levels must be achieved

▶ **TABLE 11–3**. Selected Internet Resources (Websites) on Immunization Indications, Administration, Safety, and Effective Interventions

Organization	Websites
American Academy of Family Physicians	*http://www.aafp.org/*
American Academy of Pediatrics	*http://www.aap.org/*
American College of Physicians	*http://www.acponline.org/aii/*
Food and Drug Administration	*http://www.fda.gov/*
Immunization Action Coalition	*http://www.immunize.org/*
National Immunization Program	*http://www.cdc.gov/nip/*
National Medical Association	*http://www.nmanet.org/*
	National_Programs_Adult_Immunization.htm
Network for Immunization Information	*http://www.immunizationinfo.org/*
National Partnership for Immunization	*http://www.partnersforimmunization.org/*

▶ **TABLE 11–4.** Strategies and Recommendations to Reduce Health Disparities in Routine Childhood Vaccination Schedule and Influenza and Pneumococcal Vaccination of At-Risk Adults

Overall Strategies	
Vaccination	**Strategy**
Routine childhood schedule	• Confirm findings of increased childhood vaccination gap found in National Immunization Survey (NIS) • Identify and understand causes of remaining disparities in childhood vaccinations • Assess implementation level of dual strategy to improve childhood vaccinations (see Table 11–1) • Identify potential interventions to eliminate disarities in childhood vaccination and to achieve full implementation of dual strategy (see Table 11–1)
Influenza and pneumococcal vaccination of at-risk adults	• Identify factors for differential race- and ethnic-specific vaccination rates, (eg, physician practices and patients beliefs) • Expand vaccination services to limit cost and improve access • Increase vaccination levels among Medicare beneficiaries through collaboration of private and public providers with Center for Medicare and Medicaid Services • Encourage local public health agencies to enroll Medicare providers, implement programs, and file claims for reimbursement

Specific Recommendations from Task Force on Community Preventive Services[a]

• Client recall-reminder systems
• Multicomponent interventions with education
• Vaccination requirement for child care and school attendance
• Reducing out-of-pocket costs
• Multicomponent interventions for expanding access in health-care settings
• Vaccination programs in WIC settings
• Home visits
• Provider reminder-recall systems
• Assessment and feedback for vaccination providers
• Standing orders for adults

WIC, The Special Supplemental Nutrition Program for Women, Infants, and Children.
[a]Recommended or strongly recommended.

among all populations. A dramatic example of this principle was seen with the 1989 to 1991 measles resurgence, in which children acquiring measles were four to seven times more likely to be African American or of Hispanic ethnicity. This disparity in burden of disease was caused by inequality in vaccination levels, in which white preschool children had higher vaccination rates than did African American or Hispanic children. As a direct result of the measles resur-

gence, a concerted programmatic effort was undertaken during the 1990s to raise vaccination levels among all preschool-aged children. Within several years, a long-standing difference in coverage levels between African American children and white children of up to 20 percentage points was essentially eliminated for receipt of individual vaccines[63] and substantially narrowed for receipt of multiple vaccines, and endemic measles was eliminated from the United States. Likewise, a difference in vaccination levels for individual vaccines between white children and children from other racial and ethnic minority groups is virtually nonexistent.[65] The campaign to raise coverage levels required substantial federal, state, and local resources to purchase vaccines and expand the immunization delivery and public health infrastructure of state and urban area immunization programs.

Childhood vaccination programs have demonstrated the feasibility of achieving high vaccination coverage levels and substantially reducing racial and ethnic disparities in disease and coverage levels. However, the childhood programmatic successes with individual vaccines have not been realized for all childhood vaccines for all populations or by adult vaccination programs. The situation for adults today is similar to the situation of 20 years ago for childhood individual vaccines, in which overall coverage was less than 60%, and large racial and ethnic disparities in coverage were seen. Studies are needed to examine the contribution of factors such as racial and ethnic differences in the administration of vaccines by adult health-care

▶ **TABLE 11–5**. Summary of Major Findings Regarding Childhood and Adult Immunization

Childhood Immunization
- High vaccination levels must be achieved among all populations to achieve full benefits of immunizing agents
- Inequality in vaccination levels between white preschool children and African American and Hispanic children resulted in a four- to seven-fold higher risk for acquiring measles during 1989–1991 measles resurgence
- A concerted programmatic effort during the 1990s using a dual strategy consisting of interventions likely to impact majority of children combined with additional interventions more likely to reach subgroups with higher proportions of children from racial and ethnic minority groups eliminated endemic transmission of measles in United States and long-standing disparities in vaccination levels
- National vaccination efforts must remain vigilant to maintain high vaccination levels and further close remaining immunization gaps

Adult Immunization
- Influenza and pneumococcal infections are responsible for thousands of deaths and hospitalizations among older persons each year, despite availability of effective protective vaccines
- Risk for invasive pneumococcal infections is several-fold or more higher among blacks, Alaska Natives, and American Indians
- Overall vaccination against influenza and pneumococcal infections has been below national health objectives for all adult groups and substantial racial and ethnic disparities in vaccination coverage have persisted over time (Hispanics and non-Hispanic blacks compared with whites)
- Large disparities in influenza and pneumococcal vaccinations are evident even among individuals above poverty level, with more than a high school education, and reporting multiple contacts with physicians during the year
- Non-Hispanic whites are more likely to report influenza and pneumococcal vaccination than non-Hispanic blacks at all levels of income, education, and frequency of care with health-care providers
- Multiple factors influence vaccination of African Americans and Hispanics, including patient and physician beliefs and attitudes toward vaccination, physician practice patterns, missed opportunities, and limited English proficiency
- Known successful strategies to improve adult vaccination must be widely implemented, and research is needed on less-well-understood contributors to low vaccination

providers and in the acceptance of vaccines by adult patients. Known successful strategies to improve vaccination of at-risk populations must be more widely implemented. An important challenge will be to replicate the successes of the childhood program with similar successes in adult vaccination to reduce the unacceptably high annual death toll through effective immunization programs. Additional information on vaccine indications, safety, administration and effective interventions is available (Table 11–3). A summary of strategies and recommendations to further reduce disparities in routine childhood vaccination and influenza and pneumococcal vaccination of adults appears in Table 11–4. A summary of the main points of this chapter appears in Table 11–5.

▶ REFERENCES

1. Impact of vaccines universally recommended for children—United States, 1990–1998. *MMWR Morb Mortal Wkly Rep* 1999;48(12):243–248.
2. Coffield AB, Maciosek MV, McGinnis JM, et al. Priorities among recommended clinical preventive services. *Am J Prev Med* 2001;21(1):1–9.
3. Centers for Disease Control and Prevention. *National Immunization Program. Childhood and Adolescent Immunization Schedule, 2004.* Available at: http://www.cdc.gov/nip/recs/child-schedule.htm#Printable.
4. Orenstein W, Rodewald L, Hinman A. Immunization in the United States. In: Plotkin S, Orenstein W, eds. *Vaccines,* 4th ed. Philadelphia, Pa: Saunders; 2004:1359–1361.
5. Simpson DM, Ezzati-Rice TM, Zell ER. Forty years and four surveys: How does our measuring measure up? *Am J Prev Med* 2001; 20(4 suppl):6–14.
6. Atkinson W, et al. Measles. In: *Epidemiology, Control and Prevention of Vaccine-Preventable Diseases,* 17th ed. Atlanta, Ga: Centers for Disease Control and Prevention; 2002. Available at: http://www.cdc.gov/nip/publications/surv-manual/measle.pdf.
7. Hutchins SS, Jiles R, Bernier R. Elimination of measles and of disparities in measles childhood vaccine coverage among racial and ethnic minority populations in the United States. *J Infect Dis* 2004;189(suppl 1):S146–152.
8. Centers for Disease Control and Prevention, National Center for Health Statistics. *Health, United States, 1993,* with Chartbook. p 33 (Chartbook). Available at: http://www.cdc.gov/nchs.
9. Centers for Disease Control and Prevention, National Immunization Program. *National Immunization Survey.* Available at: http://www.cdc.gov/nip/coverage/default.htm#NIS.
10. Chu SY, Barker LE, Smith PJ. Racial/ethnic disparities in preschool immunizations: United States, 1996–2001. *Am J Public Health* 2004; 94(6):973–977.
11. Barker LE, Chu SY, Smith PJ. Disparities in immunizations. *Am J Public Health* 2004;94(6):906.
12. The measles epidemic. The problems, barriers, and recommendations. The National Vaccine Advisory Committee. *JAMA* 1991;266(11):1547–1552.
13. Robinson CA, Sepe SJ, Lin KF. The president's child immunization initiative—a summary of the problem and the response. *Public Health Rep* 1993;108(4):419–425.
14. Strebel P, Papania M, Halsey N. Measles vaccine. In: Plotkin S, Orenstein W, eds. *Vaccines,* 4th ed. Philadelphia, Pa: Saunders; 2004:418–424.
15. Recommendations regarding interventions to improve vaccination coverage in children, adolescents, and adults. Task Force on Community Preventive Services. *Am J Prev Med* 2000; 18(1 suppl):92–96.
16. Woods DR, Mason DD. Six areas lead national early immunization drive. *Public Health Rep* 1992;107(3):252–256.
17. Robinson CA, Evans WB, Mahanes JA, et al. Progress on the childhood immunization initiative. *Public Health Rep* 1994;109(5):594–600.
18. Orenstein WA, Bernier RH. Toward immunizing every child on time. *Pediatrics* 1994;94(4 pt 1):545–547.
19. Fairbrother G, Kuttner H, Miller W, et al. Findings from case studies of state and local immunization programs. *Am J Prev Med* 2000; 19(3 suppl):54–77.
20. Johnson KA, Sardell A, Richards B. Federal immunization policy and funding: A history of responding to crises. *Am J Prev Med* 2000;19(3 suppl):99–112.
21. Standards for pediatric immunization practices. Recommended by the National Vaccine

Advisory Committee. *MMWR Recomm Rep* 1993; 42(RR-5):1–10.

22. Dini EF, Chaney M, Moolenaar RL, et al. Information as intervention: How Georgia used vaccination coverage data to double public sector vaccination coverage in seven years. *J Public Health Manag Pract* 1996;2(1):45–49.

23. Hutchins SS, Sherrod J, Bernier R. Assessing immunization coverage in private practice. *J Natl Med Assoc* 2000;92(4):163–168.

24. Use of a data-based approach by a health maintenance organization to identify and address physician barriers to pediatric vaccination—California, 1995. *MMWR Morb Mortal Wkly Rep* 1996;45(9):188–193.

25. Strategies to sustain success in childhood immunizations. The National Vaccine Advisory Committee. *JAMA* 1999;282(4):363–370.

26. Fairbrother G, Friedman S, Hanson KL, et al. Effect of the vaccines for children program on inner-city neighborhood physicians. *Arch Pediatr Adolesc Med* 1997;151(12):1229–1235.

27. Santoli JM, Rodewald LE, Maes EF, et al. Vaccines for Children program, United States, 1997. *Pediatrics* 1999;104(2):e15.

28. Bernier R, Orenstein W, Hutchins S, et al. Do vaccines reach those who most need them? *Vaccination and World Health*. West Sussex, England: Wiley; 1994.

29. Measles prevention. *MMWR Morb Mortal Wkly Rep* 1989;38(suppl 9):1–18.

30. Green L, Kreuter M. *Health Promotion Planning: An Educational and Environmental Approach*. Mountain View, Calif: Mayfield; 1991.

31. Flannery B, Schrag S, Farley M, et al. *Reducing Racial Disparities in Pneumococcal Disease With a New Childhood Vaccine—United States, 1998–2001*. Infectious Diseases Society of America; 2003. Available at: http://www.idsociety.org.

32. Stokley S, Santoli JM, Willis B, et al. Impact of vaccine shortages on immunization programs and providers. *Am J Prev Med* 2004;26(1):15–21.

33. Institute of Medicine. *Financing Vaccines in the 21st Century: Assuring Access and Availability*. National Academies Press; 2003. Available at: http://books.nap.edu/books/0309089794/html/R1.html#pagetop.

34. Centers for Disease Control and Prevention NIP. *Adult Immunization Schedule, 2004*. Available at: http://www.cdc.gov/nip/recs/adult-schedule.htm.

35. Prevention of pneumococcal disease: Recommendations of the Advisory Committee on Immunization Practices (ACIP). *MMWR Recomm Rep* 1997;46(RR-8):1–24.

36. Robinson KA, Baughman W, Rothrock G, et al. Epidemiology of invasive *Streptococcus pneumoniae* infections in the United States, 1995–1998: Opportunities for prevention in the conjugate vaccine era. *JAMA* 2001;285(13):1729–1735.

37. Cortese MM, Wolff M, Almeido-Hill J, et al. High incidence rates of invasive pneumococcal disease in the White Mountain Apache population. *Arch Intern Med* 1992;152(11):2277–2282.

38. Racial/ethnic disparities in influenza and pneumococcal vaccination levels among persons aged > or = 65 years—United States, 1989–2001. *MMWR Morb Mortal Wkly Rep* 2003;52(40):958—962.

39. Influenza and pneumococcal vaccination levels among persons aged > or = 65 years—United States, 2001. *MMWR Morb Mortal Wkly Rep* 2002;51(45):1019–1024.

40. Public health and aging: Influenza vaccination coverage among adults aged > or = 50 years and pneumococcal vaccination coverage among adults aged > or = 65 years—United States, 2002. *MMWR Morb Mortal Wkly Rep* 2003;52(41):987–992.

41. Singleton JA, Greby SM, Wooten KG, et al. Influenza, pneumococcal, and tetanus toxoid vaccination of adults—United States, 1993–1997. *MMWR CDC Surveill Summ* 2000;49(9):39–62.

42. Influenza and pneumococcal vaccination levels among persons aged > or = 65 years—United States, 1999. *MMWR Morb Mortal Wkly Rep* 2001;50(25):532–537.

43. Pneumococcal and influenza vaccination levels among adults aged > or = 65 years—United States, 1995. *MMWR Morb Mortal Wkly Rep* 1997;46(39):913–919.

44. Fiscella K, Franks P, Doescher MP, et al. Disparities in health care by race, ethnicity, and language among the insured: Findings from a national sample. *Med Care* 2002;40(1):52–59.

45. US Dept of Health and Human Services. *Healthy People 2010,* 2nd ed. Washington, DC: USDHHS; 2000.

46. *Influenza and Pneumococcal Immunization: A Qualitative Assessment of the Beliefs of Physicians and Older Hispanics and African*

Americans. Available at: http://www.cdc.gov/nip/Flu/flu_qualresearch.htm

47. Missed opportunities for pneumococcal and influenza vaccination of Medicare pneumonia inpatients—12 western states, 1995. *MMWR Morb Mortal Wkly Rep* 1997;46(39):919–923.

48. Fedson DS. Improving the use of pneumococcal vaccine through a strategy of hospital-based immunization: A review of its rationale and implications. *J Am Geriatr Soc* 1985;33(2):142–150.

49. Crouse BJ, Nichol K, Peterson DC, et al. Hospital-based strategies for improving influenza vaccination rates. *J Fam Pract* 1994; 38(3):258–261.

50. Egede LE, Zheng D. Racial/ethnic differences in influenza vaccination coverage in high-risk adults. *Am J Public Health* 2003;93(12):2074–2078.

51. Nichol KL, Zimmerman R. Generalist and subspecialist physicians' knowledge, attitudes, and practices regarding influenza and pneumococcal vaccinations for elderly and other high-risk patients: A nationwide survey. *Arch Intern Med* 2001;161(22):2702–2708.

52. Marin MG, Johanson WG Jr, Salas-Lopez D. Influenza vaccination among minority populations in the United States. *Prev Med* 2002;34(2):235–241.

53. Mark TL, Paramore LC. Pneumococcal pneumonia and influenza vaccination: Access to and use by US Hispanic Medicare beneficiaries. *Am J Public Health* 1996;86(11):1545–1550.

54. Fedson DS. Adult immunization. Summary of the National Vaccine Advisory Committee Report. *JAMA* 1994;272(14):1133–1137.

55. US Dept of Health and Human Services. Adult immunization action plan: Report of the Workgroup on Adult Immunization. Washington, DC: USDHHS, CDC; 1997. July 18, 2000. Available at: http://www.dhhs.gov/nvpo/pubs/adult4.htm

56. Local data for local decision making—selected counties, Connecticut, Massachusetts, and New York, 1997. *MMWR Morb Mortal Wkly Rep* 1998;47(38):809–813.

57. Adult immunization: Knowledge, attitudes, and practices—DeKalb and Fulton Counties, Georgia, 1988. *MMWR Morb Mortal Wkly Rep* 1988; 37(43):657–661.

58. Nichol KL, Mac Donald R, Hauge M. Factors associated with influenza and pneumococcal vaccination behavior among high-risk adults. *J Gen Intern Med* 1996;11(11):673–677.

59. Adult immunization programs in nontraditional settings: Quality standards and guidance for program evaluation—a report of the National Vaccine Advisory Committee and use of standing orders programs to increase adult vaccination rates. *MMWR Recomm Rep* 2000;49(RR-1): 1–13.

60. Vaccine-preventable diseases: Improving vaccination coverage in children, adolescents, and adults. A report on recommendations from the Task Force on Community Preventive Services. *MMWR Recomm Rep* 1999;48(RR-8):1–15.

61. Gyorkos TW, Tannenbaum TN, Abrahamowicz M, et al. Evaluation of the effectiveness of immunization delivery methods. *Can J Public Health* 1994;85(suppl 1):S14–30.

62. Fontanesi J, Shefer AM, Fishbein DB, et al. Operational conditions affecting the vaccination of older adults. *Am J Prev Med* 2004;26(4):265–270.

63. Sisk JE, Whang W, Butler JC, et al. Cost-effectiveness of vaccination against invasive pneumococcal disease among people 50 through 64 years of age: Role of comorbid conditions and race. *Ann Intern Med* 2003; 138(12):960–968.

64. Nichol KL, Margolis KL, Wuorenma J, et al. The efficacy and cost effectiveness of vaccination against influenza among elderly persons living in the community. *N Engl J Med* 1994;331(12):778–784.

65. Barker LE, Luman ET, McCauley MM, et al. Assessing equivalence: An alternative to the use of difference tests for measuring disparities in vaccination coverage. *Am J Epidemiol* 2002;156(11):1056–1061.

CHAPTER 12

Obesity and Nutrition

DAVID SATCHER, MD, PhD

KATHI A. EARLES, MD, MPH

▶ INTRODUCTION

The Surgeon General's Call to Action to Prevent and Decrease Overweight and Obesity, released in December 2001,[1] reported 300,000 deaths per year related to obesity and 430,000 from smoking. A March 2004 Centers for Disease Control and Prevention (CDC) report indicated that obesity was expected to overtake smoking as the number one preventable cause of death in this country, citing some 400,000 obesity-related deaths per year.[2] Findings from more recent research conducted by the CDC and the National Institutes of Health (NIH) suggested that obesity results in 112,000 American deaths each year instead of 400,000. The discrepancy in numbers has been attributed to the statistics and methodology used in the first study. While the CDC leadership agreed that they may have overestimated the number of obesity-related deaths, they did not agree with the 112,000 annual obesity-related deaths and downgraded their number from 400,000 to 365,000 as reported in January 2005. Notwithstanding the controversy over the disparate figures, the CDC stands by its conclusions that "tobacco use and poor diet and physical inactivity contributed to the largest number of deaths, and the number of deaths related to poor diet and physical inactivity is increasing."

Based on the National Health and Nutrition Examination Survey III (NHANES), the increase in obesity has been seen in all racial, ethnic, gender, and age groups in the United States. However, this epidemic is affecting minorities disproportionately—especially women and girls of African American and Latino heritage. Children especially have been affected, with a doubling of overweight and obesity since 1980 and a tripling for adolescents. Today over 65% of US adults are overweight as well and almost 31% are obese. In 1980, there was no state in which more than 20% of the population was obese. Today the opposite is true for most states.[3]

Concern about overweight and obesity relates not simply to appearance but to health. Obesity is a leading cause of death in the United States, significantly increasing the risk for diabetes, cardiovascular disease, and cancers of the colon, breast, and prostate. There are many other concerns associated with obesity, including problems related to stigma, low self-esteem, and depression. Among children, type 2 diabetes has increased 10-fold since 1980.

▶ ROLE OF THE SURGEON GENERAL

The Surgeon General of the United States has two major functions. The first is the responsibility to oversee the 6000-member Commissioned Corps of the US Public Health Service (PHS). The second responsibility is to communicate directly with the American people to assist in protecting and advancing the nation's health and safety. One primary way is through the issuance of Surgeon General's reports—reports that are based on the best available public health science, not politics, religion, or personal opinion. The credibility of Surgeon General's reports is due in large part to this historic commitment and practice.

The first official report from the Office of the Surgeon General was published in 1964 by Surgeon General Luther Terry and dealt with smoking and health.[4] This was a landmark report in the history of public health in that it put to rest for most people the long-standing debate about the safety or harm of tobacco and smoking. In preparing the report, Surgeon General Terry put together an outstanding panel of scientific advisors who reviewed all the existing studies related to smoking and health and concluded that smoking was indeed harmful to health and, among other things, that it significantly increased the risk for lung cancer.

It is important to note that according to unofficial sources, including surviving members of the panel, not only was Surgeon General Terry a smoker during the time the report was being prepared but so were 9 of the 10 members of the scientific advisory panel. However, they did not allow personal opinions or behavior to prevent them from releasing a report based on the best available public health science. According to Dr Terry's son, Michael,[5] who attended the release of the report on *Reducing Tobacco Use,* his father not only quit smoking after releasing the 1964 report, but wore a lapel pin for the rest of his life that said: "Thank you for not smoking." January 11, 2004 marked the 40th anniversary of that first Surgeon General's report. Today, the credibility of these reports is still high. Since the release of the first report, many lives have been saved because individuals decided not to begin smoking or decided to quit smoking.[6] We now have the opportunity to save many more lives by applying the best available science in our efforts to attack the epidemic of overweight and obesity.

▶ SURGEON GENERAL'S CALL TO ACTION TO PREVENT AND DECREASE OVERWEIGHT AND OBESITY[1]

The decision to produce a Surgeon General's report on overweight and obesity was born out of growing concern with the epidemic and its potential impact on the nation's health. In our report, we stated that "left unabated obesity would overtake tobacco as the leading preventable cause of death in this country." As with other reports from the Surgeon General, the intent was to educate, motivate, and mobilize the American people against this epidemic. We described the problem in vivid and dramatic terms consistent with the best available science and best available public health data, including the nature, magnitude, and distribution of the problem. We also examined the major risk factors seemingly contributing to the epidemic. These risk factors coalesce around two major forces in our society: (1) forces that have facilitated and encouraged the consumption of increasing amounts of foods and calories by the American people over the past three decades, and (2) forces that have combined to discourage and decrease physical activity among the American people.

Overweight and obesity are defined by a formula, known as the body mass index (BMI), that relates a person's weight in kilograms to his or her height in meters squared: BMI = weight (kg)/height (m^2). The BMI is a measure of body fat and can also be derived by relating pounds to height in inches with an adjusted formula. Although the BMI is not perfect, it has been found to be fairly accurate in predicting health risks, including risk of death when applied to populations globally by the World Health Organization. Using this formula, a BMI in the range of 18 to 25 is considered within normal limits; 25 to 30 is overweight, and 30 and higher is obese. The BMI can be artificially high in persons who engage in muscle-building activities, thus incorrectly categorizing them in the overweight category. By the same token, an older person who loses muscle may appear to have lower-than-normal BMI despite an elevation in body fat. But while the BMI is not perfect, it is still an excellent predictor of future health risks.[7]

By the same token, BMI cannot be applied to children in the same way as in adults. Because children grow at different rates, it is difficult to separate overweight from obesity in children, and the BMI must be plotted along growth curves as was done in the Surgeon General's report. The CDC has developed a BMI growth curve for children, which is illustrated in Figure 12–1A and B.

▶ EPIDEMIC OF CHILDHOOD OVERWEIGHT

The past decade has seen a dramatic shift in the weight patterns of children. Recent studies demonstrate that 10% of children aged 2 to 5 years and 15% of children 6 to 9 years are overweight.[8] Data from NHANES III illustrated that approximately 14% of all children residing in the United States are overweight.[9] This dramatic increase is seen at a greater rate in the minority pediatric community. Rates among minority children and adolescents are nearly 50% higher than those in the Caucasian population.[10] NHANES III data (1988–1994) demonstrated that the prevalence of overweight had increased to 21.5% in African American children and 21.8% in Hispanic children, whereas the prevalence in Caucasian children had increased to a rate of 12.3%. Of these minority groups, it appears that girls are disproportionately affected compared with boys. In addition to the disparity of excess weight within the minority pediatric population, children residing in impoverished communities are more overweight than their economically advantaged peers.[11] Multiple studies have demonstrated an increased incidence of subsequent adult obesity in adolescents who are overweight. The risk of an overweight toddler developing into an obese adult rises approximately 20%. This statistic increases in overweight adolescents, who have an 80% greater risk of developing into an obese adult.[12] Persistent overweight status in children has been associated with greater morbidity and mortality than adult-onset obesity.

Reasons contributing to the recent rise in weight gain in the pediatric population are multifactorial. Although genetics alone cannot explain obesity, it plays a significant role in excessive childhood weight gain. Children who reside in families with an overweight parent are more likely to be overweight.[13] Further supporting the role of genetics, infants born to diabetic mothers are also more likely to develop into overweight children.[14]

Although the role of genetics suggests an inherent predilection, lifestyle factors such as breast-feeding, parental modeling, television viewing, dietary trends, and physical activity also serve as significant factors. Breast-feeding appears to have a protective effect against pediatric obesity.[15] This has been demonstrated by previous studies; however, the exact mechanism remains unknown.

Parental choices pertaining to dietary habits, food preferences, and attitudes toward physical activity are powerful tools in determining the behavior of children.[16] Parents who consume an unhealthy diet and place a low priority on physical activity and fitness validate this behavior to their offspring. Likewise, healthy parental dietary behaviors and physical activity influence similar patterns in children.[17]

Children and adolescents consume large quantities of television. The Nielsen Media Research study indicates that the average child watches 2 or more hours of television per day.[18] When other forms of media are included, such as video games and computer use, the average child spends approximately 6.5 hours per day in sedentary activities. Recent studies have demonstrated a link between excessive television viewing and excessive childhood weight gain and decreased energy expenditure.[19,20] Additional studies have broken out the relationship between television viewing and excessive weight in terms of four variables: content analysis:

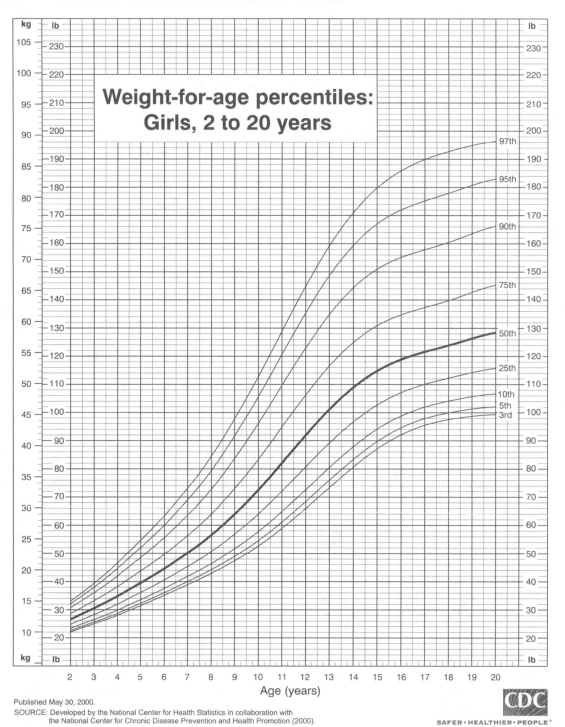

Weight-for-age percentiles: Girls, 2 to 20 years

Published May 30, 2000.
SOURCE: Developed by the National Center for Health Statistics in collaboration with the National Center for Chronic Disease Prevention and Health Promotion (2000).

SAFER · HEALTHIER · PEOPLE™

Figure 12–1A. BMI growth curve for girls aged 2 to 20 years. (*Source: Centers for Disease Control and Prevention, 2000.*)

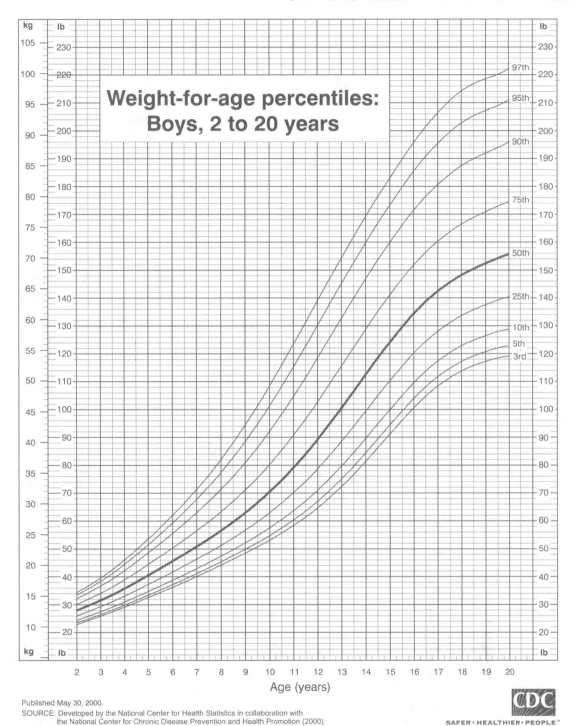

Published May 30, 2000.
SOURCE: Developed by the National Center for Health Statistics in collaboration with
the National Center for Chronic Disease Prevention and Health Promotion (2000).

Figure 12–1B. BMI growth curve for boys aged 2 to 20 years. (*Source: Centers for Disease Control and Prevention, 2000.*)

television advertising and food-related behavior; dietary intake and physical activity; and food consumption patterns.[21] Content analysis studies have demonstrated that food items are the most highly advertised product on television. Vegetables and fruits are frequently neglected options as advertisers focus on snacks high in fat, sugar, and salt content. Children repeatedly choose advertised products over unadvertised ones.[22] Purchase request studies have demonstrated a relationship between quantity of television viewing, request for specific advertised foods, and subsequent presence in the home.[23] Excessive television viewing has been associated with higher consumption of sweets, fats, carbonated beverages, and salty snacks. Conversely, excessive television viewing has also been associated with lower consumption of vegetables and fruits. Studies demonstrating a link between television viewing and excessive weight gain have been duplicated in other countries. The Institute of Nutrition and Food Safety at the Chinese Center for Disease Control and Prevention performed a study of approximately 9000 Chinese children designed to assess the association between the quantity of television viewed and obesity. The study concluded that the prevalence of obesity increased by 1% to 2% with each hourly increment of television viewed.[24]

NHANES III demonstrated the effect of increased television viewing on BMI (Fig. 12–2).

According to the data presented by NHANES III, there is a positive correlation between the number of hours of television viewed and the BMI. As the quantity of television increases, the BMI also increases. This is also true when controlling for socioeconomic and ethnic differences.

The greater percentage of obesity in the minority population is also mirrored in the patterns of television viewing by this same population. In 2000, the CDC found that 65% of African American and 53% of Hispanic youth studied watched television for 3 or more hours compared with 37% of their Caucasian peers. Compared with Caucasian children, three times as many African American children and 1.5 as many Hispanic children watch 5 or more hours of television per day.[25] Additionally, a recent study found that prime-time television programs oriented toward African American audiences presented more commercials for high-fat, low-nutrient products.[26] Characters in these television shows were frequently overweight, further reinforcing the stereotype that excessive weight is pervasive and acceptable in the minority community.

Over the past decade, there has been a trend towards consuming foods higher in fats, sodium, and cholesterol. At present, the average intake of fat, saturated fat, sodium, and cholesterol by adolescents and children is higher than current recommendations. The US Department of Agriculture found that total fat and saturated fat comprised 35.8% and 12.5%, respectively, of daily calories consumed by children.[27] In the population studied, 80% of the participants exceeded the total fat recommendations and 70% exceeded the saturated fat recommendations. Additional studies conducted by the National Food Consumption Survey demonstrated a sharp decline in the consumption of lean meats and eggs, along with an increase in the consumption of grains by adolescents from 1965 to 1996. The increase in grain, however, was attributed to high-fat products such as pizza, macaroni and cheese, and certain fast food items. As indicated previously, there is a direct link between products advertised and products consumed in the pediatric population. As highly

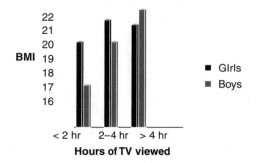

Figure 12–2. Relationship between television viewing and body mass index (BMI) in boys and girls.

advertised snacks are consumed in greater quantities than unadvertised fruits and vegetables, the fat percentage has also increased in many snack products. The proportion of fat in snacks increased from 17% to 22% of total fat from 1977 to 1996.[28] The US Adolescent Food Intake Survey further demonstrated an increase in sweet beverages consumed and a decrease in milk and raw fruits. The increase in fat and caloric consumption is greater in the minority community. NHANES III illustrated a higher percentage of energy from fat for African American and Hispanic girls and African American boys than for Caucasian boys or girls.[29] The disparity between racial groups was noted in girls as early as 6 to 9 years of age and in boys as early as 10 to 13 years of age.

Economic differences may influence the development of pediatric obesity indirectly. "Food insecurity" implies that adequate quantities and nutritional quality of foods are not available for contribution to a healthy and active life. Recent evidence suggests that nearly 12 million children reside in households defined as "food insecure,"[30] which means that they lack consistent access to enough food for active, healthy living at some point throughout the year. Recent research indicates that women residing in food-insecure households had significantly greater BMI.[31] Because parental behavior regarding dietary choices influences the behavior of children, it could be deduced that obesity related to moderately food-insecure homes can affect the excessive weight status of children through the impact on the caretakers. Of note, there is a greater prevalence of food insecurity in homes headed by single women, homes with children, and households qualifying for public assistance and residing below the poverty level. As indicated in Figure 12–3, there is an inverse correlation between income and obesity level, with differing effects on the African American and Caucasian communities.

Recent budgetary restraints and emphasis on increasing standardized test scores have led to a decline in physical education programs within the school system. According to a study con-

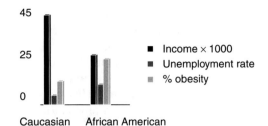

Figure 12–3. Relationship among income, unemployment, and obesity in Caucasian and African American populations.

ducted by the CDC, physical education participation decreased from 79% in the 9th grade to 37% by the 12th grade. Excluding organized physical education courses, vigorous physical activity, including intramural and team sports, declined from 73% in 9th grade to 61% in 12th grade. As with television viewing, minority children participate less often in physical activity than do their Caucasian peers. Conversely, Caucasian adolescents were less physically inactive than African American adolescents. Minority youth are less likely to participate in regular physical activity. The highest incidence of physical activity has been noted in Caucasian boys (73%), and the lowest, in African American girls (41.8%).

Obesity has devastating effects on the quality of life and contributes significantly to overall morbidity and mortality. The rise in cardiovascular disease, diabetes, certain types of cancer, and psychological disturbances is linked to the recent surge in the rate of obesity. Although cardiovascular disease is primarily a disease of adulthood, risk factors are present in childhood. The presence of fatty streaks in the aorta and fibrous plaques in the coronary vessels of children are believed to indicate progressive atherosclerosis.[32] These fatty streaks are found at a greater rate in children with elevated BMI, therefore contributing to the disproportionate share of adult-onset cardiovascular disease in this population. Hypertension, elevated plasma lipid levels, and obesity experienced in childhood are associated with asymptomatic coronary heart disease and aortic atherosclerosis.[33] The Bogalusa Heart Study further emphasized the association between childhood obesity and the development of cardiovascular disease.[34] In the children studied, an overweight youth was 7.1 times more likely to have a high triglyceride level and 2.4 times more likely to have a high total cholesterol level than his normal-weight peers. Additional studies demonstrated that obesity at age 13 years was associated with an elevated total cholesterol level at age 21 years.[35] Children with a BMI greater than 25 that persists into adulthood have a significantly greater risk of adult-onset myocardial infarction, congestive heart failure, and angina in part due to elevated lipid levels and hypertension beginning in the pediatric period.

According to NHANES data, type 2 diabetes has increased to a rate of 4.1 per 1000 among US children.[36] In another study, the rate of newly diagnosed cases of non–insulin-dependent diabetes mellitus (NIDDM) increased from approximately 2% to 4% of newly diagnosed cases of diabetes in 1992 to greater than 15% in 1996.[37] Mirroring the disparity of obesity in the minority pediatric community, 94% of all youth with NIDDM are minority.[38] Factors contributing to the development of NIDDM in the pediatric population are identical to those contributing to the rise in obesity in the pediatric community: sedentary lifestyle and high caloric consumption of fat. It is believed that over 83% of all youth diagnosed with NIDDM meet the qualifications of obesity.[39] Further linking obesity and diabetes, insulin resistance at age 21 years as measured by glucose utilization was greater among youth who were obese at age 13 years. Youth who are overweight are at a significantly greater risk for developing type 2 diabetes and the associated complications: diabetic retinopathy, cardiovascular disease, renal damage, and neuropathy.

Although obesity in the pediatric population has not demonstrated an association with pediatric forms of cancer, persistence into adulthood has been shown to be associated with certain forms of cancer. Endometrial, breast, colon, gallbladder, prostate, and kidney cancers are at increased risk in the adult obese population as compared with normal-weight adults.[40] As relates specifically to breast cancer, women who gain more than 20 pounds beginning at 18 years through midlife are twice as likely to develop postmenopausal breast cancer compared with those whose weight remains constant.[41]

The most emergent consequence of obesity as perceived by the pediatric population is the social stigma and isolation attached to being overweight. Weight-based teasing has been associated with poor self-esteem, depressive symptoms, and suicidal ideation in many adolescents.[42] These associations remained constant despite controlling for racial, ethnic, and actual weight of the adolescents studied. Data obtained from studying the behavior of a group of 8- to 11-year-olds demonstrated an association between pediatric obesity and behavior problems even after controlling for race, sex, academic history, income, and maternal education [43] A growing body of evidence links adult obesity to mental health. Although adult obesity is also frequently related to poor self-esteem, the association is less intense in the obese male population. Obese adult women were noted to have a higher prevalence of depression than their normal-weight peers.[44] This relationship increases with greater income and perceived socioeconomic status. The relationship between obesity and depression becomes even greater as weight increases. Severely obese adults have a greater rate of depressive symptoms than average-weight adults.[45]

Additional consequences of obesity include an increase in obstructive sleep apnea, osteoarthritis, and reproductive complications. Overweight children are more likely to experience sleep disturbances requiring surgical correction than children who are within normal weight for age and height.[46] Additional studies have suggested a correlation between obesity and asthma. The risk of developing arthritis has been demonstrated to increase for every 2-pound weight gain by 9% to 13% in the adult population.[47] Obesity in premenopausal women has been associated with irregular menses, infertility, and pregnancy complications, such as gestational diabetes and increased risk of birth defects.[48]

The significant comorbid features associated with obesity and the apparent epidemic rates within the adult and pediatric community make combating obesity a primary health concern. Treatment options for obesity are centered around behavior modification; physical activity, including decreasing sedentary behavior; and altering eating habits. Behavior modification designed to promote life-long changes focused on healthy behaviors has proven to be most effective when the entire family becomes involved. The initial step should be assisting caretakers in accepting their role as role models whose attitude toward physical activity and eating habits directly affects their children's behavior.[49] Caretakers should be encouraged to practice eating balanced meals, exercise regularly, and watch television sparingly, thereby modeling behavior conducive for weight modification and physical fitness.

Effective physical activity as incorporated to promote a life-long commitment to health and physical fitness has been proven to assist in weight modification and maintenance. Physical education as a regular portion of the academic setting is an effective method of introducing structured and consistent activity. Caretakers may act as effective models for establishing consistent physical activity. Activities that call for participation by the entire family should be encouraged. A guide published by the American Alliance for Health, Physical Education, Recreation, and Dance recommends that young children participate in 30 to 60 minutes of structured physical activity a day.[50] In addition, the same guidelines recommend that children participate in at least 60 minutes of unstructured activity per day. Physical activity should be incorporated into the daily routine and could include such activities as walks, playground time, walking the dog, and taking the stairs whenever possible. Older children may be encouraged to participate in organized sports, which have the combined benefit of promoting physical fitness,

group dynamics, and leadership ability. Reducing sedentary activities such as Internet usage, computer game playing, and excessive television viewing has also been shown to increase total energy expenditure.[51] Consuming snacks should be avoided during television viewing and, if necessary, should be confined to fruits and vegetables of previously designated quantities. Television time should be reduced to 1 to 2 hours daily in children over 2 years of age and avoided totally in children younger than 2 years of age.[52] Activities in the 2-year-and-under group should be focused on cognitive development, including singing and reading.

In families with young children, healthy habits that focus on nutritionally sound meals should be emphasized. Suggestions such as inclusion of fruits or vegetables with each meal; elimination of high-salt, -fat, and sugary snacks; limitation of fast foods; and eating at a communal table without the television may be effective in initiating healthy eating habits.[53] A routine that incorporates three balanced meals a day and two healthy snacks should be established. Portion sizes appropriate for the age and recommended weight and height of the child should be emphasized, and the practice of encouraging eating until full should be avoided. Emphasis on "cleaning the plate" and rewards of candy should be replaced with verbal praise. A variety of healthy choices should be allowed, because multiple studies indicate that dietary restrictions by parents lead to excessive consumption of such restricted foods in adulthood.[54] The cornerstone for weight control in all age groups has concentrated on a low-fat and reduced-caloric intake. An increase in dietary fiber (eg, fruits, grains, and vegetables) and complex carbohydrates has also proven to be effective. Meal replacement, including replacing one meal a day with commercially available products that are high in nutritional value and low in calories, has been suggested as an alternative option for adults.[55]

Pharmacotherapy and surgery are reserved for a subset of overweight individuals. Medications, when utilized, should be part of a comprehensive strategy designed to promote weight reduction. Orlistat and sibutramine are agents that have proven effective; however, there has been insufficient research into their use within the pediatric population. Orlistat, an inhibitor of fat absorption, is approved for individuals beginning at age 18 and has demonstrated a weight loss of 4% body weight within 3 months in morbidly obese patients.[56] Sibutramine, an inhibitor of norepinephrine and serotonin uptake, has demonstrated a reduction of 8.5% (7.8 kg) in BMI in severely obese individuals after 6 months of treatment when combined with behavior modification.[57] These results are in contrast to a weight reduction of 4% (3.2 kg) with behavior modification alone. The role of surgery, primarily utilized in the adult population, is reserved for a unique subset of adults and is beyond the scope of this text.

▶ HEALTHY PEOPLE 2010

Healthy People 2010, the nation's health plan for this decade, lists overweight and obesity as one of the 10 leading health indicators for monitoring and evaluation of the health of the American people. Measurable objectives are included in *Healthy People 2010* for the purpose of program development.[58] Overweight and obesity are also important as they relate to the two goals of *Healthy People 2010.* The first of the two goals is to increase the years and quality of healthy life and the second is the elimination of disparities in health among different racial and ethnic groups. Overweight and obesity interfere with quality of life across the life span, and disparities in obesity by race are major contributors to disparities in health among different racial and ethnic groups.[1]

The epidemic of obesity also threatens to reverse much of the progress the nation has made over the past 40 years in the control of cardiovascular disease, diabetes, and several forms of cancer.[59] These decades saw a dramatic decline of more than 60% to 70% in deaths from cardiovascular disease, believed to be due to reduction in tobacco use, the control of hypertension, lowering cholesterol and other lifestyle changes. Likewise, over the past 10 to 15 years, we have witnessed a decline in cancer mortality due to changes in lifestyle, environment, and early diagnosis and treatment of many forms of cancer, including breast and cervical cancer. But the increase in rates of overweight and obesity threatens to increase cardiovascular and cancer deaths and is already dramatically increasing the incidence of diabetes and its complications.

The Surgeon General's report identified ways in which we in the United States—as a society, as communities, and as individuals—can counteract the forces driving the epidemic of obesity. The actions needed are included in a strategy embodied in the acronym CARE, which stands for Communication, Action, Research, and Evaluation.[60] Some of the most appropriate settings in which this strategy can take place include the home and family, communities, schools, work sites, the health-care arena, and media and communications outlets.

To date the setting that has received the most organized attention has been the school. In October 2002, the National Healthy School Summit was convened, with First Lady Laura Bush serving as honorary chair and the former Surgeon General as working chair. Leaders in education, health, government, sports, and the food industry were invited to discuss how schools could become environments that are conducive in helping children develop lifetime habits of physical activity and good nutrition. Teams were organized for each state and the District of Columbia with the charge of helping schools move forward in meeting these requirements. Schools are also important because of their relationship to homes, families, and communities. Not all parents are equal in their ability to educate or model healthy behaviors such as physical activity and good nutrition for their children. But if schools create environments that are conducive to helping children develop lifetime habits of physical activity and good nutrition, all children can benefit, just as public education has benefited children from diverse family backgrounds over the years. Schools can also influence the behavior of families by the messages that children take home and by direct interaction through organizations such as the Parent Teachers Association (PTA).

The Surgeon General's report also recommended the workplace as an appropriate setting for preventing and reducing overweight and obesity, again using the CARE approach. Programs developed by the CDC and Home Depot were referred to as models when the report was released.[1]

Health care is another important setting for preventing and reducing overweight and obesity. Physicians, in association with other healthcare providers, can educate patients and potential patients about the importance of good nutrition and regular physical activity. Unfortunately, our disease-oriented health system is not helpful here. For example, physicians cannot be reimbursed for time spent helping patients lose weight because obesity is not defined as a disease. However, when obesity is so morbid as to be life threatening, physicians can be reimbursed for performing gastric bypass surgery and other operations. We recommend that obesity be considered a disease for the purpose of physician reimbursements.

The media were recommended as another site or setting for the CARE approach. The media must help first to communicate that obesity is not a cosmetic but a health issue. Obesity increases the risk for chronic diseases and must be attacked as a way of reducing health risks. Using some of the lessons learned from the first Surgeon General's report, we can begin to make serious strides now with overweight and obesity that will prevent a 40-year delay before the nation witnesses a downward turn in this trend. We must also communicate that we are not helpless in the face of the epidemic of obesity. We can intervene to develop better health-related policies. We can improve community and school support for physical activity and good nutrition. We can also educate, motivate, and mobilize individuals and families toward healthy lifestyles.

▶ REFERENCES

1. US Dept of Health and Human Services. *The Surgeon General's Call to Action to Prevent and Decrease Overweight and Obesity.* Rockville, Md: USDHHS, Public Health Service, Office of the Surgeon General; 2001. Available from: US Government Printing Office, Washington, DC.
2. Cigarette smoking–attributable morbidity–United States, 2000. *MMWR Morb Mortal Wkly Rep* 2003;52(35):842–844. Available at: http://www.cdc.gov/mmwr/preview/mmwrhtml/mm5235a4.htm.
3. National Center for Chronic Disease Prevention and Health Promotion. *Obesity Trends: U.S. Obesity Trends 1985–2003.* Atlanta, Ga: Centers for Disease Control and Prevention. Available at: http://www.cdc.gov/nccdphp/dnpa/obesity/trend/ maps/index.htm.
4. US Dept of Health, Education, and Welfare. *Smoking and Health: Report of the Advisory Committee to the Surgeon General of the Public Health Service.* Rockville, Md: USDHEW, Public Health Service, Communicable Disease Center; 1964. DHEW Publication No. 1103.
5. Satcher, David. Personal conversation with Michael Terry; 9 Aug 2000.
6. 40th anniversary of the first Surgeon General's report on smoking and health. *MMWR Morb Mortal Wkly Rep* 2004;53(3):49. Available at: http://www.cdc.gov/mmwr/preview/mmwrhtml/mm5303a1.htm.
7. US Dept of Health and Human Services. *The Surgeon General's Call to Action to Prevent and Decrease Overweight and Obesity.* Rockville, Md: USDHHS, Public Health Service, Office of the Surgeon General; 2001:4.
8. Ogden CL, Flegal KM, Carroll MD, et al. Prevalence and trends among US children and adolescents, 1999–2000. *JAMA* 2002;288(14):1728–1732.
9. Kant AK. Reported consumption of low-nutrient-density foods by American children and adolescents: Nutritional and health correlates, NHANES III, 1988 to 1994. *Arch Pediatr Adolesc Med* 2003;157(8):789–796.
10. Bray GA, Popkin BM. Dietary fat affects obesity rate. *Am J Clin Nutr* 1999;70(4):572–573.
11. Laitinen J, Power C, Jarvelin MR. Family social class, maternal body mass index, childhood body mass index, and age at menarche as predictors of adult obesity. *Am J Clin Nutr* 2001;74(3):287–294.

12. Guo SS, Chumlea WC. Tracking of body mass index in children in relation to overweight in adulthood. *Am J Clin Nutr* 1999;70(1):145S–148S.

13. Whitaker RC, Wright JA, Pepe MS, et al. Predicting obesity in young adulthood from childhood and parental obesity. *N Engl J Med* 1997;337(13):869–873.

14. Gillman MW, Rifas-Shiman S, Berkey CS, et al. Maternal gestational diabetes, birth weight, and adolescent obesity. *Pediatrics* 2003;111(3):e221–226.

15. von Kries R, Koletzko B, Sauerwald T, et al. Does breast-feeding protect against childhood obesity? *Adv Exp Med Biol* 2000;478:29–39.

16. Hertzler AA, Vaughan CE. The relationship of family structure and interaction to nutrition. *J Am Diet Assoc* 1979;74(1):23–27.

17. Eck LH, Klesges RC, Hanson CL, et al. Children at familial risk for obesity: An examination of dietary intake, physical activity and weight status. *Int J Obes Relat Metab Disord* 1992;16(2):71–78.

18. American Academy of Pediatrics. Children, adolescents, and television. *Pediatrics* 2001;107(2):423–426.

19. Grund A, Krause H, Siewers M, et al. Is TV viewing an index of physical activity and fitness in overweight and normal weight children? *Public Health Nutr* 2001;4(6):1245–1251.

20. Klesges RC, Shelton ML, Klesges LM. Effects of television on metabolic rate: Potential implications for childhood obesity. *Pediatrics* 1993;91(2):281–286.

21. Villani S. Impact of media on children and adolescents: A 10-year review of the research. *J Am Acad Child Adolesc Psychiatry* 2001;40(4):392–401.

22. Coon KA, Tucker KL. Television and children's consumption patterns. A review of the literature. *Minerva Pediatr* 2002;54(5):423–436.

23. Coon KA, Goldberg J, Rogers BL, et al. Relationships between use of television during meals and children's food consumption patterns. *Pediatrics* 2001;107(1):E7.

24. Ma GS, Li YP, Hu XQ, et al. Effect of television viewing on pediatric obesity. *Biomed Environ Sci* 2002;15(4):291–297.

25. Crespo CJ, Smit E, Troiano RP, et al. Television watching, energy intake, and obesity in US children: Results from the third National Health and Nutrition Examination Survey, 1988–1994. *Arch Pediatr Adolesc Med* 2001;155(3):360–365.

26. Tirodkar MA, Jain A. Food messages on African American television shows. *Am J Public Health* 2003;93(3):439–441.

27. Cavadini C, Siega-Riz AM, Popkin BM. US adolescent food intake trends from 1965 to 1996. *Arch Dis Child* 2000;83(1):18–24.

28. Jahns L, Siega-Riz AM, Popkin BM. The increasing prevalence of snacking among US children from 1977 to 1996. *J Pediatr* 2001;138(4):493–498.

29. Winkleby MA, Robinson TN, Sundquist J, et al. Ethnic variation in cardiovascular disease risk factors among children and young adults: Findings from the Third National Health and Nutrition Examination Survey, 1988–1994. *JAMA* 1999;281(11):1006–1013.

30. Andrews M, Nord M, Bicker G, et al. *Household Food Security in the United States, 1999.* Washington, DC: Food and Rural Economics Division, Economic Research Services, US Dept of Agriculture; 1999. Report No. 8.

31. Townsend MS, Peerson J, Love B, et al. Food insecurity is positively related to overweight in women. *J Nutr* 2001;131(6):1738–1745.

32. Hickman TB, Briefel RR, Carroll MD, et al. Distributions and trends of serum lipid levels among United States children and adolescents ages 4–19 years: Data from the Third National Health and Nutrition Examination Survey. *Prev Med* 1998;27(6):879–90.

33. Berenson GS, Srinivasan SR, Bao W, et al. Association between multiple cardiovascular risk factors and atherosclerosis in children and young adults. The Bogalusa Heart Study. *N Engl J Med* 1998;338(23):1650–1656.

34. Freedman DS, Dietz WH, Srinivasan SR, et al. The relation of overweight to cardiovascular risk factors among children and adolescents: The Bogalusa Heart Study. *Pediatrics* 1999;103(6 pt 1):1175–1182.

35. Steinberger J, Moran A, Hong CP, et al. Adiposity in childhood predicts obesity and insulin resistance in young adulthood. *J Pediatr* 2001;138(4):469–473.

36. Type 2 diabetes in children and adolescents. American Diabetes Association. *Diabetes Care* 2000;23(3):381–389.

37. Pinhas-Hamiel O, Dolan LM, Daniels SR, et al. Increased incidence of non-insulin-dependent diabetes mellitus among adolescents. *J Pediatr* 1996;128(5 pt 1):608–615.

38. Fagot-Campagna A, Pettitt DJ, Engelgau MM, et al. Type 2 diabetes among North American

children and adolescents: An epidemiologic review and a public health perspective. *J Pediatr* 2000;136(5):664–672.

39. Callahan ST, Mansfield MJ. Type 2 diabetes mellitus in adolescents. *Curr Opin Pediatr* 2000;12(4):310–315.

40. Pan SY, Johnson KC, Ugnat AM, et al. Association of obesity and cancer risk in Canada. *Am J Epidemiol* 2004;159(3):259–268.

41. Stephenson GD, Rose DP. Breast cancer and obesity: An update. *Nutr Cancer* 2003;45(1):1–16.

42. Eisenberg ME, Neumark-Sztainer D, Story M. Associations of weight-based teasing and emotional well-being among adolescents. *Arch Pediatr Adolesc Med* 2003;157(8):733–738.

43. Lumeng JC, Gannon K, Cabral HJ, et al. Association between clinically meaningful behavior problems and overweight in children. *Pediatrics* 2003;112(5):1138–1145.

44. Roberts RE, Deleger S, Strawbridge WJ, et al. Prospective association between obesity and depression: Evidence from the Alameda County Study. *Int J Obes Relat Metab Disord* 2003;27(4):514–521.

45. Dixon JB, Dixon ME, O'Brien PE. Depression in association with severe obesity: Changes with weight loss. *Arch Intern Med* 2003;163(17):2058–2065.

46. Must A, Strauss RS. Risks and consequences of childhood and adolescent obesity. *Int J Obes Relat Metab Disord* 1999;23(suppl 2):S2–11.

47. Felson DT, Lawrence RC, Dieppe PA, et al. Osteoarthritis: New insights. Part 1: The disease and its risk factors. *Ann Intern Med* 2000;133(8):635–646.

48. Rosenberg TJ, Garbers S, Chavkin W, et al. Prepregnancy weight and adverse perinatal outcomes in an ethnically diverse population. *Obstet Gynecol* 2003;102(5 pt 1):1022–1027.

49. Golan M, Weizman A. Familial approach to the treatment of childhood obesity: Conceptual mode. *J Nutr Educ* 2001;33(2):102–107.

50. Physical fitness and activity in schools. American Academy of Pediatrics. *Pediatrics* 2000;105(5):1156–1157.

51. Epstein LH, Valoski AM, Vara LS, et al. Effects of decreasing sedentary behavior and increasing activity on weight change in obese children. *Health Psychol* 1995;14(2):109–115.

52. Dennison BA, Rockwell HL, Baker SL. Excess fruit juice consumption by preschool-aged children is associated with short stature and obesity. *Pediatrics* 1997;99(1):15–22.

53. Ariza AJ, Greenberg RS, Unger R: Childhood overweight: Management approaches in young children. *Pediatr Ann* 2004;33(1):33–38.

54. Birch LL, Fisher JO. Development of eating behaviors among children and adolescents. *Pediatrics* 1998;101(3 pt 2):539–549.

55. Heymsfield SB, van Mierlo CA, van der Knaap HC, et al. Weight management using a meal replacement strategy: Meta and pooling analysis from six studies. *Int J Obes Relat Metab Disord* 2003;27(5):537–549.

56. McDuffie JR, Calis KA, Uwaifo GI, et al. Three-month tolerability of orlistat in adolescents with obesity-related comorbid conditions. *Obes Res* 2002;10(7):642–650.

57. Berkowitz RI, Wadden TA, Tershakovec AM, et al. Behavior therapy and sibutramine for the treatment of adolescent obesity: A randomized controlled trial. *JAMA* 2003;289(14):1805–1812.

58. US Dept of Health and Human Services. *Healthy People 2010: Understanding and Improving Health,* 2nd ed. Washington DC: US Government Printing Office; 2000.

59. US Dept of Health and Human Services. *The Surgeon General's Call to Action to Prevent and Decrease Overweight and Obesity.* Rockville, Md: USDHHS, Public Health Service, Office of the Surgeon General; 2001:xiii.

60. US Dept of Health and Human Services. *The Surgeon General's Call to Action to Prevent and Decrease Overweight and Obesity.* Rockville, Md: USDHHS, Public Health Service, Office of the Surgeon General; 2001:16.

CHAPTER 13

HIV Infection and AIDS

ERIC P. GOOSBY, MD*

► INTRODUCTION

Global Overview of HIV/AIDS

Over 21 million people have died as a result of infection with human immunodeficiency virus (HIV) or its sequela, acquired immunodeficiency syndrome (AIDS), since statistics were first collected in 1981. In 2003, there were 5 million new cases worldwide,[1,2] the greatest number of new cases reported in any year since the epidemic began.

The AIDS epidemic has continued to expand across the globe, affecting millions of individuals, their families, and communities. At the close of 2003, UNAIDS estimated a global burden of 38 million adults and children living with HIV and AIDS.[1] The epidemic varies in size within different regions of the world as well as within specific countries. Twenty-five million cases are centered in sub-Saharan Africa, 6.5 million in South and Southeast Asia, 1.6 million in Latin America, 1.3 million in Eastern Europe, 1 million in North America, and approximately 600,000 in Western Europe.[2] In addition, each country's epidemic shows wide variation among populations living in different states or provinces, and within different areas of individual cities.

Looking at the distribution of HIV across different populations gives a clearer picture of the impact HIV and AIDS have on societies. Twelve million children were orphaned in sub-Saharan Africa between 1981 and 2003. Women accounted for nearly 50% of all people living with HIV worldwide, and 57% of the infected lived in sub-Saharan Africa. Young people 15 to 24 years old account for half of all new HIV infections worldwide, and more than 6000 are infected with HIV every day. An estimated 5 million people in low- and middle-income countries who need antiretroviral medications lack the money to purchase them. Finally, the global number of persons infected with HIV continues to increase despite the fact there are preventive interventions that have been shown to be effective.[2]

HIV/AIDS Epidemic in the United States

The United States, on a smaller scale, reflects many of the characteristics for specific populations that are seen on a global level. The distribution of HIV outbreaks has centered in specific high-risk populations in specific geographic areas. Preventive strategies have been episodic, not sustained, and the availability of treatment has been hampered by access barriers such as

*The McGraw-Hill Companies acknowledge the substantial editorial contributions of Donna M. Frassetto and Nancy N. Woelfl in preparation of this chapter.

cost, transportation, stigma, and cultural perceptions of medical services. This has resulted in inequities in the populations affected by HIV, availability and utilization of medical treatment, and retention of patients in systems of care.

HIV/AIDS is a major health crisis for African Americans of all ages, geographic locations, socioeconomic status, and sexual orientations. The convergence of poverty, sexually transmitted diseases (STDs), and substance abuse compounds the impact of HIV/AIDS on the African American community.

Impact of AIDS and HIV on African Americans

The impact of AIDS and HIV on African Americans provides working definitions of AIDS and HIV. African Americans make up 12.3% of the US population but account for 39% of the cumulative AIDS cases diagnosed and reported since the epidemic began in 1981.[3,4] This corresponds to 347,000 cases diagnosed in African Americans out of the 886,000 reported AIDS cases. The Centers for Disease Control and Prevention (CDC) reported that at the close of 2002, more than 185,000 African Americans had died from AIDS.[3,4] In 2002, the most recent year for which data are available, HIV/AIDS was among the top three causes of death for African American men aged 25 to 54 years and African American women aged 35 to 44 years. Data for the same year show 21,000 of the 42,000 estimated AIDS cases in adults (50%) were among African Americans. This translates into an African American AIDS diagnosis rate 11 times higher than that of Caucasians. African American women have a 23 times greater diagnosis rate than white women, and African American men have a 9 times greater rate of an AIDS diagnosis than white men.[5]

HIV shows a similar picture. African Americans accounted for more than 50% of the new HIV diagnoses reported in the United States in 2002. A 2002–2003 study looking at late versus early testing of HIV at 16 sites through-out the United States found that 56% of the delayed-testing patients who developed AIDS within 12 months were African Americans. Late identification of HIV positivity results in delayed referral into treatment and more rapid progression of disease in any population. The majority of children born to HIV-infected mothers in 2002 were African American (62%). The leading cause of HIV infection in African American men is sexual contact with other men, followed by injection drug use, and heterosexual contact. In African American women, HIV infection is caused by heterosexual contact followed by injection drug use.[4]

These statistics describe a picture of HIV progression in the black community that is disproportionate and entrenched. It will require a high level of awareness on the part of health professionals, particularly physicians, to make prevention, timely diagnosis, and treatment of STDs and HIV a priority in order to have an impact on this chronic, expanding infection in the African American community.

▶ HIV: AN OVERVIEW OF CARE

Indications for HIV Testing

A history of sexual activity (current or remote), injection drug use (current or remote), blood transfusion, or patient incarceration creates the necessity of voluntarily counseling the patient about HIV testing and the relative risk of infection. At-risk patients should be counseled about potential consequences of not knowing their serostatus, including implications for future pregnancy and for their current and future sexual partner(s). Counseling should also include discussion of HIV transmission, safe sexual practices, and the potential impact of HIV-positive status on insurance coverage.

Testing should be offered to patients who are sexually active with partners who do not know or will not reveal their current HIV serostatus (prior 3 months). This includes those in monogamous relationships. Most patients do not know their current serostatus and the health-care provider should err on the side of testing to establish it. Persons who have received a blood transfusion in the United States before 1984 or in a foreign country at any time should be tested. The 3- to 6-month period before a person develops antibody to HIV creates a "window period" in which a contaminated unit of blood could be inadvertently given to a patient. This window was narrowed to 7 to 14 days in 1995 when a P_{24} antigen was substituted as a screening tool for all blood donations in the United States. In general it is recommended that anyone who has received a blood transfusion, regardless of date, should be tested for HIV.

HIV Staging

Once identified, HIV-positive patients should be staged to determine the amount of damage that may have occurred to the immune system. Staging is done by taking a complete history focused on identifying the most likely time of exposure to HIV, presence or absence of symptoms consistent with acute viral syndrome, opportunistic infections or malignancies, and past medical history. A CD4+ count and viral load should be obtained, along with baseline laboratory values for liver and kidney function, fasting glucose, cholesterol, and a complete blood count. It is also important to establish whether patients have had prior infections with *Mycobacterium tuberculosis;* hepatitis A, B, or C; or *Toxoplasma gondii.* Attempts should be made to vaccinate patients for hepatitis A and B as early in their infection as possible to ensure a maximal immune response.

The Department of Health and Human Services (DHHS) guidelines for antiretroviral therapy recommend initiating this therapy in persons with CD4+ cell counts lower than 350 cells/mm^3 or a viral load greater than 100,000 copies/mL.[6] The predictive ability of a CD4+ count is more sensitive than a viral load for progression of disease. The decision to initiate therapy is also dependent on a clear understanding of what a patient is willing and able to undertake at that time in his or her life. Care and attention

to identifying lifestyle and social barriers to care must be actively pursued by the provider in partnership with social service professionals to give the patient a supportive environment in which to begin a therapy that will, in most instances, be lifelong. A prior history of antiretroviral use and the possibility that the patient has been infected with resistant HIV should also be taken into account.

The importance of compliance cannot be overemphasized. Patients must maintain greater than 95% adherence to their antiretroviral regimen to achieve optimal results for the duration of their treatment. Even a 5% decrease in adherence produces a dramatic reduction in efficacy and corresponding development of resistance.[6]

Therapeutic Options

There are four classes of antiretroviral drugs: nucleosides and nucleotides; nonnucleotide reverse transcriptase inhibitors (NNRTIs); protease inhibitors (PIs); and fusion inhibitors. The nucleosides were the first class to be identified in the late 1980s when monotherapy began. Research showed a prolongation of life expectancy by 14 to 18 months with the use of azidothymidine (AZT; now zidovudine) alone. The development of didanosine (DDI) and zalcitabine (DDC), followed by lamivudine (3TC) and stavudine (d4T) in the late 1980s and early 1990s allowed for dual therapy with two nucleoside medications. This approach, in combination with prophylaxis and treatment for opportunistic infections, became the mainstay of therapy until 1994, when research produced a new class of drug called *protease inhibitors.* These were the first highly effective antiretroviral medications and, in combination with the two nucleosides, showed a profound drop in viral replication and a slowing of progression. The discovery of a nucleotide reverse transcriptase inhibitor (tenofovir), NNRTIs (efavirenz, nevirapine, delavirdine), and fusion blockers (enfuvirtide) completed the current antiretroviral armamentarium.

Effective Combinations

More than 28 different formulations of antiretroviral therapies are currently available. The appropriate choice of therapy for each patient is complex and requires an understanding of the patient's social setting and medical requirements to make an appropriate match. Consideration of pill number, dosing frequency, side effects profile, and cost is often necessary. Among the beliefs that have dominated HIV treatment is one favoring a class-sparing approach. Maintaining patients on only one class of drugs such as nucleosides, thereby sparing NNRTIs and PIs, or starting them on nucleosides plus an NNRTI, thereby sparing PIs, have been favored in various clinical trials. Studies showing a longer or shorter duration of virologic suppression with immune reconstitution, and thereby slower progression to AIDS, have favored the two nucleosides in combination with an NNRTI or a PI. The recognition that the dose of a PI could be lowered when the drug was given in combination with ritonavir has resulted in a therapeutic approach that minimizes PI-related side effects while potentiating viral suppression for long periods of time.

The relative advantages and disadvantages of antiretroviral drug choice and a complete discussion of short and long-term side effects and drug interactions are beyond the scope of this chapter. A useful review is provided in the DHHS guidelines cited earlier.[6]

Comprehensive care of the HIV-infected patient requires a knowledgeable provider as well as a medical system that responds to the needs of a chronic, progressive disease. Integrating many of the care opportunities into the community with both professional and peer supports has been shown to result in the best results for increasing longevity and decreasing use of emergency department and inpatient services. The open acknowledgment of multiple comorbidities is essential to the development of an effective treatment plan that keeps the patient functioning at the highest possible level for the longest period.

▶ FACTORS THAT CONTRIBUTE TO HIV CONTAGION

Sexually Transmitted Diseases

STDs increase the chance that exposure to HIV will result in an infection by three to five times. Ulcerative STDs that result in genital lesions (eg, syphilis, chancroid, and herpes simplex virus II) increase the likelihood of infection by increasing portals of entry, whereas nonulcerative STDs (eg, gonorrhea, *Trichomonas vaginalis,* bacterial vaginosis, and *Chlamydia trachomatis*) increase the risk of contracting HIV by providing more cells in genital secretions that can serve as targets for HIV (eg, $CD4^+$ lymphocytes), thereby presenting an added risk to the uninfected partner.[7,8]

The highest STD rates in the nation are in the African American community. Therefore, clinicians must be both aware of the connection and aggressive in diagnosis and treatment of all STDs in their patients and their patients' partners.[7] In light of the higher incidence of STDs and the relative predominance of heterosexual transmission in African American women, it is critical that clinicians encourage annual Pap smears with wet mounts for the diagnosis of bacterial vaginosis, *Trichomonas vaginalis*, and *Candida* species as routine practice. In addition, the Pap smear should be used to look for abnormal cells containing human papillomavirus, which affords an increased risk for the development of in situ and invasive squamous cell carcinoma of the external genitalia in HIV-infected patients.[6,9]

Substance Abuse

The African American community is burdened by the comorbidities of alcohol abuse, cocaine, crack, and injection drug use. Injection drug use remains the second leading cause of HIV infection in both African American men and women. The impact of alcohol in lowering inhibitions and increasing sexual activity is well documented. The addition of stimulants in the form of crack-cocaine, cocaine, and methamphetamine has resulted in a surge of HIV infection that has devastated many inner-city communities, neighborhood by neighborhood. The use of injection drugs and the sharing of equipment allows HIV, hepatitis C virus (HCV), and hepatitis B virus (HBV) to spread rapidly through these communities.[10] The presence of poverty and a paucity of available social support systems have allowed the drug-using culture, and the behaviors associated with it, to become real options for young people in their pursuit of hope and economic relief. The phenomenon of sex for drugs not only takes a social and economic toll, but spreads STDs and HIV more rapidly and contributes to rising teen pregnancies.

It is critical that health-care providers understand the important role substance abuse plays in fueling the HIV and STD epidemics in the African American community. The scenario of a young woman going to her first prenatal examination, having a routine test for HIV, and finding out she is positive from a partner who was infected as a result of a remote history of injection drug use, must be stopped. Physicians must become skilled at creating opportunities for patients to feel safe enough to reveal their current or remote history of injection drug use. Once a history is identified, establishing the serostatus for HIV, HCV, and HBV, and screening for STDs, must become routine practice.

Stigmas: Injection Drug Use, Men Who Have Sex With Men, Prison

People who use injection drugs participate not only in a behavior that is illegal but one that is widely shunned by the black community. Men who have sex with men are often unwilling to admit their homosexuality to their family, friends, or wives. Prisons continue to have a disproportionate population of young African American men. Incarcerated men often find themselves participating in sexual contact with other men or sharing equipment for injection drug use, at the same time denying they are at risk for contracting HIV. Too often a young man who becomes infected in prison infects his girlfriend or wife upon release or during a conjugal visit. This revolving door of inmates moving between prison and the community must be acknowledged and targeted to enable preventive interventions and a more realistic approach to addressing and containing high-risk behaviors during incarceration.

The use of crack-cocaine and heroin is universally denounced by society, with little thought given to identification of treatment options. This reality—coupled with low availability of drug treatment programs; organized, functioning Alcoholics Anonymous (AA) programs; or needle exchange and harm-reduction services—presents formidable obstacles to individuals who attempt to stop participating in high-risk behaviors. Community leaders must assess the messages they convey to individuals: messages that encourage clandestine behaviors, forestalling a process that might lead them to decide to stop using drugs or give them the support they need to return to a drug-free life. Social institutions must see themselves as conduits through which individuals burdened by addictions and other negative behaviors can access services that begin to create a support system that allows them to move away from destructive patterns of behavior.

The first step toward achieving this goal is to begin treating drug use and abuse as a medical disease, not a crime. This step requires treating individuals with respect rather than condemning them for past behavior. A next, important step is to create a system of care and services that links drug treatment, needle exchange, and harm reduction with quality medical, psychiatric, and social support services. This means not focusing on the failed attempts of the past but, rather, encouraging patients to try again. Physicians and community leaders of all races and ethnicities, at every level of society, must meet this challenge head on and proactively advocate these measures in their communities. Society can no longer afford the consequences of failing to embrace all its members despite the stark realities of human behavior, nor can it remain silent and allow governments to rely on interdiction as the sole and definitive response.

Poverty

The US Census Bureau, reporting on the status of the US population in 2000, indicated that nearly one in four African Americans lives in poverty.[11] The link between poverty and an increased incidence of STDs and HIV has been shown repeatedly in studies dating back to the mid-1960s. The increased incidence of AIDS associated with poverty correlates with limited access to quality health care, lack of HIV preventive education targeted to high-risk populations within the black community, as well as lack of sustained preventive messages over time. Poverty is also associated both with an increased incidence of tuberculosis and STDs, and as with other chronic, progressive medical diseases with a lower level of entry and retention in medical care. The result is a group of patients who have identified medical problems that largely go untreated. Long-term outcomes for this group are reflected in morbidity and mortality rates for most common diseases (coronary artery disease, hypertension, diabetes mellitus type 2, stroke, chronic renal failure, and cancer) that are much worse for African Americans than whites.

Self-Perception

Social and cultural factors external to the individual can increase the chances of contracting disease, and several of these must be recognized if effective strategies for combatting the HIV/AIDS epidemic are to be developed. The development of corrective strategies is the responsibility of government at all levels and the communities that bear the burden of these diseases. However, other factors exist that, if we are honest, must be acknowledged and require us to look at ourselves and the communities in which we live.

We must explore as a community the reasons why African Americans do not access medical services. Survey data from random population samples looking at HIV cost and service utilization in minority communities showed that African Americans entered care at a later stage of disease and were less likely to be retained in care over time.[12–14] The factors that allow African Americans to decide not to access available health care and, once enrolled, to decide not to continue, must be explored if we are to develop meaningful strategies to combat this situation.

Finally, as African Americans, we must examine how we perceive ourselves, our willingness to endure symptoms for long periods of time, and the barriers we create for ourselves that preclude taking advantage of readily available medical services. In so doing, we will better understand the impact we have on our own health status and the effect this mindset has on the larger black community. Understanding the relative impact of all the factors that influence our perception of HIV—how having HIV affects the way people feel about you and how you feel about yourself—are all areas worthy of self-reflection.

▶ REFERENCES

1. *UNAIDS Report on the Global AIDS Epidemic, 2004.* Available at: http://www.unaids.org.
2. UNAIDS Fact Sheets by Regions. Available at: http://www.unaids.org/html/pub/publications/fact-sheets.
3. National Center for Health Statistics. Death: Leading causes for 2000. *National Vital Statistics Report* 2002;50(16). 86 pp. Available at: http://www.cdc.gov/nchs/data/nvsr/nvsr50/nvsr50_16.pdf.
4. Centers for Disease Control and Prevention. Cases of HIV infection and AIDS in the United States, 2002. *HIV/AIDS Surveillance Report* 2002;14. Available at: http://www.cdc.gov/hiv/stats/hasrlink.htm.

5. Hader S, Smith D, Moore J, et al. HIV infection in women in the United States: Status at the millennium. *JAMA* 2001;285(9):1186–1192.

6. Public Health Service Task Force. Recommendations for the use of antiretroviral drugs in adolescents and adults. Available at: http://www.aidsinfo.nih.gov/guidelines/arch.

7. Centers for Disease Control and Prevention. *Sexually Transmitted Disease Surveillance Report,* 2002. Available at: http://www.cdc.gov/std/stats02/.

8. Fleming DT, Wasserheit JN. From epidemiological synergy to public health policy and practice: The contribution of other STDs to sexual transmission of HIV infection. *Sex Transm Infect* 1999;75: 3–17.

9. Goosby E. *Living with HIV/AIDS: The Black Person's Guide to Survival.* Roscoe, Ill: Hilton Publishers; 2004.

10. Leigh B, Stall R. Substance use and risky sexual behavior for exposure to HIV: Issues in methodology, interpretation, and prevention. *Am Psychol* 1993;48(10):1035–1045.

11. US Census Bureau. *Poverty Status of the Population in 1999 by Age, Sex and Race and Hispanic origin.* Washington, DC: USCB; 2000.

12. Andersen R, Bozzette S, Shapiro M, et al. Access of vulnerable groups to ARV among persons in care for HIV disease in US. *HCSUS Health Services Res* 2000;35(2):389–416.

13. Cunningham WE. Ethnic an racial differences in long-term survival from hospitalizations for HIV infection. *J Health Care Poor Underserved* 2000;11(2)163–178.

14. Cunningham WE, Andersen RM, Katz MH, et al. The impact of competing subsistence needs and barriers on access to medical care for persons with human immunodeficiency virus receiving care in the United States. *Med Care* 1999;37(12): 1270–1281.

CHAPTER 14

Sickle Cell Disease and Hemoglobinopathies

KRISTY F. WOODS, MD, MPH
SAMIR K. BALLAS, MD

▶ INTRODUCTION

With more than 500 hemoglobin variants identified to date, sickle cell disease (SCD) is the most common hemoglobinopathy worldwide. It affects people in Africa, the Middle East, East India, the Mediterranean, South and Central America, the Caribbean, and North America. In the United States, SCD is most common in Americans of African ancestry, with more than 70,000 Americans affected. Other qualitative and quantitative disorders of hemoglobin occur with less frequency in minority populations. This chapter provides an overview of the biochemical and molecular basis, genetics, and epidemiology of SCD. A summary of the historical landmarks in research and clinical care for SCD in the United States is given, followed by highlights regarding disease pathophysiology, common clinical manifestations, and clinical management.

Americans with SCD are subject to multiple disparities in their medical care, and the unique challenges in caring for this population are explored. In addition to race, a conglomerate of factors that include poverty, unemployment, health insurance status, disease chronicity, dependence on opioids, lack of provider education, and provider bias render individuals with SCD a vulnerable population with decreased autonomy. Because of these factors, this population is subjected to increased scrutiny of their medical care and often lacks protection from inequalities associated with a complex medical system. In concluding this chapter, we present a system of targeted education, comprehensive management, legislation, advocacy, and research to address and ameliorate the disparities in the care of patients with SCD.

▶ BACKGROUND

Normal human hemoglobin, hemoglobin A (HbA; $\alpha_2\beta_2$) is composed of two α-globin chains, two β-globin chains and four heme molecules that bind oxygen in red blood cells. The term *sickle cell disease* refers to a group of inherited disorders of hemoglobin (Hb) synthesis and includes the four most common forms: sickle cell anemia (HbSS), hemoglobin SC disease (HbSC), and the sickle β-thalassemias (HbS β^+-thalassemia and HbS β^0-thalassemia). All forms are characterized by the production of abnormal hemoglobin (HbS), chronic hemolytic anemia, and ischemic tissue damage resulting from vascular obstruction. Unlike many diseases, the molecular and genetic basis for SCD has been well established for more than 50 years.

Before the advent of modern medicine, people in West Africa realized the hereditary nature of SCD. In Nigeria there was felt to be a connection between SCD and reincarnation beliefs. The term "reincarnated child," or *Ogbanje* (Ibo tribe) and *Abiku* (Yoruba tribe), referred to a child destined to die and be born repeatedly into the world as their own siblings.[1] The reincarnated child was normal at birth but soon developed signs and symptoms similar to the clinical picture of what we now know to characterize SCD (failure to thrive, yellow eyes, large abdomen, recurrent fever, and body aches) and died at ages 5 to 10 years. The disheartened parents often inflicted a physical mark on the dead child before burial to enable identification if he or she was reborn. Children preceded in death by two to three siblings were ritualistically treated by amputating the distal phalanges of the left fifth digit, and were referred to as *Obanje* children. Native medicine men in some tribes marked patients with limb-girdle tattoos for rapid diagnosis when they presented writhing in pain.[2] And SCD was given African tribal names signifying the excruciating pain associated with the disease. The most likely English meaning for some of these names includes "body chewing" (*Nuidudui;* Ewe tribe), "I will die" (*Nwiiwii;* Fante tribe), "body biting" (*Hem kom;* Adangme tribe), and "beaten up" (*Adep;* Banyangi tribe, Cameroon).

In 1619, the first contingent of black Africans was brought to the coast of Virginia on the Dutch ship *Man of War.* Although a couple of medical autopsy reports in the mid-late 1800s are suggestive of SCD, it is likely that patients with frequent pain were misdiagnosed with rheumatism or growing pains. Dr James B. Herrick, a Chicago physician, first described SCD in the US medical literature in 1910.[3] He reported on the unusual sickle shape of red blood cells on a peripheral smear from a dental student from Grenada who presented with cough, fever, and anemia. The name "sickle cell anemia" thus was coined. Diggs et al reported on many of the clinical manifestations of the disease and, in 1934, postulated that a blockage of small blood vessels might be responsible for the painful episodes of SCD.[4] During the 1940s, others speculated on the role of oxygen and fetal hemoglobin (HbF; $\alpha_2\gamma_2$) in the sickling of red blood cells.[5,6]

The concept of SCD as a "molecular disease" was first established in 1949 when Linus Pauling demonstrated by electrophoresis that the abnormality in SCD resides in the hemoglobin protein molecule.[7] Around the same time, Neel and Beet independently identified the inheritance pattern of SCD as autosomal recessive.[8,9] The mutation in sickle hemoglobin was elucidated as a mutation at position 6 on the β-hemoglobin protein chain in 1957,[10] and the three-dimensional structure of the hemoglobin protein was deciphered and the functional elements clarified by Muirhead and Perutz in 1963.[11] Over the next 20 years, federally funded research in laboratories across the country improved our understanding of the disease from a molecular and pathophysiologic perspective.

In SCD, the α-globin chains of hemoglobin are normal; however, there is a point mutation in the DNA at triplet codon 6 of the β-globin gene (GAG $\rightarrow$ GTG). The base exchange, thymine (T) in place of adenine (A), results in a single amino acid substitution at the sixth position on the β-globin chain. A polar, hydrophilic amino acid, glutamic acid, is replaced by a nonpolar, hydrophobic amino acid, valine (glutamic acid $\rightarrow$ valine) resulting in an abnormal β^S globin chain (Fig. 14–1). When fully oxygenated, there are few structural distinctions between normal hemoglobin (HbA) and sickle hemoglobin (HbS; $\alpha_2\beta_2^S$). In the deoxygenated state, however, a conformational change occurs that decreases the solubility of sickle hemoglobin. The HbS molecules form rigid polymers within the red blood cell (erythrocyte).[12] This process, hemoglobin

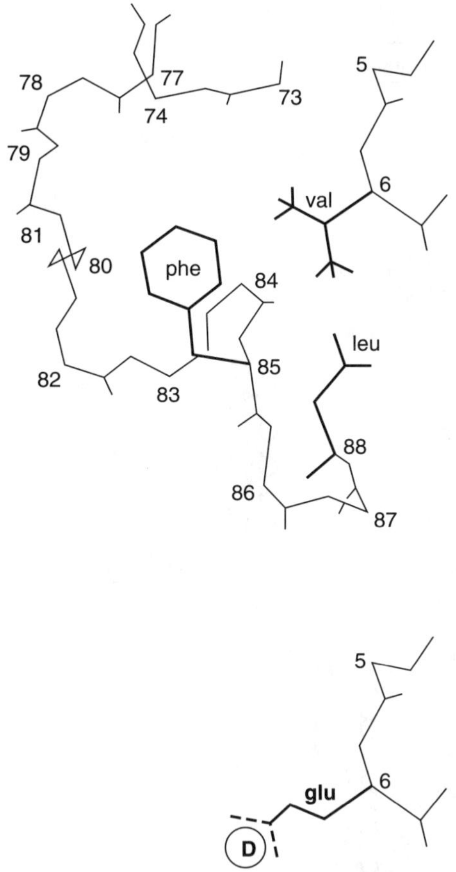

Figure 14–1. The molecular structure of hemoglobin demonstrating intermolecular contact regions between the mutant β^{6val} globin and the normal β^{6glu} globin. (From Stamatoyannopoulos, George. The Molecular Basis of Blood Diseases. Philadelphia, Pa: Saunders; 1987, with permission.)

polymerization, distorts the normal, biconcave shape of the erythrocyte causing it to assume a sickle shape (Figs. 14–2 and 14–3).

An estimated one in eight African Americans carries the asymptomatic gene for sickle hemoglobin, a condition known as sickle cell trait (AS). Individuals with sickle cell anemia (HbSS) are homozygous for the sickle globin gene, whereas those with HbSC disease and the HbS β-thalassemias have a mixed heterozygous inheritance pattern. They inherit both the sickle globin gene (β^S) and the gene for HbC ($\beta^{C[6 \text{ lysine}]}$) or thalassemia, respectively. Individuals with sickle thalassemia produce HbS and either a decreased amount (HbSβ^+thal) or no (HbSβ^0thal) normal β-globin chains. There are an estimated 72,000 Americans with SCD, and the prevalence in African Americans is as follows: HbSS (sickle cell anemia), 1:375 live births; HbSC disease, 1:835 live births; HbS β-thalassemias, 1:1667 live births.[13] Hispanics and Latinos of Caribbean or Latin American origin (ie, Puerto Rican and Cuban Americans) have SCD rates approaching rates in the black population. Those of Mexican origin (ie, Mexican American) have lower rates, closer to those in the white population (mean prevalence of 1.72 to 1.9 per 100,000).

▶ RESEARCH AND CLINICAL CARE: AN HISTORICAL PERSPECTIVE

Despite full characterization of SCD at the molecular and DNA level, not as much was known about the clinical spectrum and clinical course of the disease in the 1970s. Few advances in therapeutic and preventive approaches to care had been achieved, and the mean life expectancy was approximately 14 years.[14] In 1971, during a special message to Congress proposing a national health strategy, President Richard Nixon made research on SCD a national priority. He noted, "It is a sad and shameful fact that the causes of this disease have been largely neglected throughout our history. We cannot rewrite this record of neglect, but we can reverse it. To this end, this administration is increasing its budget for research and treatment of sickle cell anemia. . . ." The National Sickle Cell Anemia Control Act (P.L. 92-294) was signed into law in 1972. It provided for the establishment of voluntary SCD screening and counseling programs, information and education programs for health professionals and the public, and research training in the diagnosis and treatment of SCD.[15]

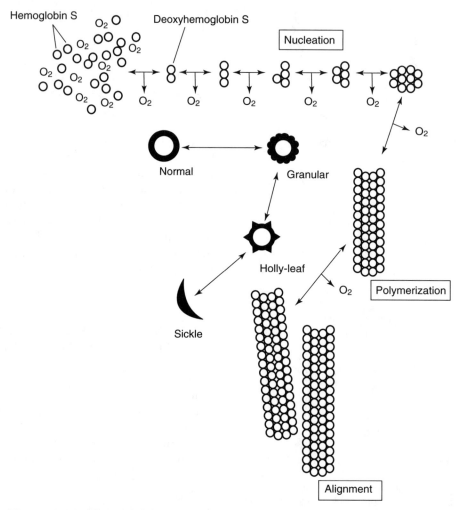

Figure 14–2. The polymerization process of sickle hemoglobin (HbS). With deoxygenation, the HbS molecule polymerizes. The polymers consist of 14-strand fibers that distort the shape of the erythrocyte membrane, changing its normal biconcave disk shape to a number of other shapes, such as granular, holly-leaf, and the classic sickle shape. *(From Besa AC. Hemoglobin and Hemoglobinopathies in Hematology. Philadelphia, Pa: Harwal; 1992, with permission.)*

Shortly thereafter, the National Sickle Cell Program was established at the National Heart, Lung and Blood Institute (NHLBI) to develop, support, and coordinate programs in SCD research. The program funded 10 Comprehensive Sickle Cell Centers at academic medical centers across the country. Despite these efforts, widespread implementation of compre-

hensive programs for screening and clinical management of individuals affected by SCD lagged behind. Fewer than 14 states offered or provided neonatal screening for SCD by the late 1970s. In 1978, the NHLBI launched the multicenter, 4000-patient Cooperative Study of Sickle Cell Disease (CSSCD). In addition to providing critical epidemiologic data regarding

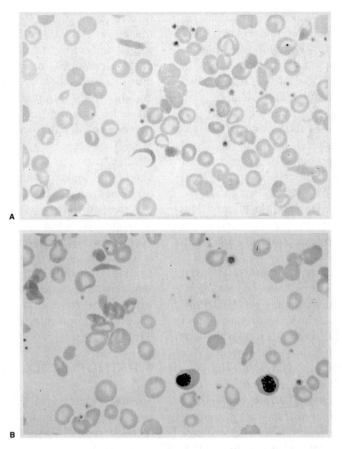

Figure 14–3. A. Peripheral smear with sickle erythrocytes. **B.** Reversibly sickled cells photographed with a Phillips 525 scanning electron microscope (1500X). (Courtesy of Drs. Kristy Woods and Samir Ballas.)

demographic characteristics and the clinical course of the disease, this landmark study created an important infrastructure for the implementation of previously lacking SCD clinical trials.[16]

In 1985 the National Institutes of Health (NIH) released the first edition of a comprehensive guide for pediatric management entitled *Guidelines for the Management of Sickle Cell Disease*. In 1986, the first multicenter clinical trial, Penicillin Prophylactic in Sickle Cell Disease Study (PROPS), established the effectiveness of penicillin in preventing deadly *Streptococcus pneumoniae* sepsis in infants and tod-

dlers. The results were pronounced, with an 84% reduction in the incidence of this life-threatening complication, and set a new standard of care for infants with SCD.[17] Prior to the study, no effective treatment had demonstrated the ability to decrease morbidity and mortality in SCD. The PROPS study presented undeniable evidence that early diagnosis of SCD and prompt administration of prophylactic penicillin could save lives. It resulted in widespread change in public health policy regarding newborn screening efforts.

The NIH convened the Consensus Conference on Newborn Screening for Sickle Cell

Disease and Other Hemoglobinopathies in 1987, which recommended that "every child should be screened for hemoglobinopathies to prevent the potentially fatal complications of SCD during infancy." The conference group further recommended that, because reliable, simple, and cost-effective techniques for screening were available and valid, universal screening should be mandated by state law and coupled with comprehensive programs for the care of sickle cell patients and their families.[18] Presently, universal screening for hemoglobinopathies is provided in 44 states, the District of Columbia, Puerto Rico, and the Virgin Islands, with screening on request available in the other 6 states.

Comprehensive care for infants, children and families with SCD involves access to continuous, quality medical care, genetic counseling, psychosocial support, and rehabilitation services. In 1993, the Agency for Health Care Policy and Research (now the Agency for Healthcare Research and Quality) issued a Clinical Practice Guideline entitled *Sickle Cell Disease: Screening, Diagnosis, Management and Counseling in Newborns and Infants*.[13] As a result of widespread newborn screening and advances in comprehensive pediatric management over the past two decades, life expectancy has improved dramatically. Individuals with SCD are now living well into adulthood with mean life expectancies of 44 years (sickle cell anemia) and 64 years (HbSC disease).[19]

Researchers had noted in the late 1940s that the adverse effects of SCD were ameliorated in very young infants who had circulating red blood cells with persistence of fetal hemoglobin (HbF; $\alpha_2\gamma_2$), which inhibits polymerization of sickle hemoglobin. But it was not until the mid 1980s that several investigators independently demonstrated that hydroxyurea and other compounds (ie, 5-azacytidine and butyrate) increased levels of fetal hemoglobin.[20–23] In 1991, Platt and the CSSCD conclusively reported the major effect of fetal hemoglobin level on severity of disease in SCD in 1991, and the NHBLI began its Multicenter Study of Hy-

droxyurea in Sickle Cell Anemia (MSH). The trial ended early in 1995 because of compelling results indicating an almost 50% reduction in painful episodes, hospitalizations for painful episodes, episodes of acute chest syndrome, and the need for transfusion.[24] In 1998, hydroxyurea became the first agent approved for the prevention of painful episodes in adults with SCD. A subsequent NHLBI study confirmed the efficacy and safety of hydroxyurea in children aged 5 to 15 years, and it is being evaluated for benefit and safety in infants (aged 6 to 24 months). In the past few years, guidelines for management of SCD patients with acute painful episodes have been issued.[25,26] Despite remarkable advances, persistent morbidity for both children and adults, new clinical challenges, and long-term care issues for those with SCD require sustained research and health-care vigilance to minimize complications and improve quality of life.

▶ PATHOPHYSIOLOGY

The historical view of SCD pathophysiology was based largely on the cycle of hemoglobin polymerization and stasis theorized by Ham and Cassel in 1940.[5] In this prototype, deoxygenated HbS polymerizes and, upon reoxygenation, the rigid hemoglobin polymers are dispersed and the reversibly sickled cell assumes the normal erythrocyte shape. As a result of repeated conformational changes with oxygenation and deoxygenation, the cell membrane becomes permanently damaged, the erythrocyte irreversibly sickled, and hemolysis occurs.[27] Whereas the life span of a normal erythrocyte (with HbA) is 120 days, sickle erythrocytes have a life span of approximately 10 days; thus the hemolytic anemia of SCD.

In the old theory, the circulating sickle erythrocytes also resulted in a change in blood viscosity, leading to obstruction of the microvasculature and subsequent tissue hypoxia. This model easily explained the two dominant pathophysiologic features of SCD, hemolytic anemia and vascular obstruction

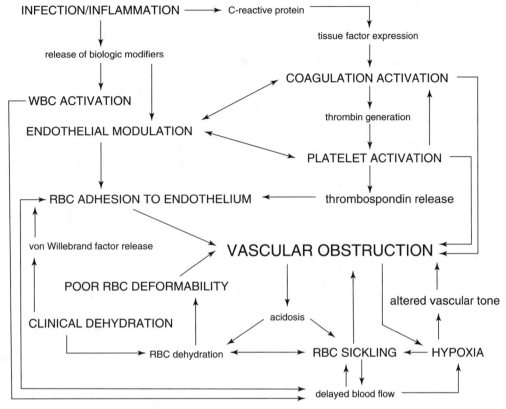

Figure 14–4. The interrelated and numerous mechanisms of vasoocclusion. *(From Embury S, Hebbel R, Mohandas N, et al, eds.* Sickle Cell Disease: Basic Principles and Clinical Practice. *New York, NY: Raven; 1994, with permission.)*

(vasoocclusion). We now understand that the mechanism for vasoocclusion is more complex, being influenced by multiple genetic, vascular, cellular, membrane, and environmental factors. In 1979 Hoover et al showed that red blood cells from patients with SCD adhere to the lining of blood vessels (vascular endothelium) more readily than red blood cells from controls.[28] And Hebbel et al showed that the extent of the stickiness of the red blood cells might be a determinant of disease severity in SCD.[29] Platelet and coagulation system activation and the release of acute inflammatory mediators, such as interleukin 6, tissue necrosis factor (TNF-α), and C-reactive protein have been documented to contribute to the process of vasoocclusion. And the elevation of inflammatory mediators at base-

line suggests a chronic inflammatory state in SCD[30–35] (Fig. 14–4).

Although vasoocclusion results in ischemic damage to organs throughout the body, the vascular system (or the vascular endothelium) is considered the primary organ damaged in SCD. In addition to adhering to the endothelium and causing vascular obstruction, sickle erythrocytes directly damage blood vessel walls in a number of ways that contribute to further disease exacerbation. Injury to the delicate endothelial cells may lead to intimal impairment and a disturbance in the balance of vasoactive peptides and mediators that control local vascular tone. Several studies have recently demonstrated higher levels of circulating plasma endothelin-1, a potent vasoconstrictor, in patients with SCD

▶ **TABLE 14-1.** Major Types of Sickle Cell Syndromes and Their Typical Hematologic Parameters

Disease	Abbreviation	Genotype	Hb (g/dL)	Retic (%)	MCV (fL)	HbA (%)	HbA$_2$ (%)	HbS (%)	HbF (%)
							Hemoglobin Composition		
Sickle cell anemia									
No α-gene deletion	SS	$\beta^s/\beta^s; \alpha\alpha/\alpha\alpha$	7.0–8.0	10–20	85–110	0	2.5–3.5	75–96	1–20
Deletion of 2 α-genes	S, α-thal	$\beta^s/\beta^s; -\alpha/\alpha$	9.0–10.0	6–12	70–80	0	3.0–4.5	75–94	1–20
Sickle β⁰-thalassemia	S, β⁰-thal	β^s/β^0 thal	7.0–10.0	6–15	60–70	0	4.0–6.0	70–90	1–20
Sickle β⁺-thalassemia	S, β⁺-thal	β^s/β^+ thal	> 10.0	5–10	60–70	10–20	4.0–6.0	65–85	1–15
HbSC disease	SC	β^s/β^c	> 10.0	5–10	75–85	0	45–50	50	1–6
Sickle cell trait	AS	β^A/β^s	12–16	1.0–2.0	>82	55–57	2.5–3.5	40	< 1.0

Hb = hemoglobin; MCV = mean corpuscular volume; retic = reticulocyte count.

* HbA$_2$ and HbC have the same electrophoretic mobility at alkaline pH and are not separable on routine analysis.

compared with controls.[36–38] Concentrations for a metabolite of nitric oxide, a potent vasodilator, have been shown to be significantly higher during steady state in patients with SCD compared with controls, with further increases during acute painful episodes.[39,40] Presently, the exact role of vascular endothelial dysfunction in SCD pathophysiology is not completely understood.

▶ CLINICAL MANIFESTATIONS AND MANAGEMENT

Most patients with sickle cell anemia (HbSS) develop hemolytic anemia within the first 6 months of life. The hemoglobin level decreases further during the second year, after which it generally stabilizes. Hemoglobin levels usually range from 6.5 to 8.5 g/dL. Reticulocyte counts are elevated and are usually in the range of 10% to 15% at baseline. The mean cell volume ranges between 85 and 110 fL, but interpretation can vary with age. The mean corpuscular hemoglobin concentration is usually within normal limits unless concomitant iron deficiency or thalassemia exists. Sickle cell anemia is associated with leukocytosis, and the mean white blood cell count is approximately 11.7×10^9/L. Although neutrophil count may be elevated (average 59%), band forms are usu-

ally not increased at baseline. Platelet count may also be elevated during asymptomatic periods in sickle cell anemia. Routine hematologic findings for various genotypes are provided in Table 14–1.

Pain is the hallmark of SCD, and the acute painful episode (acute vasoocclusive episode) is the most common cause of health-care encounters.[41] These episodes are caused by vasoclusion of small blood vessels supplying richly innervated periosteal bone and resultant ischemia. Painful episodes are debilitating, intermittent, and unpredictably interrupt the lives of patients with SCD. These episodes generally begin at about 6 months of age, when fetal hemoglobin decreases and is replaced by sickle hemoglobin, and occur throughout patients' lives. Most patients have between one and three painful episodes per year requiring hospitalization. However, a small percentage of patients have more frequent painful episodes, high health-care utilization patterns, and are at risk of early death.[19]

The frequency of painful episodes may vary between genotypes, within genotypes, and within individual patients over time. Precipitating factors such as infection and dehydration are identified in only 33% of painful episodes.[42] Based on clinical and biochemical parameters, the duration of the acute vasoocclusive event has been determined to last between 7 and 14 days.[43] The painful episode is a discrete

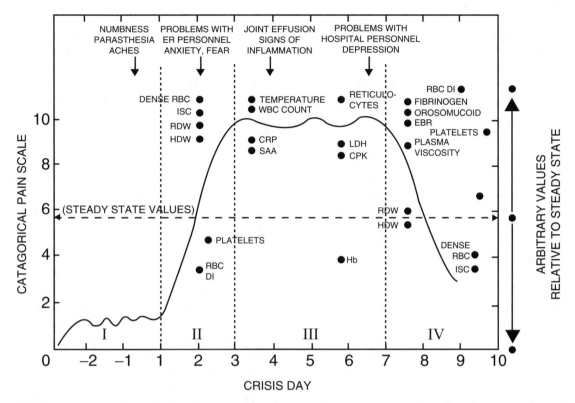

Figure 14–5. Atypical profile of events that develop during the evolution of a severe sickle cell painful crisis in an adult in the absence of overt infection or other complication. CPK = creatinine phosphokinase; CRP = C-reactive protein; ER = emergency room; ESR = erythrocyte sedimentation rate; Hb = hemoglobin; HDW = Hb distribution width; ISC = irreversibly sickled cells; LDH = lactate dehydrogenase; RBC DI = red cell deformability index; RDW = red cell distribution width; SAA = serum amyloid A.   *(From Ballas SK. The sickle cell painful crisis in adults: Phases and objective signs. Hemoglobin 1995;19:323–333, with permission.)*

event, with prodromal, initial, established (or steady state), and resolving phases identified (Fig. 14–5). Once the painful episode has begun, the process cannot be reversed and the resolution phase cannot be accelerated. Hospitalization is recommended to exclude complications and when pain is severe and not alleviated by oral opioids. The mean duration of hospitalization for uncomplicated painful episodes is approximately 3 to 4 days, in order to obtain adequate analgesia.[44] At this time, patients can be safely discharged with a prescription for an adequate dose of oral opioids to last for the duration of the episode.

Bacterial infections remain the most common cause of death in infants and children with sickle cell anemia, and a significant cause of mortality in adults. Septicemia due to *Streptococcus pneumoniae* and *Haemophilus influenzae* is four times as likely in children younger than 5 years of age with SCD than in children without the disease. In children older than 10 years, pneumonia and septicemia caused by *Escherichia coli, Salmonella* species, other gram-negative enteric bacteria, and *Staphylococcus aureus* are more common. Meningitis resulting from *Streptococcus pneumoniae* may occur in infants and children. Osteomyelitis caused by *Salmonella* species, gram-negative enteric organisms, and *Staphylococcus aureus* is also more frequent in individuals with SCD. Although there is no increased propensity for viral infections, viral illness may precipitate other clinical complications in SCD (ie, acute painful episodes) or lead to unique clinical scenarios (ie, severe anemia or aplastic crisis due to parvovirus B19).

Splenic atrophy secondary to infarction generally occurs by age 6 to 12 months. Hypersplenism may occur in young children who maintain splenic function but is more common in older children and adults with heterozygous forms of SCD. It is characterized by chronic splenomegaly, anemia, leukopenia, thrombocytopenia, and marrow hyperplasia of all the elements reduced in the blood. Splenomegaly may cause abdominal discomfort, and individuals are at risk for traumatic injury, rupture, or both. Splenic sequestration is an uncommon but life-threatening complication that occurs in patients with splenomegaly. These episodes frequently follow infection and may result in hypovolemic shock in children or splenic rupture. It carries a 15% to 20% mortality rate and a 50% risk of recurrence among survivors.[45]

Acute chest syndrome is characterized by fever, chest pain, leukocytosis, hypoxia, and new pulmonary infiltrates. It is a potentially life-threatening condition that can rapidly progress to respiratory failure. Acute chest syndrome has been reported in 15% to 43% of patients with SCD and has a high recurrence rate. The exact etiology is unclear; however, infectious agents, pulmonary vasooclusion, bone marrow and fat embolization, and rib and sternal infarction have been implicated.[46] Chronic sickle lung disease with hypoxemia, pulmonary fibrosis, and pulmonary hypertension is a progressive condition that can result in early adult mortality in some patients.

Stroke, a devastating complication of SCD, occurs most often during childhood with reported prevalences ranging from 8.5% to 17% and a high recurrence rate.[47] Most strokes are due to cerebral infarction (70% to 80%), with approximately 20% due to intracerebral hemorrhage. Transcranial Doppler screening of infants and children with SCD detects increased stroke risk based on blood flow velocity. Transfusion therapy (to decrease sickle hemoglobin to less than 30% to 50%) is recommended as primary stroke prevention in high-risk children.[48-50] An increased incidence of cerebral aneurysm, hearing loss, and neuropathy has also been reported in SCD.

The chronic hemolysis of SCD leads to the development of bilirubin gallstones during childhood, and most patients have had a cholecystectomy by adulthood. The incidence of avascular necrosis (osteonecrosis) of the humeral and femoral heads generally increases with age and can occur in all genotypes. It occurs most frequently, however, in patients with sickle cell anemia and concomitant α-thalassemia and in HbS β^+-thalassemia.[51] Early detection by magnetic resonance imaging is critical, because core decompression can arrest progression of necrosis and limit joint destruction and immobility.

Ophthalmic complications are common in SCD, and 67% of patients (any genotype) have nonproliferative retinopathy. Vasoocclusion of the peripheral retina is characterized by salmon patches (small intraretinal hemorrhages), iridescent spots, and black sunburst lesions. These findings rarely result in visual loss but can initiate events leading to severe, proliferative changes. The characteristic lesion of proliferative retinopathy is the sea-fan malformation. These fragile, new blood vessels can bleed into the vitreous chamber, giving the sensation of "floaters" or "cobwebs" in the visual field, and may eventually lead to retinal detachment. Proliferative retinopathy is most common in HbSC disease (33%) and HbS β-thalassemia (14%).[52]

In the United States, leg ulcers occur spontaneously or following trauma in approximately 25% of patients with SCD. They are typically located at the medial or lateral malleolar (ankle) areas and may take months to years to heal. Failure to heal may occur in up to 60%, and the recurrence rate is high. Priapism (painful and sustained penile erections) represents an urgent situation for patients with SCD. It can occur spontaneously in children and adults and is not associated with sexual excitation. Failure of detumescence is thought to result from either venoocclusion, excessive release of neurotransmitters, or prolonged relaxation of the cavernous muscles. Repeated episodes can cause intrapenile scarring and fibrosis and can lead to erectile dysfunction.

Beneath the threshold of clinical detectability, vasooclusion and ischemia damage organs throughout the body, and about 20% of deaths in SCD are due to chronic organ failure.[53] A compensatory cardiomyopathy of severe anemia is almost always present in adults with SCD. It is characterized by left atrial and biventricular enlargement, tachycardia, and a systolic murmur of mitral insufficiency.[54] Other factors, such as iron overload, may affect cardiac function in SCD. Arrhythmias, cor pulmonale, and congestive heart failure are becoming more common long-term complications of SCD as the population ages. Chronic hepatic insufficiency may have multifactorial causes, including hepatic ischemia due to vasoocclusion, acetaminophen or other drug toxicity, viral hepatitis, and intrahepatic stasis. Ischemic damage to the renal medullary vessels results in enuresis (bedwetting) in children and eventual inability to concentrate the urine (hyposthenuria) during times of water deprivation. Renal papillary necrosis with gross hematuria and renal tubular acidosis may also occur. Glomerular disease and chronic renal insufficiency have been reported in 4% to 18% of patients with SCD.[55] It is associated with proteinuria, aging, and the Bantu β-globin gene haplotype.

Many patients with SCD are found to be well adjusted and psychologically healthy; however, similar to patients having other chronic conditions they are at increased risk for psychosocial maladjustment. Studies in children indicate an increased risk for depression, social isolation, low self-esteem, dissatisfaction with body image, and poor peer and family relationships.[56] In one survey of well-being and health status in adults with SCD, the patients reported low scores in the areas of social functioning, emotional well-being, and mental health. The scores for adult patients with SCD were comparable to and in some cases lower than the scores of patients with congestive heart failure, diabetes, and low back pain.[57]

Iatrogenic complications from the treatment of SCD deserves a special mention. Any group of chronic or intermittent pain sufferers is at risk for opioid addiction or psychological dependency on opioids. Appropriate monitoring and prescribing of opioids analgesics lessens the likelihood of this complication. Iron overload in adults is often the result of a lifetime of injudicious administration of packed red blood cell transfusions. Improved life expectancy calls for more caution regarding such long-term treatment complications. Iatrogenic pulmonary edema is not uncommon as a result of overly aggressive management of painful episodes with intravascular volume replacement. Adults are at particular risk for this complication because of their underlying compensatory cardiomyopathy.

Clinical management for the majority of patients with SCD is primarily palliative in nature. Palliative care is the total comprehensive care of patients whose disease is not responsive to curative therapy.[58] It targets the numerous complications of SCD during the life of patients from childhood through adulthood. A major goal of palliative care is the achievement of the best quality of life for patients and their families. This means the prevention or early diagnosis of complications and maximizing both physical and psychological functioning. Palliation in SCD specifically includes (1) general supportive care, including immunizations and prophylactic medications; and (2) targeted symptomatic management of SCD-related medical complications. Although discussion of specific management for all SCD-related complications is outside of the scope of this chapter, evidence-based approaches to clinical care are available.[59]

It is the hope of those with SCD and their families that there will be, in the near future,

▶ **TABLE 14–2.** Current Approaches to Management of Sickle Cell Disease

Supportive Therapy
Folic acid, immunization
Psychosocial support

Symptomatic Treatment
Analgesics, blood transfusion
Antibiotics, surgery

Preventive Therapy
Prophylactic antibiotics (infants and children)
Immunization
Avoidance of known precipitating factors
HbF induction (hydroxyurea)
Cellular rehydration (investigational)

Curative Therapy
Bone marrow transplantation
Gene therapy (experimental, transgenic, etc)

therapy that will either cure or markedly alter the natural course of this disease. With better understanding of the pathology of SCD and the coordination of multiple therapies that attack different pathologic mechanisms of the disease, this goal seems likely. Table 14–2 lists current approaches that have the potential to ameliorate or cure SCD. Although the long-term safety and efficacy of these novel therapies have not been well studied, there is good potential for them to reach phase III clinical trials in the near future.

▶ SICKLE CELL DISEASE AND HEALTH DISPARITIES

Because SCD affects primarily African Americans in the United States, we do not have data on racial disparities in health outcomes for this population. A few small studies have compared outcomes and management in SCD to other inherited conditions (ie, cystic fibrosis), chronic illnesses (ie, juvenile diabetes, juvenile rheumatoid arthritis, cancer, and heart disease), or diseases associated with chronic pain (ie, low back pain).[57,60–65] However, the history of research and clinical care for SCD raises questions about the impact of race (or poverty) in a number of areas. For years, large sums of federal dollars were devoted to SCD research, while patients and their families could often not receive basic services and comprehensive, quality medical care at the same institutions or SCD centers. Although care of children with SCD is usually managed by pediatric hematologists, it is not unusual for the same centers to lack a coordinated transition program to adult care.[66] Some centers still do not have hematologists or experts in adult SCD management, and well-intentioned pediatric hematologists may continue to manage adult patients.

Outside of the province of the sickle cell centers, the prospect of the patient finding an adult provider trained in SCD management can be even more daunting. This is true in both urban and rural settings. One statewide study of utilization patterns found that either a general internal medicine or family medicine physician, as opposed to a hematologist, managed most hospitalizations for adults with SCD.[67] Yet in many medical school curricula, SCD is studied predominantly during the basic science years (ie, biochemistry and genetics), and there remains little formal education of students during the clinical training years. Some hematologists have little training or experience in sickle hemoglobinopathy diagnosis and management. As comprehensive, chronic disease management programs for diabetes, heart disease, and cancer have expanded at most medical facilities, such programs for the sickle cell population are often lacking or incomplete.

Patients with SCD, particularly adults, experience multiple disparities at different levels in their medical care. As a group they are forgotten in the labyrinth of bureaucracy and lost in the crevices of managed care. Their care is disparate not only because they are African Americans but also because they are often poor, not highly educated, and unemployed. Patients with SCD often lack lucrative medical coverage and require large amounts of opioid analgesics to manage their pain. Their disease entails frequent encounters with providers, most of whom have neither knowledge nor interest in the clinical diversity of SCD. A physician bias toward treating patients who suffer from chronic pain or a medical illness that has no cure has been observed.[68] Many patients with SCD are trapped in a microcosm of pain, suffering, depression, loneliness, poverty, and dependence on a system that grants them second- or third-class citizenship status. Thus, patients with SCD seem to be on the lowest rung of the totem pole of disparity.

Numerous examples of disparities in the care of patients with SCD have been described previously.[69–72] These examples cover a spectrum that extends from neglect all the way to profiling, in which "hit lists" of so-called difficult or problem patients are kept in some facilities with instructions not to treat or admit them to the hospital unless in life-threatening situations. Ironically, the writers of these lists do not realize that patients who experience frequent acute painful episodes have higher mortality rates than other patients.[40] Instead of "problem" patients, a more appropriate label might be "high-risk" patients; and rather than abandonment, a focused comprehensive plan addressing medical, psychological, and social issues affecting disease management should be considered to improve quality of life for these individuals.

The magnitude of the disparities problem for patients with SCD is illustrated by the following examples. The first pertains to a patient who reported that he obtained prescriptions for opioid analgesics from a physician other than his primary care physician (PCP) in urgent situations. In response, the PCP decided not to write any future prescription for opioids due to alleged "maladaptive behavior." The PCP stated that he would continue taking care of the patient but would never write him prescriptions for opioids. This scenario is akin to a diabetic patient whose PCP refuses to write prescriptions for insulin or other antidiabetic agents.

The second example pertains to a patient who, on his way to the hospital's sickle cell center, decided to go to the restroom at the end of a corridor a few feet behind him. A female security officer who was walking in the opposite direction saw the patient turning back and, perceiving this as suspicious behavior, called four fellow officers, all male, who appeared promptly and forced their way into the restroom. They searched the patient and the bathroom thoroughly only to find no hidden drugs, weapons, or other incriminating evidence. The officers then accompanied the patient to the sickle cell center to verify that he had a scheduled appointment.

In our experiences, we have also observed converse examples of disparities in medical care related to pain management for patients with SCD. Although the acute painful episode is the most common clinical complication, all pain in SCD is not due to an acute vasoocclusive event. Yet it is not uncommon for providers to focus on the acute painful crisis to the neglect of other related or unrelated medical complications (ie, "It's only a crisis"). This callous and superficial approach can result in a critical delay in accurate diagnosis of potentially life-threatening conditions.

In one example, a 32-year-old woman with sickle cell anemia was admitted to the hospital with abdominal pain assumed to be a crisis. After 3 days on intravenous morphine she failed to improve and went into shock. Only at that time were other diagnoses for her pain considered, and she was found to have a ruptured ectopic pregnancy. In another case, a 24-year-old woman with SCD developed persistent and severe arm pain. Over a 3-week period, she presented to and was repeatedly turned away from a local emergency department and labeled as having "drug-seeking behavior." At the sickle cell center, she was diagnosed with advanced osteomyelitis and necrotizing fasciitis. Another vignette involves an 18-year-old college student with SCD admitted for left upper quadrant pain. He explained to the admitting physicians that he had been diagnosed with hypersplenism only to be told that hypersplenism was "impossible in someone his age." He was managed as a "pain crisis." Thirty-six hours after admission, the patient's blood pressure dropped precipitously and his hemoglobin was noted to be 2 g/dL; an autopsy revealed a ruptured spleen.

These are but a few examples of how stereotyping of SCD patients and the trivializing of clinical symptoms can result in increased suffering and poor medical outcomes. Every step in pain management is full of examples of inequities in care or lack of adherence to standard pain management principles.

▶ SUMMARY AND RECOMMENDATIONS

Because patients with SCD suffer from a chronic disorder associated with multiple complications and vast heterogeneity in the clinical picture, they experience greatly diminished autonomy and, hence, require increased surveillance and protection. We believe that disparities in medical care for SCD can best be addressed by (1) targeted education, (2) comprehensive management, (3) legislation, (4) advocacy, and (5) research. Recommendations in each of these areas are provided below and summarized in Table 14–3.

Targeted Education

Education should target providers who take care of patients with SCD. This includes attending physicians, primary care providers (general pediatricians, general internists, family medicine physicians), hematologists, emergency department physicians, students, residents, fellows, nurses, and social workers. These providers who care for children or adults with SCD should be required to attend a course, seminar, or workshop given on a regular basis by an expert in SCD management. This educational activity should include not only the pathophysiology, clinical picture, complications, and approaches to management of SCD, but also a comprehensive review of sickle cell pain and its management. We highly recommend that

▶ **TABLE 14–3**. Summary of Recommendations to Ameliorate Current Disparities in the Management of Patients with Sickle Cell Disease

- **Targeted Education of Care Providers on a Regular Basis:** The goal is to keep new providers up to date on current aspects of the disease
- **Legislation:** The goal is to garner the prestige of the legal system to enforce certain requirements in the management of patients with sickle cell disease
- **Advocacy and Support Groups:** To monitor the quality of care patients receive and provide suggestions for improvement
- **Basic and Clinical Research:** To link the bench to the bedside in order to unmask the pathophysiology of the clinical manifestations and recommend specific therapeutic approaches

providers have an informal meeting with the patients when they are not experiencing painful episodes and in the steady-state phase of their illness. When this is done, particularly with emergency department personnel, they are surprised by the difference in appearance and behavior of the patients that they previously saw only when in acute pain. This experience helps providers to realize that, like the rest of us, individuals with SCD have other concerns in life, including individual goals, jobs, spirituality, personal relationships, bills, taxes, and so on. The broader perspective that is gained may greatly improve the quality of management of patients in the emergency department.

Comprehensive Management

Comprehensive management should also include the availability of a hematologist, a general pediatrician, or an internist experienced in the care of patients with SCD. Ideally this individual should be the primary care provider, and if not, the availability of a specialist for consultation is greatly desirable. Several guidelines and standards of care for patients with SCD are available today.[23,25,40,73,74] The providers mentioned above must have free access to these resources, some of which are available in Palm-PDA format. The best among these is the booklet published by the NIH and entitled *Management and Therapy of Sickle Cell Disease.*[74] This booklet can be downloaded free of charge from the Internet, or purchased in hard copy form. We recommend that any provider who takes care of individuals with SCD have a copy of this booklet. Physicians who have no interest in SCD should not be coerced by their institution or department to take care of these patients; otherwise the quality of care of the patients will not be optimal and the physicians will experience frustration and burnout syndrome.

Legislation

Legislation can greatly improve the quality of care of individuals with SCD. Individuals with SCD should be aware of and utilize existing laws that provide them and their families with protection from job loss due to medical illness (ie, American with Disabilities Act, Family Leave Act). Importantly, there is a need for federal and state policies that curtail the use of opioids, specifically for patients with chronic pain syndromes. However, laws and policies that restrict opioid use, such as multiple copy prescription programs, discourage physicians from legitimately prescribing opioids for analgesia.[75,76] A desirable policy would be legislation that prohibits and punishes profiling of patients, as practiced by individual providers or a medical facility. Another desirable policy would be legislation to control the expulsion of minorities from programs or medical facilities (eg, for increased utilization of services). Currently, expulsion of patients with SCD from programs is haphazard and whimsical in nature. Efforts should be made to avoid expulsion, which should be a last resort after review by internal and external observers and after securing an alternative facility that will accept the patient in question. So-called

problem or "high-risk" patients should be counseled and rehabilitated, not punished. The current practice, by some, of punishment by expulsion stigmatizes patients and hurls them into a vicious cycle of disparity associated with progression of their pain and suffering.

Advocacy

Improvement in the care of patients with SCD entails the presence of self-support and advocacy groups. Self-support groups should be organized by the patients themselves with the help and encouragement of empathic providers, facilities, and the community. With the help of these groups, patients should know their rights and responsibilities in negotiating the medical system. Advocacy groups should include any individuals interested in the quality of care of minorities; the community should be a major participant in this group, including the local chapter of the Sickle Cell Disease Association of America (SCDAA), if available. Examples of desirable members of advocacy groups include, but are not limited to, care providers, lawyers, journalists, politicians, family members and friends of patients with SCD, and members of the local chapter of the SCDAA. Support and advocacy groups should communicate and share information. These groups can function as resources for patients who seek to report grievances or complaints. These groups should also be able to communicate with providers and institutions targeted by the complaints in order to resolve grievances. They may also conduct visits to institutions that have programs for individuals with SCD and may conduct surveys to assess patients' satisfaction with their care.

Research

Most of the research on SCD has been basic in nature, focusing on the pathophysiology of sickling and approaches to reverse or prevent vasoocclusion. Salutary advances in this area include the finding that hydroxyurea decreases the frequency of acute painful episodes in some patients who meet the indications for its use.[23] Research continues to find additional treatments, preventive measures, and an acceptable cure (eg, in-vitro fertilization with preimplantation genetic diagnosis, bone marrow transplantation, and gene therapy). Research on sickle pain and its related issues, however, is almost nonexistent. Future research should include the effect of race and ethnicity on the metabolism of opioids and the effect of gender on the response to certain analgesics. Recent studies suggest that the response to analgesics is not uniform among patients but is sex dependent.[77] Whether this is operative in patients with SCD is still unknown. Moreover, research is needed to determine the effect of a chronic painful disorder such as SCD on consumption of analgesics, cognition, psychological functioning, and attitudes and behavior of those suffering from this illness. Advances in this area may lead to better understanding of patients' experiences and, hence, a more compassionate attitude and approach from healthcare providers.

In closing, we wish to emphasize that the care of patients with SCD has improved in recent years, although further progress is needed. We believe the approach we have outlined— of targeted education, comprehensive management, legislation, advocacy, and research— provides five milestones that can ameliorate and, we hope, abolish the disparities in the care of patients with SCD and, similarly, of any other minority group of patients with chronic disease.

► Case Scenarios

Case 1

A social worker was consulted to resolve a dispute between the nursing staff and a 36-year-old African American man with sickle α-thalassemia who was hospitalized for an acute painful episode involving shoulders, arms, low back, and legs. His pain had an intensity score of 10/10 using a 0-to-10 verbal scale anchored at one end with no pain (0/10) and at the other end with the worst possible pain. He was treated with meperidine, 125 mg IM every 2 hours as needed. Complications of his disease had included avascular necrosis of the left shoulder, leg ulcers, recurrent thrombophlebitis, pneumonia, and priapism. Physical examination revealed a well-developed, muscular young man in moderate distress. Hemoglobin concentration ranged from 11 to 13 g/dL.

The nursing staff indicated that he exhibited uncooperative, hostile, and disruptive behavior. He had a stable family life, was employed as a contractor by a construction business, and was anxious to leave the hospital to resume his nor-mal duties. It was also mentioned that he was verbally abusive, loud, and demanded medication before it was due. The patient indicated that his medications were usually delayed.

Further evaluation, discussion, and observation revealed a discrepancy between the time when the injection was given and the time it was recorded; for example, an injection given at 2 PM would be recorded at 2:30 PM when the nurse returned to the nursing station after lengthy rounds to many patients. Consequently, the patient expected another injection at 4 PM, but the record indicated it should be 4:30 PM. Repetition of this scenario escalated the problem, which could have been avoided by giving the medication on a fixed schedule (around the clock) or by patient-controlled analgesia (PCA). Unfortunately, the patient was discharged home before a change could be instituted.

COMMENT

This case illustrates a series of misunderstandings that may culminate in unrelieved pain, a hostile patient, and a frustrated nursing staff. Ethnic tension and friction seem to be most acute between young male patients with sickle cell disease and Caucasian female nurses of comparable age group. In other countries where the nursing staff and patients are of the same ethnicity, the nurses share the patients' fears and concerns and realize that their own families are susceptible to the same disease process. Finally, "clock-watchers" are neither addicts nor innately hostile. They seek pain relief. This case also demonstrates that inadequate pain management is one cause of seemingly aberrant behavior.

Case 2

A 34-year-old African American woman with sickle cell anemia presented to the emergency department complaining of sudden onset of severe abdominal pain that began 4 hours earlier. The pain was located in the lower abdominal region (left > right). The pain was constant, 10/10 in severity, did not radiate, and was not relieved with hydrocodone-ibuprofen at home. She denied a history of fever, chills, shortness of breath, chest pain, dysuria, nausea, and vomiting. Her past medical history was remarkable for avascular necrosis of the femoral head, history of cholecystectomy, and infrequent pain crises (since starting hydroxyurea 5 years ago). Medications included hydroxyurea, 1000 mg/day; folic acid, 1 mg/day; and hydrocodone, 7.5 mg, with ibuprofen, 200 mg, every 6 hours, as needed. The patient reported no history of cigarette, alcohol, or illicit drug use. No other history was obtained.

Physical examination revealed an alert and oriented woman who was uncomfortable and writhing in pain. The patient was tachycardic but other vital sign were stable, with no orthostasis. Mild scleral icterus was present. Abdominal examination revealed normal bowel sounds, and the liver span was 8 cm in the midclavicular line. There was marked suprapubic tenderness with no guarding or rebound. The rest of the examination was unremarkable. Hemoglobin concentration was 7.0 g/dL. The

patient was admitted with a diagnosis of sickle cell pain crisis.

The patient was placed in a private room and started on intravenous hydration ($^1/_2$ normal saline). Pain management consisted of intravenous morphine, 2.0 mg every 2 hours, as needed. Over the next 24 hours, the patient requested pain medications 12 times with poor analgesia (pain remained at 9/10 in severity). During the second hospital day, the lower abdominal pain persisted, and the patient was found by nurses to be somnolent, with a pulse of 120 beats/min and blood pressure that was 70/palpable. An emergent blood count revealed hemoglobin concentration of 3.5 g/dL, and emergent laparoscopy showed gross blood in the abdominal cavity. The patient suffered a cardiac arrest, and resuscitation was unsuccessful. Consent was obtained for postmortem examination, which confirmed a ruptured ectopic pregnancy.

COMMENT

This case depicts a typical example of pain escalation in a sickle cell patient, the cause of which was not identified because of misdiagnosis of the presenting clinical picture. For sickle cell patients, it is not uncommon for any pain to be attributed to sickle cell disease. Persistence or exacerbation of pain should raise the possibility of progressive tissue damage (due to the disease itself) or a comorbid condition (non–sickle cell related; in this case, an ectopic pregnancy). This case underscores the necessity of a complete history and physical examination and an inclusive differential diagnosis in patients with an underlying hemoglobinopathy. Other conditions that are often misdiagnosed as "crisis pain" (vasoocclusive episode) include appendicitis, osteomyelitis, peptic ulcer disease, septic arthritis, splenic hemorrhage, infarction or sequestration (in adults), gout, and pancreatitis.

Case 3

A 21-year-old African American woman with sickle cell anemia presented to the emergency department with sudden onset of back pain, localized to the lumbar (L1 through L3) spine. She rated her pain as 10 out of 10 in severity and typical of previous painful episodes. She denied dysuria, nausea, shortness of breath, fever or chills, and all other complaints. Her past medical history was remarkable for pneumonia, cholecystectomy, and frequent pain episodes. She had one child, and her last menstrual period was 10 days ago. The patient was taking Tylenol with Codeine at home without relief of her symptoms. Physical examination revealed a thin young woman, who appeared to be in acute distress. She was afebrile with a pulse of 100 beats/min, blood pressure of 120/80 (no orthostasis), and respirations of 12 breaths/min. She had mild scleral icterus. The lungs were clear, and auscultation of the heart showed a II/VI systolic ejection murmur. A right upper quadrant abdominal scar was present, but abdominal examination was otherwise benign. Point tenderness was present over the spinous processes of lumbar (L1 through L3) vertebrae. Extremities revealed no tenderness, ulcers or clubbing. The hemoglobin concentration was 10.2 g/dL, reticulocyte count was 11%, and other hematologic values, kidney profile, and electrolytes were within normal limits. Pulse oximetry readings showed 97% oxygen saturation.

The patient was admitted with the diagnosis of an uncomplicated, acute vasoocclusive episode (pain crisis). She was started on morphine using a patient-controlled analgesia (PCA) pump at the following dose: 1 mg PCA dose, 7-minute lockout interval, 4-hour dose limit of 30 mg. Orders also included as-needed nursing boluses of 1 mg of morphine IV every 30 minutes. Intravenous normal saline was started at rate of 100 mL/h. Twenty-four hours after admission, the patient had used a total of 90 mg of morphine and reported a pain score of 5/10 in severity. However, she reported shortness of breath. Vital signs indicated a respiratory rate of 20 breaths/min, and the pulse oximetry reading was 90%. The nurse notified the house staff that the patient was in respiratory distress, and the PCA pump was immediately discontinued.

A chest X-ray was consistent with pulmonary edema.

COMMENT

This case illustrates appropriate pain management and resultant pain relief. However, aggressive hydration (with normal saline) in a patient with an uncomplicated pain crisis is not indicated and is a common cause of iatrogenic pulmonary edema. Chronic anemia is usually associated with a chronic increase in cardiac output, which, by early adulthood, may result in a compensatory cardiomyopathy (enlargement of the heart). Thus, patients may not have the cardiovascular reserve needed to handle rapid volume expansion.

This patient had no signs of volume depletion on admission, yet was given normal saline (2400 mL over 24 hours). There are no clinical trials indicating that aggressive hydration shortens the duration of a painful episode or has a role in alleviating pain. Despite the lack of evidence, this practice is common in the management of sickle cell painful episodes. Vigorous hydration requires caution and close monitoring in patients with sickle cell anemia, particularly in adults. Because this patient was euvolemic, proper management should consist of oral fluids or maintenance intravenous fluids ($^1/_2$ normal saline at approximately 70 mL/h).

This case also demonstrates how pulmonary complications (ie, shortness of breath) may be incorrectly attributed to opioid analgesics, further complicating pain management. Respiratory suppression is a well-known side effect of opioids, but usually causes hypoventilation. Opioid analgesics were discontinued in this patient with hyperventilation, which was secondary to aggressive hydration and pulmonary edema.

▶ REFERENCES

1. Onwubalili JK. Sickle-cell anaemia: An explanation for the ancient myth of reincarnation in Nigeria. *Lancet* 1983;2(8348):503–505.

2. Konotey-Ahulu FI. The sickle cell diseases. Clinical manifestations including the "sickle crisis." *Arch Intern Med* 1974;133(4):611–619.

3. Herrick JB. Peculiar elongated and sickle-shaped red blood corpuscles in a case of severe anemia. 1910. *Yale J Biol Med* 2001;74(3):179–184.

4. Diggs LW, Chin RE. Pathology of sickle cell anemia. *So Med J* 1934;27:839–845.

5. Ham TH, Castle WB. Relationship of increased hypotonic fragility and of erythrostasis to the mechanisms of hemolysis in certain anemias. *Trans Assoc Am Phys* 1940;55:127–132.

6. Watson J. Study of sickling of young erythrocytes in sickle cell anemia. *Blood* 1948:465–469.

7. Pauling L, Itano HA. Sickle cell anemia a molecular disease. *Science* 1949;110(2865):543–548.

8. Neel JV. The inheritance of the sickling phenomenon, with particular reference to sickle cell disease. *Blood* 1951;6(5):389–412.

9. Beet EA. Observations on African children. *Arch Dis Child* 1951;26(126):119–133.

10. Ingram VM. Gene mutations in human haemoglobin: The chemical difference between normal and sickle cell haemoglobin. *Nature* 1957;180(4581):326–328.

11. Muirhead H, Perutz MF. Structure of haemoglobin. A three-dimensional Fourier synthesis of reduced human haemoglobin at 5·5A resolution. *Nature* 1953;199:633–638.

12. Besa E. Hemoglobin and hemoglobinopathies. In: Besa E, Kant J, Catalano P, eds. *Hematology.* Philadelphia, Pa: Harwal; 1992:123–136.

13. *Sickle Cell Disease: Screening, Diagnosis, Management and Counseling in Newborns and Infants.* Clinical Practice Guideline No. 6, Publication No. 93-0562. Washington, DC: US Dept of Health and Human Services, Public Health Service, Agency for Health Care Policy and Research; 1993.

14. Leikin SL, Gallagher D, Kinney TR, et al. Mortality in children and adolescents with sickle cell disease. Cooperative Study of Sickle Cell Disease. *Pediatrics* 1989;84(3):500–508.

15. *Sickle Cell Research for Treatment and Cure.* Washington, DC: US Dept of Health and Human Services; National Institutes of Health; National Heart, Blood and Lung Institute; September 2002. NIH Publication No. 02-214.

16. Gaston M, Smith J, Gallagher D, et al. Recruitment in the Cooperative Study of Sickle Cell Disease (CSSCD). *Control Clin Trials* 1987; 8(4 suppl):131S–140S.

17. Gaston MH, Verter JI, Woods G, et al. Prophylaxis with oral penicillin in children with sickle cell anemia. A randomized trial. *N Engl J Med* 1986;314(25):1593–1599.

18. Consensus Conference. Newborn screening for sickle cell disease and other hemoglobinopathies. *JAMA* 1987;258(9):1205–1209.

19. Platt OS, Brambilla DJ, Rosse WF, et al. Mortality in sickle cell disease. Life expectancy and risk factors for early death. *N Engl J Med* 1994; 330(23):1639–1644.

20. Galanello R, Veith R, Papayannopoulou T, et al. Pharmacologic stimulation of Hb F in patients with sickle cell anemia. *Prog Clin Biol Res* 1985;191:433–445.

21. Platt OS, Orkin SH, Dover G, et al. Hydroxyurea enhances fetal hemoglobin production in sickle cell anemia. *J Clin Invest* 1984;74(2):652–656.

22. Dover GJ, Charache S, Boyer SH, et al. 5-Azacytidine increases HbF production and reduces anemia in sickle cell disease: Dose-response analysis of subcutaneous and oral dosage regimens. *Blood* 1985;66(3):527–532.

23. Letvin NL, Linch DC, Beardsley GP, et al. Influence of cell cycle phase-specific agents on simian fetal hemoglobin synthesis. *J Clin Invest* 1985;75(6):1999–2005.

24. Charache S, Terrin ML, Moore RD, et al. Effect of hydroxyurea on the frequency of painful crises in sickle cell anemia. Investigators of the Multicenter Study of Hydroxyurea in Sickle Cell Anemia. *N Engl J Med* 1995;332(20):1317–1322.

25. Benjamin LJ, Dampier CD, Jacox A, et al. *Guideline for the Management of Acute and Chronic Pain in Sickle Cell Disease.* Glenview, Ill: American Pain Society; 1999.

26. Ballas SK, Carlos TM, Dampier C, et al. *Guidelines for Standards of Care of Acute Painful Episodes in Patients with Sickle Cell Disease.* Philadelphia, Pa: DIS Graphic Services, Thomas Jefferson University, sponsored by the Pennsylvania Department of Health; 2000.

27. McCurdy PR, Sherman AS. Irreversibly sickled cells and red cell survival in sickle cell anemia: A study with both DF32P and 51CR. *Am J Med* 1978;64(2):253–258.

28. Hoover R, Rubin R, Wise G, et al. Adhesion of normal and sickle erythrocytes to endothelial monolayer cultures. *Blood* 1979;54(4):872–876.

29. Hebbel RP, Boogaerts MA, Eaton JW, et al. Erythrocyte adherence to endothelium in sickle-cell anemia. A possible determinant of disease severity. *N Engl J Med* 1980;302(18):992–995.

30. Malave I, Perdomo Y, Escalona E, et al. Levels of tumor necrosis factor alpha/cachectin (TNF alpha) in sera from patients with sickle cell disease. *Acta Haematol* 1993;90(4):172–176.

31. Hedo CC, Aken'ova YA, Okpala IE, et al. Acute phase reactants and severity of homozygous sickle cell disease. *J Intern Med* 1993;233(6):467–470.

32. Singhal A, Doherty JF, Raynes JG, et al. Is there an acute-phase response in steady-state sickle cell disease? *Lancet* 1993;341(8846):651–653.

33. Taylor SC, Shacks SJ, Mitchell RA, et al. Serum interleukin-6 levels in the steady state of sickle cell disease. *J Interferon Cytokine Res* 1995;15(12):1061–1064.

34. Kuvibidila S, Gardner R, Ode D, et al: Tumor necrosis factor alpha in children with sickle cell disease in stable condition. *J Natl Med Assoc* 1997;89(9):609–615.

35. Bourantas KL, Dalekos GN, Makis A, et al. Acute phase proteins and interleukins in steady state sickle cell disease. *Eur J Haematol* 1998;61:49–54.

36. Rybicki AC, Benjamin LJ. Increased levels of endothelin-1 in plasma of sickle cell anemia patients. *Blood* 1998;92(7):2594–2596.

37. Werdehoff SG, Moore RB, Hoff CJ, et al. Elevated plasma endothelin-1 levels in sickle cell anemia: Relationships to oxygen saturation and left ventricular hypertrophy. *Am J Hematol* 1998;58(3):195–199.

38. Graido-Gonzalez E, Doherty JC, Bergreen EW, et al. Plasma endothelin-1, cytokine, and prostaglandin E2 levels in sickle cell disease and acute vaso-occlusive sickle crisis. *Blood* 1998;92(7):2551–2555.

39. Rees DC, Cervi P, Grimwade D, et al. The metabolites of nitric oxide in sickle-cell disease. *Br J Haematol* 1995;91(4):834–837.

40. Lopez BL, Barnett J, Ballas SK, et al. Nitric oxide metabolite levels in acute vaso-occlusive sickle-cell crisis. *Acad Emerg Med* 1996;3(12):1098–1103.

41. Ballas SK. *Sickle Cell Pain.* Seattle, Wash: International Association for the Study of Pain; 1998.

42. Koshy M, Leikin J, Dorn L, et al. Evaluation and management of sickle cell disease in the emergency department (an 18-year experience): 1974–1992. *Am J Ther* 1994;1(4):309–320.

43. Ballas SK. The sickle cell painful crisis in adults: Phases and objective signs. *Hemoglobin* 1995;19(6):323–333.

44. Benjamin LJ, Swinson GI, Nagel RL. Sickle cell anemia day hospital: An approach for the management of uncomplicated painful crises. *Blood* 2000;95(4):1130–1136.

45. Yam L, Li C. The spleen. In: Embury S, Hebbel R, Mohandas N, et al, eds. *Sickle Cell Disease: Basic Principles and Clinical Practice.* New York, NY: Raven; 1994;555–566.

46. Vichinsky EP, Styles LA, Colangelo LH, et al. Acute chest syndrome in sickle cell disease: Clinical presentation and course. Cooperative Study of Sickle Cell Disease. *Blood* 1997;89(5):1787–1792.

47. Ohene-Frempong K. Stroke in sickle cell disease: Demographic, clinical, and therapeutic considerations. *Semin Hematol* 1991;28(3):213–219.

48. Adams RJ, McKie VC, Hsu L, et al. Prevention of a first stroke by transfusions in children with sickle cell anemia and abnormal results on transcranial Doppler ultrasonography. *N Engl J Med* 1998;339(1):5–11.

49. Russell MO, Goldberg HI, Hodson A, et al. Effect of transfusion therapy on arteriographic abnormalities and on recurrence of stroke in sickle cell disease. *Blood* 1984;63(1):162–169.

50. Cohen AR, Martin MB, Silber JH, et al. A modified transfusion program for prevention of stroke in sickle cell disease. *Blood* 1992;79(7):1657–1661.

51. Milner PF, Kraus AP, Sebes JI, et al. Sickle cell disease as a cause of osteonecrosis of the femoral head. *N Engl J Med* 1991;325(21):1476–1481.

52. Goldberg MF. Retinal neovascularization in sickle cell retinopathy. *Trans Sect Ophthalmol Am Acad Ophthalmol Otolaryngol* 1977;83(3 pt 1):OP409–431.

53. Reed W, Vichinsky EP. New considerations in the treatment of sickle cell disease. *Annu Rev Med* 1998;49:461–474.

54. Covitz W. Cardiac disease. In: Embury S, Hebbel R, Mohandas N, et al, eds. *Sickle Cell Disease: Basic Principles and Clinical Practice.* New York, NY: Raven; 1994;725–738.

55. Powars DR, Elliott-Mills DD, Chan L, et al. Chronic renal failure in sickle cell disease: Risk factors, clinical course, and mortality. *Ann Intern Med* 1991;115(8):614–620.

56. Treadwell M, Gill K. Psychosocial aspects. In: Embury S, Hebbel R, Mohandas N, et al, eds. *Sickle Cell Disease: Basic Principles and Clinical Practice.* New York, NY: Raven; 1994:517–530.

57. Woods K, Lambert C, Miller M, et al. Health status in adults with sickle cell disease, *JCOM* 1997;4(5):15–21.

58. Von Gunten CF, Muir JC. Palliative medicine: An emerging field of specialization. *Cancer Invest* 2000;18(8):761–767.

59. Embury S, Hebbel R, Mohandas N, et al, eds. *Sickle Cell Disease: Basic Principles and Clinical Practice.* New York, NY: Raven; 1994.

60. Anderson LP, Rehm LP. The relationship between strategies of coping and perception of pain in three chronic pain groups. *J Clin Psych* 1984;40(5):170–177.

61. Seigel WM, Golden NH, Gough JW, et al. Depression, self-esteem, and life events in adolescents with chronic diseases. *J Adolesc Health Care* 1990;11(6):501–504.

62. Bennett DS. Depression among children with chronic medical problems: A meta-analysis. *J Pediatr Psychol* 1994;19(2):149–169.

63. Britto MT, Garrett JM, Dugliss MA, et al. Preventive services received by adolescents with cystic fibrosis and sickle cell disease. *Arch Pediatr Adolesc Med* 1999;153(1):27–32.

64. Perry DF, Ireys HT. Maternal perceptions of pediatric providers for children with chronic illnesses. *Matern Child Health J* 2001;5(1):15–20.

65. Chernoff RG, Ireys HT, DeVet KA, et al. A randomized, controlled trial of a community-based support program for families of children with chronic illness: Pediatric outcomes. *Arch Pediatr Adolesc Med* 2002;156(6):533–539.

66. Telfair J, Myers J, Drezner S. Transfer as a component of the transition of adolescents with sickle cell disease to adult care: Adolescent, adult, and parent perspectives. *J Adolesc Health* 1994;15(7):558–565.

67. Woods K, Karrison T, Koshy M, et al. Hospital utilization patterns and costs for adult sickle cell patients in Illinois. *Public Health Rep* 1997;112(1):44–51.

68. Groves JE. Taking care of the hateful patient. *N Engl J Med* 1978;298(16):883–887.

69. Ballas SK. Treatment of pain in adults with sickle cell disease. *Am J Hematol* 1990;34(1):49–54.

70. Ballas SK. Attitudes toward adult patients with sickle cell disease: Silent prejudice or benign neglect? *J Assoc Acad Minor Phys* 1996;7(3):62.

71. Ballas, SK, Brandon Z. Misinterpretation of pain escalation in an adult patient with sickle cell anemia defers accurate diagnosis. *Pain Digest* 1997;7:208–210.

72. Ballas SK. Ethical issues in the management of sickle cell pain. *Am J Hematol* 2001;68(2):127–132.

73. The Sickle Cell Information Center; Georgia Comprehensive Sickle Cell Center at Grady Health System. Available at: http://www.scinfo.org.

74. *The Management and Therapy of Sickle Cell Disease,* 4th ed. Washington, DC: National Institutes of Health; 2002. NIH Publication No. 02-2117. Available at: http://www.nhlbi.nih.gov/health/prof/blood/sickle/index.htm.

75. Joranson DE, Gilson AM, Dahl JL, et al. Pain management, controlled substances, and state medical board policy: A decade of change. *J Pain Symptom Manage* 2002;23(2):138–147.

76. Joranson DE, Gilson AM. Regulatory barriers to pain management. *Semin Oncol Nurs* 1998;14(2):158–163.

77. Fillingim RB. Sex, gender, and pain: Women and men really are different. *Curr Rev Pain* 2000;4(1):24–30.

CHAPTER 15

Mental Health

HENRY W. DOVE, MD
TANYA R. ANDERSON, MD
CARL C. BELL, MD

▶ INTRODUCTION

This chapter addresses mental health and its impact on the overall health status of US non-white populations. Because of untreated physical problems, difficulties accessing care, lack of insurance, and a myriad of other factors, non-white mentally ill patients with physical illness are unlikely to receive adequate treatment for their physical and mental problems, thus contributing to the problem of health disparities. As a consequence of these concurrent disparities, nonwhites experience higher disability levels. Despite the fact these disparities and their effects are a major public health concern, the literature contains little research that systematically studies and identifies factors leading to the associated negative outcomes of mental illness on physical health, especially in nonwhite populations.

This chapter outlines interventions that could lead to greater utilization of the nation's health-care system by nonwhites. Findings that suggest US nonwhite populations are disproportionately subjected to trauma in childhood that not only increases future mental illness in adulthood, but also significantly increases the likelihood of physical illness, are also discussed. Finally, potential solutions that address the relationships between trauma, mental and physical health, and the role each assumes in defining health disparities are presented. We hope this discussion will stimulate research into mitigating factors that may identify specific interventions or preventative measures to decrease the problems of physical and mental health disparities as outlined by the Institute of Medicine (IOM)[1] and former Surgeon General David Satcher, MD.[2]

▶ UNTREATED PHYSICAL PROBLEMS IN THE MENTALLY ILL

▶ Illustrative Case Histories

Case 1

Mr X, a 65-year-old African American man with a history of paranoid schizophrenia, is brought to the local emergency department of a major university teaching hospital accompanied by family. Mr X's caretakers report that over the past 2 weeks, he has become confused and combative, and he is responding to auditory and possibly visual hallucinations. Significant laboratory results in the emergency department include a BUN of 50 and creatinine of 3.4. Mr X is admitted to the psychiatry service with a presumptive diagnosis of relapsing paranoid schizophrenia. The morning after admission, the attending psychiatrist (suspecting organic mental disorder rather than schizophrenia) insists that Mr X be reevaluated by the internal medicine service, whereupon a diagnosis of subacute renal failure is made. Mr X is transferred to the medical service for a comprehensive evaluation.

Case 2

Mr Y, a 56-year-old African American man with a history of psychotic symptoms, is admitted to a general hospital psychiatric service due to a worsening of his depressive symptoms. The initial history and physical examination obtained by the family practice intern assigned to psychiatry do not reveal any physical complaints or symptoms. A few days after admission, due to a subsequent complaint of hemoptysis, pleuritic chest pain, and dyspnea, an internal medicine consultation is requested. The internist's consultative note suggests that the patient's symptoms are due to side effects caused by the antipsy-

chotic medication being taken by the patient in the hospital. Understanding the propensity for mentally ill patients who are physically ill to be written off as somatizing, the attending psychiatrist decides to obtain a more detailed medical history from the patient. Upon asking the patient if he had ever had similar symptoms in the past, the patient reported that "about 2 years prior I had 'blood clots' in the veins in the back of my right knee that caused blood clots to go into my lungs which caused the exact same problem." He further reported he did not tell anyone his past history because no one had asked him.

COMMENT

Similar scenarios are acted out daily in the nation's hospitals, community health facilities, and the offices of medical-care providers. Despite improvements in the health of the general population as a result of progress in technology, treatments, and preventative interventions, the health status of individuals with mental illness lags significantly behind that of the general population.[3] Persons with mental illness on average die 10 to 15 years earlier than the general population.[4]

Relationship Between Mental Illness and Physical Illness

Individuals with mental illness have significantly higher comorbidity and mortality rates when matched diagnostically with persons sharing similar demographics and risk factors for common diseases (eg, cardiovascular diseases, renal disease, hypertension, and diabetes).[4] This trend exists despite significant improvements in the quantity and quality of mental health services available for individuals living with severe mental illness (SMI). Some studies conclude that for individuals with SMI, high rates of comorbidity and premature mortality are normative health outcomes.[5] Although the health gap is

more marked in individuals with severe mental illness, it is evident in all who have mental illness. Data reveal that approximately 50% of all individuals with mental illness have diagnosed comorbid medical conditions, while another 35% are estimated to have undiagnosed and untreated medical disorders.[6]

Published studies in both the medical and psychiatric literature show sharp, contrasting distinctions between the physical and mental health of African Americans and other nonwhite ethnic groups when compared with that of the Caucasian population. In 2002, the IOM studied the effects of race and ethnicity on health and health-care disparities. The report generated was significant in its documentation that despite monumental gains in health-care delivery and consequent improvement in health-care status for most Americans, nonwhite ethnic groups benefited far less.[7] Another conclusion drawn by this report affirms that when factors such as age, gender, condition, and socioeconomic status are controlled, African Americans and other nonwhite ethnic groups continue to receive disparate health care, leading to worse health outcomes.[7] In the landmark document titled *Unequal Treatment: Confronting Racial and Ethnic Disparities in Healthcare,* many factors were found to contribute to the disparities in health care and resulting health status.[1] Health-care providers bring to health-care delivery systems their total humanity and life experiences. Unfortunately this includes their stereotypes, prejudices, biases, and insensitivities toward individuals that are perceived to be different. Compounding these difficulties is a tendency to deny participation and complicity with a system that delivers persistently and consistently disparate health care.

Direct clinical service providers do not exist or practice in isolation. As a part of larger health-care systems, providers are vulnerable to the demands, goals, and missions of the organizations for which they work. Forces and assumptions other than quality health care to all drive many health-care organizations. These organizations reflect the attitudes and assumptions of the people who work within them. Finally, all health disparities that exist within racial and ethnic minority groups should be interpreted against the broader context of racial, social, economic, and environmental inequalities—long a historical part of the American landscape. Permanent solutions have remained elusive despite evidence of progress having been made.[2]

Health-care organizations contribute to disparities in health care that exist between white and nonwhite populations by contributing to and perpetuating those factors that contribute to different rates of access, utilization, and prescribed health-care services.[8] It is against this backdrop of a health-care delivery system with known disparities that mental health and its impact on the overall health of nonwhite ethnic populations must be understood.

As a group, individuals with mental illness suffer disproportionately from negative outcomes when a comorbid health issue is evident.[9] When an individual with a mental illness identifies as being African American or another ethnic or racial minority, the morbidity associated with a comorbid medical illness is confounded significantly because dual disparities exist and overlap. Being nonwhite clearly creates disadvantage in the US health-care system. Being non-Caucasian with comorbid mental illness and physical health issues places the individual at greater risk for increased disability, poverty, lower educational achievement, and greater mortality from both natural and unnatural causes.[10]

Failure to Seek Health Care for Mental Illnesses

Being African American or belonging to a nonwhite ethnic group combines the category of having a mental illness with the notion of stigma. Stigmatization is associated with prejudice, avoidance, fear, rejection, and ultimately discrimination.[2] It can be such a formidable force that individuals with the stigmatized characteristic frequently identify with and internalize the public's perceptions and attitudes. In those with mental illness, the burden of stigmatization can lead to an individual being so ashamed and embarrassed that he or she denies the illness, fails to seek treatment, or fails to comply with prescribed treatments.[2] Stigmatization can also lead to decreased access to housing and employment opportunities as well as social isolation. All these factors may lead to diminished self-esteem, which further complicates the patient's mental condition, creating the potential for negative health outcomes due to diminished insight and judgment. Individuals with severe mental disorders frequently lack the social skills and resources that allow for maximal utilization of the health-care system. Underutilization, like diminished access, noncompliance, and stigmatization, is associated with increased morbidity and mortality for all mentally ill populations regardless of race or ethnicity.

Rates of mental illness for African Americans, Hispanic Americans, and Caucasians approximate one another. Data for Native Americans is less available; accurate comparison rates are highly speculative. Of note for some nonwhite populations, especially for African Americans, is high representation in "high-need" populations, defined by social factors that predispose a population to developing mental illness and needing mental health services. Individuals in high-need groups, by virtue of their typically being housed in the inner city, psychiatric hospitals, jails, prisons, or rural communities, are not accurately represented in research studies; thus the prevalence rates for mental illness may be inaccurate.[2] What is clearly not inaccurate is the association between mental illness and the increased prevalence of morbidity and mortality due to physical health problems in nonwhite populations. African Americans and Native Americans appear to have the highest associated morbidity and mortality rates for nonwhites with comorbid mental illness and physical health issues.[11] The higher morbidity and mortality rates reflect associated poverty and perhaps higher rates for alcohol abuse and substance dependency.

Nonwhite patients, like their white counterparts, experience many impediments to medical care by virtue of having mental illness. The presence of mental illness can compromise the ability of patients to provide adequate historical data that would be useful in diagnosing physical illness. Mentally ill patients being treated with psychotropic medications can experience side effects that interfere with their ability to communicate effectively and cause symptoms of physical illness that cloud diagnostic clarity. Suicidality, as a symptom, evokes significant anxiety in all clinicians but especially nonpsychiatrists. For many nonpsychiatric clinicians, it can be the "deal breaker" that leads to cursory evaluations and examinations in a quick

attempt to get the patient out the door and into the hands of a mental health professional. Likewise, depending on severity, hallucinations, delusions, and confusional states can lead to similar outcomes for the patient—inadequate evaluation and treatment of comorbid medical conditions.

Sternberg identifies categories of patient-centered, physician-centered, and disease-centered reasons as contributing factors to missed diagnoses in the mentally ill,[12] but there is nothing in the literature to delineate these reasons along racial or ethnic lines. They appear to be common and valid for all who have mental illness.

Patient-centered factors would encompass all factors that the patient brings to the physician–patient encounter that impede interpersonal connection, prevent accurate history taking, and ultimately reduce the comprehensiveness of the diagnostic evaluation and physical examination. Physician-centered reasons comprise the most important factor leading to negative evaluation outcomes for the mentally ill and include incomplete history taking, cursory physical examinations, failure to obtain or repeat laboratory tests, premature closure of differential diagnosis, and the blind-faith acceptance of collateral information and consultative advice. Finally, disease-centered reasons for missed diagnoses and potential negative outcomes include medical disorders that masquerade as missed medication and substance-induced mental disorders. Clearly, the attitudes, assumptions, prejudices, and other cognitive assessments being made by patients and clinicians alike have an impact on the success of the physician–patient relationship and thereby influence outcomes.[11]

According to the Surgeon General's report on mental health, when urban nonwhites are compared with whites, the following trends are evident.[2] Nonwhites have less access to and availability of mental health services. They are less likely to obtain needed or recommended mental health services.[13] When treatment is available and received, it is often of poorer quality than similar services received by whites. Finally, nonwhite patients are underrepresented in mental health research.[14] These disparities are significant in that they suggest mental illness is less well understood and inadequately treated in nonwhite populations. All data suggest these factors lead to negative outcomes for mental illness. Negative mental illness outcomes are intimately tied to higher levels of morbidity and mortality for comorbid physical illnesses.

Disparities in mental health care and physical health care place a significant burden on racial and ethnic nonwhite groups. As a consequence of these dual disparities, nonwhites experience higher disability levels.[1,2]

It is well known that individuals with mental illness exhibit and engage in behaviors that place them disproportionately at risk for negative physical health outcomes. Six of the 10 leading causes of death are behaviorally based and seen in those with mental illness at a greater rate than in those without. These include obesity, physical inactivity, affective instability, and negative social and environmental variables (eg, low socioeconomic status, high stress environment, and lack of social support). All of these factors, frequently seen in those with mental illness, are associated with the development, progression, or clinical manifestation of physical illnesses, including coronary artery disease, hypertension, asthma, viral infections, autoimmune disorders, and diabetes.[15]

Key to finding solutions for mental health and physical care disparities is understanding how the availability, accessibility, and utilization of services; compliance; education; cultural competence; and prevention influence outcomes. The lack of health-care service availability manifests through the absence of culturally competent services that include individuals familiar with the cultural belief systems, language, and culturally determined stigma around seeking treatments for given nonwhite ethnic populations. A dearth of nonwhite health professionals, especially psychiatrists, increases the likelihood that service availability will be limited, especially in urban and poverty-stricken communities. Outreach programs geared toward increasing the numbers of underrepresented nonwhite ethnic groups in the ranks of the health-care profession are essential.

The role of mental illness in creating physical health morbidity and influencing disparity is readily apparent. Finding ways to better treat mental illness will have a simultaneous positive impact on the physical health of the same patient population.

Even when there is adequate availability of mental health services, nonwhite populations experience lower rates of accessibility. Cost, lack of insurance, lack of parity, attitudes about receiving care and about caregivers, in association with stigma decrease the likelihood that African Americans and other nonwhite populations will seek mental health services. Creative ways of financing mental health care for those who are disqualified from governmental programs and unable to afford private insurance coverage need to be explored and implemented. The "face" of the caregiver also influences lack of availability and access. Access is improved when the face of the caregiver is the same as the face of the consumer in many nonwhite populations. White caregivers must be educated about the social norms, beliefs, and attitudes of the nonwhite members that appear in their caseloads. They must be challenged to confront their own stereotypes, especially those about patients with comorbid mental illness.

Nonwhites tend to use mental services at rates far less than their majority counterparts. This discrepancy is especially apparent in utilization rates of African Americans when services are accessed. African Americans typically access emergency services, members of the clergy, or services provided by primary care physicians. All are characterized by brevity, low rates of follow-up, and high levels of recidivism. Education that focuses on the benefits of mental health services in reducing morbidity and mortality and countering negative attitudes about participating in treatment is a powerful tool that must be implemented in nonwhite communities.

Treatment compliance issues are endemic to the practice of medicine. Whether due to stigma, associated fears and anxieties mobilized by therapeutic interventions, or because of side effects of pharmacologic treatments, lack of compliance contributes significantly to morbidity in mental illness. Programs that emphasize primary medical care and its integration into a primary psychiatric care model where both medical and psychiatric needs can be addressed during the same visit should be the model of the future (ie, one-stop shopping). Efforts to address patients' concerns and to educate them about risks inherent in noncompliance can be effective in enhancing participation in treatment and thereby reducing morbidity.

Developing outreach programs that rely on telemedicine and telepsychiatry programs and networks are viable options for extending health-care services into underserved communities. Such programs can be facilitated by the development of partnerships between underserved communities, their local health-care agencies, and universities with affiliated medical centers. University medical centers are ideally positioned to provide technical support and training to local community agencies. This type of collaboration would potentially facilitate the development of workforces equipped with evidenced-based knowledge and skills to address the general health and psychiatric health needs of underserved communities.

Finally, prevention must be discussed as the paradigm having the most potential for reducing morbidity and mortality associated with mental illness across the life span of individuals. Ethnic and racial nonwhites are exposed to violence, poverty, racism, and discrimination at rates significantly greater than other populations.[2] Poverty is a highly associated indicator for increased rates of mental illness. Nonwhites, especially African Americans, are disproportionately represented in poverty by low income, educational disadvantage, and community of residency. Measures that address the need to reduce poverty, improve community quality of life, and promote educational opportunity

may ultimately lead to a reduction of morbidity associated with mental illness.

▶ SIGNIFICANT CHILDHOOD TRAUMA CONTRIBUTING TO POOR ADULT HEALTH OUTCOMES

Adverse Childhood Experiences

The association between childhood trauma and its impact on adult health outcomes is well established by the Adverse Childhood Experience (ACE) Study.[16] This pivotal study linked 7 categories of adverse experiences in childhood (physical abuse; psychological abuse; sexual abuse; violence against the respondent's mother; living with household members who have been mentally ill or suicidal; and living with a household member who reported ever being imprisoned) to 10 risk factors and 8 disease conditions of adulthood. Risk factors include behaviors such as smoking and high numbers of sexual partners; increased incidence of ischemic heart disease, diabetes, and sexually transmitted diseases represent linked disease conditions of adulthood, respectively. Analysis revealed significant correlation between all categories of adverse childhood experiences cited, health risk, and health status outcomes reviewed.[16] Individuals having multiple categories of adverse childhood exposures were more likely to also have numerous health risk factors and negative health outcomes. Specifically, persons who experienced four or more categories of childhood exposure, contrasted with those who had experienced none, had a 7.4-fold increased risk for alcoholism, 10.3-fold increased risk for drug abuse, 4.6-fold increased risk for depression, and 12.2-fold increased risk for suicide attempts. Persons who experienced four or more categories had a 2.2-fold increased risk for smoking, 2.2-fold increased risk for poor self-rated health, 3.2-fold increased risk for 50 or more sexual partners, and 2.5-fold increased risk for having a sexually transmitted disease history compared with persons who experienced none of the adverse childhood experiences. Respondents who experienced four or more categories had a 1.4-fold increased risk for physical inactivity and a 1.6-fold increased risk for severe obesity compared with those with no adverse childhood experiences. Likewise, individuals who were exposed to four or more adverse childhood experiences had a 2.2-fold increased risk of ischemic heart disease, 1.9-fold increased risk of cancer, 3.9-fold increased risk of chronic lung disease (eg, bronchitis or emphysema), 1.6-fold increased risk for skeletal fractures, and 2.4-fold increased risk for liver disease (eg, hepatitis or jaundice) compared with their counterparts.[16] The correlation between adverse life experiences in childhood and adult adverse health outcomes is clearly established and should be addressed via evidence-based public health interventions.[17]

Public Health Implications for Nonwhite Children Exposed to Trauma and Violence

Trauma and victimization looms large in nonwhite ethnic populations as a cause of significant psychiatric morbidity, with the long-term potential for increased mortality. Because nonwhites are overrepresented in high-need populations (eg, foster care, homeless, drug addicted, inner-city resident, imprisoned), they are at greater risk of being traumatized or witnessing traumatizing events.[2] When a traumatizing event occurs in childhood, early intervention is essential in reducing long-term morbidity.[17]

Prevention and intervention strategies must be directed toward two important areas in the life of a child: the home and the health-care system in which the child is treated. Home-centered strategies that can potentially lead to positive health outcomes need to be implemented. Comprehensive home assessments designed to identify maladaptive and pathological systems that expose children to risky behaviors must be developed and implemented. As

one example, nurse home visitation programs have been found to be successful in preventing children's risky future health behaviors.[18] Interventions aimed at strengthening family process, decision-making, communication, within-family support, and organization; parental skills, supervision, and monitoring practices; and youth skills, peer-pressure negotiation skills, and communication have also been shown promise as human immunodeficiency virus (HIV) prevention tools in African American and Hispanic American youth.[19] Parents and caregivers need help to identify community support systems for themselves (separate from those for their children) to enable them to learn better coping strategies, develop blueprints for managing their lives, and promote adaptive family functioning. Emphasis on community-centered resources (ie, child care, support groups, socialization groups) and education can lead to reduction in family disintegration and correction of behavioral patterns that potentially expose children to high-risk situations that lead to overt trauma and victimization. For example, multisystemic therapy has been shown to be effective in decreasing risky youth health behaviors that potentially led to adverse health consequences.[20]

Health-care system strategies include routine, comprehensive psychosocial and physical assessments of all children living in high-risk situations. Extensive training for health-care professionals, clergy, and teachers must be developed to improve their capacity to overcome bias, look beyond stigmatization, and remain vigilant to covert and overt signs of trauma or victimization. For children living in violent and disruptive home environments, skillful, culturally informed evaluations, interventions, and treatments are an imperative.[21] Interventions that promote prevention and wellness through use of evidence-based strategies are crucial to the reduction of negative health outcomes over the life span of at-risk individuals. These strategies are in keeping with the goals established by the office of the Surgeon General to improve mental health services for children.[22]

Primary, secondary, and tertiary interventions in the home, schools, communities, and health service systems will be essential to enhanced participation of nonwhite consumers, relative to their white counterparts, in the health-care system.[22] This includes but is not limited to actions that address issues of health-care affordability; lack of cultural sensitivity in service providers; misdiagnosis, resulting in overreliance on the juvenile and criminal justice systems rather than the mental health system to address behavioral offenses; lack of accessibility to health-care services; high environmental stress; poor schooling; and high rates of unemployment.[23]

▶ SUMMARY AND RECOMMENDATIONS

Being a member of a racial or ethnic nonwhite group while having a co-occurring illness is literally hazardous to one's health. Membership in either group carries a high level of stigmatization in society and the medical community; inclusion in both groups simultaneously exacerbates the risk for health disparity. Stigmatization translates into increased rates of morbidity and mortality for medical illnesses that the majority population does not experience, when all other demographics are controlled. Faced with undeniable disparity in what many consider one of the inalienable rights of US citizens, the need to find corrective measures for disparities in both

▶ **TABLE 15–1.** Corrective Measures for Mental Health Disparities

- Reduce stigmatization of mental illness through education
- Enhance communication-based social skills training for those with mental illness
- Improve access to and availability of mental health services in underserved communities
- Enhance numbers of providers to the underserved through targeted recruitment
- Increase education to improve treatment compliance

▶ **TABLE 15–2.** Corrective Measures for Physical Health Disparities in Patients with Mental Illness

- Correct educational deficits on the part of health-care deliverers
- Improve cultural competence of health-care providers
- Provide "health-care extenders" to address shortages of providers in underserved communities
- Provide "one-stop shopping" for medical and psychiatric interventions
- Emphasize evidence-based preventions and effective interventions

mental and general health care must be forthcoming. Tables 15–1 and 15–2 outline corrective measures to address these needs. The presence of mental illness predicts adverse physical health outcomes. Addressing disparities in mental health care can also address general health outcomes for those suffering from mental illness.

There is strong evidence linking exposure to adverse childhood experiences to negative health outcomes in adults. The relationship appears to be cumulative and requires interventional strategies that can be widely implemented as well as promotion of strategies to protect children from exposure to early life trauma (Table 15–3).

▶ **TABLE 15–3.** Corrective Measures for Nonwhite Children at Risk for Poor Adult Health Outcomes

- Implement culturally informed evaluations, interventions, and treatments
- Use home-centered strategies to address maladaptive family systems and behavior
- Reduce reliance on the juvenile justice system to address behavioral problems in youth
- Enhance utilization of the mental health system to address behavioral problems in youth
- Implement evidence-based public health interventions for children diagnosed as trauma survivors

Society will benefit from taking action on the compelling evidence linking mental health status to physical health. Only through continued study, resource allocation, and education of consumers, caregivers, and the general public will the morbidity and mortality associated mental and physical health disorders be reduced.

▶ REFERENCES

1. Smedley BD, Stith AY, Nelson AR, eds. *Unequal Treatment: Confronting Racial and Ethnic Disparities in Healthcare*. Washington, DC: National Academies Press; 2003.

2. US Public Health Service. *Mental Health: Culture, Race, and Ethnicity: A Supplement to Mental Health: A Report of the Surgeon General*. Rockville, Md: US Public Health Service; 2001.

3. Berren MR, Hill K, Merikle E, et al. Serious mental illness and mortality rates. *Hosp Comm Psychiatry* 1994;45(6):604–605.

4. Felker B, Yazel J, Short D. Mortality and medical co-morbidity among psychiatric patients: A review. *Psychiatr Serv* 1996;47(12):1356–1363.

5. Segal SP, Kotler PL. A ten-year perspective of mortality risk among mentally ill patients in sheltered care. *Hosp Comm Psychiatry* 1991;42(7):708–713.

6. Farnam CR, Zipple AM, Tyrrell W, et al. Health status and risk factors of people with severe and persistent mental illness. *J Psychsoc Nurs Ment Health Serv* 1999;37(6):16–21.

7. Bentacourt JR. Unequal treatment: The Institute of Medicine's findings and recommendations on health care disparities. *Harv Health Pol Rev Archiv* 2002;3. Available at: http://www.hcs.harvard.

8. Desai M, Rosenheck R. Trends in discharge, disposition, mortality and service use among long stay psychiatric patients in the 1990s. *Psychiatr Serv* 2003;54(4):542–548.

9. Byrne C, Issacs S, Voorberg N. Assessment of the physical health needs of people with chronic mental illness: One focus for health promotion. *Can Mental Health J* 1991;39:7–12.

10. DeNoon O. Minorities suffer most from lack of mental health care. WebMDhealth, 2004. Available at: http://my.webmd.com/content/article/35/1728_87643.

11. Hogue C, Hargraves M, Colins K, et al. *Minority Health in America: Findings and Policy Implications from the Commonwealth Fund Minority Health Survey*. Baltimore, Md: Johns Hopkins University Press; 2000.

12. Sternberg D. Testing for physical illness in psychiatric patients. *J Clin Psychiatry* 1986;47(1Suppl): 3–9.

13. Richardson J, Anderson T, Flaherty J, et al. The quality of mental care for African-Americans. *Cult Med Psychiatry* 2003;27(4):487–498.

14. Bell C, Williamson J. Articles on special populations published in psychiatric services between 1950 and 1999. *Psychiatr Serv* 2002;53(4):414–424.

15. American Psychological Association. *Racial and Ethnic Health Disparities: A Fact Sheet on Racial and Ethnic Health Disparities*. APA; 2004. Available at: http://www.apa.org/ppo/isssues/phealthdis.html.

16. Felitti VJ, Anda, RF, Nordenberg D, et al. Relationship of child abuse and household dysfunction to many of the leading causes of death in adults. The Adverse Childhood Experiences (ACE) Study. *Am J Prev Med* 1998;14(4):245–258.

17. Anderson TR, DeCarlo A, Bell C, et al. Trauma and violence in childhood: A US perspective. *Psychiatr Times* 2003;20(10):91.

18. Olds DL, Hill PL, Mihalic SF, et al. Book seven: Nurse–family partnership (NFP). In: Elliott DS, series ed. *Blueprints for Violence Prevention*. Boulder, Colo: Center for the Study and Prevention of Violence, Institute of Behavioral Science, University of Colorado at Boulder; 1998.

19. Bell CC, Mckay M. Constructing a children's mental health infrastructure using community psychiatry principles. *J Legal Med* 2004;25(1): 5–22.

20. Henggeler SW, Melton GB, Smith LA, et al. Family preservation using multi-systemic therapy: An effective alternative to incarcerating serious juvenile offenders. *J Consult Clin Psychol* 1992;60(6):953–961.

21. US Dept of Health and Human Services. *Youth Violence: A Report of the Surgeon General*. Rockville, Md: USDHHS; 2001.

22. US Public Health Service. *Report of the Surgeon General's Conference on Children's Mental Health: A National Agenda*. Washington, DC: Dept of Health and Human Services; 2000.

23. Snowden LR. Barriers to effective mental health service for African Americans. *Mental Health Serv Res* 2001;3(4):181–187.

CHAPTER 16

Dentistry and Oral Health

Jeanne Craig Sinkford, DDS, MS, PhD
John W. Reinhardt, DDS, MS, MPH

▶ INTRODUCTION

The United States has one of the best oral health care systems in the world. Americans are living longer, they are retaining their teeth for longer periods of time, and their interest in oral health has increased as indicated by the increased number of annual visits to the dentist for preventive care. The effective reduction in dental caries through community water fluoridation has significantly contributed to the overall oral health of both adults and children. Because of scientific evidence of relationships between chronic oral infections and systemic disorders, oral health is increasingly perceived as an integral and important part of overall health. The evidence-based connection between oral and systemic diseases continues to emerge as newer technologies are utilized in clinical research investigations.

Dental Practice

The American Dental Association (ADA) currently reports 155,716 practicing dentists in the United States. The ratio of dentists to population is 56:100,000 or one dentist for every 1786 persons. Eighty percent of dentists are in general practice, and 15.6% are women. Six percent of dentists are from underrepresented minority groups, including African Americans, Hispanics, and Native Americans. Unlike medicine, dentistry has not been subjected to overspecialization. Dental services are delivered, in general, through private practices that operate on a fee-for-service basis with increasing numbers of individuals having access to private dental insurance. In this system, the poor, the aged, the rural, and the disadvantaged have substantially less access to the dental care than needed. A disturbing trend in the dental workforce is the aging of American dentists. It is estimated that over the next 10 years, between 22% and 25% of current professionally active dentists will retire. Current projections show that by 2014, the number of dental graduates will not be sufficient to replace the number of dentists leaving the workforce. This estimate is based on the assumptions that, from the year 2000, the number of graduates each year will be in the area of 4050 to 4100 and that all dentists for any year of graduation will have left the workforce by the age of 65. On these assumptions, about 81,600 dentists will enter the workforce, while 84,500 will leave it.[1] Also, the underrepresentation of minorities poses a challenge to the profession, especially as immigration trends contribute to increasing numbers of minorities in the US population. Of the 154,000 active dentists reported in 1999, 3.3% were black, 3.36% were Hispanic, 7.0% were Asian or Pacific Islander, and less than 1.0% were Native American.

Allied Dental Personnel

There are three recognized allied dental professions: dental hygiene, dental assisting, and dental laboratory technology. There are 266 dental hygiene, 259 dental assisting, and 25 dental laboratory technology programs in the United States. In 2003, there were 12,972 dental hygiene students, 6150 dental assisting students, and 888 dental laboratory technology students. Approximately 5000 new dental hygienists and 5000 new dental assistants are graduated each year. The availability of dental hygienists and chairside dental assistants is a perceived problem by many dentists. Underrepresented minority (URM) enrollment in allied dental education programs for 2002–2003 was as follows: Dental hygiene, 11%; dental assisting, 25%; and dental laboratory technician, 30%. The dental hygiene URM enrollment presents a similar challenge as that found in dental student enrollments.

Dental Licensure

The right to practice dentistry in the United States is granted by states through their licensing boards based on written and clinical examinations. The National Board examination provides the written portion of the licensing examination for most states. Individual states, regional boards, and regional testing agencies administer clinical examinations. Regional examinations provide mobility of dentists within regions, for example, the North Eastern Regional Board (NERB), the Central Regional Dental Testing Service (CRDTS), the Western Regional Examining Board (WREB), and the Southern Regional Testing Agency (SRTA). Reciprocity licensure requirements are determined and granted by each state on an individual basis.

Dental Education

Dental schools in the United States have a tripartite mission of education, research, and service. They also have a tradition and commitment to prevention and general practice that has positioned them to serve as a "safety net" for patients who do not have access to care in the private sector. Between 1986 and 2001, seven dental schools closed as the result of a number of factors, including a perceived oversupply of dentists. This trend has ended with the opening of three new dental schools: Nova Southeastern University (Florida), University of Nevada Las Vegas, and the Arizona School of Dentistry and Oral Health. At present, 56 dental schools and 727 dental residency training programs (424 specialty programs, 208 general dentistry programs, and 95 programs offering advanced education in general dentistry) operate in the United States. Dental schools are located in 33 states, Puerto Rico, and the District of Columbia. Each state has at least one dental hygiene program or dental residency training program.

The total enrollment in US dental schools during 2002–2003 was 17,657, which included 7410 women (41.9%). Dental schools graduate approximately 4200 dentists per year. In 2002–2003, 63.7% of dental school students were white, 5.1% were African American, 6.0% were Hispanic, 0.5% were Native American, 22.9% were Asian, and 1.8% did not specify race or ethnicity. The URM enrollment data presents a challenge to dental education and to the dental profession (Fig. 16–1). URM student enrollment has remained relatively stable despite major efforts to increase diversity in dental enrollments.

As of 2004, there were approximately 250 vacant full-time faculty positions in dental schools, representing a steady increase in reported faculty vacancies since 1992. There is widespread concern the dental faculty shortage may be worsening, and this may present an acute

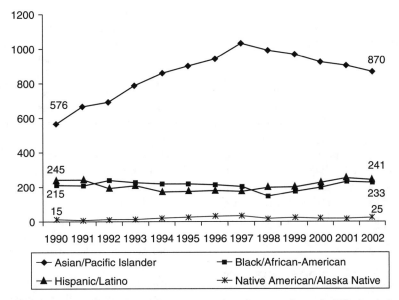

Figure 16–1. First-time, first-year minority enrollees in US dental schools: 1990–2002. *(Source: American Dental Education Association.)*

problem in the near future. In addition, the average educational debt of graduating dental students in 2002 was $107,503, ranging from $85,840 for public universities to $136,060 for private schools. Faculty vacancies and rising educational debt present two major challenges for the dental profession. Of the 4805 full-time dental faculty in 2002–2003, 267 were African American (5.5%); 233 were Hispanic or Latino (4.84%), and 16 were Native American (0.3%).

Dental Research

The dental research enterprise in the United States is built on federal appropriations to the National Institute for Dental and Craniofacial Research (NIDCR). Research funding from NIDCR supports biomedical and behavioral research and training through institutional, individual, and training grants and contracts with research partners, including other government agencies, universities, philanthropic foundations, and industry.

Dental research has led to advances in disease prevention and diagnosis, and newer treatment modalities. In the recent past, there has been a shift from an approach based on treatment of disease to one based on prevention of disease. Dentistry's research base has contributed to its stature as a health profession and has helped improve the oral health of the nation.

National research objectives are now being formulated related to the 2010 National Oral Health Objectives.[2] The NIDCR research agenda includes a wide range of research needs and potential for new discovery. In addition to basic biomedical and behavioral research, NIDCR supports investigations related to health services delivery and reimbursement, occupational health issues, biomaterials development and testing, disease etiology and prevention, epidemiologic studies of health promotion, studies to reduce health disparities, and molecular and genetic research. NIDCR is also engaged in multidisciplinary and interdisciplinary research involving partnerships among investigators in the life and physical sciences and in the area of knowledge and technology transfer.

NIDCR continues to partner with educational institutions to train future oral health researchers, with approximately 6% of its budget devoted to extramural research training. Concern regarding US dental research capacity was addressed by the NIDCR Blue Ribbon Panel on Research Training Career Development. Included among the barriers to research careers cited in the report were a relative lack of workforce diversity, misconceptions about the rewards of a career in research, and lack of a diverse pool of mentors.

Dental Health Professions Shortage Areas (D-HPSAs)

A critical issue related to this chapter is the distribution of the dental workforce and the relationship to eliminating disparities in access to oral health care. Dental shortage areas are widely distributed throughout the United States and include underserved areas ranging from inner cities to rural locations and borderline communities. The number of D-HPSAs had increased to 2112 by 2003, encompassing more than 41 million people. It is now estimated that 8481 dentists are needed to achieve a ratio of 3000 patients per dentist in the designated D-HPSAs.

▶ DENTAL DISEASE CLASSIFICATION

The two most common diseases that dentists work to prevent and treat are dental caries and periodontal disease. Dental caries constitute an infectious bacterial disease that destroys enamel and dentin, the hard tooth structure. Periodontal disease, also caused by bacteria, affects the bone and soft tissue structures that hold teeth in place. Both caries and periodontal disease can

lead to tooth loss, and both are preventable with regular professional treatment and home care.

Beyond the diseases of teeth and their direct supporting structures, dentists deal with broad problems in the craniofacial complex such as traumatic injuries to the teeth and jaws; developmental anomalies (eg, missing or malpositioned teeth, cleft lip and palate); cosmetic dental concerns; pathologic soft and hard tissue lesions, including oral and pharyngeal cancer; and acute and chronic pain of the orofacial region, such as that emanating from the temporomandibular joint. The mouth is the portal for life-sustaining food, fluids, and oxygen, as well as the primary vehicle of communication and a major factor in an attractive appearance. Consequently, good oral health is vital to overall general and psychological health. Recent research and technologic advances have greatly improved the diagnosis, treatment, and prevention of oral health problems in the United States and throughout the world.

▶ ORAL AND SYSTEMIC HEALTH

The association between oral infections and systemic diseases has been suspected for many years. A growing body of scientific evidence suggests an association between oral bacteria, viruses, and yeast and systemic diseases, including cardiovascular disease, atherosclerosis, cerebrovascular disease, preterm and low birth weight, pulmonary diseases and disorders, human immunodeficiency virus (HIV) infection, diabetes, and osteoporosis.[3-6]

Opportunistic and transmissible microorganisms are responsible for both dental caries and periodontal diseases. In periodontal disease, the microbially induced infections cause a substantial infectious burden to the entire body when untreated. Microorganisms associated with periodontal disease release toxins that stimulate an inflammatory response. Bacteria, toxins, localized cytokines, and other inflammatory mediators enter the vascular circulation and thereby activate a systemic response. The pathogenesis of the disease process reflects gene–gene and gene–environment interactions. The causal relationship between oral and systemic disease has not yet been established, but the risk factors provide evidence for an exquisite association between oral infections and systemic disease.

► SCOPE OF ORAL HEALTH DISPARITIES

Despite the US infrastructure for distribution of oral health care and preventive services, recent national studies have identified oral health disparities.[7–12]

Oral Health in America: A Report of the Surgeon General (2000),[7] the first Surgeon General's report on dentistry, identified oral health as integral to general health, stating: "Oral health is a critical component of health and must be included in the provision of health care and the design of community programs." "Silent epidemic" were the words used by former Surgeon General David Satcher to describe the unfavorable oral health of minorities and the poor. Socioeconomic status was identified in the report as a key determinate of oral health. Studies among minorities indicate that disparities in oral health care are reduced once socioeconomic status is taken into account.

The social impact of oral disease is reflected in the 51 million lost school hours for children related to dental illness and 164 million hours lost from work for adults each year due to dental disease or dental visits. A comprehensive listing of the burden of oral diseases and disorders, derived from the Surgeon General's report, is contained in Appendix 16-A.

The General Accounting Office (GAO) report[10] on oral health identified dental disease as a chronic problem for low-income people and noted the specific burden that low-income children suffer from poor dental health (eg, 80% of untreated caries in permanent teeth are found in roughly 25% of children 5 to 17 years old,

mostly from low-income and other vulnerable groups). The GAO report also identified disparities in oral health in many vulnerable populations: homeless people, minorities, and some rural residents. The report based its findings on data collected by the federal government through four national health surveys from 1988 through 1997: the National Health and Nutrition Examination Survey III (NHANES III), the National Health Interview Survey (NHIS), the Medical Expenditures Panel Survey (MEPS), and the Behavioral Risk Factor Surveillance System (BRFSS).

Barriers to Oral Health Care

The disproportionate burden of oral disease reported indicates that specific population groups are in greater need of oral health care. Variance in need for oral care is based on whether an individual requires clinical care to maintain functions such as chewing and speaking. Variance in demand for dental service is significantly responsive to gradients in dental fees—the higher the fee, the lower the demand. Other factors that influence the level of demand include income, family size, education levels, insurance coverage, health history, ethnicity, and age. The value that an individual places on good oral health influences both demand for dental insurance and demand for dental care. The value that an individual places on oral health is influenced primarily by income, education, and cultural factors.

The extent of oral health care disparities in the United States indicates that many of those in need of oral health care do not seek it. Barriers to oral health care as identified in previous reports of the Surgeon General, American Dental Education Association (ADEA), and ADA include knowledge and values, availability of care, lack of insurance, regulatory conditions, systemic barriers within health care delivery, and workforce diversity. Following is a brief synopsis of how each of these barriers affects access.

Knowledge and Values

Those in need of oral care lack knowledge about the prevention of oral diseases and the relationship of oral health to general health. In turn, public policy makers do not value or understand the value of oral health as a part of general health and health care, thereby marginalizing oral health to a lower priority.

Availability of Care

Many in need of dental care do not have access to a provider because of the maldistribution of dentists. Many underserved groups lack access because some providers are unwilling to care for them due to low reimbursement rates, lack of insurance, and other factors. Much of the dental workforce is unprepared to render culturally competent care to racially and ethically diverse populations, people with complex medical or psychosocial conditions or disabilities, the very young, and the aged.

Lack of Insurance

Numerous surveys have demonstrated that the cost of dental services is a significant barrier to receiving dental care, particularly in underserved or low-income areas. Surveys have also shown that more than 100 million US children and adults lack either private or public dental insurance.[7] This number greatly exceeds the number of people lacking medical insurance, which is about 44 million.[13] Nearly 75% of dentists do not treat Medicaid-insured patients. Most underserved groups lack dental insurance of any kind. Low reimbursement rates for public programs such as Medicaid and State Children's Health Insurance Program (SCHIP) dissuade dentists from providing care to the poor and to children. Dental care is not covered by Medicare, which limits access to dental care in the elderly population.

Regulatory Conditions

Many state laws and regulations restrict access by imposing restrictive supervision requirements on allied dental personnel. These state regulations control which professionals (dentists and allied dental personnel, such as dental hygienists) can legally provide independent basic oral health care. The restrictiveness of state regulations can contribute to the access problem. Some states have begun to consider innovative ways of providing preventive and other basic oral health services with less direct supervision by a dentist. One concern about these innovations, however, is that patients must be protected from possible malpractice by those who have less professional training.

Individual states also control dental licensure, which some believe creates unnecessary restrictions on dentists' interstate mobility and compounds access problems. In an effort to improve access, the California legislature passed regulations to allow graduates of a Mexican dental school to serve specified underserved communities in rural agricultural regions.[14]

Systemic Barriers Within Health Care Delivery

The traditional model of oral and dental care, the solo-practice dentist assisted by allied personnel providing care under the dentist's supervision, is no longer adequate to meet the oral health needs of the expanding and increasingly diverse US citizenry. Group dental practice models, though increasing in numbers, contain similar systemic barriers.

Workforce Diversity

Lack of access to dental careers has helped create a dental profession that does not reflect the diversity seen in the US population (Table 16–1). Population trends indicate the lack of diversity among dentists will become even worse over the next 50 years. By the middle of this century, the African American population is projected to increase from 12.1% to 13.6% percent; the Hispanic and Latino population from 10.8% to 24%; the Native American population from 0.7%

▶ **TABLE 16-1.** US Dentist-to-Population Ratios by Race and Ethnicity of the Dentist, 1996

	Total	Black	Hispanic	Asian or Pacific Islander	American Indian	White
US population	265,189,000	31,933,000	28,092,000	9,181,000	1,954,000	194,029,000
Active dentists	154,900	5201	5178	10,693	194	133,634
Number of dentists per 100,000 population	58.4	16.3	18.4	116.5	9.9	68.9
Number of people per dentist	1:1712	1:6140	1:5425	1:859	1:10,072	1:1452

Source: Oral Health in America: A Report of the Surgeon General. Rockville, Md: National Institutes of Health, National Institute of Dental and Craniofacial Research, US Dept of Health and Human Services; 2000.

to 0.9%, and the Asian and Pacific Islander population from 3.5% to 8.2%. The white or Caucasian population, by comparison, will decline from 73% to 53%.

Recent medical literature has reported on access to care as related to health disparities and patient treatment. The important role of black and Hispanic physicians and dentists in providing health care for underserved populations is well documented.[15-17] ADA surveys of dental practice have consistently reported practice characteristics that reflect the racial and ethnic differences of providers and their patient profiles; for example, white practitioners have a majority of white patients and the same is true for African American and Hispanic providers with regard to their patient groups. Planned practice locations by race and ethnicity[18] indicate that African American and Hispanic and Latino senior dental students plan to practice in inner cities or with underserved populations in higher percentages than white seniors. In 2002, whereas 68.7% of African American and 44.7% of Hispanic and Latino seniors anticipated the major portion of their patients would be from inner-city or underserved populations, only 20% of white seniors did.

Changing population demographics, practice trends, and practice plans all emphasize the critical need for the dental profession to increase efforts toward URM recruitment for all three as-

pects of the profession: practice, education, and research. Increasing the diversity of those entering dental careers will produce providers who ultimately improve access to care and reduce current disparities in oral health.

▶ PROGRAMS THAT ADDRESS ACCESS ISSUES

Federal Programs

Federal programs play a significant role in addressing oral health disparities and a declining dental workforce. These programs serve as a major catalyst for dental institutions to provide access to primary oral health care to underserved populations, fund training, support graduate dental education and research, expand preventive services, and increase loan repayment and scholarship programs.

The Health Professions Education Partnerships Act of 1998, Titles VII and VIII, provides funding for general and pediatric dentistry residency training programs and dental public health training programs, Health Careers Opportunity grants (HCOPs), Centers of Excellence (COEs), federal student scholarship and loan programs, and scholarships and loans for disadvantaged students. HCOPs and COEs are major institutional grants to support recruitment and reinforcement for URM and low-income students. In 2003, six dental schools had HCOP* grants and four had COEs.[†]

Medicaid: Early Periodic Screening, Diagnostic, and Treatment (EPSDT) Services

EPSDT is a federally mandated service within Medicaid for medical and dental services for enrolled children. Under EPSDT, states must provide comprehensive medical and dental services for all enrolled children even if the services are not normally covered by a state's Medicaid program.

The Oral Health Initiative (OHI), a multifaceted approach to increase oral health services for low-income children, has the potential to enhance SCHIP services and technical assistance to states. SCHIP was created as Title XXI of the Social Security Act to provide health coverage for children from low-income families whose income was not low enough to qualify for Medicaid. In 1999, nearly 2 million children were enrolled in 53 SCHIP programs. The Children's Health Act of 2000 provides a variety of approaches to address unmet oral health needs in children, including an extramural NIH Pediatric Research Loan Repayment Program that provides up to $35,000 per year to qualified health-care professionals.

Medicaid is the largest public program of health insurance for low-income people. It finances coverage for about 40 million people, over half of whom are children. Dental services for adults are optional under state Medicaid programs, and as of 2004, less than 50% of states provided adult Medicaid dental coverage.

The National Health Service Corps (NHSC) places providers in underserved inner-city, rural, and frontier communities. Over the past 30 years, NHSC has placed more than 20,000 providers in underserved areas through scholarship and loan repayment programs, but only a few have been dentists. At present, only 293 dentists and 18 dental hygienists are serving in the NHSC.

The Indian Health Service (IHS), an agency within the US Public Health Service, provides care for more than one million Native Americans and Alaska Natives. IHS dental programs are located in more than 280 hospitals and clinics across 35 states and staffed by approximately 400 dentists. Approximately 95 dentist positions in the IHS program were vacant in 2004.[19]

Under Section 752 of the Public Health Service Act, Health Education Training Centers (HETCs) and Area Health Education Centers (AHECs) are academic–community partnerships that train health-care providers in response to local needs. AHECs are designed to improve the supply, distribution, diversity, and quality of the health workforce, ultimately increasing access to health care in medically underserved areas. All US states except Iowa, Kansas, Michigan, North Dakota, and South Dakota have AHEC programs. Nine have AHECs with a dental component.*

The National Institute of Dental and Craniofacial Research (NIDCR) continues to generate discoveries that yield new knowledge and improve public health. NIDCR, in partnership with the National Center on Minority Health and Health Disparities (NCMHHD), now funds five Centers for Research to Reduce Oral Health Disparities. The major hallmark of these centers is national research and training networks to reduce health disparities. Center grants may not exceed 7 years each. Centers are currently located at Boston University, New York University, University of California at San Francisco, University of Michigan, and University of Washington.

---

*The dental schools with HCOP grant programs in 2003 were Baylor College of Dentistry, University of California at San Francisco, University of Michigan, Temple University, University of North Carolina at Chapel Hill, and University of Connecticut.

[†]The dental schools with COEs in 2003 were University of Texas Health Science Center at San Antonio, Meharry Medical College, University of Oklahoma, and University of Puerto Rico.

*The nine states with dental AHECS are Arizona, Georgia, Hawaii, Louisiana, Maryland, Michigan, Nevada, Pennsylvania, and South Carolina.

State, Private, and Other Programs

Other programs and major activities that address dental access issues include, but are not limited to, state regulations that allow for less restrictive supervision of dental hygienists, dental school satellite clinics, private sector support, and state models.

One of the major challenges to allied dental personnel utilization is state laws and regulations that limit practice settings and impose restrictive supervision requirements for dental hygienists. States that permit less restrictive supervision of dental hygienists include California, Colorado, Connecticut, New Mexico, Oregon, and Washington.

All dental schools maintain at least one on-site dental clinic, and approximately 70% of US dental schools have school-sponsored off-site satellite clinics. Many provide care to underserved and disadvantaged populations. More than two thirds of patients visiting dental school clinics are from families whose annual income is estimated to be $15,000 or less. About half these patients receive Medicaid or Medicare benefits, and more than one third have no insurance or government assistance to help pay for their dental care. Dental schools provide a national safety net for patients who cannot afford care in the private sector.

The Robert Wood Johnson Foundation, W.K. Kellogg Foundation, and California Endowment Pipeline Grants receive direction and technical assistance from the Center for Community Health Partnerships at Columbia University. W.K. Kellogg Foundation/ADEA Access to Dental Careers (ADC) grants are administered by ADEA in collaboration with the Robert Wood Johnson Foundation and California Endowment Pipeline Grants. Fifteen dental schools participate in this 5-year program to establish community-based dental education, revise curricula, and implement initiatives to increase recruitment and retention of URM and low-income students. These schools extend services to underserved urban and rural communities. ADC grants supplement the Pipeline grants by supporting direct educational costs for URM and low-income students.

The Crest Cavity-Free Zones (*www.crest.com/healthy_smiles/smileshoppes.htm*) partnership between Boys & Girls Clubs of America and the Procter & Gamble Company is an example of private-sector programming to improve access to dental care and understanding of the importance of oral health. Boys & Girls Clubs of America, founded in 1860, now serves more than 3 million youth annually in 2600 clubs across the country. The Procter & Gamble partnership provides both dental curriculum implementation and dental treatment. Ten community-based dental clinics (Crest Smile Shoppes) provide care to the children of St Louis, Cincinnati, Los Angeles, the Bronx, Denver, Houston, Chicago, Broward County, Phoenix, and Appleton, Wisconsin. The Crest program adds a dimension to the guidance-oriented character development programs traditionally offered in the Boys & Girls Club centers. Crest also provides fully equipped mobile dental vans that provide oral health screenings, treatments, and oral care tools to underserved children and their families in New York, San Bernardino, California, and San Antonio, Texas.

Community Campus Partnerships for Health (CCPH) is a national nonprofit organization that promotes health through community-based research, community service, and other strategic partnerships. CCPH is a growing network of over 1000 communities and higher educational institutions. These partnerships are powerful tools for improving health professional education, civic responsibility, and the general health of communities. Their goal is to eliminate health disparities and to achieve a workforce that is both diverse and responsive to community needs. CCPH works to improve K through 12 education and pathways for students of color from high school to the successful pursuit of health careers.

W.K. Kellogg Foundation/ADEA Minority Dental Faculty Development (MDFD) grants represent a pilot program for URM and low-income academic career development by dental schools. The 5-year grants are administered by ADEA's Center for Equity and Diversity. MDFD grants provide funding for direct educational costs for advanced training. Academic partnerships among dental and other higher education institutions, mentoring, recruitment, community involvement in diverse settings, and faculty career development are components of grants that have been awarded to seven dental schools.*

The Community Dental Care Network of Columbia University School of Dental and Oral Surgery in partnership with NewYork-Presbyterian Hospital (the hospital center for Columbia University) is a model program that includes dentistry as one of the health services offered at the School of Pregnant and Parenting Teens (SPPT) in northern Manhattan. The dental clinic at SPPT is one of eight school-based dental clinics operated by the Community DentCare Network in northern Manhattan. This type of partnership serves as a model that provides services in neighboring communities, allows subcontracting with independent community health centers for a range of services, and expands the capacity of the school to conduct community-oriented clinical research trials.

State Models

New Mexico has enacted legislation that provides a model to improve access through what has been termed *collaborative practice*. This legislation allows dental hygienists to treat patients in a variety of settings according to a protocol with a consulting dentist. California and Alaska are experimenting with ways to improve access through the licensing of foreign dentists. Minnesota, New Mexico, and Oregon changed their practice acts in 2003 to permit dental hygienists to exercise some degree of supervision over dental assistants, and California now allows hygienists to supervise assistants in certain settings.

West Virginia recently changed its state practice act to include a rule detailing a comprehensive list of expanded functions for dental auxiliaries, and Virginia and Washington now allow hygienists to place antimicrobial agents and administer topical antibiotics.[20]

▶ STRATEGIES AND POTENTIAL SOLUTIONS

1. The removal of major barriers to access to oral health care, including dental licensure and restrictive practices for allied dental personnel, is paramount. Dentistry should hasten efforts to improve validity, reliability, uniformity, and universal acceptance of clinical licensing examinations by state licensing boards. Major efforts are needed to eliminate statutes and regulations that restrict productivity of allied dental personnel. New and revised regulations that are consistent with the education and training of such personnel are required to meet the oral health needs of the changing US population and to assist dentists in meeting those needs.

2. Recruitment to the dental profession must become a national priority, with increased resources, infusion of energy at the national and local levels, and early introduction to the pipeline beginning as early as grade school. This effort should include academic, federal, community, professional, and other partnerships to attract a diverse cadre of students to careers in dentistry.

The recruitment effort should include career tracks to produce dental educators to alleviate the current and pending shortage of dental faculty, and dental researchers who possess the knowledge and collaborative skills needed to conduct complex multidisciplinary health research. Dental practitioners are needed to replace the current aging dental workforce and meet the emerging needs of the military and US public health service. These efforts should result in a dental profession that reflects the racial,

*These schools are University of Michigan, University of Illinois at Chicago, University of Alabama at Birmingham, Howard University, University of Oklahoma, Texas A&M University System Baylor College of Dentistry, and New York State Academic Dental Centers (NYSADC).

ethnic, and gender demographics of the US population. The recruitment effort should also include allied dental personnel to meet the emerging needs of an increasingly diverse US population and the changes in the oral health care delivery system anticipated for the future.

3. Dentistry must participate in the growing mandate to achieve universal and continuous health coverage for all Americans. The recently released Institute of Medicine report, *Insuring America's Health: Principles and Recommendations*, proposed a clear and compelling overall rationale for universal health insurance.[21] The report recommends universal coverage by 2010 and urges the President and Congress to act immediately by establishing a firm and explicit plan to reach this goal. The approach envisioned will promote better overall health for individuals, families, communities, and the nation by providing financial access to necessary, appropriate, and effective health services for all. Dental services should be included in legislation related to universal and continuous health coverage.

In the absence of universal health insurance, oral health should be included in all primary care deliberations. A basic package of preventive and primary care benefits should be provided to all Americans and delivered in both community and individual settings. The dental package should include the diagnostic, preventive, and treatment services that have proven effective in preventing and controlling tooth decay, gum infections, pain, soft tissue pathology, trauma, and oral and facial defects. Special patient groups should be included: those with developmental disabilities, birth defects, genetic disorders, and acquired medical disabilities, including HIV infections. Oral health services are some of the least costly health services available. It is estimated that every dollar invested in preventive dentistry saves between $8 and $50 in treatment costs.

4. Increased research activity on the reduction of oral health disparities is needed. The five NIDCR Centers for Research to Reduce Oral Health Disparities provide the cornerstone for a national collaborative network for research investigations, training, outcomes assessment, and knowledge and technology transfer related to oral health disparities and health promotion. The centers create a broad network of partnerships that focus on a variety of populations at risk for oral health disparities. NIDCR should continue its collaborations with academic institutions, Health Resources and Services Administration (HRSA), the Agency for Healthcare Research and Quality, and other federal and nonfederal agencies to extend its research and training efforts and transform new scientific knowledge into useful clinical applications and outcomes.

5. Efforts must be made to increase public information about and public policy makers' awareness of the relationship of oral health to systemic health and the benefits of preventive oral health behaviors and services. The beneficial effects of community water fluoridation in the reduction of tooth decay are well established. Yet half of the children in the United States reside in nonfluoridated communities. The media, civic and community groups, professional organizations (eg, National Dental Association, Hispanic Dental Association, Society of American Indian Dentists), corporate organizations, academic institutions, ADA, NIDCR, ADEA, and the American Association for Dental Research (AADR) should be involved in the dissemination of information regarding behaviors that promote positive oral health and improve quality of life. Community-related networks such as CCPH and AHECs should be partners in this national effort to address oral health information and behavior modification.

6. Those within and outside the profession must advocate for continued and increased investment of federal funding in programs that promote diversity within the health professions, such as Health Careers Opportunities grants (HCOPs), Centers of Excellence (COEs), health professions scholarships and loans, faculty loan repayment programs, scholarships and loans for disadvantaged students, AHECs, National Health Service Corps, Indian Health Service,

HRSA's Kids into Health Careers Program, and NIH research developmental and supplemental awards. These programs provide critical support for recruitment, education, and training that are fundamental to the nation's ability to produce and sustain a diverse dental workforce.

7. Finally, the academic preparation of dental and allied dental students must be enhanced with regard to competencies that affect treatment outcomes for an increasingly diverse patient population. Cultural and linguistic competencies must be incorporated in experiential patient care settings and included as a core component of the curriculum. Evaluation mechanisms must be developed to ensure the cultural competency of graduates, especially related to attitudes, behaviors, treatment outcomes, and quality of care. The Commission on Dental Accreditation should include cultural competency in its accreditation criteria for all dental and allied dental educational institutions.

▶ SUMMARY AND RECOMMENDATIONS

The strategies and potential solutions discussed in this chapter reflect the need for changes, including a paradigm shift from treatment to prevention, educational reform with regard to cultural competency, dental licensure revisions, and collaborative research initiatives, as well as a recommitment to educating the public about the value and relationship of oral to systemic health, improvement of access to oral health care for all Americans, and major efforts to increase diversity within the dental profession.

These solutions are within the parameters of the social contract dentistry has with society. Society gives professions a monopoly over the use of a body of knowledge and the privilege of self-regulation. In return, the profession owes society professional competence, integrity, and the provision of altruistic services.[22] The ADA affirms the concept of a social contract in its report on the future of dentistry: "Dentistry is known and celebrated for its high ethical standards and awareness of its social responsibilities

and public trust. Whatever actions the profession takes in response to future challenges, that trust must be preserved. To do so, the profession must find ways to provide care for those in need, regardless of their financial wherewithal or the challenges they present."[23]

▶ REFERENCES

1. Valachovic RW, Weaver RG, et al. Trends in dentistry and dental education. *J Dent Educ* 2001;65:546–547.
2. US Dept of Health and Human Services. *Healthy People 2010,* conference ed. Washington, DC: USDHHS; 2000.
3. Offenbacher S, Beck JD, Lieff S, et al. Role of periodontitis in systemic health: Spontaneous preterm birth. *J Dent Educ* 1998;62(10):852–858.
4. Beck JD, Offenbacher S. Oral health and systemic disease: Periodontitis and cardiovascular disease. *J Dent Educ* 1998;62(10):859–870.
5. Diehl SR, Wu T, Burmeister JA, et al. Evidence of a substantial genetic basis for IgG2 levels in families with aggressive periodontitis. *J Dent Res* 2003;82(9):708–712.
6. Slavkin HC. First encounters: Transmission of infectious oral diseases from mother to child. *J Am Dent Assoc* 1997;128(6):773–778.
7. *Oral Health in America: A Report of the Surgeon General.* Rockville, Md: National Institutes of Health, National Institute of Dental and Craniofacial Research, US Dept of Health and Human Services; 2000.
8. Haden NK, Catalanotto FA, Alexander CJ, et al. Improving the oral health status of all Americans: Roles and responsibilities of academic dental institutions: The report of the ADEA President's Commission. *J Dent Educ* 2003;67(5):563–583.
9. Warren RC. *Oral Health for All: Policy for Available, Accessible,* and *Acceptable Care.* Washington, DC: Center for Policy Alternatives; 1999.
10. *Oral Health. Dental Disease Is a Chronic Problem Among Low-Income Populations.* GAO/HEHS-00-72. Washington, DC: US General Accounting Office/Health Education, and Human Services Division; 2000.
11. *Future of Dentistry. Today's Vision: Tomorrow's Reality.* Chicago, Ill: American Dental Association, Health Policy Resources Center; 2001.

12. *Dental Education at the Crossroads: Challenges and Change.* Washington, DC, Committee on the Future of Dental Education, Division of Health Care Services, Institute of Medicine, National Academy Press; 1995.

13. Mills R, Bhandari S. *Health Insurance Coverage in the United States: 2002.* Washington, DC: US Dept of Commerce, Economics and Statistics Administration, US Census Bureau; 2003:60–223.

14. Slavkin HC. The failure of dentistry's social contract with America and California's search for legislative solutions? *J Dent Educ* 2003;67(10):1076–1077.

15. Smedley BD, Stith AY, Nelson AR. *Unequal Treatment: Confronting Racial and Ethnic Disparities in Health Care.* Washington, DC: Institute of Medicine, National Academy Press; 2002.

16. Komaromy M, Grumbach K, Drake M, et al. The role of black and Hispanic physicians in providing health care for underserved populations. *N Engl J Med* 1996;334(20):1305–1310.

17. Solomon E, Williams C, Sinkford J. Practicing location characteristics of black dentist in Texas. *J Dent Educ* 2001;65:571–578.

18. Weaver RG, Haden NK, Valachovic RW. Annual ADEA survey of dental school seniors: 2002 graduating class. *J Dent Educ* 2002;66(12):1388–1404.

19. Indian Health Services: 2004. Available at: http://www.ihs.gov/JobsCareerDevelop/CareerCenter/Vacancy/Index.cfm.

20. State Legislative Report: The American Dental Association. vol 12, 2003.

21. Institute of Medicine. *Insuring America's Health: Principles and Recommendations.* Washington, DC: National Academy Press; 2004.

22. Cruess SR, Johnston S, Cruess RL. Professionalism for medicine: Opportunities and obligations. *Med J Aust* 2002;177(4):208–211.

23. American Dental Association. *Future of Dentistry—Executive Summary.* Chicago, Ill: American Dental Association, Health Policy Resources Center; 2002:1.

APPENDIX 16-A

The Burden of Oral Diseases and Disorders: From the 2000 Surgeon General's Report on Oral Health*

Oral diseases are progressive and cumulative and become more complex over time. They can affect our ability to eat, the foods we choose, how we look, and the way we communicate. These diseases can affect economic productivity and compromise our ability to work at home, at school, or on the job. Health disparities exist across population groups at all ages. Over one third of the US population (100 million people) has no access to community water fluoridation. Over 108 million children and adults lack dental insurance, which is over 2.5 times the number who lack medical insurance. The following are highlights of oral health data for children, adults, and the elderly. (Refer to the full report for details of these data and their sources.)

* Source: *Oral Health in America: A Report of the Surgeon General*. Rockville, Md: National Institutes of Health, National Institute of Dental and Craniofacial Research, US Dept of Health and Human Services; 2000.

Children

- Cleft lip and palate, one of the most common birth defects, is estimated to affect 1 out of 600 live births for whites and 1 out of 1850 live births for African Americans.
- Other birth defects, such as hereditary ectodermal dysplasias, where all or most teeth are missing or misshapen, cause lifetime problems that can be devastating to children and adults.
- Dental caries (tooth decay) is the single most common chronic childhood disease— 5 times more common than asthma and 7 times more common than hay fever.
- Over 50% of 5- to 9-year-old children have at least one cavity or filling, and that proportion increases to 78% among 17-year-olds. Nevertheless, these figures represent improvements in the oral health of children compared to a generation ago.
- There are striking disparities in dental disease by income. Poor children suffer twice

as much dental caries as their more affluent peers, and their disease is more likely to be untreated. These poor–nonpoor differences continue into adolescence. One out of four children in America is born into poverty, and children living below the poverty line (annual income of $17,000 for a family of four) have more severe and untreated decay.

- Unintentional injuries, many of which include head, mouth, and neck injuries, are common in children.
- Intentional injuries commonly affect the craniofacial tissues.
- Tobacco-related oral lesions are prevalent in adolescents who currently use smokeless (spit) tobacco.
- Professional care is necessary for maintaining oral health, yet 25% of poor children have not seen a dentist before entering kindergarten.
- Medical insurance is a strong predictor of access to dental care. Uninsured children are 2.5 times less likely than insured children to receive dental care. Children from families without dental insurance are 3 times more likely to have dental needs than children with either public or private insurance. For each child without medical insurance, there are at least 2.6 children without dental insurance.
- Medicaid has not been able to fill the gap in providing dental care to poor children. Fewer than one in five Medicaid-covered children received a single dental visit in a recent year-long study period. Although new programs such as the State Children's Health Insurance Program (SCHIP) may increase the number of insured children, many will still be left without effective dental coverage.
- The social impact of oral diseases in children is substantial. More than 51 million school hours are lost each year to dental-related illness. Poor children suffer nearly 12 times more restricted-activity days than children from higher-income families. Pain and suffering due to untreated diseases can lead to

problems in eating, speaking, and attending to learning.

Adults

- Most adults show signs of periodontal or gingival diseases. Severe periodontal disease (measured as 6 mm of periodontal attachment loss) affects about 14% of adults aged 45 to 54.
- Clinical symptoms of viral infections, such as herpes labialis (cold sores), and oral ulcers (canker sores) are common in adulthood, affecting about 19% of adults 25 to 44 year of age.
- Chronic disabling diseases such as temporomandibular disorder, Sjögren syndrome, diabetes, and osteoporosis affect millions of Americans and compromise oral health and functioning.
- Pain is a common symptom of craniofacial disorders and is accompanied by interference with vital functions such as eating, swallowing, and speech. Twenty-two percent of adults reported some form of oralfacial pain in the past 6 months. Pain is a major component of trigeminal neuralgia, facial shingles (postherpetic neuralgia), temporomandibular disorder, fibromyalgia, and Bells palsy.
- Population growth as well as diagnostics that are enabling earlier detection of cancer means that more patients than ever before are undergoing cancer treatments. More than 400,000 of these patients will develop oral complications annually.
- Immunocompromised patients, such as those with HIV infections and those undergoing organ transplantation, are at higher risk for oral problems such as candidiasis.
- Employed adults lose more than 164 million hours of work each year due to dental disease or dental visits.
- For every adult 19 years or older without medical insurance, there are three without dental insurance.

- A little less than two thirds of adults report having visited a dentist in the past 12 months. Those with incomes at or above the poverty level are twice as likely to report a dental visit in the past 12 months as those who are below the poverty level.

Older Adults

- Twenty-three percent of 65- to 74-year-olds have periodontal disease (measured as 6 mm of periodontal attachment loss). Also, at all ages men are more likely than women to have more severe disease, and at all ages people at the lowest socioeconomic levels have more severe periodontal disease.
- About 30% of adults 65 years and older are edentulous, compared with 46% 20 years ago. These figures are higher for those living in poverty.
- Oral and pharyngeal cancers are diagnosed in 30,000 Americans annually; 8000 die from these diseases each year. These cancers are primarily diagnosed in the elderly. Prognosis is poor. The 5-year survival rate for white patients is 56%; for blacks, it is only 34%.
- Most older Americans take both prescription and over-the-counter drugs. In all probability, at least one of the medications will have an oral side effect—usually dry mouth. The inhibition of salivary flow increases the risk for oral disease because saliva contains antimicrobial components as well as minerals that can help rebuild tooth enamel after attack by acid-producing, decay-causing bacteria. Individuals in long-term care facilities are prescribed an average of eight drugs.
- At any given time, 5% of Americans aged 65 and older (currently some 1.65 million people) are living in a long-term care facility where dental care is problematic.
- Many elderly individuals lose their dental insurance when they retire. The situation may be worse for older women, who generally have lower incomes and may never have had dental insurance. Medicaid funds dental care for the low-income and disabled elderly in some states, but reimbursements are low. Medicare is not designed to reimburse for routine dental care.

CHAPTER 17

Tobacco, Alcohol, and Drugs

Beny J. Primm, MD
Lawrence S. Brown, Jr., MD, MPH, FASAM
Annelle B. Primm, MD, MPH
John S. Friedman, PhD

▶ INTRODUCTION

Disparities dominate the landscape of substance abuse. Psychological, social, and economic disparities lead to drug, alcohol, and tobacco abuse. Disparate physical and psychological effects result from substance abuse. Race, gender, age, geography, and cultural differences influence treatment disparities.

This chapter examines substance abuse disparities affecting racial and ethnic minorities, including African Americans, Hispanics, Native Americans, and Asian and Pacific Islanders. The definitions for each category are those used by the National Institute on Drug Abuse (NIDA) and by the Census Bureau.[1] The term *African American* refers to a person having origins in any of the black racial groups of Africa; *Hispanic* refers to a person of Mexican, Puerto Rican, Cuban, central or South American, or other Spanish culture or origin, regardless of race; *Native American* refers to a person having origins in any of the original peoples of North, South, or Central America who maintains cultural identification through tribal affiliation or community recognition; and *Asian or Pacific Islander* refers to a person having origins in any

of the original peoples of the Far East, Southeast Asia, the Indian subcontinent, or the Pacific Islands.

Using criteria from the American Psychiatric Association's *Diagnostic and Statistical Manual of Mental Disorders* (DSM-IV), substance abuse refers to a pattern of substance use leading to significant impairment in functioning.[2] Substance dependence refers to substance use history that includes substance abuse, continuation of use despite related problems, increase in tolerance, and withdrawal symptoms. The term *illicit drugs,* as used by the National Household Survey on Drug Abuse (NHSDA), refers to marijuana, hashish, cocaine (including crack), inhalants, hallucinogens, heroin, and prescription-type drugs used nonmedically.[3]

During the next decade, a significant shift will occur in the population of the United States. The Hispanic population is expected to increase by about 22%.[4] The African American population is expected to increase by about 3%, and the Asian American population by about 26%.[4] By 2050, non-Hispanic whites will no longer be the majority population in the United States.[4] These population changes will have a profound effect on public health interventions.

If the racial and ethnic demographics of substance abuse match the changes in population, treatment providers will have to tailor their services to the specific needs of an increasing number of minority clients.

Dr Alan Leshner, former director of NIDA, recently pointed out that there remain "significant gaps in knowledge about the effects of drug abuse and addiction in minority populations."[5] These gaps are reflected in surveys of substance abuse which primarily determine use—whether alcohol, tobacco, or illegal drugs. Both NHSDA, now called the National Survey on Drug Use and Health (NSDUH), and the National High School Senior Survey determine the use of various substances over the last year, past month, or other recent time periods. Although this is useful epidemiologic information, clinical utility is limited. Dependence and addiction, which are more difficult to ascertain, are of greater importance to clinical care and more closely related to the medical and social consequences of substance abuse.

Based on available research findings, the following questions are considered in this chapter: What are the prevalence and characteristics of substance abuse in minority populations compared with the white majority population? What health effects do racial and ethnic minorities suffer from the various forms of substance abuse? How does treatment for substance abuse among minorities compare with treatment for the white majority? Finally, what recommendations can be made to reduce treatment disparities?

▶ SUBSTANCE ABUSE

The numbers tell the story. In 2001, almost 17 million Americans 12 years of age or older abused or were dependent on either alcohol or illicit drugs.[6] Of the 17 million, rates of dependency on alcohol or illicit drugs were highest among Native Americans (14%), followed by Hispanics (8%), then whites (8%), African Americans (6%), and Asians (4%).[6] But what is true for the overall group may not be true for

subgroups. For example, Hispanic illegal drug use during the month preceding a recent NIDA survey varied from just under 4% for Cuban Americans to 10% for Puerto Ricans.[1] Such variations also apply within the Asian American community. The Chinese subgroup had the lowest past month drug use (1%), yet Korean illegal drug use (7%) was much higher.[1]

Regarding drug dependency alone, excluding alcohol, the percentage of current use is only slightly higher among African Americans than whites. According to the 2002 NSDUH survey, current illicit drug use is highest among people reporting two or more races (11.4%), followed by Native Americans (10.1%), then African Americans (9.7%), whites (8.5%), Hispanics (7.2%), and finally Asians (3.5%).[7] Some of the misleading impressions about African Americans as the dominant drug abusers in the United States are based on partial evidence, racial profiling, and administrative practices that lead to the overrepresentation of African Americans in criminal justice statistics and in public drug treatment programs where admissions draw heavily from the courts.

As for teenagers, a survey of 12th graders about illicit past year drug use found that more whites (42.8%) than African Americans (32.6%) used illicit drugs.[8] According to a recent survey, current illicit drug use among teenagers is 12.6% for whites and 10% for African Americans.[7] However, these statistics may be skewed because they do not take into account school dropouts. The dropout rate among African Americans and Hispanics is higher than that of their white counterparts, and dropout rates correlate with higher risks for deviation.[9] African American youth might be less willing to participate in surveys and less likely to provide accurate information about their drug-using history. Therefore, the illegal drug-taking experiences of African American high school seniors might be disproportionately underrepresented in surveys. Because drug abuse is an illegal act and along with alcohol abuse is stigmatized by society, many young people, in particular, are often reluctant to admit to any form of substance use or abuse. They may be hesitant to admit the magnitude of their addiction and may tell researchers that they have "kicked the habit" when, in fact, they have not. In any case, it cannot be denied that drug addiction is a serious problem in the African American community.

Regarding alcohol abuse alone, according to a 2000–2001 NHSDA survey, whites, among people aged 12 years and older, had a higher prevalence rate of current heavy alcohol use (6.3%) than blacks (4%).[10] Another study, documenting the 50- to 59-year-old age group, showed that rates of heavy drinking were substantially higher among whites than blacks by almost five to one.[11] The highest prevalence of current heavy alcohol use was among Native Americans (7.2%).[10] In contrast, Asian Americans have the lowest rates of heavy alcohol use, with the Chinese subgroup reporting only 0.3%.[10]

As with illicit drugs and alcohol, the data for tobacco reflect similar disparities. Among people aged 12 years and older, Native Americans had the highest current use of any tobacco product (44.9%).[12] The white population reported 31.3%, whereas African Americans reported 27.7%, followed by Hispanics, at 22.9%.[12] Asian Americans reported the least use (14%).[12] For smokeless tobacco, Native Americans again were the highest users, followed by whites.[13] Regarding high school seniors, a study showed that one third reported having smoked in the past 30 days, with the percentages varying from the highest (46.1%) among Native Americans to the lowest (only 14.3%) among African Americans.[8] The differences for heavy smoking (at least half a pack a day) followed a similar pattern.[6]

What conclusions can be drawn? First, contradicting popular belief, the percentages of African Americans who abuse illicit drugs, alcohol, and tobacco is the same or lower than the percentages of whites, but with a caveat: A number of African Americans are not counted by many researchers. Second, the overall percentages of Hispanics who abuse and use illicit drugs, alcohol, and tobacco are almost the same or lower than that of whites and African Amer-

icans. Third, Native Americans are the greatest users and abusers of illicit drugs, alcohol, and tobacco. Fourth, Asian Americans, except for the Koreans and Japanese, abuse substances the least. A final conclusion is that if substance abuse treatment is to be effective, interventions must take into account the disparities of abuse by specific subgroups within minority populations.

▶ ADVERSE HEALTH EFFECTS

Minorities suffer more adverse health effects from substance abuse, particularly from illicit drugs, than the white population. These disparities have been documented.[14] Human immunodeficiency virus (HIV) infection and acquired immunodeficiency syndrome (AIDS), in particular, have hit the minority communities disproportionately. Again, the numbers tell the story. In 2000, 78% of new drug-related AIDS cases reported to the Centers for Disease Control and Prevention were among ethnic minority groups.[15] Minority women were especially vulnerable. African American and Hispanic women represented 77% of reported cumulative drug-related AIDS cases among women through 2001.[16]

Between 1985 and 1999 more than twice as many blacks (95,000) as whites (37,000) developed AIDS through injection drug abuse, even though there are only one fourth as many black injection drug users.[5] Roughly the same number of Hispanics (35,000) and whites developed AIDS through injected drugs, even though there are only one eighth as many Hispanic injection drug users.[5] Minority injection drug users report a disproportionately high prevalence of hepatitis B, hepatitis C, and tuberculosis.[15] In fact, the prevalence of hepatitis C infection is much higher among African Americans and Hispanics than among whites. Between 1988 and 1994, for instance, the prevalence of antibodies to hepatitis C was 3.2% for African Americans, 2.1% for Hispanic Americans, and 1.5% for non-Hispanic whites.[15] It is important to note that the presence of hepatitis C, often found among drug abusers, increases the risk of liver damage if alcohol is also abused.

In New York City methadone maintenance treatment clinics, Brown et al assessed the race of patients with medical disorders.[9] Over 90% were African American or Latino, and 40% were female. Although this study used chart reviews as the source of data and therefore had potential ascertainment limitations, it represented one of the few systematic reviews of drug abusers in an ambulatory setting. Histories of gonorrhea, hepatitis B infection, pneumonia, and anemia were found in 28%, 23%, 21%, and 21% of the patients, respectively. This suggests that a considerable portion of African American drug users sustain a considerable range of medical disorders during their lives. These disorders include fatal and nonfatal overdoses, premature births, low birth weight, intentional and unintentional injuries, premature death, and other conditions.

Drug-related morbidity and mortality as reflected in emergency department visits and medical examiner reports also show disproportionate health consequences suffered by racial and ethnic minorities. In 1999, for example, 44% of the drug episode cases in emergency departments involved nonwhites (Hispanics, Asians, Native Americans), among whom 24% were black.[17,18] Medical examiner records of drug-related deaths in 1999 reveal that 39.6% of the decedents were nonwhite and 25.9% were black.[17,18] The substances mentioned most frequently by black and Hispanic patients in emergency department visits were cocaine, alcohol in combination, and heroin or morphine.

Although mortality rates for Hispanic Americans are lower than those for non-Hispanic whites, Hispanics have higher rates of diabetes, HIV/AIDS, and cirrhosis of the liver, all of which can be related to alcohol and drug abuse.[15] There is a strong correlation between death rates from liver cirrhosis, regardless of cause, and drinking levels. Deaths from liver disease and cirrhosis are about four times more common among Native Americans than among the general US population.[19] Hispanics are approx-

imately twice as likely as whites to die from cirrhosis despite a lower prevalence of drinking and heavy drinking.[19] The reason for this discrepancy is unclear although evidence exists that Hispanics tend to consume alcohol in higher quantities per occasion than whites, resulting in a higher cumulative overdose.[19] Among some African Americans, genetically determined variability in another alcohol metabolizing enzyme, alcohol dehydrogenase-2, appears to affect the degree of vulnerability to alcoholic cirrhosis and alcohol-related fetal damage.[16]

Alcohol and tobacco abuse threaten minorities disproportionately through other health-related consequences, including cancer, cardiovascular diseases, stroke, and tuberculosis. Cigarette smoking is a major cause of disease and death in each of the four major racial and ethnic groups, with African Americans having the greatest risk, according to the Surgeon General.[20] Since the 1970s, African American men have had consistently higher lung cancer incidence rates that white men.[20]

Of course, many other factors are associated with substance abuse. These include genetic predisposition, education, unemployment, underemployment, hopelessness, dysfunctional families, psychiatric problems, and poverty. Yet none of these factors has been unequivocally shown to be causal. Indeed, there is evidence that some, if not all, are instead consequences of substance abuse. Such social and economic dislocations are not the only causes of substance abuse, as discrimination, particularly against the African American community, plays a part as well.

▶ TREATMENT

In their monumental study, *An American Health Dilemma: A Medical History of African Americans and the Problem of Race,* W. Michael Byrd and Linda Clayton observe that:

> By the late 1980s, the deleterious effects of
> more than a decade and a half of health policies

emphasizing privatization, commercial and cutthroat competition had eroded hard won progress African Americans had made during the 1960s Civil Rights Era in health care. Contemporary evidence of the African American health crisis generated by this competitive era in health policy manifests today as wide, deep, race-based health disparities and an erosion of African American longevity for the first time in the twentieth century.[21]

Other health-care researchers concur that disparities in the treatment of minorities are an accepted fact.[22] Although the relationship between race or ethnicity and treatment decisions is complex and may also be influenced by gender, physicians' attitudes toward their patients often vary by the patient's race or ethnicity. For example, one study found that different doses of painkillers were given to patients depending on their ethnicity or race.[23] Male physicians prescribed twice the level of analgesics for white patients than for black patients; while female physicians, in contrast, prescribed higher doses of analgesics for black patients than for white patients, suggesting that male and female physicians may respond differently to racial cues. Further research is needed to discover whether physicians are recommending or not recommending narcotic painkillers to patients of different races based in part on perceived or undiagnosed vulnerability to substance abuse.[24]

The federal government has thrown some support behind attempts to reduce racial and ethnic health disparities. The *Report of the Secretary's Task Force on Blacks and Minority Health,* issued during the Reagan administration, was a comprehensive study of the health status of disadvantaged minorities. The announcement by President Clinton in 1998 that the United States was committed to the elimination of racial and health disparities in six key areas by the year 2010 placed the federal government squarely behind efforts to change the imbalances.

Regarding drug abuse treatment specifically, some studies have found that minorities fare no better or worse than nonminorities,[25] while other research suggests that ethnic and racial minorities are less likely than whites to seek substance abuse treatment, less likely to complete treatment, and less likely to reduce or eliminate substance abuse during or after treatment.[25] Still other research reveals ethnic disparities in access to care, unmet need for care, and quality of treatment.[26]

African Americans were about 12% of the US population in 1999 and represented 23% of admissions to publicly funded substance abuse treatment facilities, almost two thirds of which were for alcohol or cocaine abuse, or both.[27] It should be noted that the white population often uses private as opposed to public treatment facilities, and therefore the percentages of minorities in public facilities are higher. Hispanics were 12% of the population and accounted for 13% of the admissions to publicly funded substance abuse treatment in 1999.[28] Alcohol was the most common substance of abuse among Hispanic admissions.[28] Although Native Americans and Alaska Natives represent less than 1% of the population, they accounted for 2.4% of all publicly funded substance abuse admissions,[29] and a higher proportion of Native American females were admitted to treatment (35%) than the percentage of female admissions in the total treatment population (30%).[29]

African Americans and Hispanics were least likely to have successful treatment outcomes (42% each) compared with whites, for whom 55% of treatment outcomes were successful.[30] Clearly, more must be done to tailor treatment programs to fit the needs of special populations, particularly African Americans and Hispanics. Asian American treatment needs are detailed in a study by Davis Y. Ja and Bart Aoki.[31]

An important treatment issue is whether African American patients respond more favorably, all other factors being equal, to a therapist of similar background. Some studies conclude that the ethnicity of a counselor or clinician may not be a dominant factor. On the other hand, more recent studies conclude the opposite. As a case in point, a Midwestern residential and outpatient program that had served a clientele that was almost entirely white and middle-class found that the population of its African American clients had climbed between 35% and 40%.[25] At the same time, the African American clinical supervisor began to notice that many black clients were signing out against medical advice. Upon closer inspection, the staff found that their failure to understand these clients' cultural values was in large measure responsible for the high discharge rate.

In her assessment of the mental health treatment of African American patients, Dr. Annelle B. Primm describes a number of ways in which the patient may not relate to the therapist and vice versa: "The potential risk in cross-cultural situations is a mismatch in preferred distance giving the African-American patient a sense of being rejected by the therapist, and the therapist a sense of being crowded. Such a situation could result in difficulties in establishing a therapeutic alliance, early termination by the patient, or misdiagnosis."[32] This description applies as well to therapists and clinicians in substance treatment settings. To be successful, treatment programs should be staffed by bilingual, culturally competent clinicians who can respond flexibly to a wide variety of social, educational, and health needs. To improve cross-cultural communication, government agencies as well as private groups need to recruit more minority candidates for training as substance abuse counselors and clinicians.

As the number of racial and ethnic minorities seeking treatment increases in the next decades, providers must become more culturally competent. If treatment providers are unsure how to work effectively in cross-cultural situations, they might seek advice from the minority community. Programs themselves must be adjusted for the needs of specific minorities. For example, a program that is designed for use in a white suburb or in the inner city may encounter a cool reception on an Indian reservation. Within a minority, treatment may vary for different subgroups. Different approaches may be required, say, in treating Cuban American youth as compared with Mexican American youth.

► SUMMARY AND RECOMMENDATIONS

Racial and ethnic disparities in the substance abuse treatment of minorities cannot be evaluated without considering the mental health problems of high-risk populations. Half the people with serious mental illnesses develop alcohol or drug abuse problems at some time in their lives.[33] Such comorbidity is associated with the exacerbation of symptoms, treatment noncompliance, more frequent hospitalization, greater depression and likelihood of suicide, incarceration, family friction, and high service use and cost. Treatment for substance abuse is a critical element of treatment for mental disorders and, conversely, treatment of mental disorders is a critical element of treatment for substance abuse. Yet, only about 20% of affected individuals are treated for both types of disorders.[34] Ideally, fully integrated programs should be established in which the drug or alcohol problem and the psychiatric disorder are treated at the same location by the same therapist or treatment team. Most successful models of combined treatment include case management, group interventions, and assertive outreach. But access to such treatment remains limited and needs to be expanded, particularly for minorities. The Epidemiological Catchment Area study of the 1980s[35] and, more recently, the National Comorbidity Survey[36] found that the rates of mental illness among African Americans are similar to those of whites. Yet, as stated earlier, many people in high-risk populations are not accessible to researchers. By counting members of these high-risk groups, higher rates of mental illness among African Americans might be detected.

A 2003 study found a strong connection between drinking dependence and smoking dependence. The authors note that alcohol and tobacco tend to be gateways to illicit drug use. They suggest that targeting earlier-stage substance abuse (alcohol and tobacco) could reduce the likelihood of advancing to later stage illicit drugs.[37]

Additional research is needed to reveal what prompts dependent minority individuals to seek treatment, what their treatment choices are, how long people remain in treatment, and what their relapse rate is. Nor should research overlook ethnopsychopharmacologic factors. These include racial and ethnic disparities in vulnerability or resilience to substance abuse, as well as the neurotoxin and neurobiologic processes underlying tolerance, dependence, and relapse.

A recent study in *Preventive Medicine* found that approximately three out of four African American adult smokers used menthol cigarettes compared with one out of four white smokers.[38] Among black youths who smoke, nine out of ten choose menthols. African Americans continue to suffer disproportionately from chronic and preventable disease compared with white Americans. Of the three leading causes of death—heart disease, cancer, and stroke—smoking and other tobacco uses are major contributors. The authors of the study conclude: "One possible explanation for greater occurrence of chronic disease and the greater difficulty in quitting is because African American smokers predominantly smoke mentholated cigarettes."[38] Health authorities and other public officials need to take notice. They should prevent tobacco companies from advertising and promoting menthol cigarettes to African Americans.

Environmental risks and protective factors leading to substance abuse need to be addressed. Of special relevance to migrant farm workers, mainly Hispanics, and their children is the impact of pesticides and herbicides on drug use.[39] Additional research into early nutrition, social isolation, and environmental impoverishment will help in understanding substance abuse in socioeconomically disadvantaged minorities and immigrant populations, which, of course, include many Hispanics and Asians. Of added importance is the role of prenatal, perinatal, and early childhood environmental factors in influencing later substance abuse behavior.[39]

There are many reasons why minorities who need treatment do not receive it. These include lack of health-care coverage or coverage that does not include treatment for alcohol or drug use, unwillingness to stop using illicit drugs or alcohol, lack of knowledge about where to go for treatment, lack of transportation to treatment centers that are far away, inability to find a program that offers the type of treatment or counseling needed, and fear that neighbors, employers, police or social services may find out.[3] All these concerns must be addressed. One way to begin is for treatment providers to reach out to other groups, such as faith-based organizations, some of which are involved in substance abuse treatment.

Another way is to try to influence the criminal justice system. Nearly half of all prisoners in state and federal prisons are African Americans.[40] Instead of sentencing people to jail, the courts should divert them to drug treatment programs. Since minority populations are disproportionately affected by HIV and AIDS, often as a consequence of injected drug use, prevention and intervention must be specifically directed at behaviors that place these groups at risk. African American women, in particular, need to know the steps they can take to prevent contagion. Relapse prevention services need to focus on social support.[41] Often African Americans face more difficult social situations following treatment, including high-stress and low-support environments. Additional prevention programs are needed to reach minority populations in high-risk settings and neglected areas. These include people in correctional facilities (disproportionately African Americans and Hispanics), people in rural areas (particularly poor blacks in the South), and migrant or seasonal farm workers (who are often Hispanics and Haitians). Appropriate intervention strategies must be developed for reducing risks for such people and others who are particularly vulnerable—the homeless and homosexuals.

Any truly successful, long-term solution to changing health disparities relating to substance abuse will require attention at many points, targeting minorities and low income populations that have suffered from chronic underservice, if not outright neglect. Just as the minority AIDS Initiative was successfully approved by the federal government in 1999, new initiatives to lessen disparities for minority substance abusers

▶ **TABLE 17-1.** Summary of Recommendations

- There is a need for a universal health insurance program in the United States
- Increased health-care and substance abuse treatment services need to be provided for all Americans, especially underserved groups; this particularly applies to Native Americans, who abuse substances the most and often have the least access to treatment. This also means the achievement of health-care parity whereby access to substance abuse treatment is equivalent to access to treatment for other medical disorders
- Preventive efforts must be expanded; drug abuse prevention must begin as early as kindergarten and, when necessary, include families in which there is a history of substance abuse
- Treatment facilities must be expanded to cover more people
- Treatment specifically tailored for chewing tobacco must be expanded to include settings beyond school such as the workplace, health-care service sites, and dentists' offices. A comprehensive study concluded that "chewing tobacco showed a continued onslaught throughout adulthood."[42] Prevention and cessation programs for chewing tobacco should be targeted to high-risk groups, including older, rural, and low-income African Americans
- Treatment for the indigent must be comprehensive, "one-stop shopping" and cover a multiplicity of social, psychological, vocational, and medical problems
- Treatment must be culturally appropriate for each minority group
- New treatment modalities such as buprenorphine should be tried
- Treatment must be readily available and accessible
- Treatment providers need to do more outreach to their communities and criminal justice systems

are required today. Policy, research, and practice must all be brought together and funded adequately.

Table 17–1 outlines recommendations that should be adopted to reduce and eliminate disparities. A final recommendation cannot be emphasized enough: Additional funding is essential. As long as substance abuse treatment funding remains at current levels, health disparities will continue. Addiction treatment is cost-effective in reducing substance abuse and the associated health and social costs. Treatment is less expensive than the alternatives—not treating addicts or simply incarcerating them. For example, the average cost for 1 year of methadone maintenance treatment is approximately $4700 per person, whereas 1 year of imprisonment costs about $18,400 per person.[43] According to conservative estimates, every $1 invested in addiction treatment programs yields a return of between $4 and $7 in reduced drug-related crime and criminal justice costs.[43] When savings related to health care are included, total savings can exceed costs by a ratio or 12 to 1.[43]

The complex scientific and sociological, psychological, and economic issues that need attention require more than a single effort. A long-term commitment is needed by the federal government, state governments, and the private sector. Although society has developed a paradigm of condemnations as its primary method of dealing with substance abuse, policy makers must accept the fact that substance abuse is a symptom of other problems faced by minority Americans such as poverty, discrimination, lack of education, and unemployment. If substance abuse disparities are to be reduced and eventually eliminated, these other disparities must be addressed.

▶ **REFERENCES**

1. National Institute on Drug Abuse. *Drug Use Among Racial/Ethnic Minorities.* 2003. Available at: http://www.nida.nih.gov/pdf/minorities03.
2. American Psychiatric Association. *Diagnostic and Statistical Manual of Mental Disorders,* 4th ed. Washington, DC: APA; 2000.

3. Substance Abuse and Mental Health Services Administration. *Reasons for Not Receiving Substance Abuse Treatment.* The National Household Survey on Drug Abuse. Washington, DC: SAMHSA, US Dept of Health and Human Services; 2003.

4. US Bureau of the Census. *Projections of the Resident Population by Race, Hispanic Origin, and Nativity.* Available at: http://www.census.gov/population/projections/nation/summary.

5. National Institute on Drug Abuse. *NIDA Notes* 2001;16(1):1–3.

6. Substance Abuse and Mental Health Services Administration. *National Household Survey on Drug Abuse.* The NHSDA Report. Washington, DC: SAMHSA, US Dept of Health and Human Services; 2002.

7. Substance Abuse and Mental Health Services Administration. *National Survey on Drug Use and Health.* 2002. Available at: http://www.samhsa.gov/oas/nhsda/2k2nsduh/overview.

8. Wallace JM Jr, Bachman JG, O'Malley PM, et al. Tobacco, alcohol, and illicit drug use: Racial and ethnic differences among U.S. high school seniors, 1976–2000. *Public Health Rep* 2002;117 (suppl 1):S67–75.

9. John S, Brown L, Primm B. African Americans: Epidemiologic, prevention, and treatment issues. In: Lowinson J, Ruiz P, Millman R, et al, eds. *Substance Abuse; A Comprehensive Textbook,* 3rd ed. Baltimore, Md: Williams & Wilkins; 1997:699–705.

10. Substance Abuse and Mental Health Services Administration. *National Household Survey on Drug Abuse.* Washington, DC: SAMHSA, US Dept of Health and Human Services; 2000 and 2001: Table 2.65B.

11. Caetano R, Clark C, Tam T. Alcohol consumption among racial/ethnic minorities. *Alcohol Health Res World* 1998;22(4):233–241.

12. Substance Abuse and Mental Health Services Administration. *National Household Survey on Drug Abuse.* Washington, DC: SAMHSA, US Dept of Health and Human Services; 2000 and 2001: Table 2.25B.

13. Substance Abuse and Mental Health Services Administration. *National Household Survey on Drug Abuse.* Washington, DC: SAMHSA, US Dept of Health and Human Services; 2000 and 2001: Table 2.35B.

14. Herd D. The epidemiology of drinking patterns and alcohol related problems among U.S. African Americans. In: Spiegler D, Tate D, Aitken S, et al, eds. *Alcohol Use Among US Ethnic Minorities.*

Washington, DC: National Institute on Alcohol Abuse and Alcoholism; Research Monograph No. 18 (DHHS Pub. No. CADMJ 89-1435). Washington, US Government Printing Office; 1989:3–50.

15. Jones D, Mills A, Francis H. *Drug Use, HIV/AIDS, and Health Outcomes Among Racial and Ethnic Populations.* Suppl 1, Report No. 117, 2002.

16. U.S. HIV and Aids Cases Reported Through December 2000. *HIV/AIDS Surveill Rep* 2001;12(2): 18,20.

17. Amaro H, Raj A, Vega RR, et al. Racial/ethnic disparities in the HIV and substance abuse epidemics: Communities responding to the need. *Public Health Rep* 2001;116(5):434–448.

18. Substance Abuse and Mental Health Services Administration. *Midyear 2000 Preliminary Emergency Department Data from the Drug Abuse Warning Network.* 2001. Available at: http://www.samhsa.gov/oas/dawn/dawnmidyr/00mid_year.

19. National Institute on Alcohol Abuse and Alcoholism. *Alcohol Alert* No. 55; 2002:1–6.

20. Centers for Disease Control and Prevention. *Tobacco Use Among Racial/Ethnic Minority Groups. A Report of the Surgeon General.* Atlanta, Ga: CDC; 1998.

21. Byrd W, Clayton L. An American health dilemma. In: *A Medical History of African Americans and the Problem of Race: Beginnings to 1900.* New York, NY: Routledge; 2000.

22. Fiscella K, Franks P, Gold MR, et al. Inequality in quality: Addressing socioeconomic, racial, and ethnic disparities in health care. *JAMA* 2000;283(19):2579–2584.

23. Smedley B, Stith A, Nelson A, eds. *Unequal Treatment: Confronting Racial and Ethnic Disparities in Health Care.* Washington, DC: National Academy Press; 2001.

24. Meier B. The delicate balance of pain and addiction. *New York Times* 2003.

25. Finn P. Addressing the needs of cultural minorities in drug treatment. *J Subst Abuse Treat* 1994; 11(4):325–337.

26. Wells K, Klap R, Koike A, et al. Ethnic disparities in unmet need for alcoholism, drug abuse, and mental health care. *Am J Psychiatry* 2001;158(12): 2027–2032.

27. Substance Abuse and Mental Health Services Administration. *Black Admissions to Substance Abuse Treatment, 1999.* The DASIS Report.

Washington, DC: SAMHSA, Dept of Health and Human Services; 2002.

28. Substance Abuse and Mental Health Services Administration. *Hispanics in Substance Abuse Treatment, 1999.* The DASIS Report. Washington, DC: SAMHSA, Dept of Health and Human Services; 2002.

29. Substance Abuse and Mental Health Services Administration. *American Indians and Alaska Natives in Substance Abuse Treatment, 1999.* The DASIS Report. Washington, DC: SAMHSA, Dept of Health and Human Services; 2002.

30. Substance Abuse and Mental Health Services Administration. *Treatment Completion in the Treatment Episode Data Set (TEDS).* The DASIS Report. Washington, DC: SAMHSA, Dept of Health and Human Services; 2003.

31. Ja DY, Aoki B. Substance abuse treatment: Cultural barriers in the Asian-American community. *J Psychoactive Drugs* 1993;25(1):61–71.

32. Primm A. Issues in the assessment and treatment of African American patients. In: Lim R, ed. *Cultural Psychiatry for Clinicians: A Handbook for Working with Diverse Patients.* Baltimore, Md: John Hopkins University Press; in press.

33. Substance Abuse and Mental Health Services Administration, Office of the Surgeon General. *Mental Health: A Report of the Surgeon General.* Washington, DC: SAMHSA, Dept of Health and Human Services; 1999.

34. Dual diagnosis. Part II. A look at old reliable and promising new approaches to the treatment of mental illness with substance abuse. *Harv Ment Health Lett* 2003;20(3):1–5.

35. National Institute of Mental Health, US Dept of Health and Human Services. *The Epidemiologic Catchment Area Study, 1980–1985.* Washington, DC: USDHHS.

36. Kessler RC. National Comorbidity Survey, 1990–1992. Conducted by University of Michigan, Survey Research Center, Ann Arbor, Michigan. Inter-University Consortium for Political and Social Research [producer and distributor], 2002. See also: Kessler RC, Berglund P, Demmler O. *The U.S. National Comorbidity Survey Replication: An Overview of Design and Field Procedures.* Cambridge, Mass: Harvard; 2003. Available at: http://www.hcp.med.harvard.edu/cpe/overview.

37. Jackson KM, Sher KJ, Wood PK, et al. Alcohol and tobacco use disorders in a general population: Short-term and long-term associations from the St. Louis epidemiological catchment area study. *Drug Alcohol Depend* 2003;71(3):239–253.

38. Garten S, Falkner RV. Role of mentholated cigarettes in increased nicotine dependence and greater risk of tobacco-attributable disease. *Prev Med* 2004;38(6):793–798.

39. Trujillo K, Castaneda E, Martinez D, et al. Neuroscience research on Hispanic drug abuse. In: Amaro H, Cortes D, eds. *National Strategic Plan on Hispanic Drug Abuse Research.* Boston, Mass: National Hispanic Science Network and Northeastern University; 2003:43–66.

40. Substance Abuse and Mental Health Services Administration, Office of the Surgeon General. *Mental Health: Culture, Race, Ethnicity Supplement to Mental Health: Report of the Surgeon General.* Washington, DC: SAMHSA, Dept of Health and Human Services; 2001.

41. Walton MA, Blow FC, Booth BM. Diversity in relapse prevention needs: Gender and race comparisons among substance abuse treatment patients. *Am J Drug Alcohol Abuse* 2001;27(2):225–240.

42. Howard-Pitney B, Winkleby MA. Chewing tobacco: Who uses and who quits? Findings from NHANES III, 1988–1994. National Health and Nutrition Examination Survey III. *Am J Public Health* 2002;92(2):250–256.

43. National Institute on Drug Abuse. *Principles of Drug Addiction Treatment: A Research-Based Guide.* NIH Publication No. 99-4180 Washington, DC: NIH, 1991.

CHAPTER 18

Injury and Violence Prevention

Christine M. Branche, PhD

Alex E. Crosby, MD, MPH

▶ INTRODUCTION

Injury (both unintentional and intentional in nature) is a leading cause of death in the United States. Unintentional injuries kill more persons aged 1 through 34 years than any other cause and in 2002 comprised the fifth leading cause of death among persons of all ages.[1] Homicide and suicide are among the leading 20 causes of death in the United States for persons of all ages.[1] Injuries produce a substantial burden on society in terms of medical resources used for treating and rehabilitating injured persons, productivity losses caused by nonfatal (ie, morbid) injuries, and premature death. The burden is exacerbated by the pain and suffering of injured persons and their caregivers.[2]

Although injuries are an important public health problem, they do not affect all segments of the US population equally (see Appendix A, Fig. A–12).* Fatal and nonfatal injuries occur disproportionately by age, race, and ethnicity regardless of whether the injuries are violence-related or unintentional in nature. Race and ethnicity data are inconsistently reported in both fatal and nonfatal databases for injury, even at the

national level.[3] The data that are available currently are reported here. African American and Hispanic populations sustain a disproportionately heavy toll of most of the types of injuries documented in the United States.[1] Native Americans (American Indians and Alaska Natives) aged 19 years and younger are at greater risk of preventable injury-related deaths than others in the same age group in the United States. Compared with African Americans and whites, Native Americans had the highest injury-related death rates for motor vehicle crashes, pedestrian events, and suicide. Rates for these causes were two to three times greater than rates for whites of the same age.[1] Furthermore, for almost every injury category, males outnumber females in both fatal and nonfatal events, with one exception. Males and females attempt suicide in almost equal proportions.[4]

Scientific evidence suggests that current racial categories (eg, white, African American, and Native American) are more alike than different in terms of biologic characteristics and genetics.[5] Although racial and ethnic disparities have been described for many years, only recently has research shown that the most important factors that contribute to disparities are determinants other than racial differences.[6] The factors, which are often termed *determinants,*

* Figures illustrating statistical information presented in this chapter are included in Appendix A at the end of this book.

331

are as follows: income and social status, social support networks, education, employment and working conditions, social environments, physical environments, personal health practices and coping skills, healthy child development, health services, gender roles, and culture.[7] Often communities of color are disproportionately represented in adverse aspects of several of these determinants, such as lower socioeconomic status, limited education, and hazardous physical environments, which contribute the major portion to their health disparities. There may be other unknown underlying factors operating as well.

There are many categories of unintentional injury (eg, motor vehicle, home, recreation) and of violence (eg, child abuse, sexual assault, intimate partner violence); however, this chapter addresses only three categories due to limitations of space and evidence. In this chapter, the importance of injury as a public health problem, its burden on society, and the disparities that occur among people of color, particularly African Americans, Native Americans, and Hispanics, are discussed. Three examples are provided for discussion: motor vehicle injuries, injuries due to youth interpersonal violence, and self-directed violence. In addition to discussing data by age, race, and ethnicity, prevention programs are also described. Points of discussion for this chapter are:

- The importance of injury as a leading public health problem in the United States
- Demonstrating that fatal and nonfatal injuries disproportionately affect racial and ethnic minorities
- Financial costs associated with fatal and nonfatal injuries in the United States
- Successful community-based injury prevention programs
- Barriers to successful implementation of model prevention programs for motor vehicle crashes and interpersonal and self-directed violence in racial and ethnic minority communities

▶ DISPARITIES IN INJURIES

Motor Vehicle Injuries

Motor vehicle crashes are the leading cause of injury death in the United States, and cost a minimum of $230 billion each year.[8] In 2002, an estimated 42,850 people died on the nation's roadways and almost 3 million were nonfatally injured.[8] All races of people are killed in motor vehicle crashes, but overall crash-related death rates differ by race. Based on the data available on race and ethnicity, generally, Native Americans have the highest rates and Asians and Pacific Islanders have the lowest rates[9]; death rates are similar for African American and White Americans.* However, overall rates mask patterns and contributing causes by age, sex, amount of exposure to the traffic environment, socioeconomic status, and alcohol (ie, drinking and driving and/or riding with a driver who has been drinking) (see Fig. A–13).

Baker et al,[10] looking at the risk of motor vehicle-related deaths to children and teenagers by both population and exposure to the traffic environment, found that differences by race using deaths per 100,000 population were minor; however, using deaths per billion vehicle miles of travel, death rates were highest among African American children (14 per billion vehicle miles for African Americans versus 8 for Hispanics and 5 for whites). There are also differences by type of victim (ie, vehicle occupant, pedestrian, bicyclist, and motorcyclist). Although African Americans and whites have similar death rates among vehicle occupants, bicyclists, and motorcyclists, African American pedestrians have higher deaths rates than white pedestrians, with more than 1000 pedestrian deaths per year occurring among African Americans.[8]

Progress has been made over time. Motor vehicle death rates have declined in the United

* Age-adjusted death rates in 1999 were 16.2 per 100,000 population among African Americans versus 15.6 per 100,000 among whites.[9]

States from 21.7 deaths per 100 vehicle miles traveled in 1923 (the first year that data were available) to 1.51 in 2002—a 93% reduction.[11] This downward trend occurred despite an increased number of vehicles, drivers, and miles traveled, and a growing population. This significant progress is due to several factors. Improvements in both roads and vehicles made for important gains in saving human lives. However, laws mandating the use of seat belts and child safety seats, stricter enforcement of laws, and child safety seat and child booster seat education and distribution programs have all helped to save lives and prevent injuries.

When used consistently, occupant protection, whether safety belts, booster seats, or child safety seats, saves lives. Data show that each year safety belt use alone saves almost $50 billion in medical care expenses, lost productivity, and other injury-related costs.[12] Research shows that use of both lap and shoulder belts reduces the risk of fatal and serious injury to front-seat passenger car occupants by 45% to 50%. In addition, we know that the safest place for children to ride in motor vehicles is in the back seat (as many as 1700 lives have been saved through this practice). Data from a national public opinion survey indicate that parents admit to placing an estimated 6% of the nation's infants to 12-year-olds in the front seat of automobiles, placing them at greater risk of serious injury or death.[13] The survey data indicated, furthermore, that African American and Hispanic families of lower income and less education were more likely to place their children in the front seat.

Implementing these interventions among communities of color has not been as successful as for predominantly white communities. Data are somewhat conflicting but generally seat belt use, for example, is lower among African American and Hispanic populations.[14–16] Information from the 1997 Behavioral Risk Factor Surveillance System, a nationwide household telephone survey of adults, found that 63% of African Americans reported always using their seat belts compared with 70% of whites. The

higher reporting of seat belts by whites was consistent across socioeconomic status. Furthermore, adult safety belt use is a strong predictor of proper child restraint use (eg, child safety seats, booster seats).[14] When used correctly, child safety seats can reduce the risk of death by 70% for infants and by as much as 54% for toddlers who are involved in motor vehicle crashes and save as much as $200 million in medical costs and $3.5 billion in other costs.[17] Ellis et al reported that 60% of African American youth were less likely than other racial and ethnic groups to be properly restrained by a child safety seat, booster seat, or safety belt.[18]

Legislation is an effective tool for increasing the use of these lifesaving interventions in motor vehicles. Recent systematic reviews of the scientific literature found that seat belt laws increased observed use by 33% and reduced fatal injuries by 9%. Enhanced law enforcement, that is, high visibility and more police presence, combined with both paid and earned media about the increased presence, increased seat belt use by 16% and reduced fatalities from 7% to 15%.[19] The precipitous increase in child safety seat use, especially, is used as a perennial example of the benefits of legislation as a means to modify behavior in the motor vehicle. On the other hand, child booster seat legislation, a relatively new approach, is either under development or in review in a number of state and local jurisdictions. The booster seat is designed for children aged 4 to 8 years who have outgrown their child safety seats but are too small to ride safely in adult safety belts.

Primary seat belt laws (a driver can be stopped for a seat belt violation alone) have been actively encouraged by researchers and advocates in the motor vehicle safety arena because they have been found to be more effective than secondary laws (a driver must be stopped for another traffic violation) in increasing belt use and reducing fatalities.[18] Recent survey data suggest that African Americans and Hispanics are supportive of laws requiring front seat passengers to wear seat belts (94% and 92%, respectively) and of primary seat belts laws (68% and 72%, respectively),[20,21] but this stated support must be followed with behavior change. Research suggests that seat belt use is lower in communities of color because information about the lifesaving benefits of seat belts has not been communicated effectively in racial and ethnic minority communities.[22] Wells et al found that in cities with primary belt laws, there were no differences in belt use by race or ethnicity; however, in cities with secondary laws, African Americans were less likely than whites or Hispanics to be belted.[15] Furthermore, the issue of differential enforcement by law enforcement officers (ie, "racial profiling") has hampered full implementation of primary seat belt laws.[20]

Data that show an increase in seat belt use and the support of primary seat belt laws may have more to do with a concern about receiving a traffic ticket for nonuse than because of the perceived benefit of the seat belt in saving lives.[15] In the African American community, the argument is that once a driver is pulled over for not wearing a seat belt, then other, sometimes questionable infractions accrue. Any effort that gives law enforcement added power is met with resistance.

Seat belt use remains one of the most important preventive strategies for African Americans. Ellis et al estimated that if all African Americans buckled their seat belts, 1300 lives would be saved and 26,000 injuries would be prevented.[18] Targeted messages and innovative approaches have improved implementation, but more progress is still needed. Researchers and advocates alike agree that expanding these intervention efforts will protect even more lives. But this is the very place where the challenge remains for minority populations.

Self-Directed Violence

Injury from self-directed violence, which includes suicidal behavior, is a major public health problem in the United States and throughout the world.[23,24] In the United States, suicide has ranked among the 12 leading causes of death since 1975. In 2001, suicide was the 11th leading cause of death overall in the United States, responsible for 30,622 deaths and an estimated 264,108 persons treated in hospital emergency departments.[25,26] Other research indicates that over 70% of people who attempt suicide never seek health services.[4] As a result, prevalence figures based on health records substantially underestimate the societal burden. The human and economic costs of suicide are enormous. One study estimated the total economic burden of suicide in the United States in 1995 to be $111.3 billion.[27] The loss of life and the emotional trauma experienced by surviving family, friends, and communities that are affected by each person's attempted or completed suicide compound the economic burden.[28]

Despite the widespread impact of self-directed violence in the United States, the problem has frequently been viewed as one that affects solely white American males and the affluent.[29,30] Native Americans, however, are ending their lives at substantially greater rates than young people of other racial and ethnic groups (see Fig. A–14). Overall, suicide ranks third among the leading causes of death for persons aged 15 to 24 years. However, among Native Americans in this age group suicide is the second leading cause of death.[31] The suicide rate for Native American males aged 15 to 24 years (29.0 per 100,000) is approximately 48% higher than the racial group with the next highest rate, non-Hispanic white males (19.6 per 100,000). The discrepancy across racial groups is even greater for females. The suicide rate among Native American females aged 15 to 24 (8.4 per 100,000) is more than twice that of the next highest group, Asian and Pacific Islander females (3.6 per 100,000).[31]

Native American youth are not a homogenous group. The population represents more than 560 different cultural communities, federally defined as sovereign entities, which speak more than 250 different languages.[32] They live in a range of communities that differ dramatically in characteristics that are likely to influence the risk for youth suicide, such as social relationships, economic conditions, and availability of support services.

Youth Interpersonal Violence

Interpersonal violence is a major cause of death and disability in the United States. In 1995, all interpersonal violence was estimated to cost the United States $426 billion in direct and indirect costs each year.[33] Of these costs, approximately $90 billion is spent on the criminal justice system, $65 billion on security, $5 billion on the treatment of victims, and $170 billion on lost productivity and quality of life. The rates of morbidity and mortality from this form of violence disproportionately affect young people.[34] In 2001, homicide was the second leading cause of death among persons aged 15 to 24 years and in 2000, approximately 750,000 persons from infancy through 24 years were seen in hospital emergency departments with injuries related to assaults.[31,35]

Minority communities, especially African American and Hispanic groups, are disproportionately affected by interpersonal violence. In 2001, among African Americans aged 15 to 24 years, homicide was the leading cause of death and rates (49.2 per 100,000) were over 2.5 times (264%) higher than the US average homicide rate among this age group.[31] In 2001, among Hispanics aged 15 to 24 years, homicide was the second leading cause of death and rates (18.6 per 100,000) were over one third (37%) higher than the US average for this age.[31] In addition to a higher-than-average burden of interpersonal violence, there are other similarities between African American and Hispanic groups. Both groups tend to be more geographically concentrated than the majority (non-Hispanic white) population, with African Americans in the South and Hispanics in the West and South. Both groups have higher percentages of their population younger than 18 years. Both groups are more likely to live in urban areas.[36,37] African Americans and His-

panics also share several health determinants that contribute to interpersonal violence: lower educational attainment; greater proportions of poverty, inequality, and unemployment than the majority; and the experience of having been victims of discrimination and racism.[38] Despite these adverse circumstances, there are protective factors within these communities, such as family orientation, cultural identity, and spirituality, that prevent youth from engaging in violent behavior.[39]

▶ PREVENTION PROGRAMS

Motor Vehicle Injury Prevention

Injury prevention programs are successful in general, but success can be boosted when tailored to the community of interest. To address directly the lower use of occupant protection among low-income and minority populations, traffic safety professionals have introduced innovative strategies tailored to the communities of interest, especially in low-income African American and Hispanic communities. For example, in the southeastern United States, traffic safety advocates created diversity programs that enabled minority community leaders and law enforcement members to have open discussions about appropriate ways to increase the use of safety belts and child safety seats. Public service announcements, workshops, and community-specific outreach activities characterize other programs.[40] Based in part on the success of programs such as these, safety belt use among African Americans in the southeast region increased to 77% in 2002, an increase of 8 percentage points from 2000. Furthermore, primary care physicians serving racial and ethnic populations have been working with law enforcement officials and community leaders to design messages and other communications tailored for African American and Hispanic communities in particular.[22]

In another example, the Center for Risk Analysis at the Harvard School of Public Health developed, implemented, and evaluated the "Kids in the Back/Niños Atrás" program in low-income Hispanic communities in western Massachusetts.[41] This 3-year, community-based intervention was designed to increase the number of children 12 years and younger who ride properly restrained in the back seat of motor vehicles. Project investigators first organized a community task force and hired a Spanish-speaking member of the community to coordinate the project. All educational materials for parents and children were developed in English and Spanish and specifically tailored for the target communities. None of the materials made available for Spanish-speaking populations in other parts of the United States were deemed appropriate because they did not address the placement of children in the back seat of motor vehicles. The Center also implemented an incentive program to further motivate parents and children to adopt these behaviors. They coordinated a number of community events and safety seat checkpoints, as well, along with a public information campaign targeting parents and caregivers of children. Researchers conducted pre- and postintervention observational surveys of seating position and restraint use among children in the intervention and two control communities. During the intervention period, the proportion of children in the intervention community who were observed riding in the back seat increased from 33% to 49% compared with control communities.[42]

Suicide and Interpersonal Violence Prevention

One model for categorizing prevention programs places them into three types based on the target population[43]: (1) indicated prevention strategies to address specific high-risk individuals (ie, those already exhibiting a risk factor, condition, or abnormality); (2) selective strategies to address sections of the population that are at risk (ie, risk of becoming ill or injured is above average); and (3) universal strategies to address the general public. Because Native American populations have suicide rates approximately 1.5 times the national average, we will focus on suicide prevention programs for that group.[31] In addressing youth interpersonal violence, we will focus on African American and Hispanic populations, both of which have rates above the national average.[34]

There are limited specific examples of each type of strategy addressing suicidal behavior that have been implemented and evaluated in Native American populations. An outline of the strategies as described by the Institute of Medicine follows.* Universal prevention strategies for self-directed violence include media campaigns, strategies aimed to reduce access to lethal means, efforts to lower access to proximal risk factors, and some school-based programs.[23] There are several types of strategies operating at the selective level that have been used for suicidal behavior prevention. These include screening programs, gatekeeper training models, support and skills training, and hotlines and crisis centers.[23,44] Indicated prevention strategies include clinical or medical interventions,[45] family support training, skill-building support groups, case management, referral resources for crisis intervention and treatment, and programs for those who are incarcerated.[23,46] There are few data on the effectiveness of these strategies in minority racial and ethnic communities; nor is there information on how to make them culturally relevant.

Several organizations have used integrated approaches. Although these are challenging to design, execute, and evaluate, activities occur on multiple levels of prevention simultaneously because they may have the best chance of success.[47,48] There are also programs designed to address other health problems that have potential for reducing suicidal behavior. These programs, though not "suicide-specific" may apply to a range of "suicide-inclusive"

---

* A detailed description of the strategies can be found in Institute of Medicine, Goldsmith SK, Pellmar TC, Kleinman AM, Bunney WE, eds. *Reducing Suicide: A National Imperative*. Washington, DC: National Academy Press; 2002.

factors (eg, factors that relate to several health issues such as early antisocial behavior, substance abuse, or child maltreatment).[46,49] Interventions for suicide-inclusive factors have the promise to bring a wider range of health benefits, in that they may reduce more than one adverse outcome.

An example of a successful program is the Natural Helpers project.[48] This program was directed by the American Indian/Alaska Native Community Suicide Prevention Center and Network from a tribe in rural New Mexico and supported by the Indian Health Service, Centers for Disease Control and Prevention, and the University of New Mexico. This was a multicomponent adolescent suicide program based on the idea of youth natural helpers who were trained to respond to other young people in crisis and notify mental health professionals as well as offer health education in the school and community. Other program components included outreach to families following a suicide or traumatic death, immediate response and follow-up for reported at-risk youth, community education about suicide prevention, and suicide-risk screening in mental health and social service programs. Evaluation data showed a reduction of suicidal acts (suicide and suicide attempts) in the target population after the program was implemented.

There are some examples of successful programs that are universal, address several factors related to interpersonal violence, and have been tested among minority ethnic communities. One such program is Life Skills Training, which addresses factors such as gateway drug use (eg, marijuana) among adolescents in the middle and high school grades. The curriculum has three major components: self-management skills, social skills, and information and skills related specifically to drug use. Teachers use a variety of techniques, including instruction, demonstration, feedback, reinforcement, and practice to train students in these three core areas. Evaluations show that the program can reduce some forms of substance use that are associated with youth interpersonal violence.[50]

Another program that includes a universal strategy focused on factors related to youth interpersonal violence and has been tested with minority populations is the Seattle Social Development Project. This program focuses on elementary school students and includes both individual and environmental change approaches and multiple components known to improve the effectiveness of violence prevention efforts.[51] The original intervention group included just over 31% African Americans. The components include classroom behavior management, child skills training, and parent training. The goal of this program is to enhance elementary school students' bonds with school and their families while decreasing a number of early risk factors for violence. Through these three components, which target prosocial behavior, interpersonal problem solving, academic success, and avoidance of drug use, the Seattle Social Development Project aims to reduce the initiation of alcohol, marijuana, and tobacco use by grade 6 and improve attachment and commitment to school. At age 18, youths who participated in the full 5-year version of this program had lower rates of violence, heavy drinking, and sexual activity (including fewer multiple sexual partners and pregnancy) and better academic performance than controls.[51] The Seattle Social Development Project has been used effectively in both general populations of youths and high-risk children attending elementary and middle school.

▶ SUMMARY AND RECOMMENDATIONS

There are numerous challenges to establishing successful unintentional injury or violence injury prevention programs in ethnic minority communities, as well as opportunities for such programs. The challenges include historical and societal factors such as discrimination or segregation, differences in economic or political power from the majority race, and community structures (eg, social disorganization, weak social controls).[52]

For example, communities of color may lack sufficient economic resources to sustain programs or political influence to gain access to resources. These factors can cause researchers, program practitioners, or community members to be less willing to have efforts directed to these communities. There have been incidents in which minority communities have been the subjects of unethical projects, which caused distrust about future participation in research activities.[53] In addition, because many of the communities are economically disadvantaged, there are limited financial resources to initiate and maintain programs. Lack of intrinsic financial resources may interrupt the continuity of the intervention, especially for resource-intensive programs. Despite these challenges, if programs are not introduced in the context of the specific communities where interventions would be implemented, then communities of color are left with having interventions translated from majority community programs, where certain applications may not be relevant.[54]

There are, however, opportunities for intervention programs. Minority communities often have well-established informal social networks.[55] Financial resource challenges may be overcome through careful inclusion of community leaders as research and intervention programs are being designed. This participation helps build avenues of endorsement of the program within the community, which leads to an increase in volunteers, participants, and program promotion, and an increased desire to see the program(s) continue.

Another opportunity exists regarding the selection of the type of prevention program. Many minority communities are more receptive to broader comprehensive or noncategorical approaches that focus on preventing a range of health problems.[56] These programs identify factors that play a role in more than one health outcome, and injury program planners can maximize the endorsement of their intervention by joining with another intervention strategy. In doing so, community members can see more than one benefit to their participation. For example, injury prevention specialists can integrate child safety seat and booster seat instruction and child abuse prevention into an existing parenting class in a local community.

Lastly, the roles of the health-care professional (ie, clinician, health counselor, trainer, and researcher) are critical.[57] Health-care professionals are often also members of the communities that they serve and protect. Physicians, nurses, and allied health staff are trustworthy messengers of vital injury prevention information,[18] and they are in a position to routinely and credibly recommend the use and practice of injury prevention strategies[22] (Table 18–1). They are also perceived as leaders. Accordingly, health-care professionals should be encouraged to not restrict their interests in injury prevention to the patients and families for whom they care, but to expand their interests to the community at large by advocating for injury prevention strategies for the community and on a wider scale.

▶ **TABLE 18–1**. Summary of Recommendations to Ameliorate Current Disparities in Injuries Among Minority Populations

Motor Vehicle Injuries
- Make a priority, for both public agencies and private organizations, broader implementation of innovative strategies that have been tailored to minority communities for increased use of seat belts, child safety seats, and booster seats

Youth Interpersonal Violence
- Implement evidence-based youth violence prevention programs in communities across the United States

Suicide
- Make a stronger commitment to community-level risk and protective factor research to better understand the influences of suicide in minority populations
- Make development and evaluation of community-based programs that focus on minority populations a higher priority for both public agencies and private organizations

▶ REFERENCES

1. Centers for Disease Control and Prevention. Web-based Injury Statistics Query and Reporting System (WISQARS) [Online] (2002). National Center for Injury Prevention and Control (producer). 2004. Available at: http://www.cdc.gov/ncipc/wisqars.

2. Centers for Disease Control and Prevention. Medical expenditures attributable to injuries—United States, 2000. *MMWR Morb Mortal Wkly Rep* 2004;53(1):1–4.

3. Hahn RA, Stroup DF. Race and ethnicity in public health surveillance: Criteria for the scientific use of social categories. *Public Health Rep* 1994;109(1):7–14.

4. Diekstra R. Epidemiology of attempted suicide in the EEC. In: Wilmott J, Mendlewicz J, eds. *New Trends in Suicide Prevention.* New York, NY: Karger; 1982:1–16.

5. House J, Williams D. Understanding and reducing socioeconomic and racial/ethnic disparities in health. In: Smedley B, Syme S, eds. *Promoting Health: Intervention Strategies from Social and Behavioral Research.* Washington, DC: National Academy Press; 2000:81–124.

6. Leon DA, Walt G, Gilson L. Recent advances: International perspectives on health inequalities and policy. *BMJ* 2001;322(7286):591–594.

7. Wilkerson R, Marmot D, eds. *Social Determinants of Health,* 2nd ed. Copenhagen, Denmark: World Health Organization; 2003.

8. Centers for Disease Control and Prevention. Web-based Injury Statistics Query and Reporting System (WISQARS) [Online]. (2001). National Center for Injury Prevention and Control, Centers for Disease Control and Prevention (producer). 2004. Available at: http://www.cdc.gov/ncipc/wisqars.

9. National Highway Traffic Safety Administration. *DOT Releases Preliminary Estimates of 2002 Highway Fatalities.* Available at: http://www.dot.gov/affairs/nhtsa1303.htm.

10. Baker SP, Braver ER, Chen LH, et al. Motor vehicle occupant deaths among Hispanic and black children and teenagers. *Arch Pediatr Adolesc Med* 1998;152(12):1209–1212.

11. National Highway Traffic Safety Administration. *Traffic Safety Facts 2002.* Washington, DC: NHTSA, Dept of Transportation (DOT No. HS809612); 2004. Available at: http://www.nrd.nhtsa.dot.gov/pdf/nrd-30/NCSA/TSF2002/2002ovrfacts.pdf.

12. Blincoe L, Seay A, Zaloshnja E, et al. *Economic Impact of Motor Vehicle Crashes, 2000.* Washington, DC: National Highway Traffic Safety Administration, Dept of Transportation (DOT No. HS809446); 2002.

13. National Safety Council. Air Bag and Seat Belt Safety Campaign. Press release; 2004.

14. National Highway Traffic Safety Administration. National Occupant Protection Use Survey, 2000. Controlled Intersection Study. Washington, DC: National Highway Traffic Safety Administration, Dept of Transportation (DOT No. HS809318).

15. Wells JK, Williams AF, Farmer CM. *Seat Belt Use Among African Americans, Hispanics, and Whites.* Arlington, Va: Insurance Institute for Highway Safety; 2001.

16. Braver ER. *Race, Hispanic origin, and Socioeconomic Status in Relation to Motor Vehicle Occupant Death Rates and Risk Factors Among Adults.* Arlington, Va: Insurance Institute for Highway Safety; 2001.

17. Zaza S, Sleet DA, Thompson RS, et al. Reviews of evidence regarding interventions to increase use of child safety seats. *Am J Prev Med* 2001;21(4S):31–47.

18. Ellis HM, Nelson B, Cosby O, et at. Achieving a credible health and safety approach to increasing seat belt use among African Americans. *J Health Care Poor Underserved* 2000;11(2):144–150.

19. Dinh-Zarr TB, Sleet DA, Shults RA, et al. Reviews of evidence regarding interventions to increase the use of safety belts. *Am J Prev Med* 2001;21(4S):48–65.

20. *Seat Belts and African Americans-2000 Report: The Facts to Buckle-Up America.* Washington, DC: Dept of Transportation (DOT No. HS808866); 2001.

21. *Seat Belts and Hispanics-2000 Report: The Facts to Buckle-Up America.* Washington, DC: Dept of Transportation (DOT No. HS809045); 2001.

22. Daniels F, Moore W, Conti C, et al. The role of the African-American physician in reducing traffic-related injury and death among African Americans: Consensus report of the National Medical Association. *J Natl Med Assoc* 2002;94(2):108–118.

23. Goldsmith SK, Kleinman AM, eds. *Reducing Suicide: A National Imperative.* Washington, DC: National Academy Press; 2002.

24. Krug EG, Dahlberg LL, Mercy JA, et al, eds. *World Report on Violence and Health.* Geneva, Switzerland: World Health Organization; 2002.

25. Arias E, Anderson RN, Hsiang-Ching K, et al. Final data for 2001. *National Vital Statistics Reports,* vol 52, No. 3. Hyattsville, Md: National Center for Health Statistics; 2003.

26. Ikeda R, Mahendra R, Saltzman L, Crosby, et al. Nonfatal self-inflicted injuries treated in hospital emergency departments—United States, 2000. *MMWR Morbid Mortal Wkly Rep* 2002;51:436–438.

27. Miller T, Covington K, Jensen A. Costs of injury by major cause, United States, 1995: Cobbling together estimates in measuring the burden of injuries. In: Mulder S, van Beeck EF, eds. *Proceedings of a Conference in Noordwijkerhout.* Amsterdam, Holland: European Consumer Safety Association; 1999:23–40.

28. Crosby AE, Sacks JJ. Exposure to suicide: Incidence and association with suicidal ideation and behavior. *Suicide Life Threat Behav* 2002;32:321–328.

29. Davis R. Black suicide in the seventies: Current trends. *Suicide Life Threat Behav* 1979;9:131–140.

30. Earls F, Escobar JI, Manson SM. Suicide in minority groups: Epidemiologic and cultural perspectives. In: Blumenthal SJ, Kupfer DJ, eds. *Suicide Over the Life Cycle: Risk Factors, Assessment, and Treatment of Suicidal Patients.* Washington, DC: American Psychiatric Press; 1990:571–598.

31. Anderson RN, Smith BL. Deaths: Leading causes for 2001. *National Vital Statistics Reports,* vol 52, No 9. Hyattsville, Md: National Center for Health Statistics; 2003.

32. Tatum BD. *Why Are All the Black Kids Sitting Together in the Cafeteria?* New York, NY: Basic Books; 1997.

33. Miller TR, Cohen MA, Wiersema B. *Victim Costs and Consequences: A New Look.* Washington, DC: US Dept of Justice, Office of Justice Programs, National Institute of Justice; 1996.

34. US Dept of Health and Human Services. *Youth Violence: A Report of the Surgeon General.* Rockville, Md: USDHHS; 2001.

35. Simon TR, Saltzman LE, Swahn MH, et al. Nonfatal physical assault-related injuries treated in hospital emergency departments—United States, 2000. *MMWR Morb Mortal Wkly Rep* 2002;51:460–463.

36. McKinnen J. The black population of the United States: March 2002. *Current Population Reports.* Washington, DC: US Census Bureau; 2003:20–541.

37. Ramirez RR, de la Cruz GP. The Hispanic population of the United States: March 2002. *Current Population Reports.* Washington, DC: US Census Bureau; 2002:20–545.

38. Hawkins DF. *Ethnicity, Race, Class and Adolescent Violence.* Boulder, Colo: Center for the Study and Prevention of Violence, Institute of Behavioral Science, University of Colorado at Boulder; 1996.

39. Hill HM, Soriano FI, Chen SA, et al. Sociocultural factors in the etiology and prevention of violence among ethnic minority youth. In: Eron LD, Gentry JH, Schlegel P, eds. *Reason to Hope: A Psychological Perspective on Violence and Youth.* Washington, DC: American Psychological Association; 1994:59–97.

40. National Highway Traffic Safety Administration Regional Diversity Outreach Team. *State and Regional Diversity Outreach: Highlight Report, September 2001.* Washington, DC: NHTSA, Dept of Transportation (DOT No. HS809339). Available at: http://www.nhtsa.dot.gov/nhtsa/whatis/regions/diversityoutreach.html.

41. Greenberg-Seth J, Hemenway D, Gallagher SS, et al. Factors associated with rear seating of children in motor vehicles: A study in two low-income, predominantly Hispanic communities. *Accid Anal Prev* 2004;36(4):621–626.

42. Greenberg-Seth J, Hemenway D, Gallagher SS, et al. Evaluation of a community-based intervention to promote rear seating for children. *Am J Public Health* 2004;94(6):1009–1113.

43. Gordon R. An operational classification of disease prevention. *Public Health Rep* 1983;98:107–109.

44. White J, Jodoin N. *"Before-the-fact" Interventions: A Manual of Best Practices in Youth Suicide Prevention.* Vancouver, Canada: British Columbia Ministry for Children and Families; 1998.

45. American Academy of Child and Adolescent Psychiatry. Summary of the practice parameters for the assessment and treatment of children and adolescents with suicidal behavior. *J Am Acad Child Adolesc Psychiatry* 2001;40:495–499.

46. National Health and Medical Research Council, Dept of Health and Aged Care. *National Youth Suicide Prevention Strategy—Setting the Evidence-based Research Agenda for Australia.* Canberra, Australia: Dept of Health and Aged Care, Commonwealth of Australia; 1999.

47. Knox KL, Litts DA, Talcott GW, et al. Risk of suicide and related adverse outcomes after

exposure to a suicide prevention programme in the U.S. Air Force: Cohort study. *BMJ* 2003;327: 1376–1380.

48. Serna P, May P, Sitaker M, et al. Suicide prevention evaluation in a Western Athabaskan American Indian Tribe—New Mexico, 1988–1997. *MMWR Morb Mortal Wkly Rep* 1998;47:257–261.

49. Durlak JA, Wells AM. Primary Prevention mental health programs for children and adolescents: A meta-analytic review. *Am J Community Psychol* 1997;25:115–152.

50. Botvin GJ, Mihalic SF, Grotpeter JK. Life skills training. In: Elliott DS, series ed. *Blueprints for Violence Prevention*. Boulder, Colo: Center for the Study and Prevention of Violence, Institute of Behavioral Science, University of Colorado at Boulder; 1998.

51. O'Donnell J, Hawkins JD, Catalano RF, et al. Preventing school failure, drug use, and delinquency among low-income children: Long-term intervention in elementary schools. *Am J Orthopsychiatry* 1995;65:87–100.

52. Hawkins DF, Laub JH, Lauritsen JL. Race, ethnicity and serious juvenile offending. In: Loeber R, Farrington DP, eds. *Serious and Violent Juvenile Offenders: Risk Factors and Successful Interventions*. Thousand Oaks, Calif: Sage; 1998:30–46.

53. Corbie-Smith G, Arriola KRJ. Research ands ethics: A legacy of distrust. In: Braithewaite RL, Taylor SE, eds. *Health Issues in the Black Community*. San Francisco, Calif: Jossey-Bass; 2001: 489–502.

54. House JS, Williams DR. Understanding and reducing socioeconomic and racial/ethnic disparities in health. In: Smedley BD, Syme SL, eds. *Promoting Health: Intervention Strategies from Social and Behavioral Research*. Washington, DC: National Academy Press; 2000:81–124.

55. Sampson RJ, Raudenbush SW, Earls F. Neighborhoods and violent crime: A multilevel study of collective efficacy. *Science* 1997;277:918–924.

56. Catalano RF, Berglund ML, Ryan JA, et al. Positive youth development in the United States: Research findings on evaluations of positive youth development programs. *Ann Am Acad Political Social Sci* 2004;591:98–124.

57. Task Force on Violence. The role of the pediatrician in youth violence prevention in clinical practice and at the community level. *Pediatrics* 1999;103:173–181.

CHAPTER 19

Assessing and Managing Pain

CARMEN RENEE' GREEN, MD

► INTRODUCTION

The literature discussing global disparities in health or the health-care experience for racial and ethnic minorities and the underserved have mostly failed to address the quality of pain care or the impact that pain has on their overall health and well-being.[1-6] Primarily, the health disparities literature has focused on health inequities due to cardiovascular disease, cancer, diabetes, osteoarthritis, and obesity.[1,7,8] Yet most chronic diseases commonly associated with disparities are also associated with acute, chronic, or cancer pain.

The health community has primarily viewed pain as a symptom and not as a disease state, with unique health considerations and socioeconomic implications.[9,10] For instance, in the Institute of Medicine's (IOM) excellent treatise documenting the literature on health disparities entitled *Unequal Treatment: Confronting Racial and Ethnic Disparities in Health Care,* the conversation regarding pain was limited to only a few pages and primarily focused on analgesic care for acute and cancer pain.[11] The lack of attention to pain in general and disparate pain care, in particular, is also missing from other well-publicized public health agendas designed to improve the nation's colloquial health-related quality of life. Federal agencies such as the National Institutes of Health (NIH), Agency for

Health Research and Quality (AHRQ; formerly the Agency for Healthcare Research and Policy [AHCPR]), and Centers for Disease Control and Prevention (CDC) have acknowledged health inequities while setting goals toward eliminating racial and ethnic disparities in health.[12-14] Yet these same agencies have not addressed the differential impact of pain among racial and ethnic minorities and the underserved on their overall health and well-being. Furthermore, proposed legislation designed to address inequities has not focused on disparate pain care (eg, Senate resolution 2091 [Closing the Healthcare Gap Act of 2004], House resolution 1483 [Pain Care Coalition Act]).[15] However, an emerging literature has begun to highlight differences in pain perception as well as disparities in pain care for racial and ethnic minorities for all types of pain (ie, acute, chronic, and cancer pain) and across all settings (ie, inpatient and outpatient settings).[16,17]

Consistent with an emerging literature that presents adequate pain relief as fundamentally a human rights issue, this chapter provides a platform to discuss pain assessment and management as a unique public health problem.[18-22] It also presents groundwork for the inadequate assessment and undertreatment of pain as both a quality of care issue and as a medical error. The chapter focuses on disparities in pain assessment, the health implications of pain, access to quality pain care, pain treatment, and health-care provider variability in pain management decision making for racial and ethnic minorities. Patient accounts are included to illustrate key points. Lastly, the chapter provides a framework to direct pain research and health-care policy toward the ultimate goal of eliminating racial and ethnic disparities in pain care.

▶ THE IMPACT OF PAIN ON OVERALL HEALTH AND WELL-BEING

The World Health Organization (WHO) defines health as "a state of complete physical, social, and emotional well-being and not merely the absence of disease and infirmities."[22-24] Pain as defined by the International Association for the Study of Pain (IASP) is an unpleasant sensory and emotional experience associated with actual or potential tissue damage.[25] Pain can further be defined by its etiology or duration as follows:

- **Acute pain.** Pain that is short-lived, usually lasting less than 3 months
- **Cancer pain.** Pain due to cancer or its treatment
- **Chronic benign or nonmalignant pain.** Persistent pain for more than 6 months that is not due to cancer[25]

Irrespective of the etiology or duration, pain, diminishes overall health (ie, physical, social, and emotional health) in many ways,[26,27] as shown in Figure 19–1.

Pain remains the third largest health problem in the world, with significant psychological, physical, and social perturbations that cause needless suffering and subsequent disability.[9,21,28-32] People with chronic pain often experience concomitant depression, anxiety, post-traumatic stress disorder, sleep disturbance, fatigue, and decreased overall physical functioning.[33-38] Other studies show that pain may lead an individual to withdraw from societal roles, leading to impaired family and career relationships.[39-43] Overall, pain diminishes health and quality of life.[26,28,44-47] It is with this in mind that WHO joined the IASP and the European Federation of IASP Chapters to host the first Global Day Against Pain in 2004 to document the tremendous disease burden associated with acute, chronic, and cancer pain.[48]

The medical advantages yielding increased longevity and quality of life for most white Americans have not been uniformly applied.[49-52] More specifically, we now have methods as well as guidelines to improve pain assessment and treatment for all Americans. Yet, estimates suggest that anywhere from 65 to 100 million Americans live with chronic pain and many more millions of people are afflicted worldwide.[53] The increasing prevalence of pain has significant and potentially devastating socioeconomic and health ramifications for both the individual and society.[53] Currently, pain leads to over 700 million lost workdays and greater than $60 billion in health-care expenditures annually.[10,53] Americans spend an additional $40 billion annually on chronic pain.[10] Chronic pain remains the most frequent cause of disability in the United States and

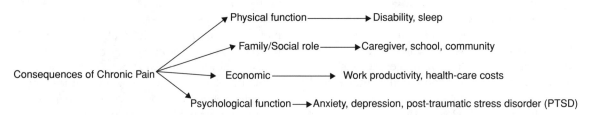

Figure 19–1. Consequences of chronic pain.

is the second leading cause for all physician visits.[10,53,54] Indeed, the increasing prevalence of chronic pain without necessary improvements in the quality of chronic pain management will have devastating socioeconomic and health ramifications as our society ages.

In light of the increasing prevalence of pain and estimates that suggest that 50% of elderly Americans currently have pain, pain threatens to interfere with their successful aging and the ability of an aging population to negotiate independently in their environments.[55–59] By the year 2030, more than 25% of the elderly population will consist of racial and ethnic minorities.[16,60–62] Yet, racial and ethnic minority elders are more likely to rate their health as poor when compared with white elders.[63] In addition to worrying about their pain and future well-being, elderly people with chronic pain avoid social activities for fear that they will not be able to meet their engagements, resulting in social isolation.[64,65] Considering the impact of accelerated aging in racial and ethnic minorities, pain may further worsen health in this population.[66–69] Thus, impoverished racial and ethnic minority elders may be particularly vulnerable to diminished health when they have pain.[70,71]

Few studies describing the impact of chronic pain on health examined an ethnically diverse population; as a consequence, the chronic pain experiences of vulnerable and underserved people have not been well described.[72] In a study of 7000 black and white Americans with chronic pain presenting to a tertiary care pain center, important differences were found in health based upon race and ethnicity.[60,61] Overall, black Americans report significantly more comorbidities, higher pain scores, increased pain severity, more suffering, and less control of pain than white Americans across the age continuum. Black Americans also reported increased physical disability (ie, impairment in activities of daily living [sexual, self-care, occupation, family life] due to pain), and more problems with sleep (ie, difficulty falling or staying asleep). The emotional health of black Americans was also severely affected by chronic pain.

Although both black and white Americans met criteria for clinical depression, the black Americans (regardless of age and gender) were significantly more depressed (consistent with moderate to severe depression). They also reported more symptoms consistent with post-traumatic stress disorder and anxiety than whites across the age continuum regardless of gender. It is unclear whether these findings reflect undertreatment, overreporting differences in pain sensitivity, or some combination of both. However, it is well documented that most individuals with depression go without treatment and that racial and ethnic minorities are often more reluctant than whites to seek treatment for mental health disorders.[71,73] Thus, it follows that pain and its sequelae are more likely to decrease the overall health and well-being of racial and ethnic minorities while further diminishing their quality of life.

▶ ASSESSMENT OF PAIN

I went to my new doctor. He checked me over pretty good. My prostate's okay and I feel pretty good. I don't believe in the flu shot—I know people who get the flu after taking the shot and I am going to take my chances. I don't get sick much anyway.

I have been hurting pretty good in my back though. So the doctor is going to get some x-rays of my back and a chest x-ray. I get around pretty good. My knees hurt. I think that it is just my arthritis. Some days I just ache and ache— I know snow is coming. My shoulder won't move—my thumb hurts and my back really hurts—it takes a while to get moving on those days. Sometimes there is no snow or rain and it just happens. I hurt every day. I don't take any pain pills but I take my blood pressure pill. When it is damp out I take some Tylenol and sometimes it gets better. You got to be careful to not take to much Tylenol. The doctor told me to take it so I do. I think it is just some cold in my back. It always hurts when I stand up and walk. Yesterday, I walked from the church to the rectory and had to stop and lean against the wall for awhile before I could go on. Sometimes I lean on the grocery basket to walk and that helps a lot. But I feel good and I am pretty lucky.... I can sit and watch my great grandson's wrestling matches. He's a good wrestler and I like sports where it is one man against another man. Anyway...I used to like to walk a lot but I don't walk much anymore.

—*Reflections on health and the impact of pain*

Despite the economic, psychological, familial, and social impact that chronic pain has on our society as well as an extensive literature documenting the benefits of optimizing pain management, guidelines designed to improve pain management are not universally used.[74–79] In fact, AHRQ sponsored the development of guidelines for pain assessment and treatment for several common conditions (eg, acute pain, chronic low back pain, and cancer pain).[74–76,78,79] An important limitation of this and other guidelines is that only one article specifically (although briefly) addresses the differential impact of pain on racial and ethnic minorities.[80] Yet, despite these guidelines developed to improve the quality of pain care, 40% of persons reported significant acute postoperative pain following surgery.[81] Among cancer patients, there are estimates that 70% die with unrelieved pain. Given clear evidence that racial and ethnic minorities suffer disproportionately more from all types of pain than do white Americans, it follows that the health status gap based on race and ethnicity is pervasive for acute, chronic, and cancer pain, as well. Thus, a pain care gap for racial and ethnic minorities also exists.

What bothers me more than anything was when you tell people that there's something wrong because I didn't have any kind of pain over here on this side and they don't listen to you. There has to be something wrong in here.

—*Reflections on the health-care experience*

Optimizing pain assessment can be problematic because pain is a subjective experience with no objective measures. The effects of pain vary substantially at the individual level. Patients with the same disease activity may report differences in pain intensity and its impact on their lives.[82–86] Both racial and ethnic minorities and women respond differently than white men to a painful stimulus.[62] In addition to race, increasing age and female gender may substantially increase the risk for physical and psychological impairment due to pain. This is an important consideration because elderly people, racial and ethnic minorities, and women often report increased pain and sequelae while being at increased risk for undertreatment.

The epidemiology of pain may be changing. New technology allowing an individual to survive significant and life-threatening trauma that would have ended in death a decade ago may also be associated with persistent and chronic pain.[87] A recent study examining intra-race differences in the chronic pain experience showed that younger blacks and whites experienced more morbidity and disability than their elders.[88] Although blacks carried a higher disease burden due to pain than whites in terms of diminished physical, social, and emotional health, this generation gap in pain has significant implications for both blacks and whites in an increasingly aging society.

I would like for them to know that I am in pain or this part of my body hurts or the other part hurts—that I am not lying about it. To examine me and to cut down on the pain...And help me out.[14]

—*Sickle cell focus group participant*

How race and ethnicity influence pain management–seeking behavior is unknown. The pain complaints of racial and ethnic minorities, the elderly, and women are often not treated similarly to the pain complaints of white men.[89–91] Disturbing racial and ethnic disparities in pain assessment and management have been identified.[72,92,93] Although the gold standard for pain assessment is patient report, physician estimates of a patient's pain intensity are lower than the patient's reports of pain intensity. Patient behavior, how patients communicate their pain complaints, physician–patient communication, and stereotyping can either complement or complicate the process. Thus, it follows that race and ethnicity are also important in assessing pain. There are clear differences in the way that women, racial and ethnic minorities, impoverished persons, and elderly people communicate their pain experiences, especially if there is a language barrier.[94–100] These differences in communication may increase the likelihood of pain complaints being discounted, especially if the patient's gender, race, or ethnicity is not congruous with the physician's. How racial and ethnic minorities present in terms of pain symptoms and whether their pain complaints differ when compared with whites remains unclear. Yet most measures used to assess pain in racial and ethnic minorities lack cultural and linguistic sensitivity and were not validated well in an ethnically diverse population.[101–105] Nonetheless, disturbing racial and ethnic disparities in pain assessment have been identified.[72,92]

Biologic, physiologic, and social mechanisms may explain differences in vulnerability to pain for racial and ethnic minorities.[53,91,92,106–109] Differences in pain-learning, culturally imposed factors, pain care beliefs, and social roles may predispose certain individuals toward multiple actions that maximize rather than minimize threats to bodily integrity or societal danger.[35,110–112] Fillingim reported wide variability in the response to a painful stimulus based on race using an experimental model.[113] From an experimental pain perspective, racial and ethnic minorities may be more vulnerable to pain-motivating circumstances.[17,92,109,114] However, these results remain controversial. Other experimental pain studies (ie, using a controlled stimulus) suggest that racial and ethnic minorities as well as women have lower thresholds for pain, greater ability to discriminate, higher pain ratings, and less tolerance to painful stimuli.[17,74–79,91,109,110,114–116] Differences in pain response have been attributed to race, ethnicity, gender, disease, age, culture, socio-economic status, past experiences, response bias, and experimental setting.[117–119] Altogether, the literature suggests that ethnic-based differences in response to experimentally induced pain may be influenced by multiple pain-modulating factors. The clinical relevance of these factors in clinical pain syndromes remains unknown.

Disability, depression, and pain intensity issues often complicate the assessment of chronic pain.[16,119,120] However, a study evaluating race, age, and gender influences among black and white clusters of patients with chronic pain (ie, chronic pain syndrome, good pain control, and disability with mild pain syndrome) upon initial presentation at a tertiary care pain center revealed important racial and age-related variability in pain symptom severity when patients presented with similar physical, emotional, and pain characteristics.[62] Again, racial and ethnic minorities had more disease burden than their white counterparts.

The first building block to quality pain care and physician pain management decision making is optimizing pain assessment.[121] Yet pain education is a neglected topic in most medical, nursing, dental, and pharmacy school curricula, further contributing to poor pain assessment for all patients.[122–127] In fact, a recent study of practicing Michigan physicians revealed that nearly 30% reported that they had not received any medical school, residency, or continuing medical education specifically directed at managing pain.[128] Thus, because of limited knowledge and education, physicians and health-care providers are ill-equipped to treat pain. In addition, health-care system factors, trust, legal factors, and health-care provider decision making influences pain assessment regardless of guidelines designed to ensure adequate pain care.

The literature supports the notion that racial and ethnic minorities are at risk for poor pain assessment when compared with non-Hispanics.[16,94,129–133] A retrospective study by Todd et al., In emergency departments found a two-fold difference in receiving analgesics based upon ethnicity in emergency room patients with acute pain secondary to isolated long bone fractures.[130] Other patient sociodemographic, substance use, or medical characteristics could not account for these differences. More specifically, 26% of non-Hispanic whites with isolated fractures of the femoral shaft, tibia, fibula, or humerus received no pain medications, whereas 55% of Hispanics received no pain medications for similar injuries.[130] In Schulman's landmark study using men and women who were black and white actors presenting similarly with acute chest pain, disturbing differences were identified, with women and racial and ethnic minorities receiving lesser quality care for their chest pain complaints.[134,135] Overall, the literature supports that physicians handle the pain complaints of racial and ethnic minorities less aggressively and there are differences in physician pain assessment and treatment based on patient characteristics regardless of the type of pain or the patient care setting. Bernabei's survey of 13,625 elderly nursing home residents with cancer showed that blacks were less likely to have their pain assessed and to have a pain score documented on their medical charts, and were 63% more likely than whites to receive no pain medications.[136] Although 40% of blacks with cancer pain reported daily pain, 25% received no analgesics whatsoever.

The emergency room used to be the worst part of my going to the hospital. The nurses didn't understand; they do all this questioning. They wanted to know why the medication was not working, why you are still in pain. If you are crying, why you are crying; if you are not crying, how can you be in pain? If you are laughing or talking, it is mental. Really you are not only experiencing your pain—the crises you are going through—but you are experiencing other peoples' opinions and feelings; that makes it worse. Dealing with your crisis and dealing with someone else who comes into your room to tell you that you can do this or, if you are doing that, something else is wrong. It's better for them to keep their opinions to themselves and just treat you.[14]

—*Sickle cell focus group participant*

For most patients with pain, it does not occur in isolation and the family is affected as well.[137–140] Sickle cell anemia provides an excellent example, because the patients are commonly children in pain who often need their parents to both advocate for them and convey their pain complaints.[141] Children with sickle cell anemia frequently miss school, owing to acute pain episodes and subsequent hospitalizations, while their parents miss work. Because there is often needless suffering, sickle cell anemia is often used as the *sine qua non* for disparities in pain care. Patients with sickle cell anemia and their families continue to provide stories documenting poor pain assessment and inadequate pain care during acute pain crises and for the chronic pain that often follows. Consider the common scenario of a sickle cell patient who presents to the emergency department (a place for universal around-the-clock access) in an acute pain crisis. The health-care provider–patient interaction in such a scenario can be challenging for racial and ethnic minorities, fraught with the potential for racial stereotyping, mistrust, and problematic physician–patient communication.[141]

In studies using patient-controlled analgesia (PCA) to examine the relationship between race and ethnicity and analgesic administration for acute postoperative pain, important findings were found. Ng found significant differences in physician prescriptions for opioid analgesics, with Hispanics receiving prescriptions less often than whites, but also found no differences in the amount of opioid analgesics that patients self-administered or in their pain intensity.[142–144] Because the health-care provider–patient interaction is minimized (prescribing of opioid analgesia is primarily the physician's responsibility whereas the amount consumed is based on the patient's request), PCA studies are important in understanding disparities in pain care.

▶ **PATIENT PERCEPTIONS AND ATTITUDES**

Patient attitudes and experiences often direct their preferences, information seeking, decision making, and health care. Several patient-related barriers exist to quality pain care that are especially problematic for racial and ethnic minority patients.[145,146] Green et al showed that black persons with chronic pain tend to believe more so than whites that race and ethnicity affected the health-care and pain care that they received.[147] Black patients also tend to believe that good patients avoid talking about pain and that pain medications could not really control pain.[147]

Health insurance coverage provides access to medical care and improves overall health but does not ensure equal health.[148] Overall, elderly black Americans with Medicare rated their health as poorer than elderly whites with similar insurance.[63] This is consistent with data provided by Green for chronic pain patients who had access to a tertiary care pain center; regardless of age, blacks had diminished physical and emotional health when compared to whites with chronic pain.[61] In another study, blacks reported increased difficulty paying for health care, compared with similar whites, despite having insurance and access to a tertiary care pain center. Blacks also reported, more so than whites, that they could not afford health care and that chronic pain was a major problem for them.[147] Black Americans also believed that race, ethnicity, culture, and gender influenced access to both health care and pain care.[147] These disparate attitudes have significant implications in a potentially vulnerable and underserved population at risk for poor pain assessment and management. It is also important to consider attitudes regarding pain and the quality of pain care in the context of racial and ethnic minorities' trust of the health-care system, since the bonds of trust are not well established (eg, Tuskegee syphilis experiments).[149] Thus, the question remains whether these perceptions or attitudes are valid or whether previous health-care experiences contributed to these beliefs.

▶ **COPING**

Passive coping and catastrophizing are detrimental to coping successfully with a pain problem.[108,150–152] Social support plays a significant role in the ability to cope with many chronic conditions, and an important role in pain management.[153] Differences in coping based on race and ethnicity have been identified. In several studies, blacks with chronic pain report more suffering due to pain than whites, regardless of age or gender.[60,61] These findings are particularly salient because differences were found in the ability to cope with pain. Older blacks reported more ability to cope with pain than younger blacks, younger whites, and older whites. Black patients also reported significantly less ability to control their pain symptoms and more impairment in their sleep due to pain. John Henryism (ie, a pattern of high-output active coping, characterized by working harder against a potentially insurmountable obstacle, that has been demonstrated in blacks and speculated to originate from slavery times) has been associated with hypertension and bodily pain.[154–156] Considering the high prevalence of hypertension in racial and ethnic minorities, further investigations are necessary to see whether or not John Henryism is actually detrimental or helpful to racial and ethnic minorities who are living with chronic pain. More research is needed regarding the relationship between pain, coping styles, environmental stressors, and comorbidities in ethnically diverse populations.

▶ **ACCESS TO PAIN CARE**

Not having a primary care physician or a usual source of medical care hinders access to quality pain care for racial and ethnic minorities.[48,147] Individuals without health insurance or a primary care physician are more likely to use emergency departments for care. In addition, racial and ethnic minorities are less likely to have a regular primary care physician and, therefore, have less access to specialty care.[63,146] Even when minorities have a primary care physician and health insurance, they may experience more difficulty in securing referrals to specialty physicians from their primary care physician. In addition, because there are close associations between race, ethnicity, and income; rising co-pays for health-care services tend to affect racial and ethnic minorities disproportionately more than whites. Overall, racial and ethnic minorities have less access to pain management specialists, receive less pain medication, and are at risk for undertreatment of their pain complaints.[16,129,136] This is particularly important considering the fact that there is also an increased disease burden for many comorbid conditions associated with pain (eg, diabetes, cancer) that additionally and differentially affect the health and well-being of racial and ethnic minorities when compared with whites.[11,50,157]

Author: Did the pain scare you?
Patient: No. I wasn't afraid. I'm never afraid of anything like that. I don't fear dying or anything like that because I know that when it happens, I won't know anything about it anyway. You're gone.... I can't worry about it. I can't fear something like that. What I fear would be anticipating that kind of pain, knowing that it was coming, and you couldn't do anything about it. I don't know if that would be fear. That would be very uncomfortable if you knew that this kind of pain was coming and you couldn't do anything about it. You look up at the clock. Now get ready, son. It's 10 minutes to 2:00p. At 2:00p Thor is going to come out and is going to try to chop his way out of your chest. That would be scary. But as long as you know there's a way to relieve the pain, it's okay.

—*Reflections on dying and pain*

On the whole, suboptimal pain assessment and treatment for all types of pain (ie, acute, chronic nonmalignant, cancer) contribute to poorer health status and quality of life for racial and ethnic minorities when compared with whites.[16] In a recent study, black patients with chronic pain believed more frequently than whites that they should have been referred to a pain center sooner, reported decreased access to health care overall, and believed that ethnicity influenced pain care.[147] Blacks with chronic pain reported that chronic pain is a major financial burden and also reported increased difficulty paying for pain care than whites with similar access to the pain center.[147] Cleeland showed that minority cancer patients were prescribed less potent analgesics, and 42% were undertreated using WHO recommendations for managing cancer pain.[27,158–160] In another study, Cleeland showed that racial and ethnic minority cancer patients treated at university centers or at centers primarily caring for racial and ethnic minorities were more likely to receive inadequate analgesia than were white patients treated elsewhere and in the community.[146,161] Anderson showed that black and Hispanic patients received insufficient care to manage their pain and that physicians underestimated severity for the majority of these patients.[70] In another study by Anderson, health-care providers in minority centers ranked lack of access to a wide range of analgesics as an important barrier to quality pain care.[145,162] A recent study by Shaya et al found racial disparities in the prescription of cyclooxygenase-2 inhibitors (COX-2) analgesics when compared with other nonsteroidal anti-inflammatory agents for black and white patients in a Medicaid managed care organization.[163] This study found that blacks were one third less likely to receive prescriptions for COX-2 analgesics than whites. Overall, these studies illustrate that racial and ethnic minority patients reported more pain, less pain relief, and were less likely to be adequately assessed for all types of pain and in all settings than white patients.

▶ PROVIDER VARIABILITY IN PAIN MANAGEMENT DECISION MAKING

Author: Tell me about the pain that you had when you had to wait for your pain medicines. What was that like?

Patient: Now that was some pain. I never had any kind of pain like that before. It felt like a little guy had a knife, trying to get out from the inside. It was tough. You all have this "1 to 10" thing. You can't measure pain like that. There was no "10" like that. That's a "35"—it isn't a "10." It's real pain. I was making noise.

Author: What do you mean you were making noise?

Patient: I was making noise! Some people grunt. I did everything but scream but I came close. I made some noise. Usually I don't make noise, I make faces with pain. But this time I made a little noise. There was some grunting and groaning going on. It came in stages. The first wave was "10." The next wave was "14." The last wave was "35."

I made up a skit for this pain about how it feels when the pain starts. It was like there was this little guy with a dagger inside my chest and he was trying to poke his way out. He comes out of my chest and pokes on my chest. Then he goes back inside my chest to see if the morphine has come yet. He said, "No. No morphine yet!" He goes outside my back to poke on my chest some more. That pain is a "10." He (the little guy) then sends Zorro out. Zorro has this knife—a sword. Zorro comes out and this pain is a little bit tougher. He goes slashing around. About that time, that pain's a "14." The "10" was the little guy. Zorro was a "14." He goes back and says, "The morphine still hasn't come. You can go out there and do what you want to do. Then they send Thor out with

the battle-ax. He comes out and he starts chopping—he's trying to chop his way out of my chest. That pain's a "35." That's the screaming and hollering pain. If that morphine don't get there in a hurry, you gonna do a lotta screaming and hollering.

That's all I'm saying about the pain medication. I think some of it has to be given—you just gotta take some pain medication if you can get it. You take it just in case the pain comes. The Vicodin is what you take when there ain't no pain and you figure it might show up in an hour. Because once the pain starts, by the time that Vicodin kicks in, you jumped out the window already! Morphine is for when that pain hits. When that pain gets to you, you got to have the morphine unless you want to scream and holler for an hour until the Vicodin kicks in.

So however long it takes, I know one thing—it (Vicodin) ain't fast enough. When you put your nurse button on to tell her you are having some pain and she shows up an hour or so later and offers you Vicodin, you say, "that Vicodin was for the 12:00 pain (when I first asked for pain medicine) and it's now 1:00." Morphine is for the 1:00 pain.

Vicodin takes too long. I don't know how long it takes, but it's too long. Now when you have that kind of pain, it wears you out. You're tired. About 20 minutes, no, within 10–15 minutes, you get tired. When it (the pain) subsides you're really, really relieved. You can really feel the relief.

—Elderly man's reflections on waiting for pain relief

Although pain is a common complaint, several studies provide documentation that health-care providers are neither knowledgeable about nor satisfied with the pain care they provide.[119,120,128,164] Despite pain management guidelines and unprecedented advances in treatment modalities, the undertreatment of pain remains problematic. Physicians' confidence in their pain management is often misplaced and not based on knowledge, while their goals for pain relief vary based on the type of pain. For instance, Michigan physicians had lesser goals for chronic pain relief, less satisfaction with their chronic pain management, and provided lesser quality pain care for chronic pain complaints than the pain care provided for acute and cancer pain. Using several clinical pain vignettes, the quality of physician-prescribed pain care for chronic pain was less than the pain care provided for acute or cancer pain. This is important, because the physicians reported seeing a higher percentage of patients with chronic pain while prescribing opioid analgesic less frequently for such patients. Consistent with Schulman's study, race, age, and gender seemed to play a role in how physicians made their decisions for similar pain problems.[135] It follows that physicians may be less likely or willing to hear chronic pain complaints, especially those of racial and ethnic minorities, contributing to suboptimal care for chronic pain. Thus, physician perceptions and goals may lead to variability and the unintentional undertreatment of pain (especially chronic pain) for all Americans and for racial and ethnic minorities, in particular.

The worker's compensation literature also provides evidence for disparate pain care.[165,166] Racial and ethnic minorities were twice as likely as whites to be disabled 6 months after occupational back injuries. In another worker's compensation study by Tait et al, blacks without legal representation received less treatment and received lower disability ratings than whites without legal representation.[167] However, when both blacks and whites had legal representation, no differences were found in disability ratings or in treatment received. In addition, for blacks in the worker's compensation system, less treatment was also associated with less satisfaction with the process, and with higher levels of post-settlement disability.[168,169] Taken together, these findings suggest that disparities in treatment are associated with disparities in disability and outcomes.

Racial and ethnic minorities face additional barriers to adequate pain management. In two pharmacy studies, pharmacies located in minority neighborhoods were less likely to carry opioid analgesics than those in nonminority neighborhoods.[170] Green also showed that blacks used less complementary and alternative medicine techniques (including acupuncture) and significantly less manipulation, biofeedback, or relaxation training than whites for chronic pain.[171] Thus, poor pain assessment, inadequate pain treatment, and decreased ability to obtain pain medications (even when prescribed) complicate appropriate and quality pain management for racial and ethnic minority persons, thereby impairing their overall health and well-being. In conjunction with the findings presented in this chapter, there is a critical need for advocacy and health-care policy to rectify these ills.

► SUMMARY AND RECOMMENDATIONS

Pain profoundly affects morbidity, mortality, quality of life, and health-care expenditures. The potential implications of poorly treated pain are devastating for the individual, and the cost to society is staggering. Therefore, ensuring optimal pain management is critically important from a public health perspective.[172,173]

There is evidence that pain (especially chronic pain) has unique health implications in racial and ethnic minorities that are often unrecognized or overlooked.[16,60,61,74] There are no longitudinal and prospective studies to examine the long-term effects of pain on overall health and well-being in an ethnically diverse population. It is clear that in addition to race and ethnicity, age, gender, and socioeconomic factors may make certain racial and ethnic minorities more vulnerable to pain. Thus, racial and ethnic minorities who are elderly, impoverished, or women are extremely vulnerable to the distressing effects of pain.[55,60–62,174–178]

Appropriate cultural and linguistic interventions must be developed to ensure quality pain assessment and management such that racial and ethnic disparities in pain care can be eliminated. The role of health-care provider variability in pain management decision making as well as health-care system factors must be examined. It is by improving pain care for the underserved and most vulnerable populations in our society that pain care will be improved for all.[148,179,180] In a climate of increasing patient safety concerns, inadequate pain assessment and treatment must be viewed as a quality-of-care issue.[181–183] In the middle of the Decade for Pain Research and Control, pain relief is fundamentally a human rights issue while inadequate pain care is fundamentally a medical error.[184,185]

► ACKNOWLEDGMENTS

The author wishes to thank Mr Frank LaMar, Jr, Ms Julian F. Posey, and Mr Donald Smith for sharing their story with you and her. She also thanks the Michigan-Pain Outcomes Study Team (M-POST), Michigan Center for Urban African American Aging Research (MCUAAAR), and Marcus A. Hatter, MD, for their inspiration and ongoing support.

► REFERENCES

1. Baquet CR, Hammond C, Commiskey P, et al. Health disparities research—A model for conducting research on cancer disparities: characterization and reduction. *J Assoc Acad Minor Phys* 2002;13(2):33–40.
2. Institute of Medicine. The Institute of Medicine's goal to eliminate health care disparities. In Swift E, ed. *Guidance for the National Healthcare Disparities Report*. Washington, DC: National Academy Press; 2002.
3. Lurie N. Addressing health disparities: Where should we start? *Health Serv Res* 2002;37(5): 1125–1127.
4. Bierman AS, Clancy CM. Health disparities among older women: Identifying opportunities to improve quality of care and functional health outcomes. *J Am Med Womens Assoc* 2001;56(4): 155–159,188.
5. James SA. Confronting the moral economy of US racial/ethnic health disparities. *Am J Public Health* 2003;93(2):189–190.
6. Association for Healthcare Research and Quality. *National Healthcare Disparities Report*. Rockville, Md: US Dept of Health and Human Services;2003:195.
7. Green CR, Tait RC, Gallagher RM. Introduction: The unequal burden of pain: Disparities and differences. *Pain Med* 2005;6(1):1–2.
8. Glanz K, Croyle RT, Chollette VY, Pinn VW. Cancer-related health disparities in women. *Am J Public Health* 2003;93(2):292–298.
9. Gunn CC. Chronic pain: Time for epidemiology. *J R Soc Med* 1996;89(8):479–480.
10. Crombie IK, Davies HT, Macrae WA. The epidemiology of chronic pain: Time for new directions. *Pain* 1994;57(1):1–3.
11. Smedley B, Stith A, Nelson A. *Unequal Treatment: Confronting Racial and Ethnic Disparities in Health Care*. Washington, DC: National Academy Press; 2003.
12. National Institutes of Health, National Institute on Neurological Disorders and Stroke. *Five-Year Plan on Minority Health Disparities. Area of Focus IV: Health Disparities in Treatment and Management of Chronic Pain Disorders.* Bethesda, Md: NIH; 2001.
13. Mueller KJ, Ortega ST, Parker K, et al. Health status and access to care among rural minorities. *J Health Care Poor Underserved* 1999;10(2):230–249.
14. Nerenz DR, Bonham VL, Green-Weir R, et al. Eliminating racial/ethnic disparities in health care: Can health plans generate reports? *Health Aff (Millwood)* 2002;21(3):259–263.
15. Frist WH. Shattuck lecture: Health care in the 21st century. *N Engl J Med* 2005;352(3):267–272.
16. Green CR, Anderson KO, Baker TA, et al. The unequal burden of pain: Confronting racial and ethnic disparities in pain. *Pain Med* 2003;4(3): 277–294.
17. Edwards RR, Fillingim RB. Ethnic differences in

thermal pain responses. *Psychosom Med* 1999; 61(3):346–354.

18. Fishman SM, Gallagher RM, Carr DB, Sullivan LW, The case for pain medicine. *Pain Med* 2004; 5(3):281–286.

19. Gallagher RM, Verma S. Managing pain and co-morbid depression: A public health challenge. *Semin Clin Neuropsychiatry* 1999;4(3):203–220.

20. Gallagher RM. Primary care and pain medicine. A community solution to the public health problem of chronic pain. *Med Clin North Am* 1999;83 (3):555–583.

21. Moore R, Brodsgarrd I. Cross cultural investigations of pain. In: Crombie IK, ed. *Epidemiology of Pain*. Seattle, Wash: IASP Press; 1999:53–80.

22. Pearl JD. Cancer pain management: Still a public health issue. *Am Soc Anesthesiol* 1998;62:17.

23. Breslow L. A quantitative approach to the World Health Organization definition of health: Physical, mental and social well-being. *Int J Epidemiol* 1972;1(4):347–355.

24. Kelly MP. The World Health Organisation's definition of health promotion: Three problems. *Health Bull (Edinb)* 1990;48(4):176–180.

25. Fields HL, ed. *Core Curriculum for Professional Education in Pain,* 2nd ed. Seattle, Wash: IASP Press; 1995.

26. Skevington SM. Investigating the relationship between pain and discomfort and quality of life, using the WHOQOL. *Pain* 1998;76(3):395–406.

27. Cleeland CS. The impact of pain on the patient with cancer. *Cancer* 1984;54(11 suppl):2635–2341.

28. Ferrell BR, Griffith H. Cost issues related to pain management: Report from the Cancer Pain Panel of the Agency for Health Care Policy and Research. *J Pain Symptom Manage* 1994;9(4):221–234.

29. Scher AI, Stewart WF, Lipton RB. Migraine and headache: A meta-analytic approach. In: Crombie IK, ed. *Epidemiology of Pain*. Seattle, Wash: IASP Press; 1999:159–170.

30. Crombie IK, ed. *Epidemiology of Pain*. Seattle, Wash: IASP Press; 1999.

31. Schmader KE. Epidemiology and impact on quality of life of postherpetic neuralgia and painful diabetic neuropathy. *Clin J Pain* 2002;18: 350–354.

32. Whelan CT, Jin L, Meltzer D. Pain and satisfaction with pain control in hospitalized medical patients: No such thing as low risk. *Arch Intern Med* 2004;164(2):175–180.

33. Feine JS, Lund JP. An assessment of the efficacy of physical therapy and physical modalities for the control of chronic musculoskeletal pain. *Pain* 1997;71(1):5–23.

34. Call-Schmidt TA, Richardson SJ. Prevalence of sleep disturbance and its relationship to pain in adults with chronic pain. *Pain Manage Nurs* 2003;4(3):124–133.

35. Kulich RJ, Mencher P, Bertrand C, Maciewicz R. Comorbidity of post-traumatic stress disorder and chronic pain: Implications for clinical and forensic assessment. *Curr Rev Pain* 2000;4(1): 36–48.

36. Buchwald D, Goldberg J, Noonan C, et al. Relationship between post-traumatic stress disorder and pain in two American Indian tribes. *Pain Med* 2005;6(1):72–79.

37. Bland CJ, Schmitz CC. Characteristics of the successful researcher and implications for faculty development. *J Med Educ* 1986;61(1): 22–31.

38. Menefee LA, Frank, ED, Doghramji K, et al. Self-reported sleep quality and quality of life for individuals with chronic pain conditions. *Clin J Pain* 2000;16(4):290–297.

39. Subramanian K, Rose SD. Social work and the treatment of chronic pain. *Health Soc Work* 1988;13(1):49–60.

40. Vasudevan S. Management of chronic pain: What we achieved in the last 25 years. In: Ghia JN, ed. *The Multidisciplinary Pain Center Organization and Personnel Functions for Pain Management*. Boston, Mass: Kluwer Academic; 1998:85–115.

41. LeResche L. Gender differences in pain: Epidemiologic perspectives. *Pain Forum* 1995;4(4): 228–230.

42. Roy R. *Chronic Pain in Old Age. An Integrated Biopsychological Perspective*. Toronto: University of Toronto Press; 1995.

43. Walls C, Zarit S. Informal support from black churches and the well-being of elderly blacks. *Gerontologist* 1991;31(4):490–495.

44. Crook J, Rideout E, Browne C. The prevalence of pain complaints in a general population. *Pain* 1984;18(3):299–314.

45. Ferrell BA. Pain evaluation and management in the nursing home. *Ann Intern Med* 1995;123 (9):681–687.

46. Nurmikko TJ, Nash TP, Wiles JR. Recent advances: Control of chronic pain. *BMJ* 1998;317 (7170):1438–1441.

47. Ryes-Gibby CC, Aday L, Cleeland C. Impact of pain on self-rated health in community-dwelling older adults. *Pain* 2002;95:75–82.

48. Green CR. Pain: Racial disparities in access to pain treatment. *Clin Updates* 2004;XII(6):1–4.

49. James SA, Keenan NL, Strogatz DS. Socioeconomic status, John Henryism and blood pressure in black adults: The Pitt County study. *Am J Epidemiol* 1992;135(1):59–67.

50. Lillie-Blanton M, Brodie M, Rowland D, et al. Race, ethnicity, and the health care system: Public perceptions and experiences. *Med Care Res Rev* 2000;57(1):218–235.

51. Williams DR, Lavizzo-Mourey R, Warren RC. The concept of race and health status in America. *Public Health Rep* 1994;109(1):26–41.

52. Williams DR. Race, socioeconomic status, and health. The added effects of racism and discrimination. *Ann N Y Acad Sci* 1999;896:173–188.

53. Loeser JD, Melzack R. Pain: An overview. *Lancet* 1999;353(9164):1607–1609.

54. Mathias SD, Kuppermann M, Liberman RF, et al. Chronic pelvic pain: Prevalence, health-related quality of life, and economic correlates. *Obstet Gynecol* 1996;87(3):321–327.

55. Roberto KA. Chronic pain in the lives of older women. *J Am Med Womens Assoc* 1997;52(3):127–131.

56. Farrell MJ. Pain and aging. *Am Pain Soc Bull* 2000;10(4):8–12.

57. Goldman B. Chronic-pain patients must cope with chronic lack of physician understanding. CAMJ 1991; 144(11):1492,1494–1495,1497.

58. Gagliese L, Melzack R. Chronic pain in elderly people. *Pain* 1997;70(1):3–14.

59. Helme RD, Gibson SJ. The epidemiology of pain in elderly people. *Clin Geriatr Med* 2001;17 (3):417–431.

60. Green CR, Baker TA, Sato Y, et al. Race and chronic pain: A comparative study of young black and white Americans presenting for management. *J Pain* 2003;4(4):176–183.

61. Green CR, Baker TA, Smith EM, Sato Y. The effect of race in older adults presenting for chronic pain management: A comparative study of African and Caucasian Americans. *J Pain* 2003;4 (2):82–90.

62. Green CR, Ndao-Brumblay SK, Nagrant AM, et al. Race, age, and gender influences among clusters of African American and white patients with chronic pain. *J Pain* 2004;5(3):171–182.

63. Collins K, Hall A, Neuhaus C. *U.S. Minority Health: A Chartbook*. New York, NY: Commonwealth Fund; 1999:161.

64. Gibson SJ, Katz B, Corran TM, et al. Pain in older persons. *Disabil Rehabil* 1994;16(3):127–139.

65. Mobily PR, et al. An epidemiologic analysis of pain in the elderly. *J Aging Health* 1994;6(2): 139–154.

66. LaVeist TA. On the study of race, racism, and health: A shift from description to explanation. *Am J Public Health* 2000;93(12):2067–2073.

67. Maynard C, Beshansky RJ, Griffith JL, Selker HP, et al. Causes of chest pain and symptoms suggestive of acute cardiac ischemia in African-American patients presenting to the emergency department: A multicenter study. *J Natl Med Assoc* 1997;89(10):665–671.

68. Goodman AH. Why genes don't count (for racial differences in health). *Am J Public Health* 2000;90(11):1699–1702.

69. Harrell JP, Hall S, Taliaferro J. Physiological responses to racism and discrimination: An assessment of the evidence. *Am J Public Health* 2003;93(2):243–247.

70. Anderson KO, Mendoza TR, Valero V, et al. Minority cancer patients and their providers: Pain management attitudes and practice. *Cancer* 2000;88(8):1929–1938.

71. Ruiz P, Venegas-Samuels K, Alarcon RD. The economics of pain. Mental health care costs among minorities. *Psychiatr Clin North Am* 1995; 18(3):659–670.

72. McCracken L, Matthews AK, Tang TS, Cuba SL. A comparison of blacks and whites seeking treatment for chronic pain. *Clin J Pain* 2001;17:249–255.

73. Kales HC, Blow FC, Bingham CR, et al. Race, psychiatric diagnosis, and mental health care utilization in older patients. *Am J Geriatr Psychiatry* 2000;8(4):301–309.

74. Green CR, Tait A. Attitudes of healthcare professionals regarding different modalities used to manage acute postoperative pain. *Acute Pain* 2002;4(1):15–21.

75. Jacox A, Carr DB, Payne R. New clinical-practice guidelines for the management of pain in patients with cancer. *N Engl J Med* 1994;330(9):651–655.

76. Carr E. How to achieve effective pain management. *Nurs Times* 1997;93(37):52–53.

77. Carr E. Myths and fears about pain-relieving drugs. *Nurs Times* 1997;93(40):50–51.

78. Carr DB, Miaskowski C, Dedrick SC, Williams GR. Management of perioperative pain in hospitalized patients: A national survey. *J Clin Anesth* 1998;10(1):77–85.

79. Carr TD, Lemanek KL, Armstrong FD. Pain and fear ratings: Clinical implications of age and gender Differences. *J Pain Symptom Manage* 1998; 15(5):305–313.

80. Ashburn M, et al. Practice guidelines for acute pain management in the preoperative setting: An updated report by the American Society of Anesthesiologist's task force on acute pain management. *Anesthesiology* 2004;100(1573–1581).

81. Bonica JJ. Cancer pain: A major national health problem. *Cancer Nurs* 1978;1(4):313–316.

82. Aguirre J, Gallardo R, Pareja JA, Perez-Miranda M. Cluster of MMPI personality profiles in chronic tension-type headache and predictable response to fluoxetine. *Cephalalgia* 2000;20(1): 51–56.

83. Buckelew SP, Shutty MS Jr, Hewett J, et al. Health locus of control, gender differences and adjustment to persistent pain. *Pain* 1990;42(3):287–294.

84. Cipher DJ, Clifford PA, Schumacker RE. The heterogeneous pain personality: Diverse coping styles among sufferers of chronic pain. *Altern Ther Health Med* 2002;8(6):60–69.

85. Cook AJ, Chastain DC. The classification of patients with chronic pain: Age and sex differences. *Pain Res Manage* 2001;6(3):142–151.

86. Corran TM, Farrell MJ, Helme RD, Gibson SJ. The classification of patients with chronic pain: Age as a contributing factor. *Clin J Pain* 1997;13 (3):207–214.

87. McCracken LM, Gross RT, Aikens J, Carnrike CL Jr. The assessment of anxiety and fear in persons with chronic pain: A comparison of instruments. *Behav Res Ther* 1996;34(11–12):927–933.

88. Baker TA, Green CR. Intrarace differences among black and white Americans presenting for chronic pain management: The influence of age, physical health, and psychosocial factors. *Pain Med* 2005;6(1):28–38.

89. Riley JL 3rd, Wade JB, Myers CD, et al. Racial/ethnic differences in the experience of chronic pain. *Pain* 2002;100(3):291–298.

90. Weisse CS, Sorum PC, Sanders KN, Syat BL, et al. Do gender and race affect decisions about pain management? *J Gen Intern Med* 2001;16(4):211–217.

91. Edwards RR, Moric M, Husfeldt B, et al. Ethnic similarities and differences in the chronic pain experience: A comparison of African American, Hispanic, and white patients. *Pain Med* 2005;6 (1):88–98.

92. Edwards CL, Fillingim RB, Keefe F. Race, ethnicity and pain: A review. *Pain* 2001;94(2):133–137.

93. Weisse, CS, Foster KK, Fisher EA. The influence of experimenter gender and race on pain reporting: Does racial or gender concordance matter? *Pain Med* 2005;6(1):80–87.

94. Todd KH, Lee T, Hoffman JR. The effect of ethnicity on physician estimates of pain severity in patients with isolated extremity trauma. *JAMA* 1994;271(12):925–928.

95. Towery S, Fernandez E. Reclassification and rescaling of McGill Pain Questionnaire verbal descriptors of pain sensation: A replication. *Clin J Pain* 1996;12(4):270–276.

96. Sist TC, Florio GA, Miner MF, et al. The relationship between depression and pain language in cancer and chronic non-cancer pain patients. *J Pain Symptom Manage* 1998;15(6):350–358.

97. Birdwell BG, Herbers JE, Kroenke K. Evaluating chest pain. The patient's presentation style alters the physician's diagnostic approach. *Arch Intern Med* 1993;153(17):1991–1995.

98. Grossman SA, Sheidler R, Swedeen K, et al. Correlation of patient and caregiver ratings of cancer pain. *J Pain Symptom Manage* 1991;6(2):53–57.

99. Closs SJ. Pain in elderly patients: A neglected phenomenon? *J Adv Nurs* 1994;19(6):1072–1081.

100. Lasch KE. Culture, pain, and culturally sensitive pain care. *Pain Manage Nurs* 2000;1(3 suppl 1):16–22.

101. Barrett B, Shadick K, Shilling R, et al. Hmong/medicine interactions: Improving cross-cultural health care. *Fam Med* 1998;30(3):179–184.

102. Nelson DV, Novy DM, Averill PM, Berry LA. Ethnic comparability of the MMPI in pain patients. *J Clin Psychol* 1996;52(5):485–497.

103. Kremer E, Atkinson JH Jr. Pain measurement: Construct validity of the affective dimension of the McGill Pain Questionnaire with chronic benign pain patients. *Pain* 1981;11(1):93–100.

104. Borkan J, Reis S, Hermoni D, Biderman A. Talking about the pain: A patient-centered study of low back pain in primary care. *Soc Sci Med* 1995; 40(7):977–988.

105. Howell JD. Ethnicity and estimates of pain by physicians. *JAMA* 1994;272(15):1168–1169.

106. Melzack R, Wall PD. Pain mechanisms: A new theory. *Science* 1965;150(699):971–979.

107. Haefner HK, Khoshnevisan MH, Bachman JG, et al. Use of the McGill Pain Questionnaire to compare women with vulvar pain, pelvic pain and headaches. *J Reprod Med* 2000;45(8):665–671.

108. Geisser ME, Roth RS, Bachman JE, Eckert TA. The relationship between symptoms of posttraumatic stress disorder and pain, affective disturbance and disability among patients with accident and non-accident related pain. *Pain* 1996;66(2–3):207–214.

109. Edwards RR, Doleys DM, Fillingim RB, Lowery D. Ethnic differences in pain tolerance: Clinical implications in a chronic pain population. *Psychosom Med* 2001;63(2):316–323.

110. Edwards R, Augustson EM, Fillingim R. Sex-specific effects of pain-related anxiety on adjustment to chronic pain. *Clin J Pain* 2000;16(1):46–53.

111. Green C, Flowe-Valencia H, Rosenblum L, Tait AR. Do physical and sexual abuse differentially affect chronic pain states in women? *J Pain Symptom Manage* 1999;18(6):420–426.

112. Green CR, Flowe-Valencia H, Rosenblum L, Tait AR. The role of childhood and adulthood abuse among women presenting for chronic pain management. *Clin J Pain* 2001;17:359–364.

113. Edwards RR, Ness TJ, Weigent DA, Fillingim RB. Individual differences in diffuse noxious inhibitory controls (DNIC): Association with clinical variables. *Pain* 2003;106(3):427–437.

114. Edwards RR, Fillingim RB, Yamauchi S, et al. Effects of gender and acute dental pain on thermal pain responses. *Clin J Pain* 1999;15(3):233–237.

115. Fillingim RB, Edwards RR, Powell T. Sex-dependent effects of reported familial pain history on recent pain complaints and experimental pain responses. *Pain* 2000;86(1–2):87–94.

116. Fillingim RB, Edwards RR, Powell T. The relationship of sex and clinical pain to experimental pain responses. *Pain* 1999;83(3):419–425.

117. Edwards RR, Fillingim RB, Ness TJ. Age-related differences in endogenous pain modulation: A comparison of diffuse noxious inhibitory controls in healthy older and younger adults. *Pain* 2003;101:155–165.

118. Edwards R, Augustson E, Fillingim R. Differential relationships between anxiety and treatment-associated pain reduction among male and female chronic pain patients. *Clin J Pain* 2003;19(4):208–216.

119. Green CR, Wheeler JR, LaPorte F, et al. How well is chronic pain managed? Who does it well? *Pain Med* 2002;3(1):56–65.

120. Green CR, Wheeler JR, LaPorte F. Clinical decision making in pain management: Contributions of physician and patient characteristics to variations in practice. *J Pain* 2003;4(22):29–39.

121. Green CR. Racial disparities in access to pain treatment. In: *Pain Clinical Updates.* Seattle, Wash: IASP Press; 2004:1–4.

122. Clarke EB, French B, Bilodeau ML, et al. Pain management knowledge, attitudes and clinical practice: The impact of nurses' characteristics and education. *J Pain Symptom Manage* 1996;11(1):18–31.

123. Weis OF, et al. Attitudes of patients, house staff and nurses toward postoperative analgesia care. *Anesth Analg* 1983;62(1):70–74.

124. Weiner D, Peterson B, Ladd K, et al. Pain in nursing home residents: An exploration of prevalence, staff perspectives, and practical aspects of measurement. *Clin J Pain* 1999;15(2):92–101.

125. Turk DC. Clinicians' attitudes about prolonged use of opioids and the issue of patient heterogeneity. *J Pain Symptom Manage* 1996;11(4):218–230.

126. Weinstein SM, Laux LF, Thornby JL, et al. Physicians' attitudes toward pain and the use of opioid analgesics: Results of a survey from the Texas Cancer Pain Initiative. *South Med J* 2000; 93(5):479–487.

127. Weinstein SM, Laux LF, Thornby JL, et al. Medical students' attitudes toward pain and the use of opioid analgesics: Implications for changing medical school curriculum. *South Med J* 2000; 93(5):472–478.

128. Green, CR, Wheeler JR, Marchant B, et al. Analysis of the physician variable in pain management. *Pain Med* 2001;2(4):317–327.

129. Bonham VL. Race, ethnicity, and pain treatment: Striving to understand the causes and solutions to the disparities in pain treatment. *J Law Med Ethics* 2001;29(1):52–68.

130. Todd K, Samaroo N, Hoffman J. Ethnicity as a risk factor in inadequate emergency department analgesia. *JAMA* 1993;269(12):1537–1539.

131. Todd KH. Pain assessment and ethnicity. *Ann Emerg Med* 1996;27(4):421–423.

132. Todd KH, Deaton C, D'Adamo AP, Goe L. Ethnicity and analgesic practice. *Ann Emerg Med* 2000; 35(1):11–16.

133. Todd KH. Influence of ethnicity on emergency department pain management. *Emerg Med (Fremantle)* 2001;13(3):274–278.

134. Chibnall J, Dabney A, Tait R. Internist judgements of chronic low back pain. *Pain Med* 2000; 1:231–237.

135. Schulman KA, Berlin JA, Harless W, et al. The effect of race and sex on physicians' recommendations for cardiac catheterization. *New Engl J Med* 1999;340(8):618–626.

136. Bernabei R, Gambassi G, Lapane K, et al. Management of pain in elderly patients with cancer. SAGE Study Group. Systematic assessment of geriatric drug use via epidemiology. *JAMA* 1998; 279(23):1877–1882.

137. Rodgers C, Levin L, Robeson M, Kunkel EJ. Pain and disability in families of chronic noncancer pain patients. *Psychosomatics* 1996;37(5):476–480.

138. Benjamin LJ, Swinson GI, Nagel RL. Sickle cell anemia day hospital: An approach for the management of uncomplicated painful crises. *Blood* 2000;95(4):1130–1137.

139. Gil KM. Coping with sickle cell disease pain. *Soc Behav Med* 1989;11(2):49–57.

140. Platt OS, Thorington BD, Branbilla DJ, et al. Pain in sickle cell disease. Rates and risk factors. *N Engl J Med* 1991;325(1):11–16.

141. Whitten CF, Waugh D, Moore A. *Unmet Needs of Parents of Children with Sickle Cell Anemia.* Detroit, Mich: Wayne State University School of Medicine; 1998:275–276.

142. Ng A, et al. Bridging the analgesic gap. *Acute Pain* 2000;3(4):194–199.

143. Ng B, Dimsdale JE, Rollnick JD, Shapiro H. The effect of ethnicity on prescriptions for patient-controlled analgesia for post-operative pain. *Pain* 1996;66(1):9–12.

144. Ng B, Dimsdale JE, Shragg GP, Deutsch R. Ethnic differences in analgesic consumption for post-operative pain. *Psychosom Med* 1996;58(2):125–129.

145. Anderson K, et al. Multi-site randomized trial of pain management education for minority outpatients with cancer pain. *Pain* 2003;4(2):95.

146. Cleeland CS, Gonin R, Baez L, et al. Pain and treatment of pain in minority patients with cancer. The Eastern Cooperative Oncology Group Minority Outpatient Pain Study. *Ann Intern Med* 1997;127(9):813–816.

147. Green CR, Baker TA, Ndao-Brumblay SK. Patient attitudes regarding healthcare utilization and referral: A descriptive comparison in African- and Caucasian Americans with chronic pain. *J Natl Med Assoc* 2004;96(1):31–42.

148. Primm BJ, Perez L, Dennis GC, et al. Managing pain: The challenge in underserved populations: Appropriate use versus abuse and diversion. *J Natl Med Assoc* 2004;96(9):1152–1161.

149. Northington-Gamble VN. Under the shadow of Tuskegee: African Americans and health care. *A J Public Health* 1997;87(11):1773–1778.

150. Riley JL 3rd, Robinson ME, Geisser ME. Empirical subgroups of the Coping Strategies Questionnaire-Revised: A multisample study. *Clin J Pain* 1999;15(2):111–116.

151. Geisser ME, Roth RS, Theisen ME, et al. Negative affect, self-report of depressive Symptoms, and clinical depression: Relation to the experience of chronic pain. *Clin J Pain* 2000;16(2):110–120.

152. Geisser ME, Roth RS, Robinson ME. Assessing depression among persons with chronic pain using the Center for Epidemiological Studies–Depression Scale and the Beck Depression Inventory: A comparative analysis. *Clin J Pain* 1997;13(2):163–170.

153. Ford M, Tilley B, McDonald P. Social support among African-American adults with diabetes, Part 1: Theoretical framework. *J Natl Med Assoc* 1998;90(6):361–365.

154. James SA, Keenan NL, Strogatz DS, et al. Socioeconomic status, John Henryism, and hypertension in blacks and whites. *Am J Epidemiol* 1987;126(4):664–673.

155. James SA, Hartnett SA, Kalsbeek WD. John Henryism and blood pressure differences among black men. *J Behav Med* 1983;6(3):259–278.

156. Strogatz DS, James SA. Social support and hypertension among blacks and whites in a rural, southern community. *Am J Epidemiol* 1986;124:949–956.

157. Mayberry RM, Mili F, Ofili E. Racial and ethnic differences in access to medical care. *Med Care Res Rev* 2000;57(suppl 1):108–145.

158. Cleeland C. Pain and its severity in cancer patients. *PRN Forum* 1982;1(2):1–2.

159. Cleeland CS, Cleeland LM, Dar R, Rinehardt LC. Factors influencing physician management of cancer pain. *Cancer* 1986;58(3):796–800.

160. Cleeland CS, Gonin R, Hatfield AK, et al. Pain and its treatment in outpatients with metastatic cancer. *New Engl J Med* 1994;330(9):592–596.

161. Cleeland CS. Undertreatment of cancer pain in elderly patients. *JAMA* 1998;279(23):1914–1915.

162. Anderson KO, Richman SP, Hurley J, et al. Cancer pain management among underserved minority outpatients: Perceived needs and barriers to optimal control. *Cancer* 2002;94(8):2295–2304.

163. Shaya FT, Blume S. Prescriptions for cyclooxygenase-2 inhibitors and other non-steroidal anti-inflammatory agents in a Medicaid managed care population: African Americans versus Caucasians. *Pain Med* 2005;6(1):11–17.

164. Green CR, Wheeler JR. Physician variability in the management of acute postoperative and cancer pain: A quantitative analysis of the Michigan experience. *Pain Med* 2003;4(1):8–20.

165. Tait RC, Chibnall JT. Physician judgments of chronic pain patients. *Soc Sci Med* 1997;45(8):1199–1205.

166. Tait RC, Chibnall JT. Work injury management of refractory low back pain: Relations with ethnicity, legal representation and diagnosis. *Pain* 2001;91(1–2):47–56.

167. Chibnall JT, Tait RC, Merys SC. Disability management of low back injuries by employer-retained physicians: Ratings and costs. *Am J Ind Med* 2000;38(5):529–538.

168. Tait RC, et al. Management of occupational back injuries: Differences among African Americans and Caucasians. *Pain* 2004;112(3):389–396.

169. Chibnall JT, Tait RC. Disparities in occupational low back injuries: Predicting pain-related disability from satisfaction with case management in African Americans and Caucasians. *Pain Med* 2005;6(1):39–48.

170. Morrison RS, Wallenstein S, Natale DK, et al. "We don't carry that"—Failure of pharmacies in predominantly nonwhite neighborhoods to stock opioid analgesics. *New Engl J Med* 2000;342(14):1023–1026.

171. Green CR, Ndao-Brumblay SK. Chronic pain and the use of alternative medicine at initial presentation to a tertiary pain care center. Paper presented at: American Academy of Pain Medicine meeting; March, 2004; Orlando, Fla.

172. Sullivan LW, Eagel BA. Leveling the playing field: Recognizing and rectifying disparities in management of pain. *Pain Med* 2005;6(1):5–10.

173. Lebovits A. The ethical implications of racial disparities in pain: Are some of us more equal? *Pain Med* 2005;6(1):3–4.

174. Baker TA, Whitfield KE. Arthritis, depression, and pain: A biobehavioral relationship in older African Americans. In: Taylor RJ, ed. *African American Research Perspectives*. 2003;60–71.

175. Clancy CM, Massion CT. American women's health care. A patchwork quilt with gaps. *JAMA* 1992;268(14):1918–1920.

176. Hopper SV. The influence of ethnicity on the health of older women. *Clin Geriatr Med* 1993;9(1):231–259.

177. Werner P, Cohen-Mansfield J, Watson V, Pasis S. Pain in participants of adult day care centers: Assessment by different raters. *J Pain Symptom Manage* 1998;15(1):8–17.

178. Hayward RA, et al. Inequities in health services among insured Americans. Do working-age adults have less access to medical care than the elderly? *New Engl J Med* 1988;318(23):1507–1512.

179. Blendon RJ, Benson JM, DesRoches CM. Americans' views of the uninsured: An era for hybrid proposals. *Health Aff* 2003;(July–December):W3-405–W3-414.

180. Reinhardt UE. Is there hope for the uninsured? *Health Aff* 2003(July–December):W3-376–W3-390.

181. Leape LL, Berwick DM. Safe health care: Are we up to it? *BMJ* 2000;320(7237):725–726.

182. Charatan F. Senators introduce bill to improve patient safety. *BMJ* 2000;320(7233):465.

183. Cooke J. *Preventing Death and Injury From Medical Errors Requires Dramatic, System-Wide Changes;* 1999.

184. The pain decade and the public health. *Pain Med* 2000;1(4):283–285.

185. Kohn LT, Corrigan JM, Donaldson MS, eds. *To Err Is Human: Building a Safer Health System.* Washington, DC: National Academy Press; 1999.

CHAPTER 20

Case Studies in Multicultural Medicine and Health Disparities

Wally R. Smith, MD

Jada Bussey-Jones, MD

Carol R. Horowitz MD, MPH

Michelle Whitehurst-Cook, MD

Alice Hm Chen, MD, MPH

▶ INTRODUCTION

Health disparities arise from a complex array of causes within and outside the control of medical practitioners. Physicians, other health-care workers, and patients may each bring to the medical encounter ignorance or apathy regarding the need to communicate with people who are unlike them. They may mistrust other races or cultures. Or, they may operate using racial or cultural stereotypes based on conscious or subconscious prejudice. They may not appreciate important cultural and language differences that impede communication between clinicians and patients and result in lower quality of care.

For example, slavery and its legacy of ongoing segregation have created a racial and cultural divide between African Americans and Caucasians in the United States, which is evident in current-day disparities in education, justice, housing, and health. Although that gap has narrowed on some fronts, it is still widespread in medical practice. In addition, new gaps will likely arise as the racial and ethnic composition of the United States becomes more diverse. African Americans, Latinos, Asian Americans, Pacific Islanders, and Native Americans currently comprise 25% of the US population[1] but this percentage may increase to 36% by the year 2020, and to nearly 50% by the year 2050.[2,3] Low-income and low-literacy populations may also experience health disparities due to cultural distance from their providers.

Health-care workers interested in reducing disparities need to understand the many likely causes of disparities. They also need skills and strategies to use during the health encounter to help reduce disparities. The cases that follow, all taken from real practice, illustrate examples of likely causes of disparities that are under the clinician's control. The discussion of each case offers advice about how clinicians may avoid such negative outcomes. The intent of these vignettes is that they be used as case material for teaching purposes. For example, teachers could present learners one of the cases, and could facilitate a group discussion afterward, using the written discussion as a guide or supplement.

▶ MISTRUST

Case Study: I'm Not Addicted

A 26-year-old African American man was admitted to the acute-care internal medicine service with a severe painful episode due to sickle cell disease. He was not known to the African American attending physician's continuity clinic, which happened to specialize in sickle cell disease. The patient reported multiple recent emergency department (ED) visits for sickle cell pain, and conflicts with ED staff regarding his requests for more opiates than they seemed willing to give for his pain. He complained to the attending physician, "Those white people just don't believe I'm in pain. A black man doesn't stand a chance of getting enough pain medicine in this Emergency Room or hospital. They think I'm addicted."

The patient's past medical history was unremarkable. He had no primary care. His social history revealed he was in a recovery program for substance abuse, primarily cocaine. His family history revealed a sister with sickle cell disease, also a street drug abuser, who had done jail time.

The patient was promised pain relief and had an uneventful hospital stay. He came to the sickle cell clinic as scheduled, and bonded with black and white caregivers there over several months to years. He began receiving substantial quantities of opiates for almost daily pain, titrated up as tolerance developed. Each prescription was photocopied, and these prescriptions and an opiate use agreement signed by the patient were placed in the chart. Hospitalizations after that were rare.

Later, during an ED visit, he tested positive for cocaine. The patient was warned he could not be prescribed opiates while using street drugs, and he agreed to be placed on a urine-monitoring program in the sickle cell clinic. On one of these clinic visits, the patient's urine was reported to be positive for codeine, when he had not been on prescribed codeine for pain relief. He vehemently denied using codeine and said the laboratory must have made an error. He was nearly discharged from the clinic based on this violation of protocol, but persistent calls to the laboratory before discharge revealed the gel pattern for the opiate profile test had been misinterpreted, and his urine was indeed appropriate. Unfortunately, after several years of care in the clinic, a urine drug screen proved positive for heroin and lidocaine, which clinicians believed was an attempt to disguise use of nonprescribed, metabolized opiates. The patient was dismissed from the clinic, with a referral for opiate treatment and an invitation to continue getting his other care in the university system.

DISCUSSION

This case illustrates how mistrust on the part of patients and physicians often arises in the care of adults with sickle cell disease, the most common and well-known genetic disease affecting African Americans. The patient described in this case was articulate and intelligent but had no college education or job skills. He reported job discrimination. His normal-appearing body habitus was unlike that of many sickle cell patients, who are underweight and have underdeveloped secondary sexual characteristics. Often, on job interviews, he was told, "You don't look sick." When he had to miss work for a crisis, he was sometime told, "You just had a crisis last week. How do I know you're having one now?" He, like other patients, sometimes hid the fact of his sickle cell disease during employment interviews. This led to his being dismissed when employers found out about his illness. His most steady job, working with a caterer, required him to set up and break down tables and chairs for banquets and other functions. He reported being forced to quit this job because of worsening pain after heavy exertion.

This patient's comment during the initial inpatient encounter illustrates how mistrust may cloud pain management. Opioid tolerance, or diminished analgesic responsiveness to usual doses of opiates, develops often by adulthood after repeated exposures to opiates; for example, during childhood in patients with sickle cell disease. Tolerant patients receiving usual doses of opiates without relief, and requesting higher doses, may come into conflict with ED staff and others, who may not trust the patient's report of pain, believing that the patient is "addicted" to opiates.[4] These conflicts are undoubtedly exacerbated by different-race relationships (white physician, black patient), but black physicians may also be opiophobic. Pseudoaddiction (ie, appropriate but misinterpreted requests for pain relief by patients with legitimate pain) may lead to undertreatment of pain.[5] Patients experiencing disputes about pain relief may develop mistrust for their caregivers and avoid future disputes by staying at home when in pain.[6,7]

Psychological addiction, manifested by dose escalation, "doctor-shopping" for opiates, "losing" medication, and recreational use of opiates, occurs in only a minority of sickle cell patients. Although substance abuse was present in this case, the abusing patient's drug of choice was not opiates, but cocaine. Clinic visits, along with prescribed opiates for his pain, were part of clinical support for him. With this care, he remained remain drug-free for several years. However, street drug abuse is a reality. It is part of the culture of poverty and may be prevalent among patients who happen to have diseases with treatment disparities. Abusing patients with pain still should have their pain treated and also receive services to address their substance abuse. However, as in this case, to protect themselves practitioners must have strict rules in place regarding the use of opioids. These must be consistently followed to avoid practitioners becoming subjects of legal inquiries or investigations by medical licensure boards. For the majority of sickle cell patients who do not use street drugs, adequately treating their pain as part of comprehensive management will reduce ED use, hospitalizations, and length of stay[8] and can build stronger, trusting relationships between physicians and patients and prevent patient job loss.

▶ STEREOTYPING

Case Study: Here Comes Another One

A 15-year-old African-American girl presented to her rural, female, African American family physician with lower abdominal pain that had begun about 6 hours earlier. The pain was localized in the right lower quadrant and suprapubic area. She described the pain as a deep, dull ache of 8/10 or 9/10 intensity, which had been constant for the last 3 to 4 hours. Nothing made it worse, but she felt better when she was supine. She had a poor appetite and felt nauseous but had not vomited. She had experienced chills, and her mother measured her temperature with an oral thermometer at 101°F (38.3°C) before coming to the office. The patient had begun menses at age 11, and her last menstrual period was 2 weeks prior to this visit. She noted no change in her daily bowel patterns. There was no history of melena or hematochezia. She also denied urgency, frequency, dysuria, or vaginal discharge. The patient, in the absence of her mother, acknowledged that she was a virgin. She had been in good health with no major illness in the past and no significant family history of inflammatory bowel disease. The family had shared meals, and no one else was sick. There had been no history of a similar illness in the small rural community.

Past medical history was also negative for surgery or past hospitalizations. The patient, an average student, was a 10th grader at the local high school, where she participated in the local marching band. Her plans were to attend college. She denied use of drugs, alcohol, or cigarettes. She lived at home with her mother, father, and 12-year-old brother. She had no allergies and took no medications except acetaminophen for her current pain, without significant relief. Review of other systems was negative. She denied a history of abdominal pain midmenstrual cycle.

At the time of initial evaluation by her family physician the patient's physical examination showed blood pressure of 110/60 mm Hg; pulse, 100/min; temperature, 101.5°F; respirations, 20/min; weight, 118 lb; height, 5 feet, 3 inches. The only significant finding on examination involved the abdomen, which was diffusely tender to palpation, especially in the right lower quadrant and suprapubic area. Rebound was positive, but there was no costovertebral angle tenderness. Pelvic examination revealed a closed cervix without exudate. The suprapubic area was tender on bimanual examination. The hymen was not intact, but prominent remnants were present.

The family physician determined the patient had an acute abdomen, most likely secondary to appendicitis. The history of virginity made the diagnosis of pelvic inflammatory disease less likely. The patient was transported by her parents to an urban emergency department 30 miles away for consultation with the on-call general surgeon for definitive treatment. The surgeon, who was then en route from treating patients at another hospital, called the emergency department, requesting that the hospital operator contact him when the patient had arrived and had the necessary blood work.

On arrival at the emergency department, the on-call surgeon ordered laboratory, urine, and sexually transmitted disease cultures. His examination corroborated the acute abdomen status, but he was impressed with the amount of suprapubic discomfort. The surgeon reviewed the lab results, which noted a white cell count of 15,000/mm^3 with a left shift of leukocytes. Results of the patient's serum pregnancy test and

urinalysis were negative. An acute abdominal x-ray series was nondiagnostic. Urinalysis was not pathologic.

The surgeon contacted the referring family physician and stated his belief that the diagnosis was pelvic inflammatory disease. The patient's hymen was not intact, and he suspected that she was not being honest about her past sexual experiences. He prescribed intravenous antibiotics and watched her overnight.

Over the next 24 hours, the patient improved slightly, with a decreased temperature and less pain, although she had persistent right lower quadrant tenderness with less suprapubic findings. A pelvic ultrasound to rule out a tubo-ovarian abscess revealed, instead, an appendicial abscess. The patient was taken to surgery, where a ruptured appendix was removed. She remained in the hospital for 2 weeks, to allow for IV antibiotic treatment and removal of the drains placed during surgery.

DISCUSSION

Current treatment for acute appendicitis usually results in a laparoscopic approach with no more than a 1- or 2-day hospital stay. Because this patient did not receive timely surgery, she had complications that resulted in a prolonged hospital stay and added cost of care.

Physicians who see patients in a hectic setting, with limited time to build rapport or to get to know the patients, often make unconscious decisions about the patient based on prior experiences with similar patients. Clinicians may use the limited information they have about a social, racial, or cultural group to stereotype patients and their behaviors, and may wrongly proceed with a treatment plan based on a false stereotype. It is imperative that physicians approach each patient's problem objectively using the best evidence available. Care is enhanced when the physician takes time to listen to the patient and makes treatment decisions based on the facts. Decisions based on stereotyping may lead to poor patient–physician communication, distrust, and disparities in care.

In this case, the general surgeon on call had seen several patients already at another hospital and was hurriedly leaving to evaluate this new patient. Based on his experience with inner-city youth, he made assumptions concerning the patient, which were later refuted. The patient's temporary slight improvement confirmed in his mind an incorrect diagnosis.

Most physicians do not consider themselves prejudiced and do not believe that their decision making based on unconscious stereotypes could exacerbate health disparities. However, prejudice and bias formulated in childhood may later have an impact on adult interactions. Clinicians need to become aware of their personal biases and unconscious prejudices and understand how these can contaminate treatment decisions. Through recognizing a tendency to revert to quick decisions based on past associations, clinicians can work to prevent unequal care based on stereotypes. Physicians must also acknowledge negative feelings when dealing with, for example, a patient who seems less than motivated, or who behaves in a hostile manner. Does this patient remind the physician of other patients? Is a patient's negative reaction related to the physician's nonverbal cues, which the patient interprets as bias? Are these nonverbal cues benign, or are they representative of unconscious prejudice or stereotyping? Is the physician able to discuss past negative exchanges with his or her patients?

▶ CULTURAL DIFFERENCES

Case Study: Just a Sore Throat

A second-year resident in internal medicine presented a case to his preceptor. He described a 74-year-old African American woman whom he had known for about 1 year, with a history of hypertension and arthritis, deemed noncompliant with medications, who complained of a sore throat for 1 month. In previous visits, her throat culture had been negative, and she did not respond to presumptive treatment for allergies. Her blood pressure was persistently elevated, and she refused to take clonidine in addition to her other antihypertensives. He described her as "fatalistic," deciding to leave things in the hands of God, not interested in pursuing medical treatment unless it was for symptoms such as her sore throat. Her physical examination was normal except for blood pressure of 146/92 mm Hg and mildly erythematous throat and nasal mucosa. The resident planned to reassure her that the sore throat would go away with time, and to leave the blood pressure medicines alone, as the patient refused to make any changes.

The preceptor briefly interviewed the patient with the resident, to determine if this was the best course of action. The preceptor ascertained that the patient had had no heat for the past month. Each evening, she turned on the gas oven in her kitchen, left the oven door open and slept in front of it to keep warm. The preceptor suspected that this dry heat was responsible for the patient's sore throat. The preceptor also explored her hesitancy to take antihypertensive medications. The patient reported that her best friend had taken clonidine and when she ran out for a couple of days, her blood pressure went up suddenly, she had a stroke, and the doctors told her this was because she had stopped the pills. The patient was afraid if she forgot to take her pills once in a while, she would have a stroke like her friend did, so she chose not to take this medication.

The patient agreed to put a pot of water in the oven to humidify the air, and the physicians contacted the clinic's social worker to help the patient with her heating situation. She also agreed to use the clonidine patch, as she was confident she would remember a weekly administration. When the patient returned to clinic 2 weeks later, her sore throat had abated, and her blood pressure was 138/86.

DISCUSSION

To effectively and efficiently treat patients, we must appreciate the impact that culture, including our biomedical culture, has on health care. Culture can be viewed as beliefs, values, and attitudes shared and perpetuated by members of a social group.[4] Culture is a complex whole that also includes shared traditions, customs, language, and norms that must be learned from families and social communities.[5] Each medical encounter provides the opportunity for the interface of several different cultures: the culture of the patient, the culture of the physician, and the culture of medicine. This interface often influences adherence to medical regimens, patient satisfaction, health-care utilization, and health outcomes.

When ignorant or unaware of their own culture, physicians can make assumptions about patients that can lead to missed diagnoses and missed opportunities for effective treatment. When patients "refuse" to take prescribed medications, they are often labeled "noncompliant," difficult, or fatalistic because they make us as clinicians feel inadequate. Particularly when working with socioeconomically disadvantaged populations, the social history may help clinicians expand their differential diagnoses to include social problems many physicians would not imagine, such as a sore throat due to a heating emergency. This patient sensibly feared that missing doses of a medication would make her more ill than not taking the medication at all. The resident assumed the patient was fatalistic, when perhaps the resident was fatalistic that his patient would not take additional steps to safeguard her health.

We practice medicine most often from a medicocentric point of view. In our role as clinicians, the tradition of medicine and the medical culture often override our own individual cultures when caring for patients. However, seeking care at physicians' offices and hospitals may be viewed as a last option by patients. Patients may seek advice from several sources, including their faith tradition, family members, friends, and herbalists or nontraditional healers. Additionally, many medical symptoms are self-diagnosed and self-treated.[9] Recognizing and addressing previous attempts at treatment can help demonstrate the course of the disease, identify potentially harmful or helpful interventions taken, and build therapeutic alliances.

One example of attempts at self-treatment is the use and nondisclosure of use of alternative medicines. An estimated 60 million Americans used alternative medical therapies in 1990, and use frequently was not disclosed to Western providers.[10–12] There are strong traditional or native healing traditions that continue to be used in the African American, Native American, Asian American, and Latino communities in the United States. For example, surveys suggest that 50% to 84% of Mexican families use folk medicine.[13,14] Although data are limited regarding the safety and efficacy of many herbal treatments, it is important to explore the use of these treatments, as well as possible risks related to interactions with traditional medicines or to impurities in products, which are not FDA regulated.[15,16] Additionally, physicians' knowledge of their patients' use of these therapies can facilitate responsible use and build partnerships with patients.[17]

▶ LANGUAGE BARRIERS

Case Study: Wait Three Days

A 13-year-old girl routinely served as her family's interpreter for medical visits. When she developed severe abdominal pain, her parents took her to the hospital. Unfortunately, she was too sick to interpret for herself, and the hospital did not provide an interpreter. After a night of observation, her Spanish-speaking parents were told, without the aid of an interpreter, to bring her back immediately if her symptoms worsened, and otherwise to follow up with a doctor in 3 days. However, what her parents understood from the conversation was that they should wait 3 days to see the doctor. After 2 days, with her condition deteriorating, they felt they could no longer wait and rushed her back to the emergency department. A ruptured appendix was diagnosed, and the patient was airlifted to a nearby medical center, where she died a few hours later.

DISCUSSION

This fairly straightforward case of appendicitis demonstrates the impact of not only cultural differences, but also language barriers, on outcomes. In this case, the daughter, who normally served as her parents' medical interpreter, needed an interpreter for herself when she became ill but did not receive one. Her parents, respectful of their medical providers, attempted to follow what they thought were appropriate instructions. The lack of accurate communication cost the patient her life.

Unfortunately, as this case illustrates, sometimes physicians see patients who have limited English proficiency without an interpreter being present. A recently published case report cites how this resulted in delayed diagnosis of one patient's obstructive uropathy and renal failure until the patient's third presentation, and subsequent loss of employment for the patient.[18] At other times, physicians rely heavily on untrained, ad hoc interpreters such as patient family members, secretarial or custodial hospital staff, or other patients for translation.[19] Ad hoc interpreters have been shown to make frequent errors, including omissions, paraphrasing, use of incorrect words, substitutions, and additions.[20,21] One investigator found that 23% to 52% of physician's questions were mistranslated or not translated at all.[22]

Minor children, in particular, should not be used as medical interpreters, given both the complexity of medical settings and the emotional valence of many health-care encounters.[23] Even when children are fluent in English, they are often not fluent in their parents' native language—and unless the provider speaks the language, the provider has no way of assessing this. In addition, even fully bilingual children are unlikely to understand and be able to adequately communicate medical terms and concepts such as risk, anesthesia, surgery, or appendix. Finally, it is inappropriate to place children in the position of relaying sensitive, important, or emotionally charged information, as they may feel responsible for the information or guilty about any miscommunication that may arise.

There is a growing body of research that shows that language barriers in health-care settings result in decreased access, diminished comprehension, reduced satisfaction, and lower quality of care.[24-27] Access to trained interpreters and bilingual or bicultural providers can address these disparities.[28-30] As a result, there are a number of state and national initiatives designed to increase the numbers of bilingual providers and trained professional medical interpreters, including the Department of Health and Human Services' National Standards for Culturally and Linguistically Appropriate Services in Health Care (CLAS).[31] Of the 14 standards, 4 are related to provision of services for patients with limited English proficiency.

Finally, individual clinicians can improve their ability to work with patients who have limited English proficiency by receiving training on how to work with both trained and untrained interpreters. Such training not only increases the use of professional interpreters, but also increases physicians' satisfaction with the medical care they provide to patients with limited English proficiency.[32]

▶ REFERENCES

1. *Resident Population Estimates for the US by Sex, Race, and Hispanic Origin: April 1, 1990 to July 1, 1999, with Short-Term Projection to November 1, 2000.* US Census Bureau; 2001. Available at: http://www.census.gov/population/estimates/nation/intfile3-1.txt. Accessed October 20, 2001.

2. *Projections of the Resident Populations by Race, Hispanic Origin, and Nativity: Middle Series, 2016 to 2020.* US Census Bureau; 2001. Available at: http://www.census.gov/population/projections/nation/summary/np-t5-e.txt. Accessed October 20, 2001.

3. *Issues Brief: Development of Healthy People 2010 Objectives.* Available at: http://odphp.osophs.dhhs.gov/pubs/HP2000/newsbit.htm.

4. Shapiro BS, Benjamin L, Payne R, Heidrich G. Sickle cell-related pain: Perceptions of medical practitioners. *J Pain Symptom Manage* 1997;14(3): 168–174.

5. Elander J, Lusher J, Bevan D, et al. Understanding the causes of problematic pain management in sickle cell disease: Evidence that pseudoaddiction plays a more important role than genuine analgesic dependence. *J Pain Symptom Manage* 2004; 27(2):156–169.

6. Murray N, May A. Painful crises in sickle cell disease—patients' perspectives. *BMJ* 1988;297 (6646):452–454.

7. Bobo L, Miller ST, Smith WR, et al. Health perceptions and medical care opinions of inner-city adults with sickle cell disease and asthma compared with their siblings. *South Med J* 1989;82: 9–12.

8. Brookoff D, Polomano R. Treating sickle cell pain like cancer pain. *Ann Intern Med* 1992;116(5): 364–368.

9. Dean K. Self-care responses to illnesses: A selected review. *Soc Sci Med* 1981;15:673–687.

10. Eisenberg D, Kessler RC, Foster C, et al. Unconventional medicine in the US—prevalence, costs, and patterns of use. *N Engl J Med* 1993;328(4): 246–252.

11. Astin J. Why patients use alternative medicine: Results of a national study. *JAMA* 1998;279(19): 1548–1553.

12. Furnham A, Forey J. The attitudes, behaviors and beliefs of patients of conventional vs. complementary (alternative) medicine. *J Clin Psychol* 1994;50:458–469.

13. Marsh WW, Hentges K. Mexican folk remedies and conventional medical care. *Am Fam Physician* 1988;37(3):257–262.

14. Hunt LM, Arar NH, Akana LL. Herbs, prayer, and insulin: Use of medical and alternative treatments by a group of Mexican American diabetes patients. *J Fam Pract* 2000;49(3):216–223.

15. Jonas W. Alternative medicine and the conventional practitioner. *JAMA* 1998;279(9):708–710.

16. Belongia E, Hedberg C, Gleich G, et al. An investigation of the cause of the eosinophilia-myalgia syndrome associated with tryptophan use. *N Engl J Med* 1990;323:357–365.

17. Eisenberg D. The invisible mainstream. *Harv Med Alum Bull* 1996:20–25.

18. Bussey-Jones J, Genao I. Impact of culture on health care. *J Natl Med Assoc* 2003;95(8):732–735.

19. Andrulis D, Goodman N, Pryor C. What a difference an interpreter makes. The Access Project; April 2002.

20. Elderkin-Thompson V, Silver RC, Waitzkin H. When nurses double as interpreters: A study of Spanish-speaking patients in a U.S. primary care setting. *Soc Sci Med* 2001;52:1343–1358.

21. Launer J. Taking medical histories through interpreters: Practice in a Nigerian outpatient department. *BMJ* 1978;2(6142):934–935.

22. Ebden P. The bilingual consultation. *Lancet* 1988; 1:347.

23. Haffner L. Cross-cultural medicine: A decade later. *West J Med* 1992;157(3):255–259.

24. Fiscella K, Franks P, Doescher MP, Saver BG. Disparities in health care by race, ethnicity, and language among the insured. *Med Care* 2002;40: 52–59.

25. Crane JA. Patient comprehension of doctor–patient communication on discharge from the emergency department. *J Emerg Med* 1997;15 (1):1–7.

26. Carrasquillo O, Orav EJ, Brennan TA, Burstin HR. Impact of language barriers on patient satisfaction in an emergency department. *J Gen Intern Med* 1999;14:82–87.

27. Ghandi TK, Burstin HR, Cook EF, et al. Drug complications in outpatients. *J Gen Intern Med* 2000;15:149–154.

28. Manson A. Language concordance as a determinant of patience compliance and emergency room use in patients with asthma. *Med Care* 1988; 26(12):1119–1128.

29. Jacobs EA, Lauderdale DS, Meltzer D, et al. Impact of interpreter services on delivery of health care to limited-English-proficient patients. *J Gen Intern Med* 2001;16:468–474.

30. Fernandez A, Schillinger D, Grumbach K, et al. An exploratory study of communication with Spanish-speaking patients. *J Gen Intern Med* 2000;19:167–174.

31. Assuring cultural competence in health care: Recommendations for national standards and an outcomes-focused research agenda. *Federal Register* December 22, 2000;65(247):80865–80879.

32. Karliner L, Perez-Stable EJ, Gildengorin G. The importance of training in the use of interpreters for outpatient practice. *J Gen Intern Med* 2004; 19:175–183.

SECTION III

Issues in Health-Care Policy and Delivery

CHAPTER 21

Cultural Competency

ANA NÚÑEZ, MD*

CANDACE ROBERTSON, MPH

▶ INTRODUCTION AND DEFINITIONS

Cultural Competence

Health-care providers aspire to attain finite sets of skills not only in clinical behaviors such as palpation and auscultation, but also in provider–patient communication. "Clinical competence" implies achievement of the level of skills needed to diagnose disease and deliver care. "Cultural competence" has come to represent the ability of health-care providers to interact with patients who are different from themselves. This difference implies ethnicity, but from a broader perspective encompasses differences that include gender, race, age, religion, culture, language, education, socioeconomic status, and permutations of these parameters.

Cultural competence has been described, variously, as knowledge, attitude, and skills (educational perspective)[1] about health-related beliefs and cultural values (socioeconomic perspective), disease incidence and prevalence (epidemiologic perspective), and treatment efficacy (outcomes perspective).[2] It has also been defined as "a set of behaviors, knowl-

edge, attitudes, and policies that come together in a system, organization, or among health professionals that enables effective work in cross-cultural situations."[3]

Health-care providers must be able to shift from a problem- or disease-focused perspective to the human and contextual perspective of the patients who present to them. They must also be able to recognize and acknowledge their own biases, prejudices, and stereotypes. This change of perspective includes considering how patients' concerns might influence communication and clinical assessments. To succeed in this more patient-centered approach, providers must enhance the communication skills necessary to negotiate effectively and collaborate with patients to optimize outcomes that work within the patients' world.

Cross-Cultural Efficacy and Cultural Humility

Cross-cultural efficacy and cultural humility provide two additional perspectives for examining the knowledge, attitudes, and skills needed in the health-care setting to bridge the gap between the science of medicine and the art of healing.

Cross-cultural efficacy focuses on the dynamic between the patient and the provider.

* The McGraw-Hill Companies acknowledge the substantial editorial contributions of Donna M. Frassetto and Nancy N. Woelfl in preparation of this chapter.

This perspective emphasizes the acquisition of skills as an ongoing process rather than the attainment of a finite set of skills at one point in time, and that neither the caregiver nor the patient culture is preferred. The traditional medical encounter involves the intersection of three cultures: the culture of the physician, the culture of the patient (which is rarely the same as that of the physician), and the medical culture that provides the context for the interaction. In the cross-cultural efficacy model, the emphasis for health-care providers is on learning to see their own culture and understand the impact of their behaviors on others whose culture is different, as well as the impact of the patients' behaviors on the provider.

Cultural humility, described by Tervalon et al,[4] sheds light on the important role of health-care provider insight and awareness in the clinical encounter. In this perspective, the provider is encouraged to engage in regular self-evaluation and self-critique. The goal is to shift the power differential in patient–physician interactions and develop balanced relationships with individuals and populations.[4]

The power differential plays a role in the provider–patient interaction. In some settings, the goal of the provider–client interaction is developmental and advocacy focused. For example, when a client initiates psychotherapy, the client is at the low end of the power scale and the psychologist at the high end. If progress is made, the client becomes more empowered and better skilled in self-care, resulting in increased power on his part and a decrease on the provider's scale. In general, the consumer movement has shifted encounters away from a paternalistic (adult–child) approach to one that is more equitable (adult–adult). Nonetheless, the provider, with his or her knowledge and skills, retains more power in the interaction.

There are advantages and disadvantages to this dynamic. However, in general, the less collaborative a provider, the more likely it is he or she will truncate communication with the patient. For example, telling patients they must take their medicine is not an unreasonable thing to do. Patients may readily consent but not,

however, change their behavior. A more collaborative approach would involve asking a patient whose condition has not improved after medication was prescribed whether he or she has taken the medicine and what problems were experienced. This approach creates an opportunity to openly discuss the matter, which may lead to greater understanding and compliance.

The consumer movement may also influence health practitioners' perceptions of the need to enhance skills in this area because insured patients have a choice as to which provider they see. If clinicians seem unresponsive, patients can go elsewhere, as described in the following example.

> A female obstetrician/gynecologist practiced in a 17-member group. She suggested to her colleagues, all of whom were male, that gender communication skills were important in care. Her colleagues were not interested until insurance coverage changed and a large number of patients left the practice. The other members of the group then quickly expressed interest in hiring a consultant to teach them gender-based communication skills.

Patients' value and belief systems, behaviors, and health-care practices are critical factors influencing the success of a clinical encounter. Differences in recognition of symptoms, health-seeking behaviors, communication and expression of symptoms, ability to understand treatment plans or instructions, expectations of care, and adherence to prevention efforts and treatment regimens contribute to disparities in health and to poor health outcomes.[5] Failure to address the cultural aspects of care that have an impact on health and health care is clearly detrimental: Patients who are minorities experience higher rates of disease, disability, and death, and often receive a lower quality of care compared with nonminorities.[6]

▶ COMPONENTS OF CULTURAL COMPETENCE

Whether one uses the term *cultural competence*, *cross-cultural efficacy*, or *cultural humility*, the ultimate goal of efforts to incorporate these approaches into practice is to better prepare health-care providers to recognize, understand, and manage sociocultural issues that emerge within the clinical encounter.[7] All three approaches require knowledge, attitudes, and skills.

Knowledge

Cultural competence efforts seek to increase providers' knowledge of cultural beliefs, practices, and changing attitudes toward health care and health-seeking behaviors. Recognizing disparities in the incidence and occurrence of disease, especially among racial and ethnic patient populations, is also an important aspect of the cultural competency knowledge base. Three examples illustrate why awareness is an important factor in reducing disparities and improving outcomes.

1. Although breast cancer occurs less often in African American than Caucasian women, African American women experience a higher mortality rate. There is debate as to the genetic and physiologic mechanisms of the disease in African American women, but delays in obtaining treatment and barriers to care may play a role in the different outcomes seen in this patient population.
2. The onset of prostate cancer may occur earlier in African American men than in men of other ethnic and racial groups. Despite recommendations for screening evaluations to begin at age 40, many African American men are not screened even though there is an opportunity to do so when they seek care for other conditions.
3. Many studies that have evaluated cardiac care have demonstrated differential care based on gender and ethnicity.[8–13] These differences persist even when controlling for income and insurance coverage.[14]

Race and ethnicity are not the only contributors to health disparities. Providers must also be familiar with gender differences in occurrence. As an example, ankylosing spondylitis was once thought to occur almost exclusively in men (10:1 ratio). Research later determined that women also developed the disease, but its manifestation was less severe and more likely to be overlooked. A male predominance still exists, but the ratio is 3:1. Both Caucasian and Native American men are at increased risk for this disease.[15]

Patient compliance with treatment regimens is influenced by health-care beliefs and group norms developed within the family system. Clinician education about health-related topics may not change the patient's core health beliefs, which are internalized. But clinicians can help patients verbalize their beliefs so they can collaborate on a mutually acceptable treatment plan. Data alone will not sway values, attitudes, or beliefs.

At times, it is not just single patients with whom clinicians negotiate. Social relationships may be linear, collateral, or individual. In medical culture, the social relationship traditionally has been individualistic; that is, clinicians prefer to relate to the patient one-to-one. In other cultures, the social relationship is one-to-many or one-to-family. With the exception of pediatricians, clinicians are not uniformly comfortable opening the examination room door to find more than one person in the room, or having a family member as the chief informant. Yet, if patients prefer that decision making occur within the family context rather than as the sole responsibility of the individual, it is beneficial to the encounter if the clinician is skilled at communicating and negotiating with more than one person and able to address the health issue with a varied audience.

Attitude

Addressing attitudinal issues (eg, enhancing self-awareness of one's attitudes toward people of different racial, religious, or socioeconomic backgrounds) can minimize the influence of stereotypes and beliefs on the recognition, diagnosis, and treatment of disease, enabling clinicians to provide better care. Attitudinal components of cultural competence are often the most challenging areas in which to educate health-care providers. Relevance and interest are important factors in learner motivation, but there is often still a great deal of provider resistance to discussing issues of culture and diversity in health care. Some health professionals experience anger toward perceived preferential treatment of minorities; conversely, others feel guilt. Still others deny differences exist or generalize that "everyone is just the same; we are all human."

Discussions of cultural issues must address racism and a "blame the victim" mentality that is sometimes seen in health care. If these issues are not discussed in a nonjudgmental context, larger attitudinal objectives are unlikely to be attained. These objectives include but are not limited to:

1. Understanding the importance of cultural issues in optimal health-care delivery;
2. Awareness of others as having both similar and dissimilar characteristics;
3. Developing comfort with issues of difference;
4. Increasing self-awareness in dealing with cross-cultural situations;
5. Developing an ability to acknowledge issues that include stereotyping and bias; and
6. Avoiding the presumption of understanding without asking.

The issue of stereotyping is particularly challenging for health-care providers. The very skills and competencies that are fostered during training may contribute to this issue. Much of the learning process in health professions education is based on identification and classification of phenomena. For example, a streptococcal infection appears as a gram-positive coccus under the microscope. Pattern recognition is integral to diagnosis, and this mindset is so well developed in health-care providers that they subconsciously look for patterns in populations and apply them to individuals.

Training in medicine oriented toward facts, evidence, and disease does not translate well into an understanding of the role individual and cultural influences play in patient behavior and the clinical encounter.

Skills

To incorporate cultural knowledge and culturally sensitive attitudes into care delivery, health professionals must be able to integrate, synthesize, and apply them in the form of skills. These skills include:

1. Integrating knowledge and attitudes by demonstrating respect and validating other cultures;
2. Applying knowledge and attitudes to discover the cultural context of the health-care problem as well as patient needs, expectations, and culturally appropriate resources;
3. Adapting communication skills to situations in which English is not the common language between health-care provider and patient;
4. Demonstrating proficiency in the use of interpreters; and
5. Considering the influence of culture on all aspects of care delivery including negotiation, problem solving, diagnosis, management, and treatment to achieve optimal health-care outcomes.

The following example illustrates the importance of these skills in everyday patient care:

A Mexican American man, who was a hospital anesthesiologist, needed to have knee arthroscopy. He was admitted to the outpatient surgery unit, where a third-year medical clerk obtained his medical history. During the examination, the *clerk* asked the patient whether he lived with his family, and the patient replied he did not. The clerk did not pursue further questions about the patient's family.

Before the procedure, the orthopedic surgeon decided to review the patient's chart. He was surprised to see the student had listed the patient as single and living alone, given that the surgeon had met the man's wife and son at hospital functions. The patient's cultural interpretation of "living with family" meant living with his parents. Since this was not true, he had answered that he did not live with family.

As this example illustrates, something as simple as the word "family" can have many meanings, with implications for health care.

Other skills that are not always included in cross-cultural effectiveness training include demonstrated ability to work as a member of a team with other health professionals and the ability to recognize situations in which patient advocacy is needed. The issues health-care providers must address in providing patient care often require resources that extend beyond the individual clinician. Some health-care providers are evaluated on their level of team performance but this is not always the case for physicians. A team approach to health service delivery not only provides more resources, but also prevents individual clinician "burn-out." For appropriate patient advocacy, the provider must be able to assess not only instances when the patient does not fit into the system, but also situations in which the system does not fit the patient.

Increasing proficiency in this area leads to improved communication skills, enabling providers to effectively ask patients questions about race or ethnicity, family, religion, relationships, immigration experiences, social support, and other life factors that may influence their health-care beliefs, practices, and health-seeking behaviors. These skills ultimately enhance the patient–provider encounter and better equip providers with the tools necessary to treat patients in a culturally appropriate manner.[6] Research has demonstrated that provider–patient communication directly influences patient satisfaction, patient compliance, and health outcomes.[7] Enhancing cultural competence among health-care providers also provides health care that is more responsive to the needs of diverse populations, enhancing the quality of this care and recipients' satisfaction with care.[6]

▶ WHY ADDRESS CULTURAL ISSUES IN CARE?

The gap between patient and provider expectations is not new. Historically the literature provides examples of disparities in care due to ethnicity and gender. Prior to introduction of the informed consent process, abuse of patients' rights often occurred as a result of what appeared to be compelling scientific questions. Physicians and scientists are motivated to find problems and solve them. Patients, on the other hand, want healers, sometimes miracle workers, and certainly desire physicians who never err. Patients often want to be heard, to be understood, and to have physicians understand the larger context of their lives. Physicians face the tension between being scientists and being healers. Armed with facts, data, and technology, they are trained to know. Experts on the working of the human body, they are less comfortable addressing aspects of the patient encounter that seem intangible and cannot be measured.

Multicultural education has emerged in response to the need to provide health professionals with the skills required to meet the needs of an increasingly diverse patient population that expects holistic care and views cultural identity as an integral component of self.

▶ HEALTH DISPARITIES

Despite improvements in the overall health of Americans and continued advances in medical and scientific research, health disparities persist for ethnic and racial minorities in the United States, particularly in regard to health promotion and prevention. Racial differences exist in the incidence and prevalence of health conditions, access to health care, health outcomes, and treatments received. Poverty, gender bias, racism, language differences, homophobia, housing status, lack of sick leave, child-care needs, health insurance, domestic violence, substance abuse, and homelessness are variables that contribute to the health disparities observed in minority populations.[16]

More than 30 million residents of the United States do not speak English as their primary language. Research has shown that Spanish-speaking patients discharged from emergency departments are less likely than their English-speaking counterparts to "understand their diagnoses, prescribed medications, special instructions, plans for follow-up care, [or to] be satisfied with their care or willing to return if they had problems."[17] Research has also shown that patients with limited English proficiency are less likely to receive eye, dental, or physical examinations as well as mammograms, breast examinations, and Pap smears.[17]

Additional variables, including stereotypes about minority women and particular health beliefs, may also lead to poor medical care and treatment outcomes.[18] Differences in the diagnostic studies and therapies prescribed for minority patients have been observed in coronary artery angioplasty, bypass surgery, and cancer treatment. Minorities are less likely to receive best-practice therapies, even when confounding variables such as insurance status, income, and severity of disease are controlled. Similar patterns have been described in the principal diagnostic procedure performed on patients, the history and physical examination. Therapeutic disparities such as these are associated with poor health outcomes.[19]

Culturally diverse populations are at increased risk for premature mortality, morbidity, and disability. These increased rates have been attributed to barriers such as lack of health insurance, inaccessible "free" clinics, language differences, cultural conflicts, and lack of trust.[20] Minorities are less likely to be screened, diagnosed, referred, treated, or insured.[21]

Table 21–1 outlines the prevalence of selected risk factors and chronic illnesses among four minority groups. Native Americans have the highest prevalence of risk factors for chronic disease, exceeding even that of other minorities. Increased incidence of obesity, smoking rates, cardiovascular disease, hypertension, high cholesterol, and diabetes are observed in Native American populations.[22] In many tribes, diabetes has become a major cause of morbidity and mortality,[23] and tobacco use is higher among American Indians and Alaskan Natives than other minority groups.[22] African Americans and Hispanic Americans continue to experience disproportionate rates of diabetes as well.

Cardiovascular Diseases and Asthma

Disparities in the occurrence of hypertension, cardiovascular disease, stroke, and asthma are seen among minorities. Hypertension occurs at higher rates among African Americans and Native Americans of both genders than among other racial and ethnic groups.[24] The prevalence of hypertension among African Americans is 40% higher than in whites. Research reports similar disparities between Hispanic populations and non-Hispanic whites. In addition to higher rates of hypertension, minorities tend to develop the disease at an earlier age and are less likely to receive treatment to control it.[25]

Death rates for heart disease are more than 40% higher among African American populations than among whites. Death rates from heart disease are generally higher overall in men than in women, but women have poorer outcomes immediately after myocardial infarction. Forty-four percent of women die within 1 year of myocardial infarction versus 27% of men. Additionally, disparities in income and education levels are associated with differences in the occurrence of heart disease. Families in the lowest income levels report limitation in activity due to chronic disease that is three times that of the highest income families. Americans who reside in rural areas have higher rates of heart disease than Americans residing in urban areas.[26]

Use of antihypertensive drugs, particularly angiotensin-converting enzyme inhibitors,

▶ **TABLE 21-1**. Prevalence of Selected Risk Factors and Chronic Diseases Among Four Miniorty Populations, by Race and Ethnicity

Risk Factor or Chronic Disease	Women			
	American Indian %(n = 1040)	Black %(n = 7735)	Hispanic %(n = 2722)	Asian %(n = 2549)
Obesity	37.7	37.6	28.4	3.1
Current smoking	36.8	20.4	11.2	3.3
Cardiovascular diseases	13.0	9.4	5.6	5.5
Hypertension	36.8	40.9	22.4	17.6
High cholesterol	33.5	34.2	28.9	23.3
Diabetes	19.7	14.5	8.4	4.7

Risk Factor or Chronic Disease	Men			
	American Indian %(n = 751)	Black %(n = 3218)	Hispanic %(n = 1535)	Asian %(n = 1655)
Obesity	40.1	26.5	26.6	2.7
Current smoking	42.6	29.3	26.8	34.4
Cardiovascular diseases	16.4	9.9	7.4	7.5
Hypertension	38.5	34.5	20.5	16.1
High cholesterol	37.1	31.4	35.7	31.4
Diabetes	16.8	11.6	7.1	4.8

Adapted from Centers for Disease Control and Prevention (CDC). Health Status of American Indians compared with other racial/ethnic minority populations—selected states, 2001–2002. *MMWR, Morb Mortal Wkly Rep* 2003;52(47):1148–1152.

increases the risk of stroke by 40% in African Americans when compared with use of diuretics alone.[27] Although stroke rates for the population at large have been declining, the decline is not as significant in the African American population. Racial differences in stroke morbidity and mortality are even greater than those for coronary heart disease. The age-adjusted stroke death rate for African Americans is almost 80% higher than that of whites, with the highest rates seen among African American women born prior to 1950.[26] Among children, African Americans have a relative risk for stroke of 2.12 when compared with white children.[28] This is explained in part by the higher incidence of sickle cell disease in African American children, an illness that has no counterpart among white children.

According to the American Heart Association, women are more likely than men to have a stroke within 6 years of a heart attack[28] and have a one-in-five lifetime risk of stroke versus a one-in-six lifetime risk for men.[29] This translates into an excess of 40,000 female deaths per year from stroke-related causes.

The rate of asthma among preschool children is increasing more quickly than that of any other age group. African American children are twice as likely to be both diagnosed with asthma and hospitalized for it.[30] A study of child Medicaid beneficiaries with asthma reported that African American children had worse asthma status based on physical and emotional health scores, symptoms, and missed days of school. Latino children also had increased school absences and, along with African American children, were less likely to use inhalers and more likely to rely on home nebulizers.[31]

Death from asthma is two to six times more likely to occur among African Americans and Hispanics than whites. The death rate from asthma among children doubled from 1979 to

1993 and was slightly higher among women than men.

Asthma hospitalization rates among children, young adults, and women are high. African American patients are hospitalized at rates three times higher than whites and along with inner-city asthma patients, use emergency departments most often. African Americans are four times more likely than white patients to visit an emergency department for asthma treatment.[26]

Boudreaux et al[32] reported that black and Hispanic patients with asthma were hospitalized more often than whites, used emergency departments more frequently, had lower mean peak expiratory flow rates, and were more likely to report severe symptoms 2 weeks after discharge. Apter et al[33] observed that race, low educational achievement, and lower household income were associated with poor patient compliance. In a study exploring the contributions of race and income to disparities in asthma prevalence among children, Akinbami et al[34] found that although there was no difference in asthma prevalence between racial and poverty groups, asthma morbidity, activity limitations, and severity of limitations were increased among African American and poor children.[34]

Organ Donation

Although notable among all groups, the problem of insufficient organ donation rates is particularly acute among minority communities. Studies of donors by race indicate that 70% of donors are Caucasian, while approximately 13% are African American; 13%, Hispanic; 2%, Asian; and 2%, other or multiracial.[35] Minorities, however, constitute approximately half of the persons on national transplant waiting lists, including almost 24,000 African Americans; 13,000 Hispanics and Latinos; and 4500 Asians and Pacific Islanders.

Various reasons have been reported for the apparent disparity in donor rates. These include lack of knowledge about organ donation, religious beliefs, distrust of the health-care community, fears about premature declaration of death, and the perception that organs of racial and ethnic minorities will not go to members of these communities who need them.[36] Callender et al[37] reported several variables that contribute to the shortage of minority donors, particularly African Americans. These include lack of community awareness regarding the great need for transplants within the African American community, religious beliefs such as "wanting to be whole when you go to heaven," awareness of the Tuskegee study and fear of being used as a guinea pig, fear that signing an organ donor card could result in premature death, and racism (ie, the belief organs donated by African Americans would go to Caucasian patients).[37]

Decreased donation rates among Hispanic donors are also a concern, given the rapid demographic growth of the Hispanic population. Frates and Garcia Bohrer explored barriers to organ and tissue donation[38] and reported deterrents similar to those for African American patients.[36,37] A common theme was reluctance to discuss dying and plans for death. Hispanic Americans also indicated lack of knowledge related to organ donation procedures; fear that declaring themselves donors meant health-care professionals would not try as hard to save them and would allow them to die so their organs could be harvested; and the wish to die with all body parts intact.

▶ EDUCATION TO REDUCE HEALTH DISPARITIES

Cultural diversity continues to present many challenges for health-care professionals. The Institute of Medicine and the Office of Minority Health recommend increasing awareness of racial and ethnic disparities by integrating cross-cultural education into the training of all current and future health professionals.[39] Health-care providers must be able to address these issues in a comprehensive manner across the life span. Patient mistrust of the health-care system, socioeconomic variables, physician bias, impaired physician–patient communication, and lack of cultural competence among health-care professionals all contribute to the disparities described in this chapter.[19]

Lack of cultural competence has been reported as a major barrier to eliminating health disparities.[40] Culturally competent care moves beyond biologic parameters to a more holistic approach, and seeks to increase knowledge, change attitudes, and hone clinical skills.[41] Culture shapes the way in which individuals rationalize their world and provides a lens through which they create meaning.[1] We are all influenced by and belong to multiple cultures that include and extend beyond race and ethnicity.[42] An examination of individual biases and effective cross-cultural communication skills are paramount to the elimination of intercultural barriers and the optimal delivery of health care to diverse people.

Cultural competence education seeks to create an understanding and appreciation of cultural differences and similarities as well as the impact of these factors on the patient. Cultural competence can enhance patient trust and communication, improving overall health outcomes.[43] The ultimate goals of culturally sensitive environments are to decrease medical errors and safety concerns,[40] to improve and increase patient compliance, and to reduce health disparities.

▶ CULTURALLY EFFECTIVE SYSTEMS OF CARE

Whether at the practice or the health system level, cultural effectiveness is difficult to achieve. The health-care environment is not inherently a respectful place. Time constraints and limited resources exacerbate this problem. Some hospitals, for example, encourage house officers to draft discharge orders at the time of admission to improve efficiency. The attitude of "not my job" plays a role as well. Young physicians often feel that asking, "Who

lives at home with you?" is the responsibility of a social worker, not a busy resident. Shrinking resources to provide ancillary services may shift the onus of responsibility back to a time-challenged provider. Civility, much less cultural competence, becomes a scarce commodity in these situations.

This mentality of scarcity can restrict providers' ability to affirm the successes of others and may even lead them to feel satisfaction at their misfortune (ie, cultural bullying). Problem-solving ability, even when there is a solution, becomes limited as well. The danger of operating under this type of mindset is the competition it fuels and the belief that, "with only so much to go around," the successes of one person always come at the expense of another. For health-care providers with a scarcity mentality, the allocation of more resources toward one person or group may be seen as leaving fewer resources for others. A generation of providers is thus created that may have trouble sharing resources, accepting change, planning positively, and believing the best about other people.[44]

Among the consequences of this mentality for medicine is the stereotyping of certain groups and strategic limitation of the resources available to them. Under the façade of limited resources, judgments regarding the provision of services are made on racial, ethnic, or socioeconomic grounds. When differences come to be viewed negatively, the opportunity to develop creative solutions to the challenges of providing care to diverse populations is lost. Some argue that health-care resources are expensive and there is a need for even more limits than currently exist. This view is not necessarily unrealistic from a national or global perspective. However, when an individual practitioner acts on the belief that denying resources to a particular group of patients is justified, the result will be negative health outcomes.

Finally, if an entire practice, hospital, or other health-care setting does not engage all staff members in the effort to enhance cultural skills, patients may never reach the health-care provider, no matter how skilled and effective he or she is. Feelings must be elicited and acknowledged so staff trainees can evaluate their impact and move beyond them to establish common goals for creation of a culturally inclusive care environment. What values, beliefs, and perceptions do the staff hold concerning a "good" patient and a "bad" one? Discussions of systematic bias within institutions, although emotionally challenging, are an essential component of the dialogue about cultural competence.

None of these steps can be accomplished in a single presentation or event related to cultural competence. The process requires leadership, commitment, and directed growth toward a plan for transforming the health-care organization into one that fully embraces the diversity of patients and dedicates itself to improving health delivery for all people. The value of this effort for institutions that undertake it will be optimization of its strengths and a high level of patient satisfaction.

Incorporating Cultural Change Initiatives into Practice

Several models have been proposed as ways to initiate cultural competency training programs. The LEARN model incorporates the following aspects: *L*isten with sympathy and understanding; *E*xplain your point of view in understandable, nonmedical language; *A*cknowledge and discuss similarities and differences to your approach and viewpoint; *R*ecommend a mutually acceptable course of action; *N*egotiate an agreement.[45] CRAASSH, an acronym for *C*ulture, *R*espect, *A*ssess, *A*ffirm, *S*ensitivity, *S*elf-Awareness, and *H*umility, is a model developed by the National Center for Primary Care at Morehouse School of Medicine that emphasizes the importance of the following components:

1. Cultural dynamics and the expression of the many variables that influence culture;
2. Demonstrating respect by asking questions, addressing patients appropriately, respecting personal boundaries and space, and expressing respect for and seeking to learn about the patient's culture;
3. Assessing health beliefs, knowledge, literacy (described in *Healthy People 2010* as "The degree to which individuals have the capacity to obtain, process, and understand basic health information and services needed to make appropriate health decisions"), care-seeking behaviors, and relevant relationships (who is important to the patient, what role that person plays in the patient's life, and how the patient would like that person to be included);
4. Affirming the positive values and characteristics of other cultures by recognizing the expertise and experience that the patient offers and reframing cultural differences to address positive characteristics that contribute to practices we may often view as different;
5. Offering sensitivity through awareness of cultural nuances, historical, political, religious, and social concerns, and differences in models of disease and health;
6. Examining one's personal attitudes and biases through identifying personal norms and values; and
7. Exhibiting a measure of humility in recognizing that cultural competence is not a finite skill set that is acquired but rather a life-long journey and commitment.[46]

Encouraging patients to talk about what they believe and how they actually behave is an essential element of cultural communications. If patients disclose broader contextual information about their lives rather than simply reiterating the health-care providers' instructions, the health professional may gain insights that lead to greater patient compliance with prescribed therapies. In clinical care, it is more important to listen to the patient than to operate from "cultural FAQs," as illustrated by the following example:

A senior medical student who worked in a health center that provided care for underserved Latinos met with a teenage mother who had come with her infant to the clinic. Around the infant's neck was a leather amulet that the student recognized from a health beliefs and practices lecture she had had. She told the mother, "I know what that is—it's a charm to keep your baby from harm." The teen responded, "No, it's just a thing my grandma put on the baby."

In this case, inquiring about the patient's belief would have been more helpful than assuming it. As a result of what the Latino woman may have perceived as stereotyping, the medical student probably lost a valuable opportunity to educate and alert the young mother to the danger of infant strangulation.

Before and After the Patient Encounter

These techniques can be incorporated into clinical practice at several points. Fundamentally, clinicians can address these issues before or after patient encounters.

Before the patient encounter, health-care providers can scan the literature for evidence-based information on disparities that highlights racial, ethnic, and gender differences. They can clarify racial and ethnic sample composition for clinical trials of new medications to assess whether it resembles their practice population. They can link to sites that give ethnically specific data and use it as a guide to formulating differential diagnoses. Clinicians can engage in continuing education that increases their knowledge base with respect to cultural issues relevant to patients in their care. If engaged in research, health-care providers can learn about community- and culturally responsive research strategies that optimize patient "buy-in" and avoid research that could be perceived as exploitative.

During the Clinical Encounter

Although some authors have suggested that a portion of the history be dedicated to cultural questions,[5] rather than marginalizing the inquiry, these issues can be incorporated into the initial examination (Tables 21–2 and 21–3). During this time, the maximal amount of information is obtained about the patient's world. Sensitive issues are often divulged later, after rapport is developed, affording another opportunity to explore the patient's beliefs, health practices, and expectations.

During Clinical Problem-Solving

Clinicians can employ additional strategies for patient encounters that involve challenges to care delivery, such as less-than-optimal compliance, failure to understand health-care instructions, or an impasse in resolving the active medical condition. Learning about the cultural context of care enhances clinician understanding of the complexity, reality, and humanity of patients. Too often, cultural issues are viewed as barriers to be overcome. Although a deficit approach to cultural issues in care undermines the value of diversity, it is important to recognize that clinicians are primarily problem solvers. Thus, in refractory cases, it is useful to explore culture and health practices as the following example shows: The blood pressure of an Asian Indian woman with hypertension and diabetes was poorly controlled using three antihypertensive agents. After multiple changes to medication schedules, patient education, consultation evaluations, and a secondary workup for hypertension, the patient made a casual comment about the difficulty she had in swallowing pills. The clinician followed up by asking how the patient compensated for this long-standing problem, to which she responded that she placed all of her pills in a candy jar and during the course of the day, as she walked around her home, she randomly took a few pills. The woman's perception of cause and effect, onset of action of medicine, and control was probably not a cultural habit, but a result of miscommunication between the provider and patient.

The clinical encounter provides several points of entry at which clinicians can include cultural influences on health care and discuss their impact with the patient. Inquiring about health practices rather than assuming behavior

▶ **TABLE 21-2.** Techniques to Incorporate Cultural Issues into Care in the Physical Exam and Care Delivery

Portion of History	Inquire About	Example
Chief complaint and history of presenting illness	What health beliefs are conveyed with the presentation, patient understanding, and expectations? What are health perceptions about risk?	"What do you think is the cause of this?" "What do you feel might work or not work?"
Past Medical and Surgical History	What has the patient's experience been in the medical system? What is the relative importance that the patient places on medical versus surgical care? Are mental health issues divulged or even addressed as health issues?	"What do you think put you at risk for the illness(es) you had?" "In your encounters in hospitals or offices, have their been good and bad experiences? if so, tell me about them."
Family history	Beyond disease-specific questions, broaden the inquiry to ask the patient about his or her ancestry, where ancestors came from, and what illnesses patient perceives he or she is at risk for based on genetics. Introducing the idea that different peoples have different opinions and approaches to health can lead to a direct question about the relationship between ethnicity or family background and health.	"I am sure that you are aware that your genes influence your health risk. What ancestry are you? (Or, "Where did your ancestors [or your family] come from?") "Do you feel that there is a relationship between your health and your ethnicity or family background?"
Social history	Address wellness and illness in questions. In terms of health habits, ask about self-care that the patient learned in the home. Inquire into social support, and obtain information about the patient's world. Specifically ask about the role of spiritually in health, as the patient may be reluctant to share this with health-care providers. Ask if the patient participates in religious practices that could influence his or her health care. When asking about smoking, drug, or alcohol usage, include questions about family of origin and current family habits as well (broaden the circle to the world beyond the individual). Inquire about self-care in stress reduction.	"What did you learn growing up about taking care of your health?" "Who all lives at home with you?" (This inquiry has more impact than, "Are you married or do you have a partner.") "Tell me about your family" "Some people who are observant of their religion perform fasts for periods of time or have traditions that are important to know about, since it may influence taking medications at certain times. Are there any cultural or religious practices that might influence your health or health care? When you are very stressed out, how do you take care of yourself? Who helps you when you need help? Who are your emergency contact people and how are they connected to you?"

▶ **TABLE 21–2.** (*Continued*)

Portion of History	Inquire About	Example
	Ask who else needs to be included in the discussion of the patient's health. This acknowledges that some patients have cultural systems that are community or group focused, so that the clinician needs to shift from a 1-to-1 orientation to a 1 to-group and needs to know how to communicate with that group in order to make progress in a clinical case.	
Nutrition	Ask the patient to describe what he or she ate the previous day. Inquire if there are changes in the patient's diet associated with festivities, customs, or traditions that you need to know about.	"Often the food we eat may have hidden salt or fat that we are unaware of—especially foods we grew up with. Are their certain types of ethnic foods or seasoning that you eat or use frequently [sofrito, curry, etc.]?"
Medications, including alternative and over-the-counter drugs	Inquire about the use of any types of supplements or medications, including over-the-counter products, home remedies and salves, and alternative or complementary therapies.	"In addition to prescription medicine, do you use any over-the-counter medicines or health aids?" "Do you use any alternative or complementary health practices, such as acupuncture, chiropractic care, herbal medicine, and so on?"
Prevention	A typical patient attitude toward prevention in the United States is, "if it isn't broken, don't fix it." Patients may bring culturally embedded attitudes and perceptions of health screening and prevention. Motivation for health screening should be framed in a positive way, avoiding fear tactics. Some health screening habits (self-breast or testicular examinations) may be viewed as immodest. Education and negotiation will facilitate progress.	"If you stop smoking, you will be able get to the bus in time, rather than miss it because you are winded." This statement is more positive than warning the patient that he or she will develop lung cancer, which, in some cultural groups, is interpreted as akin to putting a curse on the patient.
Sexual history	Extend usual questions about sexual activity, sexually transmitted diseases, and gynecologic or urologic issues to explore the status and attitudes of intimate relationships, attitudes toward sexuality and safe sex (especially as it relates to attitudes of femininity or	"Have you heard of the term 'safe sex'? What does it mean to you?" "Tell me about your relationship—are you satisfied with it? What about being intimate?"

(*Continued*)

► **TABLE 21–2.** (*Continued*)

Portion of History	Inquire About	Example
	masculinity), and gender role and expectations, and delve into screening for violence or abuse.	
Allergies	Beyond differentiating true allergies from intolerances, explore the health beliefs of the patient.	"What was it about your reaction to the medicine that made you feel you were allergic?"
Review of systems	As areas are focused on, attend to the importance or significance the patient places on the system. Some areas may be perceived as more important, as uncomfortable to discuss, or as having additional meaning.	"When I asked about constipation or diarrhea, you seemed especially uncomfortable. As clinicians, we have to ask a lot of personal questions. Is there something about this body area that concerns you? "Is there anything else you would like to tell me about?"

► **TABLE 21–3.** General Issues in the Physical Examination

Issue	Culturally Competent Provider Action	Example
Modesty	Adequately cue the patient to what will occur next in the examination, and explore areas where she or he seems reluctant.	"I need to perform a testicular [breast] examination next. First, I will [. . . .] The reason is[. . .]"
Number of people in the examination room	Inquire if the patient wants someone to be in the room with him her during the examination. There are some limitations that patients and their family may prefer in terms of discordance of genders of the patient and provider. For example, some female patients will refuse examinations, including gynecologic, if the provider is male.	"I strive to give privacy to my patients in the physical examination, but if you want someone in the room with you, please let me know." If there is no way to attend to the same-gender request of the patient and family, then inform them and negotiate whether getting care at this point in time is a higher priority than waiting for another provider. Include the dominant male family member if the female patient wishes him to be in the room.
Health care delivery	Emphasize personal interest in what the patient is actually likely to do or has done, recognizing that change happens slowly and that sharing the truth about behaviors is what is most important.	"What were you able to do or not do?" "How are you handling the medications? Any problems or questions?" "Tell me what you really are doing"

based on knowledge about culturally based health habits eliminates the danger of misattribution. One clinician, for example, told an African American patient with hypertension to cut salt pork out of her diet. The patient, a practicing Muslim woman, said nothing but left the encounter offended because she did not eat pork. The clinician was trying to convey the relationship between salt consumption and blood pressure control. Instead of noting that foods high in salt can raise blood pressure and inquiring whether there were any foods, such as salt pork or soy, that the patient ate on a regular basis, the clinician incorrectly attributed the patient's suboptimal control to a food that she did not eat.

► NATIONAL ISSUES

How does emphasis on cultural competence fit into national trends? In rulings on affirmative action, higher courts have, by and large, eliminated programming to increase the likelihood that ethnic minorities have access to education and related career opportunities. Other forces are moving away from larger social goals for racial equity, believing disparities in education, the workplace, and health care have been resolved. The group that appears to have benefited most from affirmative action was white women.[47,48] Over the past 10 years, the shareholder movement has pushed corporate boards into being more responsible, thus prompting them to "change their complexion."[49] Throughout the 1980s and 1990s, there was a rise in the inclusion of "nonnormative" individuals, although this trend may be declining.[47] As the doors of affirmative action close to women, they also close to those disproportionately affected by health disparities, leaving them without a seat at the table to influence institutional policy.

How, then, do health professionals advocate for reductions in health disparities? How do they, for example, help patients who have no insurance choose whether to take medications for cardiac problems or diabetes, when they can afford only one? These challenges speak to the larger issue of a culturally effective health-care system and move the debate from the confines of the individual provider's office to the larger arena of health-care delivery.

Cultural competence at one level can be seen to deal with the "haves" and the "have nots." As the numbers of working under- and uninsured swell and the middle class shrinks, the at-risk population becomes larger. The current "safety net" is not sufficient to help the number of under- and uninsured people in the United States who do not have health care. According to the US Census, between 15% and 30% of the population was uninsured in 2003. The segment of the population with employment-based health coverage dropped from 70.1% in 1987 to 64.2% in 2002. In 2001 and 2002, both the number and percentage of Americans covered by health insurance declined.[50]

The United States must transform its health-care financing network into a realistic and tenable health-care system that provides better access to health care for all its citizens.

► SUMMARY AND RECOMMENDATIONS

Cultural effectiveness is an essential clinical competence, a goal to be pursued rather than a discrete end point. It is an ongoing process of learning and skill building, of refining and improving upon.[1] By allowing patients to disclose their lives, experiences, and the personal factors that influence them, health professionals can develop strategies to address the whole patient, not just his or her disease. By enhancing communication between patients and clinicians, health care professionals can also elicit information that can change the course of a clinical encounter. Moreover, with added knowledge and skills, health professionals can craft solutions in a number of "languages" of cultural relevance, affording patients a number of ways to connect with care, ultimately decreasing health disparities and improving wellness in patients.

Educational objectives can be defined by beginning at the end and asking, "What do you want to achieve?" Once that is clarified, the best way to measure the objectives can be identified. There needs to be consensus among health-care providers, health industry administrators, governmental officials, and patients that health disparities need attention, education, and research. From the individual student to the largest managed care organization, a dedicated effort needs to be put into place, involving resources and measurements of impact, to train clinicians working in offices and hospitals. Organizations need to be receptive to the change needed to encourage culturally responsive and

▶ **TABLE 21–4.** Summary of Main Points Regarding Cultural Competency

Patients' value and belief systems, behaviors, and health-care practices are critical to a successful clinical encounter
Disparities in the recognition of symptoms, health-care–seeking behaviors, communication and expression of symptoms, ability to understand treatment plans or instructions, expectations of care, and adherence to prevention efforts and treatment regimens each contribute to disparities in health and poor health outcomes
World-views, family systems, and barriers to care are important aspects of knowledge-based issues for culturally effective care delivery
To provide quality health-care, providers must recognize the individual and cultural influences that affect a patient's behavior
Physicians must recognize and understand the layers of influence that culture imparts on peoples' health in order to deliver high quality care and eliminate health disparities
The entire office, hospital, or other health-care setting must include all members (office staff as well as health-care professionals) in the effort to enhance the medical encounter and provide a culturally appropriate experience

▶ **TABLE 21–5.** Summary of Recommendations

• Adoption and evaluation of health professional education and of health professional societies' principle of cross-cultural effectiveness in care, with input from the intended communities at need
• Resources for training that enable implementation of effective curricula
• Development of a system of rewards for individuals, organizations, hospitals, and systems that deliver high-quality, culturally effective care
• Annual evaluation of progress on health disparities
• Ongoing assessment of health policy issues as they affect populations and culturally effective care
• Development of a strategic plan for a health-care system crafted by stakeholders (health-care professionals, industry, government), with a realistic implementation plan
• Resources, including training for interpreter services
• Requirement of second-language training for health-care professionals
• Investment in language technology and software that aids in traversing the linguistic and literacy gaps in patient care
• Evaluation and implementation of a functional, interconnecting public health infrastructure with sufficient resources to achieve realistic goals

appropriate health care for diverse patients. Table 21–4 summarizes the main points about cultural competency that have been outlined in this chapter. Recommendations to help achieve the goal of a culturally responsive health-care system are summarized in Table 21–5.

▶ REFERENCES

1. Nunez AE. Transforming cultural competence into cross-cultural efficacy in women's health education. *Acad Med* 2000;75(11):1071–1080.
2. Lavizzo-Mourey R, Mackenzie ER. Cultural competence: Essential measurements of quality for

managed care organizations. *Ann Intern Med* 1996;124(10):919–921.

3. Cross TL, Bazron BJ, Dennis KW, Isaacs MR. *Promoting Cultural Competence and Cultural Diversity in Early Intervention and Early Childhood Settings.* Washington, DC: National Center for Cultural Competence, Georgetown University; 1989.

4. Tervalon M, Murray-Garcia J. Cultural humility versus cultural competence: A critical distinction in defining physician training outcomes in multicultural education. *J Health Care Poor Underserved* 1998;9(2):117–125.

5. Betancourt JR. Cross-cultural medical education: Conceptual approaches and frameworks for evaluation. *Acad Med* 2003;78(6):560–569.

6. Anderson LM, Scrimshaw SC, Fullilove MT, et al. Culturally competent healthcare systems. A systematic review. *Am J Prev Med* 2003;24(3 suppl):68–79.

7. Betancourt JR, Green AR, Carrillo JE, et al. Defining cultural competence: A practical framework for addressing racial/ethnic disparities in health and health care. *Public Health Rep* 2003;118(4):293–302.

8. Jha AK, Varosy PD, Kanaya AM, et al. Differences in medical care and disease outcomes among black and white women with heart disease. *Circulation* 2003;108(9):1089–1094.

9. Winkleby MA, Kraemer HC, Ahn DK, et al. Ethnic and socioeconomic differences in cardiovascular disease risk factors: Findings for women from the Third National Health and Nutrition Examination Survey, 1988–1994. *JAMA* 1998;280(4): 356–362.

10. Fiscella K, Franks P, Gold MR, et al. Inequality in quality: Addressing socioeconomic, racial, and ethnic disparities in health care. *JAMA* 2000;283(19):2579–2584.

11. Chen J, Rathore SS, Radford MJ, et al. Racial differences in the use of cardiac catheterization after acute myocardial infarction. *N Engl J Med* 2001;344(19):1443–1449.

12. Kahn KL, Pearson ML, Harrison ER, et al. Health care for black and poor hospitalized Medicare patients. *JAMA* 1994;271(15):1169–1174.

13. Pearcy JN, Keppel KG. A summary measure of health disparity. *Public Health Rep* 2002;117(3):273–280.

14. Wyatt SB, Williams DR, Calvin R, et al. Racism and cardiovascular disease in African Americans. *Am J Med Sci* 2003;325(6):315–331.

15. Arnett F. Ankylosing spondylitis. In: Kooperman WJ, ed. *Arthritis and Allied Conditions,* 14th ed. Philadelphia, Pa: Lippincott Williams & Wilkins; 2001:1311–1323.

16. Health Resources Services Administration, Bureau of Primary Health Care. *Pathways to Wellness: Women Centered Primary Care.* Washington, DC: US Dept of Health and Human Services; 2001. Available at: http:// www.bphc.hrsa.gov.

17. Betancourt JR, Jacobs EA. Language barriers to informed consent and confidentiality: The impact on women's health. *J Am Med Womens Assoc* 2000;55(5):294–295.

18. Kumanyika SK, Morssink CB, Nestle M. Minority women and advocacy for women's health. *Am J Public Health* 2001;91(9):1383–1388.

19. Geiger HJ. Racial stereotyping and medicine: The need for cultural competence. *CMAJ* 2001;164(12):1699–1700.

20. Kim-Goodwin Y, Clarke P, Barton L. A model for the delivery of culturally competent community care. *J Adv Nurs* 2001;35(6):918–925.

21. Stone C. Cultural orientation: An emerging dimension of quality in women's health services. *Qual Man Health Care* 2000;8(4):52–64.

22. Centers for Disease Control and Prevention. Health status of American Indians compared with other racial/ethnic minority populations— selected states, 2001–2002. *MMWR Morb Mortal Wkly Rep* 2003;52(47):1148–1152.

23. Lee ET, Howard BV, Savage PJ, et al. Diabetes and impaired glucose tolerance in three American Indian populations aged 45–74 years. The Strong Heart Study. *Diabetes Care* 1995;18(5): 599–610.

24. Centers for Disease Control and Prevention. Cancer mortality among American Indians and Alaska Natives—United States, 1994–1998. *MMWR Morb Mortal Wkly Rep* 2003;52(30):704–707.

25. American Medical Association. *Facts on Health Disparities.* 2003. Available at http://www.ama-assn.org/ama/pub/category/8930.html.

26. US Dept of Health and Human Services. *Healthy People 2010: Understanding and Improving Health,* 2nd ed. Washington, DC: US Government Printing Office; November 2000.

27. National Institutes of Health NHLBI News Release. NHLBI study finds traditional diuretics better than newer medicines for treating hypertension embargoed by journal 2002. Available at: http://www.nhlbi.nih.gov/new/press/02-12-17.html.

28. American Heart Association. *Heart and Stroke Statistical Update*. Dallas, Tex: 2002. Available at: http://www.womenshealth.org/0javascripts/dropinnav.htm?/press/sexdifferences /cardio.htm.

29. Peck P. Stroke is a woman's disease, too. United Press International; 2004. Available at: http://www.nlm.nih.gov/medlineplus/news/fullstory_15950.html.

30. Roberts EM. Racial and ethnic disparities in childhood asthma diagnosis: The role of clinical findings. *J Natl Med Assoc* 2002;94(4):215–223.

31. Lieu TA, Lozano P, Finkelstein JA, et al. Racial/ethnic variation in asthma status and management practices among children in managed Medicaid. *Pediatrics* 2002;109(5):857–865.

32. Boudreaux ED, Emond SD, Clark S, et al. Race/ethnicity and asthma among children presenting to the emergency department: Differences in disease severity and management. *Pediatrics* 2003;111(5 pt 1):e615–621.

33. Apter AJ, Boston RC, George M, et al. Modifiable barriers to adherence to inhaled steroids among adults with asthma: It's not just black and white. *J Allergy Clin Immunol* 2003;111(6):1219–1226.

34. Akinbami LJ, LaFleur BJ, Schoendorf KC. Racial and income disparities in childhood asthma in the United States. *Ambul Pediatr* 2002;2(5):382–387.

35. United Network for Organ Sharing, 2004. Available at: http://www.unos.org.

36. Guadagnoli E, McNamara P, Evanisko MJ, et al. The influence of race on approaching families for organ donation and their decision to donate. *Am J Public Health* 1999;89(2):244–247.

37. Callender CO, Miles PV, Hall MB. Experience with National Minority Organ Tissue Transplant Education Program in the United States. *Transplant Proc* 2003;35(3):1151–1152.

38. Frates J, Garcia Bohrer G. Hispanic perceptions of organ donation. *Prog Transplant* 2002;12(3):169–175, 2002.

39. Office of Minority Health, Office of Public Health and Science, US Dept of Health and Human Services. Assessment of state minority health infrastructure and capacity to address issues of health disparity; 2000. Available at: http://www.omhrc.gov/omh/sidebar/cossmo/EXEC_SUM.html.

40. Kritek PB, Hargraves M, Cuellar EH, et al. Eliminating health disparities among minority women: A report on conference workshop process and outcomes. *Am J Public Health* 2002;92(4):580–587.

41. Callister L. Culturally competent care of women and newborns: Knowledge, attitude and skills. *J Obstet Gynecol Neonatal Nurs* 2001;30:209–215.

42. Smedley B, Stith A, Nelson A, eds. *Unequal Treatment: Confronting Racial and Ethnic Disparities in Health Care*. Washington, DC: Committee on Understanding and Eliminating Racial and Ethnic Disparities in Health Care, Board on Health Sciences Policy, Institute of Medicine, National Academy Press; 2002.

43. Green AR, Betancourt JR, Carrillo JE. Integrating social factors into cross-cultural medical education. *Acad Med* 2002;77(3):193–197.

44. Covey S. *The Seven Habits of Highly Effective People*. New York, NY: Simon and Schuster; 1989.

45. Berlin EA, Fowkes WC Jr. A teaching framework for cross-cultural health care. Application in family practice. *West J Med* 1983;139(6):934–938.

46. Personal communication. Toolkit booklet produced under contract with the Georgia Department of Human Resources Chronic Disease Prevention and Health Promotion Branch in Partnership with the Morehouse School of Medicine.

47. *Fact Sheet 2002: Catalyst Census of Women Corporate Officers and Top Earners in the Fortune 500*. New York, NY: Catalyst; 2002. Available at: http://www.catalystwomen.org/press_room/factsheets/COTE%20Factsheet%202002.pdf.

48. *Diversity in the Executive Suite: Good News and Bad News*. Korn Ferry International; 2002.

49. Darazsd J. National Association of Corporate Directors. Available at: http://www.wherearewomen.org.

50. Fronstin P. Sources of health insurance and characteristics of the uninsured: Analysis of the March 2003 Current Population Survey. Washington, DC: EBRI, Issue Brief Executive Summary; 2003:264.

CHAPTER 22

Case Studies in Cultural Competency

Oladipo Kukoyi, MD[*]

Jason Wilbur, MD

Mark Graber, MD

Hans House, MD

▶ INTRODUCTION

Whether you are an experienced practitioner with many years' service or a student currently preparing for a health profession, you are sure to encounter diverse patients on a daily basis. The demographic trends elaborated in this book suggest that at least one of every four patients you see in the clinical setting will not share your cultural, ethnic, or linguistic heritage.

The 1985 report of the Secretary's Task Force, US Department of Health and Human Services,[1] marked the beginning of a steadily growing literature on the health status of racial and ethnic minorities. This literature now consists of over 30,000 published articles, potent evidence based on the subject.[2] Clinical best practices, many of which are incorporated in this text, are a major product of this knowledge base.

Although clinical practice guidelines[3] address the science of health-care delivery, they are not intended to address its behavioral or communication components. In an environment in which there is never enough time, simply keeping abreast of the science of care is a daunting task. What guidance is there for the student or practitioner who seeks to develop or enhance his or her transcultural or cross-cultural skills? In December 2000, the US Office of Minority Health released the National Standards for Culturally and Linguistically Appropriate Services (CLAS) in Health Care. The CLAS regulations,[4] however, are formulated as broad principles that require a coordinated institutional approach to implement. Development of cultural competence tools for individual practitioners is still a nascent field.

The case studies that follow cannot and do not try to address every variation of ethnic, racial, or cultural diversity that could occur in a patient–provider context. They are intended to complement the scientific data presented in this book with an experiential counterpoint. To

* The McGraw-Hill Companies acknowledge the substantial editorial contributions of Donna M. Frassetto and Nancy N. Woelfl in preparation of this chapter.

generalize too much about cultural norms and values using this material would not be wise. Rather, it is hoped these case studies will motivate further exploration using the "Resources for Reading" at the end of the chapter.

Case Study 1

A young Arab couple, Mr and Mrs Issa, come into your office to seek prenatal care. Mrs Issa, who was born in the Midwest, is in her first trimester as dated from her last menstrual period. She has no prior health history and no health concerns today. Her husband is a recent immigrant from the Middle East and has many questions for you.

1. Which of the following statements about Arab American demographics is *false*?
   a. Most are Christian
   b. Most are American born
   c. Most trace their ancestry to the Middle East
   d. They comprise the largest segment of Muslims in the United States
   e. They are mostly concentrated in a few states

Answer: d.

DISCUSSION

There have been two large waves of Arab immigration to the United States. The first wave began at the end of the 19th century and consisted mainly of Lebanese Christians from what was then Greater Syria. The second wave has brought more diverse populations from Iraq, Yemen, and Jordan, as a result of the liberalization of United States immigration laws in 1965. However, 80% of Arab Americans were born in the United States. The religious affiliation of Arab Americans is predominately Christian (77% Christian; 23% Muslim). The largest segment of Muslims, moreover, is African American, a large proportion of whom belong to the Nation of Islam, which is an indigenous branch of Islam. Most Arab Americans trace their ancestry to the Middle East, and although they reside in all 50 states, a handful of states have

the highest populations: California, Michigan, and New York account for one third of the population.

2. The Issas are Muslim, and you are aware there are cultural issues that may arise during your care of this couple. As you are obtaining a social history from them, they inform you that Islam worldwide is characterized by the following characteristics:
   a. Most Muslims are in the Middle East
   b. Mecca, the holy land, is in Iraq
   c. Muslims must pray five times a day
   d. All people in the Middle East are Arabs
   e. All Arabs are Muslims

Answer: c.

DISCUSSION

Islam is one of the world's three large monotheistic religions, sharing common ground as descendants of Abraham with Jews and Christians. Followers of Islam are known as Muslims and are found throughout the world, with the greatest number in Asia followed by Africa. The largest Muslim country in the world is Indonesia, which has over 170 million Muslims. In fact, not one Middle Eastern country makes the top-10 on a list of countries with the largest Muslim populations, although most Middle Eastern populations are heavily Muslim. The Middle East is very diverse and contains several non-Arab groups, including Turks, Jews, Christians, and Iranians, who can be Persian, Kurdish, or Berbers. Not all Arabs are Muslims, as the large populations of Arab Christians in Lebanon and Israel attest. Mecca, birthplace of the Prophet Mohammed, is in modern-day Saudi Arabia, not Iraq.

3. Which of the following are helpful practices in taking care of Muslim patients?
   a. Allow them to have same-sex providers if desired and if possible
   b. Provide food that is *halal*
   c. Allow wearing of coats over revealing hospital gowns

d. Provide time and space for their *salat* (prayers)

e. All of the above

Answer: e.

DISCUSSION

Islam does not encourage men and women to mix freely in public, and, for this reason and for preservation of modesty, provision of same-sex providers is an option that should be provided to Muslim patients if so desired. For similar reasons, many Muslims (and most patients I know), object to wearing hospital gowns that reveal too much in the back. Allowing patients the option of covering up is reasonable for all people. Muslims (like Jews) are forbidden to eat certain foods, and their food must be prepared by a reliable and certified *halal* food source and cooked according to the rules for *halal* cooking. One of the pillars of Islam involves prayer five times a day, and most devout Muslims will try to carry this out, even when hospitalized for an illness. Providing the space and time for this is respectful.

Suggestion: Do not be surprised if your patients refuse to eat hospital food and eat foods brought from home for this reason. Having *halal* food makes it more likely your patient will eat food that is needed for recovery at the hospital. Patients may need assistance in identifying foods that have been prepared using animal shortening or pork seasonings. They should avoid regular gelatin made with pork, marshmallow, and other confections made with pork. Avoid medicines such as cough suppressants, and extracts, such as vanilla or lemon, that contain alcohol.

4. This visit goes very well and you see the Issas 1 month later for their second prenatal visit. Mrs Issa informs you that the month of Ramadan starts next week. You know that this is the month in which Muslims are expected to fast from sunup to sundown. Which of the following groups of people are excluded from this requirement?

a. Pregnant women

b. Menstruating women

c. Nursing women

d. People on a journey

e. All of the above

Answer: e.

DISCUSSION

During the month of Ramadan, all Muslims are expected to abstain from food, drink, and sex from dawn to dusk. People excused include those mentioned in options a through e, above, and the sick and elderly. They are however expected to make up the number of days missed later in the year. If they are physically unable to do this, they must feed a needy person for every day missed.

Suggestion: Taking care of a sick Muslim patient during the month of Ramadan can be problematic. Although the Qur'an allows sick people to abstain from fasting, some may insist on observing the fast and choose to abstain from food, drink, medications, or tests. This can interfere with regular care. Asking an Imam (Muslim cleric) to help discuss this with the patient can be very helpful.

5. As part of the routine prenatal care, which of the following laboratory tests is likely to be of the lowest value?

a. Cystic fibrosis screen

b. Blood glucose

c. Glucose-6-phosphate dehydrogenase (G6PD)

d. Sickle cell anemia

e. Thalassemia

Answer: a.

DISCUSSION

Diabetes mellitus is a common condition in people of Arab descent. Other diseases prominent in the Arab countries include G6PD deficiency, sickle cell anemia, and the thalassemias. Cystic fibrosis is mostly seen in Caucasian populations.

6. When the time comes for delivery, Mr Issa insists that no male be allowed near his wife's delivery room. He answers questions that the nurses ask of his wife and, when delivery is imminent, he chooses to leave the room, with his wife screaming in the pangs of labor. Some of the nurses are concerned about this behavior and are suspicious that the husband is abusing the wife, although she has denied this repeatedly when they have asked. When the nurses bring this concern to you, you tell them:
   a. "You're right, this looks like a case of spousal abuse; let's call the authorities"
   b. "Maybe you're right, but let's wait until the baby is born before we do anything else"
   c. "It was wrong of him to leave the room with his wife in pain, but that does not make him an abuser"
   d. "I do not think he abuses his wife. I think his behavior is within cultural norms"
   e. None of the above

Answer: d.

DISCUSSION
In traditional Arab cultures, the husband is the family leader and decision maker. He may answer questions directed to his spouse and may decide when his wife should eat and bathe, or the wife may decide basic care patterns such as when to bathe, eat, and breast feed. The health-care team should ascertain how the family wants to make these decisions before the time comes to make them. Although it has been traditional for men to leave matters of birthing to the women, lately, many in the younger generation of Muslims have chosen to remain with their spouses during labor. This is often a personal choice, without a right or wrong answer. The nurses would benefit from more cultural training to recognize norms in cultural behavior and avoid unjustified suspicions of inappropriate behavior where none exists.

7. A healthy 8-lb, 1-oz boy is born. The nurses are passing the infant around and admiring his wonderful hair when the father angrily takes the infant from them. They are surprised, and unsure of what they did wrong. You know the answer, and tell them he is angry because:
   a. Women are not supposed to carry male infants
   b. The nurses might be giving the infant the evil eye
   c. The father is afraid they might call immigration services
   d. All of the above
   e. None of the above

Answer: b.

DISCUSSION
Many cultures around the world believe in a form of "evil eye." It is known in Hispanic cultures as *mal de ojo* and is also part of the belief system of many African cultures (eg, among Somalis). The basic premise is that people who envy the wealth, success, or beauty of others cause adversity by gazing at them. Newborns are particularly susceptible to the evil eye, and expressions of congratulations may be interpreted as envy. As such, it is desirable to avoid saying anything that would be interpreted as praising or admiring the infant, unless invited to do so by the family.

8. The next day, during rounds, you ask the Issas if Mrs Issa is comfortable and if she needs pain medication. She denies having any pain, but Mr Issa firmly insists that she be given pain medication. What do you do?
   a. Listen to Mrs Issa and do not order any pain medication
   b. Listen to Mr Issa and order acetaminophen
   c. Listen to Mr Issa and order intramuscular nonsteroidal anti-inflammatory agents
   d. Listen to Mr Issa and order opioids
   e. None of the above

Answer: c.

DISCUSSION

Arab culture is nonconfrontational, and members of this culture often seek to avoid conflict. Thus, a female patient will usually downplay her pain, knowing that her husband will ensure that she receives pain medication when she needs it. Arab patients also often believe that intrusive procedures such as injections and intravenous fluids are more effective than oral interventions and might prefer an intramuscular analgesic over an oral one.

Case Study 2

You are on call in the emergency department when a young Chinese couple brings in their 2-year-old son for evaluation of fever of 2 days' duration. The boy recently started day care and has been tugging at his right ear. He also has a clear discharge from his nose. You begin to perform a physical examination and notice several welts on the boy's back. They appear to be several days old and are continuous. You suspect child abuse and begin to question the family about the welts.

1. Which of the following approaches is likely to lead you to the right answer about the cause of these welts?
   a. "Did you abuse your child?"
   b. "Do you know how the welts got on your son's back?"
   c. "Have you engaged in any complementary or alternative medicine?"
   d. "I am going to have the call the authorities"
   e. "Are you the boy's biological parents?"

Answer: c.

DISCUSSION

The usage of complementary and alternative medicine is extremely common among Asian populations. Three treatments, in particular, leave welts that are difficult to distinguish from the bruises left by beatings. This has been the source of much misunderstanding between Asian parents who have recently immigrated to the United States and Western health-care providers. In some cases, parents whose children have been administered these treatments by family members or healers have been charged with child abuse and had their children taken from them. Knowing that these forms of treatment are common can help the health-care provider avoid false accusations of abuse. The three common treatments are:

- **Coining and pinching.** A treatment in which a metal coin is dipped in oil, heated, and then rubbed briskly over the skin until welts appear. These welts can also be produced by pinching the skin between the thumb and index finger. These procedures, which are thought to be a means of drawing out fever and illness, leave long lines of continuous dark bruises over the skin.
- **Cupping.** Suction produced by heating and applying small tubes or hot cups to the forehead or abdomen. The cups produce a negative pressure as they cool, resulting in a circular ecchymosis on the skin.
- **Moxibustion.** This treatment for an excess of *yin* (cold) is based on a notion of the therapeutic value of heat. Pulverized wormwood or other burning incense is heated and applied to the torso, head, or neck to produce superficial burns. Sometimes this treatment accompanies acupuncture.

2. The couple answers that their cousin, who recently came from China, did indeed apply coining but that their son did not appear to get better. That is why they have come to the emergency department. As the father tells you this, you notice that he avoids looking at you. How do you interpret this?
   a. As proof of abuse
   b. As a sign of respect
   c. As a sign of shyness
   d. As a sign of fear
   e. As a sign of disgust

Answer: b.

DISCUSSION

Etiquette is very important in traditional Asian societies, and respect for age and position are emphasized. Because of a physician's societal stature, the father was showing respect by looking away when talking to avoid meeting the physician's eye. This is not a sign of fear or shyness, just a cultural show of respect.

Suggestion: Sitting with the legs crossed, leaning on a table or desk, and pointing at anything with the foot when talking are considered signs of contempt toward the person whom one is addressing.

3. After completing your examination, you diagnose the boy with otitis media and prescribe a course of amoxicillin. Which of the following actions is most likely to improve compliance?
   a. Patting the boy on the head on your way out
   b. Ordering a CBC to assure the parents you have been thorough
   c. Asking the family if they understand how to use the medicine
   d. Asking the family to repeat what they have been told in their own words
   e. None of the above

Answer: d.

DISCUSSION

The head is considered the most sacred part of a human being, so the health-care provider should never touch it without first obtaining the parents' permission. If a provider pats a child on the head and then the child becomes ill, the provider may be blamed for taking the child's soul and causing the illness. Similarly blood is viewed as a vital element and in Asian traditional medicine, blood is not drawn for medical purposes. Some Asians believe that venipuncture not only upsets the body's natural balance but also weakens the person, because the body does not replenish lost blood. As a result, providers should minimize the number of tests they order that involve drawing blood. If blood needs to be drawn, reassurance should be given that the blood will not be administered to anyone else. Blood is believed to represent a person's essence, and the thought that one's essence may be given to someone else can cause great fear.

The concept of "face" is extremely important in Asian cultures, and to preserve harmony, patients may appear to agree with a diagnosis and treatment plan even though they have no plan to carry it out. Because of a cultural respect for harmony, Asian patients who do not understand a treatment or even disagree with it may avoid conflict and suppress negative thoughts and emotions. This is because nonacceptance of a request, especially if it is made by a physician, would disrupt harmony. Further, to maintain both their own "face" and that of the physician, Asian patients may avoid admitting that they do not understand the diagnosis or treatment plan or may pretend to accept it when they disagree with it. Physicians should learn to observe the indirect (often nonverbal) communication signs that indicate confusion or displeasure about the diagnosis or treatment plan and should make sure their patients understand the diagnosis and plan. Asking patients to describe the plan in their own words is better than asking, "Do you understand?"

Case Study 3

A young couple that just immigrated to your town from Bosnia comes to your clinic because they are expecting their first child. The wife, who is in her early 20s, is in her first trimester and has no known medical problems. She speaks no English, and her husband speaks only a little. However, using his limited English and some hand gestures, you feel that you could conduct an interview with them. You have just completed a video CME course on "Cultural Competence" to help you deal with such a situation.

1. Cultural competence is defined as:
   a. Learning about multiple cultures
   b. Being able to speak multiple languages

c. Taking diversity classes
d. Adopting a set of cultural behaviors and attitudes that enable you to deliver effective medical care to people of different cultures
e. Hiring staff from a variety of different cultures

Answer: d.

DISCUSSION

Although the other answers are laudable goals, they do not define cultural competence. Cultural competence is a set of behaviors and attitudes that aims to help health-care professionals provide better care to patients from all cultures.

2. You take a few minutes to reflect on why cultural competence is important. You remember a few ways that being culturally competent could help you. Which of the following statements is *not* one of them?
   a. It allows efficient use of time and resources
   b. It increases the chance of providing services that are consistent with patient needs
   c. It might improve health outcomes for minority patients
   d. It might improve patient retention
   e. It is less expensive in the long run

Answer: e.

DISCUSSION

The National Center for Cultural Competence at Georgetown University has identified six compelling reasons why health-care providers should incorporate cultural competency into their practice. They are:

- To respond to current and projected demographic changes in the United States
- To eliminate long-standing disparities in the health status of people of diverse racial, ethnic, and cultural backgrounds
- To improve the quality of services and health outcomes

- To meet legislative, regulatory, and accreditation mandates
- To gain a competitive edge in the marketplace
- To decrease the likelihood of liability and malpractice claims

Cultural competence allows you to use your time and resources efficiently, thus increasing the likelihood that you will provide the services your patient actually wants. This can lead to improved health outcomes for your patients and increase their satisfaction with the process, allowing you to retain more minority patients. Unfortunately, no studies so far show that it can reduce the costs of your practice.

3. Pondering this, you decide to try to provide culturally competent care to this couple. Which one of the following is *not* a step in providing culturally competent care?
   a. Understanding your own culture
   b. Understanding the cultures of others
   c. Accepting every cultural practice as equally valid even when against best medical practices
   d. Understanding how your patients' cultural beliefs affect their attitude towards health care
   e. Adapting your way of working to provide optimal care

Answer: c.

DISCUSSION

The goal of cultural competence is to provide better health care for patients from different cultures. Some of the specific things this goal calls for include:

- Being respectful of cultural differences
- Learning about other cultures
- Being aware of the health impact of cultural beliefs and practices
- Being sensitive to patients' needs
- Using interpreters when necessary
- Adapting to provide optimal care

An easy way to remember this is to use Berlin and Fowkes' LEARN model (*L*istening to the patient's perspective, *E*xplaining and sharing one's own perspective, *A*cknowledging differences and similarities between these two perspectives, *R*ecommending a treatment plan, and *N*egotiating a mutually agreed-on treatment plan).

Suggestion: Although learning and respecting the different cultural beliefs of patients is vital, providing good care does not call for accepting practices that are detrimental to your patient's health.

4. Now that you are ready to proceed with caring for your patient, the question of language arises. Should you rely on the husband as an interpreter? To help guide you, you call your hospital compliance officer who tells you that:
   a. According to federal law, you must provide an interpreter for patients who need it, at your own cost if necessary
   b. Patients must bring in their own interpreters at their own expense
   c. Most insurance companies reimburse for interpreter services
   d. Using family and staff to translate rarely leads to errors and is acceptable practice
   e. There are no privacy concerns when using nonprofessional interpreters

Answer: a.

DISCUSSION

The 2000 US census found that more than 46 million adults, approximately 14% of the US population, speak a language other than English at home, and over 10% of the US population is foreign born. When a health-care professional does not speak the primary language of the patient, loss of important information, misunderstanding of instructions, and poor shared decision-making can occur. Title VI of the 1964 Civil Rights Act requires health-care professionals to provide translation services for patients who need them, at the provider's cost if necessary. Failure to do so would qualify as discrimination and could be prosecuted. Unfortunately, most insurance companies do not reimburse for these services. Interpreters can be scarce and costly. As a result, many physicians use any help they can get for translation, including staff members and family members who are bilingual. This leaves room for error. Using a family member as an interpreter may lead patients to avoid disclosing relevant information they do not want known by the family. Professional interpreters have been trained and certified, whereas ad-hoc interpreters often have no formal training and can make translation errors.

5. What is the proper way to use an interpreter?
   a. Address all questions to the interpreter
   b. Address questions to the patient while looking at the interpreter
   c. Address questions to the patient while facing the patient
   d. Address questions to the interpreter while facing the patient
   e. None of the above

Answer: c.

DISCUSSION

The physician should communicate with, and look directly at, the patient. Remember that nonverbal communication is still important even when a common language is not shared. The physician should speak clearly and give the interpreter time to translate questions and answers. The physician should periodically pause to ensure that the patient understands the questions that are being asked. One way to do this is by asking brief, close-ended questions. Failure to look at the patient while asking questions may be perceived as rude and should be avoided.

6. The husband insists on being the interpreter, but you are not sure this is a good idea. You remember that low literacy is associated with poor outcomes. Which of the following statements is *false*?

a. Patients with low literacy have a 50% increased risk of hospitalization
b. Only 50% of patients take medications as directed
c. Low literacy is a stronger predictor of a person's health than race
d. Low literacy is only an issue among minorities and immigrants
e. None of the above

Answer: d.

DISCUSSION

Poor literacy skills are a stronger predictor of health than a person's race, age, income, socioeconomic status, or employment status. Unfortunately, up to 90 million people in the United States have low literacy skills and many are ashamed to share this with their physicians. This can lead to "noncompliance" because patients cannot read prescription and other instructions. It is not surprising, then, that low literacy patients have an increased risk of hospitalization. To help combat this problem, the American Medical Association (AMA) Foundation has launched the "Ask Me 3" program (*www.askme3.org*). This program urges physicians to ensure their patients ask and understand the answers to three simple questions: What is my main problem? What do I need to do? Why is it important for me to do this? Other strategies to improve communication include asking patients to repeat instructions back to the physician; using of basic, nonmedical lingo when talking to patients; and allowing patients to talk without interruption at the beginning of the visit.

Case Study 4

You are seeing a 67-year-old African American man for the first time in your clinic. He claims to be healthy but has not seen a physician for over three decades. He starts the interview by stating, "Doctors! Can't trust 'em. My wife made me come today." You tell him you are going to ask some questions about his history and then perform a physical examination. After completing the physical examination, you tell him you recommend age-appropriate screening examinations for colon and prostate cancer. The patient politely declines both. You try to explain the importance of screening to him.

1. Which of the following statements about screening is *false* ?
   a. Prostate cancer is a leading cause of death among African American men
   b. Colon cancer is a leading cause of death among African American men
   c. There is clear evidence that screening for colon cancer reduces mortality in African American men
   d. There is clear evidence that screening for prostate cancer among African American men saves lives
   e. Prostate cancer disproportionately affects African American men

Answer: d.

DISCUSSION

There is no firm evidence that screening for prostate cancer reduces mortality from the disease, although some findings suggest additional research is warranted. Prostate cancer is the seventh leading cause of death overall in the United States. In 2002, an estimated 189,000 new cases of prostate cancer were diagnosed in American men, and approximately 30,200 men died from the disease. The burden of prostate cancer varies among different racial and ethnic groups. African American men have about a 60% higher incidence and a twofold higher mortality rate from prostate cancer than white men. Compared with white men, mortality from prostate cancer is 35% lower in nonwhite Hispanics and 40% lower in Asian Americans and Pacific Islanders.

2. After hearing your explanation, the patient agrees to colon cancer screening but still declines prostate cancer screening. Your examination also revealed an elevated blood pressure reading of 160/90 with no abnormal cardiac, lung, or other organ system findings.

These findings are confirmed at subsequent visits, and you recommend that the patient begin taking the antihypertensive agent hydrochlorothiazide to treat his high blood pressure. The patient agrees to begin antihypertensive therapy, but he wants to know whether the research on which you based your choice included black people. You can confidently answer yes, knowing that the ALLHAT trial specifically addressed the issue of generalizability by making sure that about a third of the 33,357 subjects were black.[5] However, you know this has not always been true in scientific research. In fact, you know that minorities are underrepresented in research data on which treatment choices are based. Which of the following is *not* a reason why there are few minorities in research studies?

a. Past history of abuse leading to mistrust of the health-care system
b. Lack of representation of minorities in the medical profession
c. Discrimination
d. Overrepresentation of minorities at lower socioeconomic levels
e. None of the above

Answer: e.

DISCUSSION

All of the above are reasons why few minorities are included in research studies. Minorities' contact with the medical system has been fraught with abuse in the past. The most egregious example of this is the Tuskegee Syphilis Study in which African American men with syphilis were recruited for a naturalistic study of the disease in the 1930s. Over 400 African American men with syphilis were recruited as well as 200 men without syphilis as controls. Informed consent was not obtained, and subjects were told the lie that spinal taps (done for research) were a form of treatment. It was soon apparent that the death rate among those with syphilis was about twice as high as it was among the controls. When penicillin was found to be effective as a cure

for syphilis in the 1940s, the participants were neither informed nor offered treatment, so that the naturalistic study could continue.[6]

This and other past examples of mistreatment by the medical community is a major reason why many minority patients are less likely to participate in research. There have also been overt and subtle discriminatory barriers against minority participation in clinical trials. Minorities are more likely to be poor and undereducated, and research subjects are generally more educated and of higher socioeconomic status. Finally, there is a significant underrepresentation of minorities in the medical profession. For example, although blacks comprise 13% of the population, they are only 4% of the physician population. All these problems lead to difficulties recruiting minority participants for research trials.

3. What percentage of Americans belongs to a minority group?
a. 15%
b. 20%
c. 25%
d. 31%
e. 41%

Answer: d.

DISCUSSION

According to the 2000 US census, 31% of Americans are ethnic minorities, up from 24% in 1990. Yet, only 10% of physicians are from minority groups. This is problematic. The lack of minority physicians leads to a discrepancy in health-care access. Data indicate minority physicians are more likely to serve minority patients and are more likely to serve in urban, underserved areas (which tend to have a greater concentration of underprivileged patients).[7] Black physicians are five times more likely to treat black patients and Hispanic physicians two and a half times more likely to treat Hispanic patients, as compared with nonblack and non-Hispanic physicians, respectively. Minority physicians are also more likely to serve Medicaid patients and those without insurance. Patients of all races consistently rate their relationship with their physician better when their physician is of the same ethnic background.

4. Which of the following statements is *false*?
   a. Patients living in a disadvantaged neighborhood have an increased incidence of coronary artery disease
   b. Patients living in inner-city, disadvantaged neighborhoods have an increased incidence of asthma
   c. Minority patients who are not economically deprived have the same incidence of disease as those who are economically deprived
   d. Both a and c
   e. Both b and c

Answer: c.

DISCUSSION

Patients living in disadvantaged neighborhoods have increased incidences of coronary artery disease and asthma. Minority patients who are economically well off tend to have better health than poorer members of their ethnic group, though their health is still worse than that of comparable white populations.

5. In taking care of African American patients, all of these general principles are helpful to keep in mind *except*:
   a. Family relationships are extremely important
   b. Religion often has a role in the patient's life
   c. It is expected that physicians will call patients by their first name
   d. Food is an important part of African American culture
   e. Nonverbal communication is often as important as what is said

Answer: c.

DISCUSSION

African Americans often maintain extended family ties and view health care as a family responsibility. Therefore, physicians should consider enlisting the family's help in taking care of an ill family member.

Religion is often an important aspect of African American culture, and members of the clergy are highly respected in the community. Churches are very helpful for community outreach efforts and evidence exists that using churches to conduct preventive care services, such as immunizations and screening programs, leads to better patient compliance with preventive guidelines. Some patients may view illness as a test of their faith, and it is prudent for the physician to acknowledge and respect patients' beliefs and perception of illness to the extent that it influences their seeking or receiving health care. Patients of lower socioeconomic status have little choice but to eat what is available at a lower cost. This means advice to patients about eating a well-balanced diet with fresh fruit, lean meat, and fresh vegetables may be to no avail. Advising simple changes in diet such as substituting fish or chicken for red meat in dishes, eating inexpensive raw vegetables, modifying cooking techniques, and changing to a vegetable-based rather than a meat-based diet may be more likely to meet with success.

Communication is important, and African Americans are particularly attentive to nonverbal aspects of communication, such as body language and voice inflection. Respect is also emphasized in this culture, and patients often prefer to be addressed by their formal titles and not their first names or appellations such as "honey," "sweetie," or "dear," which many patients consider condescending. Asking patients permission to call them by their first names is appreciated.

African Americans often prefer that information be provided using real-life examples, rather than cold, dry data or written messages. A useful summary of general principles that should be kept in mind when taking care of African

Americans is found in an article by Witt et al.[8] They are:

- Gain patient trust and understand the historical distrust of the health-care system
- Understand and employ the kinship web in decisions regarding screening and treatment
- Involve the church in developing and delivering prevention and care messages
- Ask patients about the meaning of words or phrases
- Ask patients about the use of alternative medicines and herbs
- Tailor messages about prevention to depictions of real-life situations
- Pay attention to body language and other nonverbal communication

Case Study 5

Two Cuban friends come to your office seeking a family physician to take care of their general health needs. They are both Cuban, but one is white and the other, black.

1. Which of the following assumptions is correct?
   a. Hispanic people are of one race
   b. Hispanic people can all speak English
   c. Hispanic people share a common language
   d. Hispanic people are not American
   e. Hispanic people all like to be called Latino

Answer: c.

DISCUSSION

The term *Hispanic* denotes members of an ethnic group who share some cultural practices, with Spanish as their primary language. However, they comprise a significantly diverse group that may or may not speak English; may be of any race; hail from different countries of origin; and have differing histories, socioeconomic status, or cultural identity. Some members of this ethnic group feel the term *Hispanic* is derogatory, reflecting European ancestry, and may pre-

fer the term *Latino*. Thirteen percent of the overall US population is Hispanic, and they are the largest ethnic group in the United States, having experienced a 58% increase during the 1990s. Despite the diversity represented within the Latino culture, certain values are shared. As in many black cultures, family ties are strong, and families tend to be large and extended. Families serve as the main source of support and often share in decision making. Physicians with a warm beside manner who demonstrate appropriate respect (especially to the elderly) are especially appreciated. Immigrants from Latin America usually come to the United States for economic or political reasons. Hispanics represent a broad spectrum of socioeconomic backgrounds and enter a variety of living conditions in the United States; these facts have an enormous impact on immigrant and public health.

2. Which of the following statements about health issues affecting the Latino community is *false*?
   a. Infectious diseases are common
   b. Fear of deportation prevents some from seeking health care
   c. Lack of insurance can be a potent barrier to accessing health care
   d. Moving to the United States can paradoxically raise the risk for habits that lead to illness, such as obesity and diabetes
   e. Elderly Latinos have a higher mortality than their white counterparts

Answer: e.

DISCUSSION

Recent immigrants are prone to infectious diseases due to inadequate housing, sanitation, or immunizations. There are many reasons for low vaccination rates in this population. They include disbelief in the need for the vaccine, being unaware of the vaccine, lack of patient education by a health provider, lack of transportation, and financial restrictions.

Immigrating to the United States can result in poorer nutrition, obesity, a sedentary lifestyle, and an increase in smoking and risky sexual behavior in Latinas (Hispanic women). This translates, in part, into a twofold increased incidence of diabetes in Latinas. For Latino men, there is an increased risk of drug abuse, alcohol abuse, tobacco use, and driving under the influence. These risks increase the longer the patient lives in the United States.

Latinos often do not receive preventive health care. For example, they have a lower rate of screening for diabetes and hypertension than blacks or whites. Some avoid seeking health care services because they fear being discovered by immigration authorities. Others are hindered by lack of insurance. Complementary and alternative practices are also common. Although they are less likely to access health care, older Hispanics seem to have a similar or greater life expectancy than same-age whites in the United States and suffer lower mortality from cardiovascular diseases, cancer, and chronic illnesses. The risk of diabetes, however, is higher. This phenomenon has been described as "selective immigration" and implies a predilection for healthier individuals to immigrate to another country.

3. You get into a discussion of race with your new patients, and they point out several things to you that you had not thought of before. Which of the following is true about race?
   a. It is a valid biological construct
   b. It is interchangeable with ethnicity
   c. All members of a certain culture are the same race
   d. It is a purely social construct
   e. It has no importance in American history
   Answer: d.

DISCUSSION
Race is a politically and emotionally charged topic in the history of the United States. Since the late 18th and early 19th centuries, attempts have been made to validate race as biologically based to justify discriminatory practices. How-ever, the Human Genome Project demonstrated conclusively that there is no biological basis for race.[9] Humans share over 99.9% of their DNA, and one cannot tell a member of one race from another on the basis of genetics. Although the terms *race* and *ethnicity* are often used interchangeably, they are not equivalent. Race is an arbitrary social construct that is applied to people based on visual appearance, whereas ethnicity refers to people with a common country of origin, a shared ancestry, or a common historical past. Culture refers to a specific set of values, beliefs and customs shared by members of a community. People from the same culture can be of different races, as in this case scenario, which focuses on white and black Hispanics from Cuba. One need only listen to the news to see that race continues to play an important and often divisive role in American life.

4. Which of the following statements about health disparities is *false*?
   a. White Hispanics have a higher incidence of breast and colorectal cancer
   b. Clinicians may order fewer diagnostic tests if they do not understand a patient's description of symptoms
   c. Clinicians may overcompensate by ordering more tests when they do not understand what their patients are saying
   d. Minority children are more likely to be evaluated and reported for suspected abuse even after controlling for likelihood of abusive injury
   e. Blacks have the highest colorectal cancer mortality rates
   Answer: a.

DISCUSSION
The incidence of colorectal and breast cancer is actually lower in white Hispanics than in other whites and blacks. However, this does not always translate into less significant disease. There are significant disparities in health-care quality and outcomes for minorities compared with nonminorities, even when controlling for

possible confounding factors such as income, education, and insurance. So even though Hispanics have a lower incidence of the above-named cancers, they have a similar mortality when compared with non-Hispanics. The statements in b through e are correct. Of particular note, blacks have the highest colorectal cancer mortality rates. Also of note is the fact that when toddlers of different races present with similar fractures, minority toddlers are significantly more likely to be reported for suspected abuse, even after controlling for age, insurance status, and likelihood of abuse. This is a reflection of biases and stereotyping.

Minority patients are significantly less likely to have their pain treated by physicians. Additionally, few, if any, pharmacies located in poor, inner-city areas have narcotics available for patients with a prescription. This has a further adverse effect on the pain management of minority patients.

In general, mortality rates among racial and ethnic minorities are higher for cancer, heart disease, diabetes, stroke, kidney failure, human immunodeficiency virus (HIV) infection, and acquired immunodeficiency syndrome (AIDS). Minority groups are also disproportionately affected by asthma, lead poisoning, accidents, homicides, and other environmental health concerns. Some minorities experience higher infant mortality rates and are less likely to receive timely prenatal care. There are numerous other examples of health-care disparities that exist between majority and minority groups. These include but are not limited to:

- Infant death rates for blacks are twice those of whites.
- Heart disease mortality rates are 40% higher in blacks compared with whites.
- Hispanics are almost twice as likely as whites to die from diabetes and are more likely to be obese and have high blood pressure than non-Hispanic whites.
- Blacks are 13% less likely to undergo coronary angioplasty and one third less likely to receive bypass surgery than whites.

- Only 7% of black and 2% of Hispanic preschool children hospitalized for asthma are prescribed routine medications to prevent future hospitalizations, compared with 21% of white children.
- The length of time between an abnormal screening mammogram and follow-up diagnostic testing is more than twice as long for Asian American, Hispanic, and blacks women than for white women.
- Minorities are less likely to receive immunizations, mammograms, and other preventive care, even when funded by Medicare.
- Higher rates of uninsurance and a lack of physicians in minority communities result in reduced access to primary care.
- Minorities are less likely to undergo heart catheterizations, coronary artery bypass grafting, dialysis, lung cancer surgery, and organ transplantation.
- Blacks have 55% higher mortality rate and 6-year shorter life expectancy than whites.
- Several studies show the deleterious effect of discrimination on health outcomes, including increasing the risk of diabetes, hypertension, depression, and preterm birth, independent of other risk factors.

Data suggest that, although perhaps not overtly racist, unconscious biases on the part of physicians can affect the care of patients. A frequently cited study in the *New England Journal of Medicine* in 1999 found that, all things being equal, physicians were 60% less likely to refer black women for cardiac catheterization than men and whites.[10] It is our hope that raising physicians' awareness of such unconscious biases will help to mitigate their effect, resulting in the provision of better care to all patients.

▶ REFERENCES

1. US Dept of Health and Human Services, Task Force on Black and Minority Health. *Report of the Secretary's Task Force on Black and Minority Health*. Washington, DC: USDHHS; 1985.

2. National Library of Medicine, PubMed Index. Available at: http://www.ncbi.nlm.nih/entrez.

3. Agency for Healthcare Research and Quality, National Guideline Clearinghouse. Available at: http://www.guideline.gov.

4. US Dept of Health and Human Services, Office of Minority Health. *National Standards for Culturally and Linguistically Appropriate Services in Health Care.* 2001. Available at: http://www.omhrc.gov/clas.

5. US National Institutes of Health; National Heart, Lung, and Blood Institute. *The Antihypertensive and Lipid-Lowering Treatment to Prevent Heart Attack Trial—ALLHAT.* Available at: http://www.nhlbi.nih.gov/health/allhat/.

6. Gamble VN. A legacy of distrust: African Americans and medical research. *Am J Prev Med* 1993;9(6 suppl):35–38.

7. Smedley BD, Stith AY, Nelson AR. *Unequal Treatment: Confronting Racial and Ethnic Disparities in Health Care.* Washington, DC: National Academy Press; 2003. Available at: http://books.nap.edu/books/030908265X/html/.

8. Witt D, Brawer R, Plumb J. Cultural factors in preventive care: African-Americans. *Prim Care* 2002;29(3):487–493.

9. Human Genome Project Information. Available at: http://www.ornl.gov/sci/techresources/Human_Genome/home.shtml.

10. Schulman KA, Berlin JA, Harless W, et al. The effect of race and sex on physicians' recommendations for cardiac catherization. *N Engl J Med* 1999;340:618–626.

▶ RESOURCES FOR READING

American Medical Association. Cultural Competence Compendium: Section IV—Underserved and Underrepresented Racial, Ethnic, and Socioeconomic Groups. Chicago, Ill: AMA. Available at: http://wwwama-assn.org/ama/pub/category/2661.html.

Diaz VA Jr. Cultural factors in preventive care: Latinos. *Prim Care* 2002;29(3):503–517,viii.

Kreps GL, Kunimoto EN. *Effective Communication in Multicultural Health Care Settings. (Communicating Effectively in Multicultural Contexts 3).* Thousand Oaks, Calif: Sage; 1994.

Lane WG, Rubin DM, Monteith R, et al. Racial differences in the evaluation of pediatric fractures for physical abuse. *JAMA* 2002;288(13): 1603–1609.

Like RC, Steiner RP, Rubel AJ. STFM Core Curriculum Guidelines. Recommended core curriculum guidelines on culturally sensitive and competent health care. *Fam Med* 1996;27:291–297.

Lynch EW, Hanson MJ. *Developing Cross-Cultural Competence: A Guide for Working with Children and Their Families,* 3rd ed. Baltimore, Md: Paul H Brookes Publishing; 2004.

National Center for Cultural Competence. Available at: http://www.georgetown.edu/research/gudc/ncc6.html.

Paniagua FA. *Assessing and Treating Culturally Diverse Clients: A Practical Guide. (Multicultural Aspects of Counseling Series 4).* Thousand Oaks, Calif: Sage; 1994.

Qureshi B. *Transcultural Medicine: Dealing with Patients from Different Cultures,* 2nd ed. Dordrecht, Netherlands: Kluwer; 1994.

Rodriguez MA. Cultural and linguistic competence: Improving quality in family violence health care interventions. *Clin Fam Pract* 2003;5(1): 213–235.

Sirovitch BE, Schwartz LM, Woloshin S. Screening men for prostate and colorectal cancer in the United States: Does practice reflect the evidence? *JAMA* 2003;289(11):1414–1420.

Smedley BD, Stith AY, Nelson AR. *Unequal Treatment: Confronting Racial and Ethnic Disparities in Health Care.* Washington, DC: National Academy Press; 2003. Available at: http://books.nap.edu/books/030908265X/html/.

US Preventive Services Task Force. *Screening for Prostate Cancer.* 2002. Available at: http://www.ahrq.gov/clinic/uspstf/uspsprca.htm.

Witt D, Brawer R, Plumb J. Cultural factors in preventive care: African-Americans. *Prim Care* 2002;29(3):487–493.

CHAPTER 23

Diversity and the Health-Care Workforce

RUBENS J. PAMIES, MD

GEORGE C. HILL, PhD

LEVI WATKINS, JR, MD

MARY J. MCNAMEE, PhD, RN

LOIS COLBURN

▶ INTRODUCTION

Nearly 40 years ago Dr Martin Luther King, Jr, said, "Of all the forms of inequality, injustice in health care is the most shocking and inhumane."[1] This statement has haunted the health-care system since it was pronounced. It is estimated that in the mid-1960s, approximately 3% of physicians in the United States were minorities [2] and despite the push to desegregate education, there were still health professions schools that did not admit African Americans. Beginning in the late 1960s, on the heels of the death of Dr King, the health professions began the effort to increase the number of minorities entering careers in health care. Over the intervening years, there have been many initiatives—funded by the federal government and philanthropy—focused on increasing the numbers of minorities entering into health and science careers.[3,4]

Perhaps the most compelling argument for building a diverse health workforce comes from the US Institute of Medicine's (IOM) landmark report, *Unequal Treatment: Confronting Racial and Ethnic Disparities in Healthcare.*[5] Undertaken at the request of Congress, the IOM systematically studied the literature to assess differences in the kinds and quality of health care received by minorities in the United States. Part of the charge also involved providing recommendations on how to eliminate healthcare disparities. Among the legal, regulatory, and policy interventions to reduce disparities, the IOM recommended that there be an "increase in the proportion of underrepresented U.S. racial and ethnic minorities among health professionals."[5]

Although the rationale for increasing the representation of minorities in the late 1960s through the 1970s tended to focus on issues of equity and access to education, the IOM report focused on the benefits or outcomes of having a diverse health-care workforce, that is, the potential to reduce health disparities. Well-articulated arguments support the importance of having diversity in health-care manpower in the 21st century, especially in the traditional health professions. Based on the evidence examined, the IOM concluded that: (1) individuals from minority groups prefer to obtain health care in an environment in which they see minority health-care providers; (2) minority health-care providers are more likely to practice in underserved areas; (3) minorities consider pursuing professions where they see minority role models, such as faculty; and (4) minorities are more likely to participate in research studies when the research is conducted by a health-care provider from the same minority group. Increasing the number of minority health-care professionals also benefits the professions as a whole by enhancing the learning environment through a diverse group of learners and increasing the cultural competence of peers.

The purpose of this chapter is to review the demographic characteristics of the United States and the health-care workforce, including those in the educational pipeline. The chapter also reviews current challenges and barriers to building the diverse health-care workforce recommended in *Unequal Treatment.*

▶ US POPULATION CHANGES: TWO MAJOR TRENDS

Two major demographic trends are affecting the workforce in the United States—the growth of this country's minority population and the aging of the population. Both have potential to significantly alter the health-care workforce.

Over the past 30 years, the United States has become an increasingly diverse nation. In 1970, racial and ethnic minorities comprised less than 17% of the population. By 2000, 30% of the US population was minority. With each decade the number of citizens from minority groups has increased at a greater rate than the non-

minority population. Between 1970 and 2000, the population of non-Hispanic whites grew by 15%, while the number of minorities grew by over 150%.[6,7] Most of this growth was fueled by large-scale immigration from areas such as Latin America and Asia. Since 1980, the Asian and Pacific Islander population has tripled, and the Hispanic population has doubled.

By the year 2050, the US Census Bureau projects that nearly half of the US population will be minority[8] (Table 23–1). This demographic shift has already occurred in California, Hawaii, and New Mexico, as well as the District of Columbia, which have populations comprised primarily of minorities. Thirteen additional states now have minority populations of at least 30% (Table 23–2). Furthermore, even states with historically low numbers of minorities have seen dramatic shifts. For instance, in Massachusetts the nonwhite population grew from just over 4% in 1970 to 18% in 2000, and in Nebraska, from less than 5% to nearly 13%.[6,7]

Not only has the minority population of the United States changed, but so too has the way in which racial and ethnic data are collected by the US Census Bureau and the federal government.[9] The 2000 Census marked the first time that individuals could designate more than one race in addition to Hispanic ethnicity, and nearly 3% of the population did so. Individuals could select any one of 15 different race categories plus three options for writing in a more specific race. This change, coupled with Hispanic ethnicity, has the potential to yield up to 264 racial and ethnic combinations, thereby challenging the country's concept of what constitutes a minority.*

The United States has also grown older since the 1990 census, with the median age increasing from 32.9 years in 1990 to 35.3 in 2000, reflecting the aging of the baby boom population.[10] A wide variation, however, exists in the age composition for segments of the population, with those reporting two races and Hispanics having the youngest populations (22.7 and 25.8 years,

---

*There are a possible 132 different racial group categorizations, plus up to 39 Hispanic or Latino groups.

▶ **TABLE 23-1**. US Interim Population Projection by Race and Hispanic Origin, 2000–2050

Race or Hispanic Origin	2000	2010	2020	2030	2040	2050
Total population[a]	282,125	308,936	335,805	363,584	391,946	419,854
White alone	81.0[b]	79.3	77.6	75.8	73.9	72.1
Black alone	12.7	13.1	13.5	13.9	14.3	14.6
Asian alone	3.8	4.6	5.4	6.2	7.1	8.0
All other races[c]	2.5	3.0	3.5	4.1	4.7	5.3
Hispanic[d]	12.6	15.5	17.8	20.1	22.3	24.4
White non-Hispanic	69.4	65.5	61.3	57.5	53.7	50.1

[a]Population in thousands.

[b]Percentages.

[c]Includes American Indian and Alaska Native alone, Native Hawaiian and Other Pacific Islander alone, and two or more races.

[d]Hispanics may be of any race.

Source: US Census Bureau. U.S. Interim Projections by Age, Sex, Race, and Hispanic Origin; 2004. Available at: http://www.census.gov/ipc/www/usinterimproj/. Internet release date March 18, 2004.

▶ **TABLE 23-2**. Emerging Majorities—States With Minority Populations of 30% or More

State	Minority Population in 2000 (%)
Hawaii	77.1
District of Columbia	72.2
New Mexico	55.3
California	53.3
Texas	47.6
Mississippi	39.3
New York	38.0
Maryland	37.9
Louisiana	37.5
Georgia	37.4
Arizona	36.2
Nevada	34.8
Florida	34.6
New Jersey	34.0
South Carolina	33.9
Alaska	32.4
Illinois	32.2

Source: US Census Bureau. Population by Race and Hispanic or Latino Origin, for the United States, Regions, Divisions, and States, and for Puerto Rico: 2000. Available at: http://www.census.gov. Internet release date April 2, 2001.

respectively), while non-Hispanic whites have the oldest (38.6 years).

Interim population projections indicate that the US population will continue to age through 2050. In 2000, 12.4% of the population was aged 65 and older. By 2050, this figure will approach nearly 21%.[8] According to the Bureau of Labor Statistics, "by 2050 for every 100 people working, there will be 111 who are not in the labor force," and of this group, nearly three quarters will be either under 16 or over 65 years[11] (Table 23–3). Furthermore, by 2050 almost half the labor force will be minority.[11] Ultimately, as minorities constitute a larger percentage of the US workforce, the country will increasingly need to rely on these groups not only for its health care but also to support the dependent population of the young and the old.[12]

▶ THE HEALTH-CARE WORKFORCE IN THE 21ST CENTURY

The United States prides itself on being the world leader in health care and health-care research. This leadership has led to a lengthening of the life span for the population, new medications, treatments, and a health-care workforce

▶ **TABLE 23–3**. US Interim Population Projection by Age, 2000–2050

Year	Total (No.)[a]	Population (%)	Percentage Change From 2000
	Projection Population of Persons ≥ 65, 2000–2050		
2000	35,061	12.4	—
2010	40,243	13.0	14.8
2020	54,632	16.3	55.8
2030	71,453	19.6	103.8
2040	80,049	20.4	128.3
2050	86,705	20.7	147.3

[a]Population in thousands.

Source: US Census Bureau. U.S. Interim Projections by Age, Sex, Race, and Hispanic Origin; 2004. Available at: http://www.census.gov/ipc/usinterimproj/. Internet release date March 18, 2004.

that accounted for 8.5% of the national workforce in 2002.[13]

Historically, health professions such as dentistry, medicine, pharmacy, and optometry have been male dominated. Because of affirmative action as well as the women's movement, gender inequity has decreased over the past 30 years. Data from the US Census Bureau show that in 1970 women comprised 9% of physicians, 3% of dentists, 12% of pharmacists, and 3.5% of optometrists.[14] By 2000, the percentage of women in medicine had increased to 27%, in dentistry to 18%, pharmacy to 46.5%, and optometry to nearly 28%.[15] The trend toward increasing numbers of women in health professions requiring advanced degrees will continue as the older, male workforce retires. As an example, in the under-40 age group, women now account for about one third of physicians and dentists, whereas they comprise less than 15% of physicians and less than 5% of dentists in the 50 and older bracket.[15]

In those health-care fields that do not require postbaccalaureate education, women tend to be in the plurality. Women account for 90% of dietitians and nutritionists, 92% of registered nurses, 77% of audiologists, and 98% of dental hygienists.[15]

Nowhere is the gender equity transformation greater than in the group of individuals currently enrolled in health professions schools. Women comprised nearly half of new entrants into allopathic medical schools in 2003[16] and 42% of new entrants into dental schools in 2001.[17] Similar trends are also apparent in other health professions.[17]

The current racial and ethnic composition of the US national health-care workforce continues to shows a major imbalance in the number of minorities in the health professions (Table 23–4). Although the minority population in the United States has more than doubled in the past 30 years and the number of minority health professionals has increased substantially,* blacks, Hispanics, Native Hawaiians or Pacific Islanders, and American Indians or Alaska Natives remain underrepresented in those professions requiring a baccalaureate or advanced professional degree, such as pharmacy, medicine or nursing.[15]

In 2000, African Americans, approximately 12% of the US population, comprised only 5% of physicians and 9% of registered nurses, yet they accounted for nearly 21% of licensed practical nurses and 31% of health-care aides. Hispanics, the largest single minority group in 2000, are underrepresented in all health occupations (listed in Table 23–4), including professions not requiring a baccalaureate degree. American Indians, Alaska Natives, and Native Hawaiians show similar trends.

▶ MINORITIES IN HEALTH PROFESSIONS EDUCATION PROGRAMS

As noted at the beginning of this chapter, two major demographic trends are beginning to

---

*In 1970 US Census, there were only 6044 black physicians and 2384 black dentists; by 2000, the number of blacks who were physicians increased over fivefold to 31,390, and dentists more than twofold, to 5075.

▶ **TABLE 23-4.** Race and Hispanic Origin of Selected Health Professions, 2000

Selected Health Occupation	Total (No.)	Hispanic (%)	Non-Hispanic				
			White (%)	Black (%)	Asian (%)	AI/AN (%)	NH/PI (%)
Dentists	155,715	3.6	82.8	3.3	8.8	0.2	0.0
Dieticians and nutritionists	80,440	6.3	72.0	15.1	4.6	0.4	0.1
Optometrists	30,950	2.7	86.5	1.6	7.9	0.1	0.0
Pharmacists	206,360	3.2	78.9	5.1	11.2	0.2	0.0
Physicians and surgeons	705,960	5.1	73.6	4.4	14.9	0.2	0.0
Physician assistants	57,970	8.1	76.2	8.4	4.5	0.7	0.1
Podiatrists	10,950	1.7	90.0	4.6	2.8	0.0	0.0
Registered nurses	2,268,000	3.3	80.4	8.8	5.7	0.4	0.1
Clinical laboratory technologists	298,635	5.7	70.8	11.0	10.2	0.4	0.1
Dental hygienists	113,965	3.7	90.9	2.3	2.0	0.3	0.1
Diagnostic related technologists	227,720	5.9	81.7	7.5	3.2	0.4	0.1
Licensed practical nurses	596,355	5.8	68.4	20.8	2.4	0.8	0.1
Nursing and home health aides	1,802,660	10.5	51.9	31.0	3.1	1.0	0.2
Occupational and physical therapist assistants/aides	10,475	3.2	58.3	6.5	1.6	0.3	0.0
Dental assistants	22,010	2.5	58.6	2.3	6.2	0.1	0.0

AI/AN, American Indian or Alaska Native; NH/PI, Native Hawaiian or Pacific Islander.

[a]This table does not represent all races available in the EEO file. Therefore, percentages do not sum to 100%. Race data are for "race alone."

Source: US Census Bureau, EEO Tool. Employment by Occupation, Sex, Age, and Race for U.S. Total. Available at: http://www.census.gov/eeo2000/index.html.

occur in health professions schools—namely the graying and increasing diversity of the population. However, like the greater health professions workforce, the student bodies and faculties of this country's health professions educational programs do not reflect the demographic composition of the larger society.

Students

Over the decade of the 1990s, the number of minority students of all racial and ethnic groups increased in health professions schools. In 1991–1992, minorities comprised less than 30% of enrolled students; by 2000–2001, they ac-

counted for more than 30% in most health professions, a change that was the result of continued growth in the number of Asian and Pacific Islander students enrolled.[17] In allopathic medicine, Asians accounted for nearly 15% of students in 1991–1992; by 2000–2001, they comprised just over 20% of enrolled students.[18] The numbers of other underrepresented minorities—blacks, Hispanics, and Native Americans—remained relatively constant during this time (Table 23–5).

Data from baccalaureate nursing programs show a much more promising trend. In the 1993–1994 academic year, black, Hispanic, and Native American students comprised 13% of enrolled students; in 2003–2004, these same

▶ **TABLE 23-5**. Total Enrollment by Race and Ethnicity in Selected Health Professions Schools, 1991-1992 and 2000-2001

Number

Race or Ethnicity	Allopathic Medicine		Osteopathic Medicine		Dentistry		Optometry		Pharmacy		Podiatry	
	91–92	00–01	91–92	00–01	91–92	00–01	91–92	00–01	91–92	00–01	91–92	00–01
White non-Hispanic	47,094	42,242	5778	8230	11,152	11,185	3754	3634	18,242	22,565	1664	1386
Black	4334	4900	236	400	907	862	141	126	1531	3132	233	177
Hispanic	3645	3645	276	381	1187	925	295	268	867	1255	161	103
Asian	9438	13,331	685	1734	2585	4295	652	1373	2755	7392	201	290
Native American	301	519	37	72	51	112	22	27	87	137	8	12
Total	65,602	66,160	7012	10,817	15,882	17,349	4864	5428	23,482	34,481	2247	1968

Percentage

Race or Ethnicity	Allopathic Medicine		Osteopathic Medicine		Dentistry		Optometry		Pharmacy		Podiatry	
	91–92	00–01	91–92	00–01	91–92	00–01	91–92	00–01	91–92	00–01	91–92	00–01
White non-Hispanic	71.8	63.8	82.4	76.1	70.2	64.5	77.2	66.9	77.7	65.4	74.1	70.4
Black	6.6	7.4	3.4	3.7	5.7	5.0	2.9	2.3	6.5	9.1	10.4	9.0
Hispanic	5.6	5.5	3.9	3.5	7.5	5.3	6.1	4.9	3.7	3.6	7.2	5.2
Asian	14.4	20.1	9.8	16.0	16.3	24.8	13.4	25.3	11.7	21.4	8.9	14.7
Native American	0.5	0.8	0.5	0.7	0.3	0.6	0.5	0.5	0.4	0.4	0.4	0.6

Source: US Dept of Health and Human Services, Health Resources and Services Administration. United States Health Personnel Factbook. Washington, DC: USDHHS; June 2003.

groups accounted for 18.5%. Blacks alone account for over 12% of students enrolled. At the master's level, similar trends have occurred. In 1993–1994, slightly over 8% of enrolled students were black, Hispanic, or Native American; by 2003–2004, these groups comprised 15.4%[19] (Table 23–6).

Between 1993 and 2001, the percentage of health professions degrees awarded to non-Hispanic white students declined in most disciplines. In 1993, whites accounted for nearly 75% of all allopathic medicine graduates; by 2001, the percentage of whites fell to approximately 67%. Similar trends were seen in osteopathic medicine, dentistry, and optometry (Table 23–7). The primary reason behind this decline was the increase in the number of Asian and Pacific Islander students in the health professions. In 1993, Asians comprised about 15% of dentistry graduates; by 2001 the figure was nearly 24%. Throughout the 1990s the percentage of graduates who were black, Hispanic, or Native American either increased slightly or remained the same. Only in podiatry did the percentage of underrepresented minority graduates decline, from 15.3% to 9.3%.

Graduates from baccalaureate and masters level nursing programs are more likely to be black, Hispanic, or Native American. In the 2003–2004 academic year, just over 17% of baccalaureate and over 13% of masters-level graduates were underrepresented minorities (see Table 23–6).

Health Professions Faculties

Faculties at health professions schools such as dentistry, medicine, and pharmacy are still for the most part white and male. Of full-time US medical school faculty, less than 31% are female and more than 75% are non-Hispanic whites.[20] For at least one these professions, dentistry, there is concern about a shrinking pool of dental educators, resulting from retirement of current faculty and the low numbers of dental graduates entering academic dentistry. Data from a 2001–2002 survey indicated there were 335 open dental faculty positions, but only 250 of these positions were being actively recruited, and 20% had been open 1 year or longer.[21]

There is growing concern over the shortage of nursing faculty as a result of both retirement (average age was nearly 51 in 2001) and advanced degree nurses moving into clinical practice rather than academic roles.[22,23] In 2003, the American Association of Colleges of Nursing (AACN) reported nearly a 9% faculty vacancy rate for doctorally prepared nurses.[24] The shortage of nursing faculty not only compounds, but is compounded by, the shortage of nurses in the workforce. In 2003, AACN found that more than 10,000 potential baccalaureate nursing students were turned away due to faculty shortage and a lack of clinical sites and classroom space.

Although the student bodies of health professions schools have grown more diverse, particularly with the increase of Asian students, the faculties of these schools still lag in numbers of black, Hispanic, and Native American faculty (Table 23–8). About 90% of full-time nursing faculty in baccalaureate and graduate programs are white, with African American faculty comprising the largest group of minority faculty at 5.6%. Both dental and medical school faculty are more racially and ethnically diverse than nursing school faculty. The largest percentage of minority faculty are Asian, with just over 9% in dental schools and nearly 12% in medical schools. Black and Hispanics together comprise slightly more than 10% of dental faculty and 7% of medical school faculty. Native American faculty comprise a very small percentage of all faculty in nursing, dentistry, and medicine (see Table 23–8).

▶ PREPARATION FOR THE HEALTH PROFESSIONS

The pathway to a professional health-care career can be fraught with dead ends, detours, and barriers for many students, especially minorities. The barriers begin in elementary and

▶ **TABLE 23-6.** Nursing Enrollments and Graduates, 2003—2004

Race	Total Enrollment						Graduates					
	Undergraduate		Masters				Undergraduate		Masters			
	No.	%	No.	%			No.	%	No.	%		
White	89,923	76.1	27,024	78.4			24,738	78.2	7614	79.5		
Black	14,616	12.4	3635	10.5			3436	10.9	876	9.1		
Hispanic	6479	5.5	1473	4.3			1708	5.4	341	3.6		
Asian	6458	5.5	2127	6.2			1480	4.7	540	5.6		
Native American	765	0.6	202	0.6			276	0.9	57	0.6		
Total	118,241	—	34,461	—			31,638	—	9578	—		

Source: Berlin LE, Stennett J, Bednash G. Enrollment and Graduations in Baccalaureate and Graduate Programs in Nursing, 2003–2004. Washington, DC: American Association of Colleges of Nursing; 2004.

▶ **TABLE 23-7.** First Professional Degrees Awarded, 1992–1993 and 2000–2001

Number

Race or Ethnicity	Allopathic Medicine		Osteopathic Medicine		Dentistry		Optometry		Pharmacy[a]		Podiatry	
	92–93	00–01	92–93	00–01	92–93	00–01	92–93	00–01	92–93	00–01	92–93	00–01
White non-Hispanic	11,279	10,284	1359	1913	2451	2613	903	820	1263	4163	350	399
Black	900	1085	45	92	159	192	24	28	109	446	42	34
Hispanic	610	787	69	97	212	188	31	37	56	212	30	14
Asian or Pacific Islander	2001	2888	132	317	532	1036	139	328	369	1339	35	66
Native American	73	88	69	23	10	34	3	2	7	24	1	1
Total[b]	15,531	15,403	1627	2450	3605	4391	1148	1289	1904	6234	476	528

Percentage

Race or Ethnicity	Allopathic Medicine		Osteopathic Medicine		Dentistry		Optometry		Pharmacy[a]		Podiatry	
	92–93	00–01	92–93	00–01	92–93	00–01	92–93	00–01	92–93	00–01	92–93	00–01
White non-Hispanic	72.6	66.8	83.5	78.1	68.0	59.5	78.7	63.6	66.3	66.8	73.5	75.6
Black	5.8	7.0	2.8	3.8	4.4	4.4	2.1	2.2	5.7	7.2	8.8	6.4
Hispanic	3.9	5.1	4.2	4.0	5.9	4.3	2.7	2.9	2.9	3.4	6.3	2.7
Asian or Pacific Islander	12.9	18.7	8.1	12.9	14.8	23.6	12.1	25.4	19.4	21.5	7.4	12.5
Native American	0.5	0.6	4.2	0.9	0.3	0.8	0.3	0.2	0.4	0.4	0.2	0.2

[a]The increase in the number of first professional degrees awarded in Pharmacy reflects the movement to the PharmD from the BS in Pharmacy.
[b]Total also includes persons for whom no race or ethnicity data are available and nonresident aliens.

Source: US Dept of Education, National Center for Educational Statistics. IPEDS Completion Survey.

▶ **TABLE 23-8.** Racial and Ethnic Composition of Health Professions Faculty in Nursing, Dentistry, and Medicine

Race or Ethnicity	Full-time Nursing Faculty, 2003		Full-time Dental Faculty, 2002–2003		Full-time Medical School Faculty, 2003–2004	
	No.	%	No.	%	No.	%
White	9161	90.1	3724	77.0	79,540	75.3
Black	548	5.6	267	5.5	3305	3.1
Hispanic	184	1.5	233	4.8	4091	3.9
Asian or Pacific Islander	185	1.9	443	9.2	12,531	11.9
Native American	38	0.4	16	0.3	108	0.1
Multiple races	—	—	—	—	635	0.6
Other or not reported	—	—	152	3.1	5466	5.2
Total	10,116	—	4835	—	105,676	—

Sources: **Nursing schools:** Berlin LE, Stennett J, Bednash G. Salaries of Instructional and Administrative Nursing Faculty in Baccalaureate and Graduate Programs in Nursing 2003–2004. Washington, DC: American Association of Colleges of Nursing; 2004. **Dental schools:** American Dental Education Association Survey of Dental Educators, 2002–2003. **Medical schools:** Association of American Medical Colleges, Faculty Roster System. Available at: http://www.aamc.org/data/facultyroster/usmsf03/start.htm.

secondary school, and continue through college. They have many origins (socioeconomic, academic, cultural, financial, and political), are often intertwined, and work synergistically to deter students from a direct path to a health-care career.

Many studies have been undertaken by governmental agencies, professional associations, and philanthropic organizations to identify the most significant barriers deterring students, especially minority students, from the pursuit of health-care careers.[3,4] These barriers cluster around the topics of preparation, persistence, and price.

Preparation

Preparation for a health-care career has many facets: educational, socioeconomic, psychological, and financial. Educational preparation for success in college and beyond begins informally in the home with children's books, daily reading time, introduction of new words in conversation, and listening.[25] It continues formally in elementary school, where the educational building blocks of reading, mathematics, and written and oral communication are introduced, nurtured, and developed.

Students from families with inadequate income, single-parent households, or low levels of parental education are predisposed to experience academic difficulties in primary school because of family characteristics. For example, one study identified third-grade reading level as a significant predictor of student success in college, positing that by third grade, the phonetic basics of reading have been learned and students become more skilled at applying their reading skills thereafter.[25]

At the primary school level of the educational pipeline, reading and mathematics achievement gaps appear early. Whereas 41% of white students read at grade level in fourth grade, only 15% of Hispanic and 12% of African American students do.[26] The achievement gap is similar when comparing mathematics and sci-

ence scores.[27,28] These achievement gaps remain fairly constant through elementary school and serve to exclude minority children from gifted and talented programs and from placement in college preparatory curricula in high school.[29]

There are no quick fixes for the achievement gaps between and among minority and majority student groups. Educational system-wide interventions, such as Project Grad, focus on decreasing the achievement gap and have shown positive results but are difficult to implement due to the school district–wide nature of the interventions.[30]

Parental income and parental education pose socioeconomic barriers to adequate student academic preparation and future educational success. Parental income serves as a proxy for a combination of factors that have an impact on the quality of education accessible to students from primary through professional education. Income determines area of residence; available primary school options, quality of instruction, parent and faculty expectations of the students, opportunities for student enrichment, and disposable income for learning materials. As early as the seventh grade, correlations are reported between educational and occupational expectations and student socioeconomic status (SES).[31] Thus, the seeds of low expectations for educational achievement and occupational choices are sown early for poor children from both majority and minority families.

The importance of parents knowing about and requesting a rigorous high school curriculum as preparation for college and graduate education cannot be overemphasized. In one study, a college preparatory curriculum negated the effect of low SES, with 62% of those who were well prepared graduating from college whereas only 21% of poorly prepared low SES students succeeded in doing so.[32]

According to a 2003 Pew Foundation report, for majority and minority students to succeed in entry-level university courses, they need an elementary and secondary education that prepares them with "habits of the mind." The report presents a compendium of specific knowledge and skills foundations in English, mathematics (through trigonometry and statistics), natural science courses, second language, and art as the basic preparatory curriculum for college and graduate education.[33]

The importance of mastery of mathematics and science in high school was reiterated in a 2004 College Board report, which identified physics, precalculus, and calculus classes in high school as subjects associated with high SAT and ACT scores. Results reported for racial and ethnic minority groups indicated that African Americans, Mexican Americans, and American Indians had the lowest number of students who completed these courses in high school, respectively.[34]

A similar relationship between mathematics course completion in high school and future academic success is reported by Adelman,[32] who identified completing a mathematics course above the algebra II level in high school as the most important predictor of student college graduation.

The relationship between low SES and limited educational achievement in high school and college also appears in the 2001 College Board report, *Swimming Against the Tide: The Poor in American Higher Education*. This study indicated that students from the lowest SES quartile entering college demonstrated marked achievement gaps when compared with those in the upper two SES quartiles in reading (44% versus 78%), mathematics (44% versus 82%), science (39% versus 79%), and social science (45% versus 79%). These gaps translate to 20% to 25% lower ACT and SAT scores than their higher SES classmates on admission.[31]

Although the percentage of low SES majority and minority students entering college within 3 years of high school graduation is increasing,[35] the number who graduate within 6 years is discouraging. Only 54% of low SES, 46% of African American, and 47% of Latino students persist to graduation.[35] The importance of parental income on the pathway to college graduation and completion of an advanced degree in the health sciences is clear.

Parental education level is also a strong predictor of student academic success in higher education. Parental education level encompasses many subjective areas, including parent experience with and knowledge of the educational system, value placed on education, expectations of the child in school, expectations of the school, comfort in communicating with teachers regarding the child and the curriculum, and parental encouragement and support of educational achievement and the pursuit of higher education.[36]

Parents want the best for their children, but parents who have limited educational backgrounds themselves often do not know how to be active partners with their child and the school to facilitate the child's educational potential. They are not aggressive in pursuing or questioning the criteria for student selection to gifted and talented placement programs in elementary and middle schools. As a result, their children are less likely to be placed in a rigorous college preparatory program, honors, or advanced placement class in high school[37] (Table 23–9). Minority students are often advised into a vocational-technical curriculum and full-time employment after high school graduation, rather than preparation for attending college.[30]

In the past 30 years, the standard-of-living expectations for high school graduates have

▶ **TABLE 23–9.** Participation in Gifted and Talented Classes by Ethnic Group and K–12 Population, 1997

Ethnic Group	Gifted Population (%)	K–12 Population (%)
White	76.6	64.0
African American	6.6	17.0
Latino	8.6	14.3
Asian	6.6	3.1
Native American	0.9	1.1

Source: US Dept of Education, Office for Civil Rights; 1999.

changed markedly. Previously, the recipient of a high school diploma could expect to find full-time employment in a company with health benefits that would provide a reasonably comfortable lifestyle with annual raises.[38] The earnings for workers with high school diplomas versus college graduates and those with advanced degrees over the past 30 years now show static earnings growth for the high school diploma holder.[38] With outsourcing of jobs to the international markets, the importance of preparing for and completing a college education becomes more essential for students each year. Dropping out of high school or terminating education at high school graduation relegates another generation of minority students into the low-income and low-education category, with its associated barriers to pursing higher education. As the nation continues to become more diverse, this cycle of lack of expectations and lack of minority student preparation for higher education will exacerbate the shortage of minority health-care and research professionals.

Persistence

Persistence in pursuit of a goal is a characteristic that low-income, first-generation college students must possess in abundance to overcome the academic preparation barriers described earlier. They still face significant academic, psychological, and financial challenges in pursuing college and a health-care professional program.

Academic barriers to students are objective and measurable, such as grade point average and SAT and ACT scores. The psychological barriers are subjective and not easily discussed with families, friends, or advisors. Being the first individual in a family to complete high school and prepare for college puts stress on students and requires their steadfast persistence.[37] Students who are the first generation in their families to attend college have limited opportunities to learn about the variety of health-care careers available, develop a relationship with role models, participate in shadowing experiences, or learn about summer enrichment health-care and research opportunities, and they have limited social support for pursuing a professional goal.[3] These opportunities are available and part of the culture of students from professional families. It is not unusual to see several generations of children of health-care professionals pursuing health-care careers. Familiarity with a role, acquaintance with role models, and opportunities to shadow and learn more about a health-care professional role attract students to particular roles. Majority and minority students from first-generation college families must be self-directed and persistent in seeking out these opportunities. This singular focus on a goal that is outside their environmental comfort zone brings with it considerable self-reflection and self-doubt.

Reported psychological barriers identified by first-generation African-American students contemplating college include concern that college is not an option and that attending college will not be beneficial, and fear of being socially isolated and intimidated on a large, predominately white college campus.[39] Fear that college is not an option stems from many sources, including family, peers, and environment. Family members may not see the value in pursuing college and may not support this goal verbally or financially. Students whose peers are not college bound venture to a new campus without the company or support of friends; and students who have completed elementary and high school with primarily minority students know that their education was inferior to that of other majority students entering college.[40,41] It is telling that in 2000 in all the institutions of higher education in the United States, 23.6% of African American college graduates came from historically black colleges or universities.[42] These students have opted to decrease the environmental stress of college by continuing their higher education in a primarily minority environment.

Fears related to attending college prevent students from completing application materials and initiating their college education straight from high school.[37] Delaying the start of college or attending college part-time prevents students from completing prerequisites and applying for admission to health-care professional programs in a timely fashion.[36] Admission to health-care professional programs is highly competitive, and admission committees seek students who have demonstrated their academic ability when enrolled full-time. Students who persist in their pursuit of a health-care career and excel while taking prerequisite courses two or three at a time do not receive the same respect for their abilities in admission decisions.

Price

Real and perceived financial barriers also deter low-income minority and first-generation college students from pursuing their educational goals. Lack of family income can preclude students from attending high school summer math and science enrichment programs, taking standardized test (ACT, SAT) review programs, and applying for admission to 4-year institutions of higher education. These students and their families are unfamiliar with the process of "shopping" institutions of higher education for scholarships, grants, and financial aid offers. They overestimate the cost of college, are confused by the extensive financial information requested on the application forms, and are unable to balance the benefits of college with their perception of the high cost.[43] In one study, parents overestimated the cost of tuition and fees at a public university by 70%.[43] Without a realistic idea of costs, and assistance in completing application forms and navigating the higher education application process, students who are academically qualified but from low-income, poorly educated families do not persevere in completing applications and either delay their college education or select a community college to begin their education part-time.[44]

Although perceived college costs delay minority student applications to college, real costs hinder minority students entering institutions of higher education. Minority high school graduates who persist and achieve admission to a university encounter a financial aid environment that now favors merit instead of need in financial aid awards. Over the past 14 years while college costs have continued to escalate, the focus of college student financial aid has shifted from grants to loans and from need based to merit based.[45] In the 1990s, Pell grant appropriations, which provide financial assistance to low-income, full-time students, grew by 23% while institutional aid in the form of non–need- and merit-based scholarships increased 84%. As a result, more financial assistance now goes to middle-class students, while low-income students increasingly must rely on loans to meet educational costs or on employment and part-time college attendance.[45]

Educational pathway detours related to financing a college education place additional distance and hurdles between minority students and entry into a health-care career. Programs in the United States that lead to MD, DDS, PharmD, and PhD degrees are few in relation to the number of postsecondary institutions of higher education, and competition for admission to these programs is intense. Admission committees know the academic rigor required of health professional students and seek students who have demonstrated academic success when taking heavy class loads. They surmise that students who have faced academically challenging semesters in the past will be similarly successful in the future. Part-time students do not fare as well in evaluation of readiness for the challenges of health career education using this standard.

Further elaboration on the intertwined personal, academic, institutional, cultural, and political factors that actively affect minority students pursuing a health-care career is found in the 2001 IOM publication, *The Right Thing to Do; The Smart Thing to Do: Enhancing Diversity in Health Professions.*[46]

► SOCIOPOLITICAL CHALLENGES TO INCREASING DIVERSITY

Background

Lyndon B. Johnson framed the concepts underlying affirmative action nearly 40 years ago. As then-President Johnson noted in his speech, "It is not enough to just open the gates of opportunity. All our citizens must have the ability to walk through those gates."[47] While the legislative efforts of the 1960s began to pave the way for access to higher education, it was not until the turmoil resulting from the death of Dr Martin Luther King, Jr, that more immediate and dramatic gains occurred in the number of minorities enrolled in and graduating from higher education programs. This trend was also observed in health professions programs. In 1961, 803 black students were enrolled in allopathic medical schools; of this number, nearly 80% were at two schools, Howard and Meharry. By 1970, this number had nearly doubled to 1509, with most now enrolled at "majority" medical schools.[48,49]

The first significant challenge to affirmative action in admissions came in the 1970s with the *University of California Regents v Bakke*.[50] This case officially set the parameters for admissions practices in higher education for almost 25 years. The Supreme Court, in a 5-to-4 decision, upheld the right of universities to use race as one of the many admissions factors to be considered as part of a holistic review. The decision, however, specifically prohibited the use of quotas or separate admissions tracks.

New challenges to affirmative action in higher education began to unfold in the mid-1990s, and some still have an impact today. Two initiatives in California, both led by Ward Connerly, a University of California regent, reignited national debate over the use of affirmative action in admissions policy. The first, SP-1, adopted by the Regents of the University of California, prohibited consideration of race, religion, sex, color, ethnicity, or national origin as criteria for admission to any University of California school or program of study.[51] Con-

nerly, joined by then-Governor Pete Wilson, continued his efforts to eliminate the use of affirmative action through a ballot initiative in California, *Proposition 209*, which stated that "the state shall not discriminate against, or grant preferential treatment to, any individual or group on the basis of race, sex, color, ethnicity, or national origin in the operation of public employment, public education or public contracting."[52] The initiative was passed in 1996 and after court challenges went into effect in 1997. Although the Regents of the University of California system ultimately rescinded SP-1 in 2001, *Proposition 209* remains law.

Subsequent to the passage of *Proposition 209* in California, the anti–affirmative action campaign moved to the state of Washington, where a similar constitutional ballot initiative, *Initiative 200*, passed by a narrow margin in 1998.[53] In contrast to the situation in California, where *Proposition 209* had gubernatorial support, Washington's governor, in a directive about implementation of *Initiative 200*, noted:

> Diversity of all kinds—racial, gender, ethnic, socio-economic, and geographic to name a few—are [sic] vitally important to the educational experience. It is thought-provoking interaction with people different from ourselves that opens our minds, broadens our perspectives and sets a top-quality education apart from a mediocre one. I encourage our state institutions of higher education to intensify recruitment and outreach programs to maintain diversity in our state's educational system. However, preferences in admissions based on race, sex, color, ethnicity and national origin should be discontinued.

Initiative 200 currently remains in effect.

In Texas, Cheryl Hopwood and other plaintiffs brought suit against the University of Texas under the Equal Protection Clause of the Fourteenth Amendment and argued that, because the University of Texas Law School gave substantial racial preferences in admissions, they had been discriminated against and denied admission.[54,55] Rather than using race as one of many factors in

▶ **TABLE 23–10**. Underrepresented Minority Matriculants to US Medical Schools, 1995 and 2001[a]

State	1995	2001	Numerical Change, 1995–2001	Percentage Change, 1995–2001
California	179	126	−53	−29.6
Texas	218	181	−37	−17.0
Mississippi	14	5	−9	−64.3
Louisiana	46	35	−11	−23.9
Washington	14	6	−8	−57.1
All other states	1554	1433	−121	−7.8
Total	2025	1786	−239	−11.8

[a]Underrepresented minorities include African Americans, Mexican Americans, mainland Puerto Ricans, American Indians, Alaska Natives, and Native Hawaiians.

Source: Cohen JJ. The consequence of premature abandonment of affirmative action in medical schools admissions. JAMA 2003;289(9):1146.

the admissions process, the University of Texas Law School used a dual admissions process: one for majority applicants and another for minority applicants. Different procedures to evaluate prospective candidates were used by each committee. The District Court, citing *Bakke,* found that the university failed to establish a compelling state interest for its separate treatment of minority applicants and that the admissions process was not a narrowly tailored remedy to improve past discrimination. Although the District Court did not enjoin the law school from using race in admissions, a 1996 decision by the Fifth Circuit Court of Appeals did. The Court agreed that "any consideration of race or ethnicity by the law school for [the] purpose of achieving a diverse student body is not a compelling interest under the Fourteenth Amendment." This decision by the Fifth Circuit Court affected not only Texas, but also Mississippi and Louisiana. In 1997, the Texas attorney general announced that all public universities in Texas must employ race-neutral admissions criteria.[56] A recent Supreme Court decision involving a Michigan case, discussed in the next section, vacated the earlier decision by the Fifth Circuit Court.

Taken together, *Proposition 209, Initiative 200,* and *Hopwood* set the tone for the latter half of the 1990s. The impact of these events

can be seen in medical school admissions for the states involved. Between 1995 and 2001, California medical schools experienced a decline of nearly 30% in the number of underrepresented students matriculating, while Texas medical schools saw a 17% decline (Table 23–10).[57] Although it may never be possible to disentangle the effect of various challenges to affirmative action from the normal ebb and flow of the medical school applicant pool, many in the medical school community felt admissions committees were becoming more conservative for fear of possible legal action.

Affirmative Action Reaffirmed

In late 1997, the University of Michigan became the focal point of two lawsuits challenging the use of race in admissions practices in higher education. The first case, *Gratz et al v Bollinger,*[58] centered on the admissions practices of the university's undergraduate college, while the second case, *Grutter v Bollinger,*[59] challenged the law school. In both suits, the plaintiffs argued that the university's admissions practices unlawfully discriminated against applicants because the university took race and ethnicity into account as a "plus" factor in admissions. Ultimately, both cases were heard by the Supreme

Court in the fall of 2002. The Supreme Court handed down its ruling in June 2003.

In a 6-to-3 decision, the Court ruled that the admissions process of the undergraduate school at the University of Michigan was unconstitutional because it used a formula approach and did not provide individualized consideration of applicants, something deemed essential in the *Bakke* decision. The undergraduate program used a point system, with underrepresented minority applicants automatically receiving 20 points on a 150-point scale.[58]

In *Grutter v Bollinger,* in a 5-to-4 decision, the Court ruled the admissions policies used by the law school, where race was only one of many admissions factors considered, did not violate the US Constitution or other federal civil rights statutes. The majority opinion, written by Justice Sandra Day O'Connor, stated that the law school's "narrowly tailored use of race in admissions decisions" furthered "a compelling interest in obtaining the educational benefits that flow from a diverse student body."[59]

Implications of the Supreme Court Affirmative Action Decisions

The June 23, 2003 Supreme Court decision finally "lifted . . . the cloud of uncertainty that had engulfed affirmative action" since the *Bakke* decision.[60] The majority opinion, written by Justice Sandra Day O'Connor, captured the importance of the decision on affirmative action in the admissions process. She noted, "in order to cultivate a set of leaders with legitimacy in the eyes of the citizenry, it is necessary that [the] path to leadership be visibly open to talented and qualified individuals of every race and ethnicity. All members of our heterogeneous society must have confidence in the openness and integrity of the educational institutions that provide this training."[59]

In practical terms, what must health professions schools consider in designing an admissions policy to conform to the requirements of the *Grutter* decision? The following key points

are outlined in a recent document from the Association of American Medical Colleges.[60]

- Health professions schools must address why having a racially and ethnically diverse student body is educationally valuable.
- Schools must ensure there are no quotas or set-asides, and that applicants are considered in the same competitive pool, using the same policies, procedures, and admissions committee members.
- The admissions process must be holistic and individualized, with race as only one of many factors considered. If necessary, schools should hire additional admissions officers or expand admissions committees to ensure that individualized review can take place.
- Schools should adopt a definition of diversity that includes, but is not limited to, racial and ethnic diversity.
- Health professions should make good-faith efforts to consider workable race-neutral alternatives to race-conscious policies; however, not all race-neutral alternatives must be exhausted before considering race-conscious policies. A school is not required to adopt those alternatives if it deems them inappropriate or unworkable.
- There should be a periodic review process to determine whether race and ethnicity remain necessary as factors in the admissions process to the school.
- Finally, health professions schools should support research that explores the benefits of diversity.

▶ WORKFORCE DIVERSITY AND INTERNATIONAL MEDICAL GRADUATES

As the United States strives to create a diverse workforce, some advocate international medical graduates (IMGs) as an interim solution.

The debate on the role of IMGs in augmenting the health-care workforce has a long history.[61,62] The National Advisory Commission on Health Manpower was charged in 1967 to "develop appropriate recommendations for action [to improve] the availability and utilization of health manpower." Although the central focus of the commission's recommendations was to increase the supply of physicians by expanding the current capacity of US medical schools through increased class size and construction of new schools, the commission also suggested that IMGs could aid in reducing health manpower shortages.[60] Subsequently, medical schools expanded from 89 in the mid-1960's to 126 by 2002,[63] and the number of IMGs grew dramatically such that by 2002, one quarter of practicing US physicians were international graduates.[64] It should be noted that the IMG physician workforce does not consist solely of foreign-born individuals. Nearly 16% of the IMGs in residency programs in 2003 were native US citizens.[65] Recent data on practicing physicians indicate that nearly one third of foreign IMGs were from India (21%) or the Philippines (9%) and that the 10 countries listed in Table 23–11 account for more than 50% of physicians in this group.[64]

IMGs can be recruited to practice in rural and underserved areas through use of visa waivers that allow an individual to seek permanent residency after a service obligation period. The use of IMGs to address physician shortages in these vulnerable communities has raised concerns about quality of care and cultural competency within the professional community. A survey of the nine poorest neighborhoods in New York City showed that 70% of the physicians were IMGs, and that physicians from urban areas who accepted Medicaid were more likely to be IMG practitioners and to lack board certification.[66] In urban and rural underserved environments with diverse foreign-born IMGs, there is the potential that "when physicians and patients differ with respect to race, ethnicity, language, religion and values, ensuring fair, equitable and culturally sensitive care is more challenging."[67] Foreign-trained practitioners may experience very different physician–

▶ **TABLE 23–11.** Ten Most Prevalent Non-US Nationalities Among International Medical Graduates Working in the United States

Country of Birth	IMG Physicians (%)	IMG Residents and Fellows (%)
India	21.0	25.1
Philippines	9.0	3.9
Cuba	4.2	< 2.0
Pakistan	4.2	6.8
Iran	3.1	3.3
Korea	2.7	< 2.0
Egypt	2.5	2.7
China	2.4	3.9
Germany	2.0	< 2.0
Syria	2.0	2/8

IMG, international medical graduate.

Source: American Medical Association, Physician Masterfile, 2004. Reproduced with permission from McMahaon GT. Coming to America—International medical graduates in the United States. N Engl J Med 2004;350(24):2437.

patient relationships than in their country of origin, and even experience a sense of disorientation in terms of their role within the health-care team.[64] Even among those IMGs who share a common language such as Spanish, there may be vast differences between the socioeconomic backgrounds of the health-care provider and the patient that could potentially nullify the bond of a common language.[67]

Although using international graduates seems to represent an immediate solution to the physician and nursing shortage, it is not without its own potential problems for the practitioner. A study of nurses who emigrated to Australia to serve that country's growing multicultural society showed perplexing results. The foreign-trained nurses reported feelings of "isolation, alienation, anxiety, depression, and culture shock" at being away from their country of origin.[68]

There are also ethical concerns regarding the reliance on IMGs to solve workforce distribution problems in this country that center around developed countries such as the United States

▶ **TABLE 23–12**. Summary of Recommendations

- There must be continued focus by federal, state, foundation, and professional associations on the disparities in health care and research related to minority populations. Large-scale, national, data-driven initiatives from organizations such as the Institute of Medicine and the W. K. Kellogg's Sullivan Commission are needed to keep these concerns at the forefront and mobilize the many constituencies that must work together to address them
- Standards on diversity and cultural competence such as those of the Liaison Committee on Medical Education must become a formal part of the accreditation process and be rigorously enforced for all health professions educational programs
- High school and college pipeline programs must be critically reviewed, assessed for program effectiveness, and disseminated nationally to allow for wide-scale replication
- Minority and nonminority groups must be mobilized to improve K–12 curricula and counseling and promote a college preparatory curriculum for all students
- Health professions schools must build partnerships with undergraduate colleges with large minority student enrollments such as historically black colleges and universities, Hispanic-serving institutions, and tribal colleges to identify, mentor, and ultimately recruit students into health professions programs
- Health professions education associations and societies should initiate national campaigns similar to the American Association of Medical Colleges' "Project 3,000 by 2000," to mobilize schools to recruit, admit, and retain minority students
- Professional societies and health-care organizations should actively involve minority professionals in recruitment efforts through mentoring, shadowing, and participating in minority student group activities related to health careers. Programming must also include educating students about the various health professions career paths and building programs that address academics and socialization skills
- Health professions schools and health-care organizations, such as hospital systems, should collaborate to develop career ladders to move unskilled and semiskilled workers to more advanced careers, developing career paths that take an individual from a nursing aide to registered nurse
- In light of the Supreme Court *Grutter* decision, health professions education schools must establish a vigorous research agenda to investigate the educational benefit of having a diverse student body

taking "the best and the brightest from less developed nations" at the expense of those "donor" nations.[69]

Do IMGs solve the problem of the maldistribution of health-care professionals in the United States? It is not entirely clear. Some research has shown that when foreign graduates complete their residency training and postgraduate professional obligations, they pursue much the same career trajectories as graduates of US medical schools.[70,71] Others argue that IMGs do fill an important void in providing care in medically underserved areas.[72,73] However, even if states adopted aggressive policies to recruit IMGs with common cultural backgrounds to their minority populations, such as increasing the number of Latino physicians in California, the numbers would still be insufficient to meet the needs of that state's Hispanic population.[67]

▶ SUMMARY AND RECOMMENDATIONS

The population of the United States is becoming more diverse, with minorities now the plurality in several states. With continued immigration and higher minority birth rates, this demographic trend will eventually occur in all 50 states. Over the past 30 years, a variety of efforts have been initiated to increase the number of minority health professionals, including outreach programs to minority students in high school and college, affirmative action in admissions to health professions programs, and use of international medical graduates. Despite these efforts, the current US health-care workforce does not reflect these demographic changes—most practicing dentists, nurses, pharmacists, physicians, and allied health personnel are still non-Hispanic whites. Consequently the dichotomy between the racial and ethnic composition of the population and the racial and ethnic composition of the health-care workforce has continued to grow.

Ultimately, in addition to existing programs, long-term, multifaceted efforts that address the underlying causes of underrepresentation in the health professions must be devised if the United States is to have a health workforce representative of its population. Sustained multifaceted leadership will be required from the federal, educational, professional, financial, and business domains. The recommendations outlined in Table 23–12 include both short- and long-term strategies to address this issue.

▶ REFERENCES

1. King ML, speech at the Second National Convention of the Medical Committee for Human Rights, Chicago, Illinois, March 25, 1966.
2. Colburn L, ed. *Minority Graduates of U. S. Medical Schools: Trends 1950–1998.* Washington, DC: Association of American Medical Colleges; 2000.
3. Grumbach E, Coffman J, Gandara P, et al. *Strategies for Improving the Diversity of the Health Professions* [report]. California Endowment; Center for California Health Workforce Studies, University of California at San Francisco; Education Policy Center, University of California at Davis; 2003.
4. Sullivan Commission. *Briefing: Missing Persons: Minorities in the Health Professions.* Internet release date September 20, 2004. Available at: http://www.sullivancommission.org.
5. Smedley BD, Stith AY, Nelson AR. *Unequal Treatment: Confronting Racial and Ethnic Disparities in Healthcare.* Washington, DC: National Academies Press; 2003.
6. US Census Bureau, Table A-7. *Race and Hispanic Origin, for the United States, Regions, Divisions and States (1970).* Internet release date September 13, 2002. Available at: http://census.gov.
7. US Census Bureau, Census 2000 PHC-T-6. *Population by Race and Hispanic or Latino Origin for the United States, Regions, Divisions, States, and for Puerto Rico: 2000.* Internet release date April 2, 2001. Available at: http://census.gov.
8. US Census Bureau. *U. S. Interim Projections by Age, Sex, Race, and Hispanic, Origin;* 2004. Internet release date March 18, 2004. Available at: http://www.census.gov/ipc/www/userinterim proj/.
9. *Federal Register* Notice (10/30/97, vol 62, No. 210), Revisions to the Standards for the Classification of Federal Data on Race and Ethnicity. (OMB Directive 15.)
10. US Census Bureau. *Age: 2000: Census 2000 Brief.* Issued October 12, 2001. Available at: http://www.census.gov.
11. Bureau of Labor Statistics. A century of change: 1950–2050. *Monthly Labor Review* 2002;May: 15–28.
12. US Census Bureau. *Projections of the Total Resident Population by 5 Year Age Groups, Race, and Hispanic Origin with Special Age Categories: Middle Series 2050–2070.* Internet release date January 13, 2000. Available at: http://www. census.gov.
13. Bureau of Labor Statistics. Occupational employment projections to 2012. *Monthly Labor Review* 2004; February:80–105.
14. US Census Bureau. *1970 Census of the Population, Detailed Characteristics of the Population;* June 1973.
15. US Census Bureau, EEO Data Tool. *Employment by Occupation, Sex, Age and Race for U. S. Total.* Available at: http://www.census.gov/ eeo2000/index.html.
16. Association of American Medical Colleges. Available at: http://www.aamc.org/data/facts/.
17. US Dept of Education. *Digest of Educational Statistics.* Hyattsville, Md: National Center for Health Statistics; 2002.
18. Association of American Medical Colleges. *Minority Students in Medical Education: Facts and Figures XII.* Washington, DC: AAMC; 2002.
19. Berlin LE, Stennett J, Bednash G, eds. *Enrollment and Graduation in Baccalaureate and Graduate Programs in Nursing, 2003–2004.* Washington, DC: American Association of Colleges of Nursing; 2004.
20. Association of American Medical Colleges. *U. S. Medical School Faculty.* Available at: http://www. aamc.org.
21. Livingston HM, Dellinger TM, Hyde JC, Holder R. The aging and diminishing dental faculty. *J Dent Educ* 2004;68(3):345–354.
22. DeYoung S, Bliss J, Tracy J. The nursing faculty

shortage: Is there hope? *J Prof Nurs* 2002;18(6): 313–319.

23. Rodts MF. Good news, bad news about the nursing shortage. *Orthop Nurs* 2004;23(3):161–162.

24. Berlin LE, Sechrist KR. The shortage of doctorally prepared nursing faculty. *Nurs Outlook* 2002;50(2):50–56.

25. Armbruster B, Lehr F, Osborn M. *A Child Becomes a Reader*. Washington, DC: National Institute for Literacy, US Dept of Health and Human Services; 2003.

26. US Dept of Education. *The Nation's Report Card: Reading Highlights*. Washington, DC: National Center for Educational Statistics; 2003.

27. US Dept of Education. *The Nation's Report Card: Mathematics*. Washington, DC: National Center for Educational Statistics; 2001.

28. US Dept of Education. *The Nation's Report Card: Science*. Washington, DC: National Center for Educational Statistics; 2001.

29. Figueroa R, Ruiz N. Minority underrepresentation in gifted programs: Old problems, new perspectives. In: Tashakkori A, Ochoa S, eds. *Readings on Equal Education,* vol 16. *Educating Hispanics in the U. S.: Politics, Policies, and Outcomes*. New York, NY: AMS Press; 1999:119–141.

30. Gandara PC, Bial D. *Paving the Way to Postsecondary Education: K–12 Intervention Programs for Underrepresented Youth*. Washington, DC: National Center for Education Statistics, Office of Educational Research and Improvement, US Dept of Education; 2001.

31. Terenzini P, Cabrera A, Bernal E. *Swimming Against the Tide: The Poor in American Higher Education*. Research Report No. 2001-1. New York, NY: College Entrance Examination Board; 2001.

32. Adelman C. *Answers in the Toolbox: Academic Intensity, Attendance Patterns, and Bachelor's Degree Attainment*. Washington, DC: US Dept of Education, Office of Educational Research and Improvement; 1999.

33. Association of American Universities and the Pew Charitable Trust. *Understanding University Success*. Eugene, Ore: Center for Educational Policy Research; 2003.

34. *Special Report for State Education Officials and Secondary School Administrators*. New York, NY: College Entrance Examination Board; 2004.

35. Berkner L, He S, Cataldi E. *Descriptive Summary of 1995–1996 Beginning Postsecondary Students: Six Years Later*. Washington, DC: US Dept of Education, National Center for Education Statistics; 2002.

36. Cooper R. Impact of trends in primary, secondary and postsecondary education on applications to medical school. II. Considerations of race, ethnicity and income. *Acad Med* 2003;78:861–876.

37. Garcia G, Nation C, Parker N. Paper contribution A: Increasing diversity in the health professions: A look at best practices in admissions. In: Smedley BD, Butler AS, Bristow LR, eds. *In the Nation's Compelling Interest: Ensuring Diversity in the Health Care Workforce*. Washington, DC: Institute of Medicine, National Academies Press; 2004:233–272.

38. Carey K. *A Matter of Degrees: Improving Graduation Rates in Four Year Colleges and Universities*. Indianapolis, Ind: Lumina Foundation for Education; 2004.

39. Freeman K. Increasing African-American participation in higher education. *J Higher Educ* 1997;68(5):523–550.

40. Orfield G. The growth of segregation. In: Orfield G, Eaton S, eds. *Dismantling Desegration. The Quiet Reversal of Brown vs Board of Education*. New York, NY: New Press; 1996.

41. Orfield G, Yun J. *Resegregation in American Schools*. Cambridge, Mass: Harvard Civil Rights Project; 1999.

42. American Council on Education. *Nineteenth Annual Status Report on Minorities in Higher Education 2001–2002*. Washington, DC: ACE; 2002.

43. American Council on Education. *Attitudes Toward Public Education*. Washington, DC: ACE; 2002.

44. Carbrera AF, LaNasa SM. *Understanding the College Choice of Disadvantaged Students*. New Directions for Institutional Research, Vol 107. San Francisco, Calif: Jossey-Bass; 2000.

45. *Trends in Student Aid*. New York, NY: College Board; 2002.

46. Smedley BD, Stith AY, Colburn L, et al. *The Right Thing to Do; The Smart Thing to Do: Increasing Diversity in the Health Professions*. Washington, DC: Institute of Medicine, National Academies Press; 2001.

47. *Public Papers of the Presidents of the United States: Lyndon B. Johnson, 1965*. Vol II, entry 301. Washington, DC: Government Printing Office; 1966:635-640.

48. Datagram: U. S. medical student enrollments, 1968–69 through 1970–71. *J Med Educ* 1971;46: 96–97.

49. Raup RM, Williams EA. Negro students in medical schools in the United States. *J Med Educ* 1964;39:444–456.

50. *University of California Regents v Bakke,* 429 US 953 (1978).

51. *Policy on Future Admissions, Employment and Contracting Resolution Rescinding SP-1 and SP-2.* Available at: http://www.universityof california.edu/regents/policies/6031.html.

52. *California's Proposition 209.* Available at: http://www.acri.org/209/209text.html.

53. *Implementation of Initiative Measure 200.* Available at: http://www.governor.wa.gov/eo/dir98%2D01.htm.

54. *Hopwood v Texas,* 78 F3d 932 (5th Cir 1966), *cert denied,* 518 US 1033 (1996).

55. *Hopwood v Texas,* 121 S Ct 2550 (2001).

56. Effect of *Hopwood v. State of Texas* on various scholarship programs of the University of Houston. *Letter Opinion No. 97-001.* Available at: http://tarlton.law.utexas.edu/hopwood/morales. htm.

57. Cohen JJ. Consequences of premature abandonment of affirmative action in medical school admissions. *JAMA* 2003;289:1143–1149.

58. *Gratz et al v Bollinger,* 122 F Supp 2d 811 (ED Mich 2000), *rev'd* 539 US 244 (2003), *on remand to* 80 Fed Appx 417 (6th Cir Mich).

59. *Grutter v Bollinger,* 137 F Supp 2d 821 (ED Mich 2001), *stay granted,* 247 F3d 631 (6th Cir 2001), *brig en banc ordered,* 277 F3d 803 (6th Cir 2001), *rev'd* 288 F3d 732 (6th Cir 2002), *aff'd* 539 US 306 (2003).

60. *Assessing Medical School Admissions Policies: Implications of the U. S. Supreme Court's Affirmative-Action Decisions.* Washington, DC: Association of American Medical Colleges; 2002.

61. Stewart WH. Implementing the report of the national advisory commission on health manpower. *JAMA* 1969;210(10):1911–1913.

62. Iglehart JK. The quandary over graduates of foreign medical schools in the United States. *N Engl J Med* 1996;334(25):1679–1683.

63. Robinson L, ed. *AAMC Data Book: Statistical Information Related to Medical Schools and Teaching Hospitals.* Washington, DC: Association of American Medical Colleges; 2004.

64. McMahon GT. Coming to America—International medical graduates in the United States. *N Engl J Med* 2004;350(24):2435–2437.

65. Appendix II: Graduate medical education. *JAMA* 2004;292(9):1099–1113.

66. Brellochs C, Carter AB. *Building Primary Care in New York City's Low-Income Communities.* New York, NY: Community Service Society of New York; 1990.

67. Council on Graduate Medical Education. *Tenth Report: Physician Distribution and Health Care Challenges in Rural and Inner-city Areas.* Washington, DC: US Dept of Health and Human Services, Public Health Service, Health Resources and Services Administration; 1998.

68. Hofmeyer A, Cecchin M. Enactment of virtue ethics: Collaboration between nurse academics and international students in questionnaire design. *Aust J Adv Nurs* 2001;18(3):8–13.

69. Mullan F. Time capsule thinking: The health care workforce, past and future. *Health Aff* 2002; 21(5):112–122.

70. Mick SS, Lee SY. International and U. S. medical graduates in U. S. cities. *J Urban Health* 1999; 76(4):481–496.

71. Salsberg ES, Forte GJ. Trends in physician workforce, 1980–2000. *Health Aff* 2002;21(5): 165–173.

72. Baer LD, Ricketts TC, Konrad TR, et al. Do international medical graduates reduce rural physician shortages? *Med Care* 1998;36(11):1534–1544.

73. Hagopian A, Thompson MJ, Kaltenbach E, et al. Health departments' use of international medical graduates in physician shortage areas. *Health Aff* 2003;22(5):241–249.

CHAPTER 24

Diversity Management in Nursing

COLLEEN CONWAY-WELCH, PhD, RN, FAAN*
RANDOLPH F. R. RASCH, PhD, RN
MARILYN DUBREE, MSN, RN
SHARON JONES, MSN, RN

"Diversity is not a haphazard event, but is the result of a series of unique circumstances"
—*Tropical Rainforest (www.mongobay.com)*

▶ INTRODUCTION

This chapter focuses on the issue of diversity among nurse managers, nurses, and nurse-support staff, and how this issue influences their interactions. The major lesson to be learned is that little evidence-based data is available regarding the management dynamics and challenges that result when the cultures of managers and those they manage differ. As the nursing shortage worsens and the nursing workforce ages, management will need to be even more creative and thoughtful in addressing issues of diversity. Two major reasons why nurses leave

nursing are that nurse managers do not manage well and physicians do not respect them.

R. Roosevelt Thomas, Jr, president of the American Institute for Managing Diversity, supports a broad definition for diversity, including age, personal and corporate background, education, function, and personality. Diversity issues also include lifestyle, sexual preference, geographic origin, tenure with the organization, exempt or nonexempt labor status, and managerial versus nonmanagerial status.[1]

There are three overarching challenges for health-care industry leadership regarding diversity: (1) underrepresentation of persons of color in management positions, (2) persistent gaps in compensation and satisfaction between managers of color and Caucasian managers, and (3) racial and ethnic disparities in health-care

* The McGraw-Hill Companies acknowledge the substantial editorial contributions of Donna M. Frassetto and Nancy N. Woelfl in preparation of this chapter.

delivery processes and outcomes. Although diversity can be defined from a number of perspectives, including civil rights, affirmative action, reverse discrimination, quotas, racism, and sexism,[2] it can also be interpreted as working with people who are "multiracial, multicultural, multiethnic and gender-oriented as well as representing differences in age, education, economic level and tenure with the presence or absence of disabilities."[3]

► EVIDENCE-BASED MANAGEMENT

There is a surprising lack of evidence-based guidance in either the management or the nursing literature about the challenges nurse leaders, minority or majority, face in managing members of diverse groups, and there is virtually no mention of the skill sets needed.[4,5] Much theoretical and practical research needs to be done.

Evidence of the effectiveness of the few diversity management curricula that exist for both managers and those managed has not been vigorously evaluated or disseminated. One would anticipate that actions resulting from such curricula would benefit organizations from both financial and performance improvement aspects; evidence is lacking, but perhaps assumed, to support the business case that diversity among nurse managers and nurse staff contributes to quality and efficiency.

Ivancevich and Gilbert[6] stress that the business case for diversity can be proactive and is based on the operational reality that there is a need to optimize the contributions of an increasingly diverse national workforce, whereas affirmative action is relative and based on government legislation and moral imperatives.[1,7] The improper or underutilization of a diverse workforce may be a legal issue, but certainly it is a managerial and leadership issue. Some of the challenges to multicultural leadership are outlined in Table 24–1.[6]

Nurse managers who are able to build effective multicultural workgroups must by definition incorporate the skills of the multicultural leader.[1] Von Bergen et al also emphasize that diversity management includes administering social environments and systems, along with organizational climates and procedures, and entails recognizing, being open to, and utilizing human differences.[7]

Ivancevich and Gilbert[6] present thoughtful arguments supporting the need to explore four research alternatives to quasi-field experiments in the area of diversity management: (1) researcher–administrator partnerships; (2) researcher observation within organizations, (3) detailed case histories and analysis, and (4) third-party evaluations of diversity management initiatives. Evidence generated using approaches other than a quasi-field approach is sadly lacking and would be a major contribution to management curricula in schools of nursing.

► DEMOGRAPHICS

US Census Bureau statistics for 2004 indicate approximately 31% of US residents are members of racial or ethnic minority groups. Sixty-nine percent are Caucasian but, by 2050, that figure will drop to 50%. By 2030, in the western parts of the United States, almost 30% of the population will be non-Caucasian, and the US Census Bureau projects that the percentage will increase to 40% by 2050.[8] The US Bureau of Labor Statistics estimates that one of every three new jobs will be in the health-care industry. In the future, managers will face labor shortages along with an increasingly diverse workforce.[9–11] The US Department of Labor, Bureau of Labor Statistics, projects that registered nurses (RNs) will have the largest job growth (27%) among all professions in the next decade. Total RN employment is expected to grow from 2.2 million in 2002 to 2.9 million in 2012. Positions available, due to increasing need and net replacement, will total more than 1.1 million. The average age of nursing graduates today is 31 years old; the average age of the employed RN is 45; and the average age of nurse faculty

▶ **TABLE 24–1.** Differences Between Traditional and Multicultural Leaders

Element	Traditional Leader	Multicultural Leader
Participation	Egocentric frame of mind	Synergistic frame of mind
		Mentor
Goals and outcomes	Single focus	Integrated focus
Organizational structure	Layered management: individual	Expertise at point-of-care with team focus: flat
Decision making	Subjective mindset	Objective mindset
	Single focus	Multifocus
Rewards	Self-serving	Serves the people
	Individual seniority	Performance or team based
Management role	Holds onto power	Steps aside to build the "team power"
	Direct	
	Central	Coach
		Facilitate
Personal relationships	Seeks to be Number 1	Seeks to make others the center of attention
	Center of attention	
		Whole process
Job design	Narrow	Multiple task
	Single task	Shared with the team
Communication	Top-down flow	Open flow across all levels
		Open
Information flow	Central	Shared
	Limited	Team plan
Job process	Management plan	

is 57. These statistics raise red flags even before they are analyzed for diversity. The demographics warn of a troubling future of increasingly diverse patients and a nondiverse, aging staff. Equally troubling, diversity among nurses and nurse managers continues to elude the workforce.

Minorities in nursing do not begin to reflect current and future population trends (Fig. 24–1).

- Of the 2.8 million nurses in the United States, the number of RNs identifying their background as one or more racial minority groups or Hispanic/Latino was about 334,000 in 2000.
- Approximately 34,000 or 1.2% of non-Hispanic RNs identify themselves as two or more races.
- In 2000, among the total RN population, minority nurses constituted about 8%; minority representation in the general population was more than 30% in 2000.
- The number or percentage of minority nurses in management or administrative positions is not known.

▶ WHY PURSUE DIVERSITY MANAGEMENT?

While society is beginning to grapple with the problem of aging among nurses, nurse faculty, nurse managers, and patients, little attention has been devoted to the impact that diverse beliefs and practices regarding aging will also have on the diminished nurse workforce. The law of unintended consequences comes into play, too, as affirmative action, equal opportunity, the Americans with Disabilities Act, and various other rules and regulations have clouded the original vision for why society should pursue diversity,

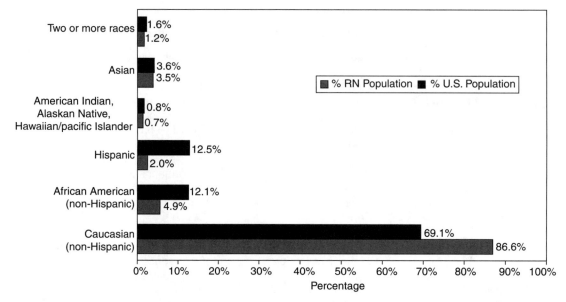

Figure 24–1. Racial and ethnic distribution of the registered nurse workforce.   *(Source: 2000 Sample Survey of RNs. Washington, DC: Health Resources and Services Administration; 2001.)*

based on morals and ethics.[12] A diverse workforce, with managers skilled in managing such a workforce, is a desirable goal because it is the right thing to do, not because federal law requires it or because it will make employers look good.[12]

Efforts to increase the diversity of the nurse workforce, as well as the diversity of nurse managers, have had limited success beyond numeric goals and compliance with existing regulatory requirements. Ethical and moral reasoning logically demands a diversified nurse staff and nurse manager workforce and poses the question, "Whose problem is it to increase the diversity of the healthcare workforce? Is it a public policy maker's problem? Academia's? Management's? All of the above?"[12]

How the issue of diversity in the nurse workforce is managed will dictate, in part, responses to these questions that range from workplace morale to worker productivity, acceptable management practices, and legal risk factors.[7] Although 85% of new entrants into the US workforce in 2000 were diverse,[7] fewer than 2% of the chief executive and chief operating officers

in the health-care system are not white males.[13] US residents speak at least 329 languages.[13] Managers are naturally ethnocentric; their first reaction is to interpret other cultures within the content and understanding of their own culture.[14] In a global multicultural workforce, managers will need to learn to work cooperatively in cross-cultural environments if they are to be successful. The fact that very few, if any, schools of nursing even require a second language is a major concern.

▶ CULTURAL RELATIVISM AND CULTURAL COMPETENCY

Competent management skills include the ability to assess and incorporate into the management team, as well as the staff being managed, an awareness of commonly held cultural beliefs and behaviors. Further, they include the ability to successfully negotiate the needed balance among the ethnocultural beliefs and practices of management, staff, patients, and the culture of the current health-care delivery system in the United States.[15]

Diversity management skills draw on the positive aspects of cultural relativism, in which all points of views are equally valid and truth is relative to the individual and his or her environment. Cultural relativism posits that the thinking and behavioral norms of every culture are valuable. Cultural relativism can provide a way to understand apparent conflicts between the expectations and definitions of "appropriate" care occurring among nurse managers, staff nurses, nonnurse support staff, patients, and families.[16] The strength of cultural relativism is that it allows a person to hold fast to his or her moral intuitions without being judgmental about other cultures that do not share them.

In a complementary manner, cultural competency can be defined as a set of cognitive behaviors, attitudes, and policies that come together in a system, agency, or among professions, enabling them to work effectively in cross-cultural situations.[14]

The American Academy of Physician Assistants has developed a model, based on four layers of diversity,[17] to build cultural competence. The academy formulated a model of training that emphasizes respect, building trust, and recognizing differences. Language, both written and spoken, is a large element of the model (Fig. 24–2).

The ability to deliver appropriate and respectful management direction to staff and patients from other cultures will be increasingly

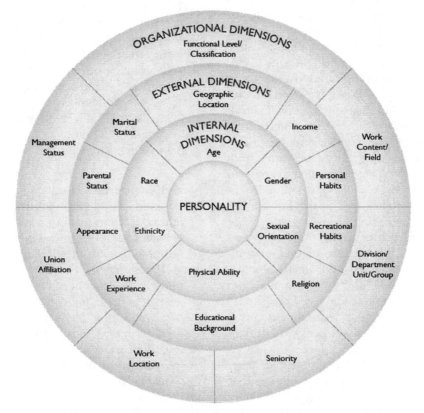

Figure 24–2. Four layers of diversity. (Internal and external dimensions are adapted from Laden M, Rosener J. *Workforce America!: Managing Employee Diversity as a Vital Resource.* Homewood, Illinois: Business One Irwin; 1991. Used with permission.)

challenging, but a diverse workforce, coupled with an innovation-focused business strategy, can provide institutions with a competitive advantage when pursuing market share and should add to the business case for increasing diversity.[18] For example, the literature suggests that, for the banking industry, racial diversity enhances an employer's performance in pursuing innovative strategies. Dansky et al[19] suggest that corporate sensitivity to diversity strongly influences strategic decision making, which, in turn, influences human resource practices such as diversity initiatives.

Svelha[20] describes diversity management as a strategically driven process with an emphasis on skill building, policy creation that enhances employee growth, and continuing assessment of the marketing issues resulting from a changing workforce and customer demographics. This is much more than simply making changes necessary to comply with affirmative action guidelines. In fact, "Retaining new employees from diverse backgrounds is essential to successfully achieving workforce diversity and cost effectiveness because tremendous financial resources are involved in recruiting and orientating new staff."[21] The cost of recruiting, orienting, and training a new staff nurse varies from $50,000 to $80,000. Thus, providing avenues to support employees in creating a culturally diverse work environment is vital. One way to achieve this is by making diversity goals part of annual job performance ratings. Although there is no evidence that mandatory attendance at diversity programs is effective, diversity fairs featuring speakers, food, and entertainment from other cultural backgrounds are well accepted.

As patients express the desire for caregivers who share the same cultural background, language competence becomes increasingly critical. It may be difficult for a nurse manager whose first language is English to counsel a staff member whose first language is not English because of nuances of meaning; it may be even more difficult to ask patient-sensitive questions through a translator who may live in the patient's neighborhood.

Pratt[22] emphasizes that, in many ways, diversity management is simply another term for good management practices that recognize each worker as a unique individual. When nurse managers represent the same diversity ratios as their staff and patients, and when staff represent the same diversity profiles as their patients, interactions and patient safety should be enhanced. When management is primarily Caucasian, and not aligned with the cultural context of the patient population and workforce, communication may suffer and patient safety could be a problem.[23]

▶ EMOTIONAL INTELLIGENCE

As both nurse managers and their staffs become more culturally diverse, their emotional intelligence quotient is enhanced (i.e., what they do, how they look, what they say, and how they say it). The concept of emotional intelligence is as important as the traditional ideas of superior intelligence or professional expertise and allows individuals to be affirmed for their uniqueness rather than discounted. Components of emotional intelligence include[24]:

- **Self-awareness.** Knowing feelings of the moment and using those preferences to guide decision making; having a realistic assessment of one's own abilities and a well-grounded sense of self-confidence.
- **Self-regulation.** Handling emotions so that they facilitate rather than interfere with the task at hand; being conscientious and delaying gratification to pursue goals; recovering well from emotional distress.
- **Motivation.** Using deepest preferences to move toward one's goals to help one take initiative and strive to improve, and to persevere in the face of setbacks and frustrations.
- **Empathy.** Sensing what people are feeling, being able to take their perspectives, and cultivating rapport and attunement with a broad diversity of people.

- **Social skills.** Handling emotions in relationships well, and accurately reading social situations and networks; interacting smoothly; using these skills to persuade and lead, negotiate and settle disputes, and facilitate cooperation and teamwork.

Factors such as quality, productivity, and job satisfaction reduce operating costs; support the investment of time, energy, and effort in developing emotionally intelligent, multicultural workgroups; and should also help make the business case for the need for diversity management. Because one strategy for dealing with the US nursing shortage is recruitment of nurses who have received their educational preparation in other countries, patient care and safety will be increasingly dependent on expanding sensitivity to the impact of globalization.[25] Sinetar[26] emphasizes that those who are increasingly able to venture into the expanding landscape of global thinking and embrace a philosophy of cultural creativity and stewardship will find innovative solutions to the challenges ahead. Gantz[27] suggests that workgroups that learn to blend cultures create a unique climate capable of generating higher efficiency. He notes that culturally competent leadership is being in the right place before the right time and knowing how to guide the multicultural workgroup to higher ground.

What makes some diversity initiatives successful and others fail? Plummer[28] suggests a focus on rules of civil behavior rather than trying to change people's beliefs. Diversity must be conceptualized using a wider cultural lens, defining issues in ways that do not victimize others, and managing interpersonal racial and gender conflict in ways that are not punitive. These are skills needed by the nurse managers of the future.

Over the years, the focus of diversity training has changed from an altruistic approach (the right thing to do) to a civil rights emphasis to a business strategy. Diversity management cannot mandate positive feelings, but it can improve cross-cultural communication and personal relationships among co-workers. However, it is unrealistic to expect that every member of a culturally diverse group should or will learn to like each other.

► COMPETENCIES

Diversity management training is most effective when it is competency based. Nurse managers must have a background in group dynamics, attitude and behavioral change, organizational development, and languages. Diversity training that incorporates these areas, along with demonstrated competencies in the affective, cognitive, and behavioral domains (including systems interactions) achieves the most success. It is important to have goals and objectives related to diversity that have evidence and metrics attached to them in order to measure outcomes. Nurse managers should focus on projects that explore and measure outcomes of diversity management strategies and then pilot promising approaches. This is an area ripe for health systems research. The issue of diversity and nursing management was highlighted by the American Association of Colleges of Nursing (AACN) when it asked members to report the following information to the Sullivan Commission on Diversity in Healthcare Workforce. The Sullivan Commission[29] was created to identify workable solutions to improve access to care for all Americans. AACN asked its member schools whether they had:

- Programs in place to attract students from diverse backgrounds.
- Formal curricula on cultural competence either as a course or integrated throughout the program.
- A monitoring program for students with minority backgrounds or actively engaged in efforts to recruit and retain faculty with diverse backgrounds.

Deans and directors of nursing programs should also be prepared to answer whether their curricula include evidence-based practices to teach both minority and nonminority nurses how to manage diverse workforces.

Nursing has yet to specifically identify measurable cultural and diversity management competencies in areas such as content, critical thinking, psychomotor skills, and communication abilities. Each role and behavior must be described in detail, with varying levels of performance identified, perhaps using Brenner's adaptation of the Dreyfus model of novice to expert.[30]

The technology of learning management systems can enable supervisors, nurse managers, nurses, and non-nurse staff to validate and track these competencies and give them aggregate and discrete data about their diversity management skills. Aggregate data can be used to assess educational gaps and needs related to

▶ **TABLE 24–2.** Summary of Major Findings Regarding Diversity Management in Nursing

- There is little evidence to guide nurse managers and their staffs regarding management issues as staff and patients become more diverse.
- The demographics of diversity in the nurse workforce are of great concern; there is a paucity of nurse managers from diverse backgrounds, and data regarding their numbers, age, and level of management position is unavailable.
- The business case for diversity among nurse managers and nurse staff has yet to be made, although it is intuitively important.
- Major efforts by nursing education institutions need to be directed toward minority recruitment and teaching the art and science of diversity management from an evidence-based perspective.
- Diversity management skills should be competency-based and present in every nursing curriculum.
- Many strategies of diversity management are simply good strategies of management that recognize the uniqueness of the individual.

the competency and to design and offer educational remediation linked to performance evaluation. Although these metrics are in the very early stages, their impact on improving diversity management skills could be profound.

▶ **SUMMARY AND RECOMMENDATIONS**

Table 24–2 summarizes key points discussed in this chapter. In addition to the Sullivan Commission,[29] the urgency of diversity in the health care professions has also been recognized by the Institute of Medicine (IOM) publication, *In the Nation's Compelling Interest: Ensuring Diversity in the Health Care Workforce*,[31] although the commission did not focus on diversity in leadership. The need for managers who can provide role models as successful diversity managers will become increasingly critical as nursing attempts to attract minorities into nursing and nursing leadership positions.

▶ **REFERENCES**

1. Morrison AM. *The New Leaders: Guidelines on Leadership Diversity in America.* San Francisco, Calif: Jossey-Bass; 1992.
2. Umiker WO. *Management Skills for the New Health Care Supervisor.* Gaithersburg, Md: Aspen; 1998.
3. Harrison DA, Price KH, Bell MP. Beyond relational demography; Time and the effects of surface and deep-level diversity on work group cohesion. *Acad Manage Executives* 1998;41:96–107.
4. Wheeler, ML. *Diversity: Business Rationale and Strategies: A Research Report.* New York, NY: Conference Board; 1995.
5. Ellis C, Sonnefeld JA. Diverse approaches to managing diversity. *Hum Resource Manage* 1994;33:70–110.
6. Ivancevich JM, Gilbert JA. Diversity management: Time for a new approach. *Public Personnel Manage* 2000;29(1):75.
7. Von Bergen CW, Soper B, Foster T. Unintended negative effects on diversity management. *Public Personnel Manage* 2002;31(2):239–244.

8. US Census Bureau. US Interim Projections by Age, Sex, Race, and Hispanic Origin, 2004. Available at: http://www.census.gov/ipc/www/usinterimproj/.

9. Cox T. *Cultural Diversity in Organizations: Theory, Research, & Practice.* San Francisco, Calif: Berrett-Koehler; 1994.

10. Dreachslin JL, Hunt PL. *Diversity Leadership.* Chicago, Ill: Health Administration Press; 1996.

11. Richard OC. Racial diversity, business strategy, and firm performance: A resource-based view. *Acad Manage J* 2000;43(2):164–177.

12. Matus JC. The movement for diversity in health care management. *Health Care Manager* 2003;April–June(2):117–122.

13. US Bureau of Census. Available at: http://www.census.gov.

14. Alexander GR. A mind for multicultural management. *Nurs Manage* 2002;33(10):30–33.

15. Pachter LM. Cultural issues in pediatric care. In: Behrman RE, Kliegman RM, Jenson HB, eds. *Nelson Textbook of Pediatrics,* 15th ed. Philadelphia, Pa: Saunders; 1996:16–18.

16. Kavanagh KH, Kennedy PH. *Promoting Cultural Diversity: Strategies for Health Care Professionals.* Newbury Park, Calif: Sage; 1992.

17. Diversity: In health care delivery. *Pfizer Journal* [serial online] 2004;8(2). Available at: http://www.thepfizerjournal.com/default.asp?ajournal&n=tpj36.

18. Richard O, McMillan A, Chadwick K, et al. Employing an innovation strategy in racially diverse workforces—Effects on firm performance. *Group Organ Manage* 2003;28(1):107–126.

19. Dansky KH, Weech-Maldonado R, DeSouza G, et al. Organizational strategy and diversity management: Diversity-sensitive orientation as a moderating influence. *Health Care Manage Rev* 2003; 28(3):243–253.

20. Svehla T. Diversity management: Key to future success. *Frontiers Health Serv Manage* 1994; 11(2):3–33.

21. Mateo MA, Smith SP. Workforce diversity in hospitals. *Nurs Leadership Forum* 2003;7(4): 143–149.

22. Pratt JR. Managing a culturally diverse work force. *Home Health Care Manage Prac* 1999; 11(4):67–69.

23. Muller HJ, Haase BE. Managing diversity in health services organizations. *Hosp Health Serv Admin* 1994;39(4):415–434.

24. Goleman D. *Working with Emotional Intelligence.* New York, NY: Bantam Books, 1998.

25. Wellins RS, Byham WC, Wilson JM. *Empowered Teams: Creating Self-Directed Work Groups That Improve Quality, Productivity and Participation.* San Francisco, Calif: Jossey-Bass; 1991.

26. Sinetar M. *Developing a 21st Century Mind.* New York, NY: Villard; 1991.

27. Gantz NR. Leading and empowering the multicultural work team. *Semin Nurse Manage* 2000;10(3):164–170.

28. Plummer DL. Approaching diversity training in the year 2000. *Consult Psychol J Pract Res* 1998; 50(3):181–189.

29. Sullivan Commission on Diversity in the Healthcare Workforce. *Missing Persons: Minorities in the Health Professions: A Report of the Sullivan Commission on Diversity in the Healthcare Workforce.* Durham, NC: Sullivan Commission; 2004. Available at: http://admissions.duhs.duke.edu/sullivancommission/index.cfm.

30. Dreyfus HL, Dreyfus SE. *Mind over Machine: The Power of Human Intuition and Expertise in the Era of the Computer.* New York, NY: Free Press; 1986.

31. Smedley BD, Butler AS, Bristow LR. *In the Nation's Compelling Interest: Ensuring Diversity in The Health Care Workforce.* Washington, DC: National Academies Press; 2004.

CHAPTER 25

Trust, Medical Care, and Racial and Ethnic Minorities

VANESSA NORTHINGTON GAMBLE, MD, PhD

▶ INTRODUCTION

Trust is the cornerstone of the provider–patient relationship and the foundation for quality health-care delivery and outcomes. It is an element of constructive relationships between investigators and participants in biomedical research. Trust also plays a role in sustaining public support for health-care professionals, biomedical research, and public health.

The American public's trust in medicine has declined over the past several decades. Reasons behind this decline include the increased penetration of managed care, limits on patient choice, the growth of for-profit medicine, the growing medical sophistication of patients, and media coverage of medical errors and research scandals.[1-3] Research suggests this lack of trust is particularly acute in racial and ethnic minority communities.[4] Thus, the erosion of trust is a significant obstacle in efforts to improve the health of minority communities that must be addressed if we are to eliminate racial and ethnic disparities in health and health care.

This chapter examines the complex relationship among trust, racial and ethnic minorities, and health care. It provides an overview of the topic, reviews the literature on the topic, and offers some recommendations on how to develop a trustworthy health-care system that benefits racial and ethnic minorities.

▶ TRUST AND HEALTH CARE

In recent years, a growing body of research has examined the concept of trust in health care: its definition, components, impact, and measurement. As of yet, there is not a universally accepted definition or conceptual model of trust. But there are definitions that provide a useful conceptualization of the topic. Rotter defines trust as "an expectancy held by a person or group that the word, promise, verbal or written statement of another person or group can be relied upon."[5] Mechanic and Schlesinger state that "trust refers to the expectation of the public that those who serve them will perform their responsibilities in a technically proficient way (competence), that they will assume responsibility and not inappropriately defer to others (control), and that they will make patients' welfare their highest priority (agency)."[6]

There are two broad categories of trust: interpersonal trust and social trust. Interpersonal trust refers to trust in individuals such as physicians and other health-care professionals. Goold cogently described the importance of trust in the physician–patient relationship when she asked, "Without trust, how could a physician expect patients to reveal the full extent of their medically relevant history, expose themselves to the physical exam, or act on recommendations for tests or treatments?"[7] Interpersonal trust usually comes as a result of direct personal experience with an individual. Social trust refers to trust in collective institutions such as hospitals, health plans, or health-care professions. Social trust usually arises not only as a result of personal interactions, but also from collective relationships, media portrayals, and historical experiences. Although the two categories are interrelated, they are not mutually exclusive. For example, an individual may trust his or her own personal physician, but not trust the generic "medical profession." Or, a person might seek care from an unknown provider affiliated with a particular hospital because he or she trusts the reputation of the facility. Trust is not a static process, but rather an ongoing, dynamic one that is created through consistent positive relationships.[8] Mechanic reminds us that trust is also fragile and can be "easily challenged by a discomforting act or by a changing social situation."[1]

Researchers have identified trust as a factor critical for positive health outcomes.[9–11] It has been associated with increased patient and physician satisfaction, improved provider–patient communications, greater adherence to medical recommendations, and continuity of primary care. Trust may also help reduce health-care costs because it may obviate the need for additional tests and referrals that patients request in order to feel reassured about physicians' recommendations and diagnoses.[12] Patients themselves have identified factors such as caring and comfort, technical competence, and good communication skills as some of the physician behaviors that engender trust.[12]

▶ RACE, TRUST, AND MEDICAL CARE

Research has demonstrated that racial and ethnic minorities have lower levels of trust in medical providers and in medical institutions than do white Americans. Distrust can lead to decreased patient satisfaction, low enrollment in clinical trials, greater reluctance to seek medical care, poorer patient adherence to treatment recommendations, and increased unwillingness to donate organs. Hence, distrust can adversely affect health outcomes and contribute to racial and ethnic disparities in health and health care.

Most of the studies that have examined trust, health care, and racial and ethnic minorities have focused on African Americans. Research has demonstrated that African Americans have lower levels of social trust toward medical institutions than do white Americans. For example, in a 2000 study that examined the attitudes of 781 African American and 1003 white cardiac patients, LaVeist et al found that patients' perceptions of the existence of racism in the medical care system and their level of medical mistrust were significant predictors of patient satisfaction. In this study, African Americans were more likely to perceive racism in the health-care system and report distrust in clinical settings, and thus expressed less satisfaction with their medical care.[4]

Research by Boulware et al underscores the need to better understand minority patients' attitudes toward the various components of the health-care system rather than the system in general. In a 2003 study, they analyzed the attitudes of 118 Maryland residents (42% non-Hispanic black and 58% non-Hispanic white) toward physicians, health plans, and hospitals.[13] Their results demonstrated that the levels of trust differed according to the object of trust. They found that African Americans were nearly half as likely to express trust in their physicians as whites and were 20% less likely than whites to express trust in hospitals. Paradoxically, African Americans were twice as likely to express trust in their health plans. The researchers hypothesize that perceptions of distrust may be more pervasive in situations where race cannot be hidden. Thus, the finding about increased trust in health plans might be explained by the fact that the respondents rarely had face-to-face interactions with health plan personnel, a situation that yields racial anonymity and perhaps less fear of racial discrimination. This research also revealed that the black participants had greater concerns about personal privacy.

Studies have also suggested that African Americans have lower levels of interpersonal trust toward physicians and have demonstrated that they fear that physicians might, because of their race, make decisions that are detrimental to them.[10,14] Still it should be noted that these analyses have demonstrated that most African Americans do trust their physicians, but a significant minority do not. When asked in a 1999 study whether they trusted their primary nephrologist's judgment about their medical care, African Americans responded "somewhat or not at all" more often (men, 22%; women, 24%) than whites (men, 11%; women, 12%).[15] Concerns about raced-based discrimination in the physician–patient relationship may affect the level of trust that minority patients initially offer physicians who are not of the same race. Research has shown that race concordance between patient and physician is positively correlated with higher perceptions of quality of care, communications, patient satisfaction, and participatory decision making.[16–19] Such research makes plain that for many African Americans, their relationship with their physicians is not solely a medical one, but a racialized one that carries with it experiences born out of this country's legacy of racism and racial discrimination. Indeed, racial bias has been demonstrated to play a role in physicians' interactions with minority patients.

Researchers have also analyzed African Americans' attitudes toward particular measures such as organ donation and have found lower levels of trust.[20,21] African Americans are less likely to be organ donors—attitudes that are based, in part, on their beliefs about their differential treatment in the medical care system and the devaluation of black lives in the United States. One study found that more African Americans (37.9%) agreed that physicians would be less likely to save their lives if they were known to be organ donors than did white Americans (21.2%).[21] African Americans disproportionately

suffer from chronic kidney disease and develop it at an earlier age than white populations. Therefore, the demonstrated paucity of live and cadaveric kidney donations from African Americans significantly contributes to the disparities in the mortality and quality of life of African Americans with kidney disease.

Participation of racial and ethnic minorities in medical and public health research studies is a critical component of efforts to eliminate health disparities. Trust is a critical factor determining whether a person will enroll in a research study.[22] However, members of minority groups express low levels of trust toward research. Using data from a national telephone survey, Corbie-Smith et al found that in comparison to white Americans, African Americans were more likely not to trust their physician to fully explain research participation (41.7% versus 23.4%); more likely to believe that they had been used as participants in an experiment without their permission (79.2% versus 51.9%) and more likely to express concerns that someone like them would be used as guinea pigs without their permission (24.5% versus 8.3%).[23] In an earlier study, Corbie-Smith et al found that a lack of trust among African Americans led to strains in the informed consent process.[24] They demonstrated that distrust led African Americans to believe that informed consent was solely geared toward persuading them to participate in clinical trials, not to protect them. Corbie-Smith et al concluded that informed consent seemed to hinge on the presence or absence of interpersonal trust.

Despite the burgeoning diversity of America's racial and ethnic minorities, most of the research into trust has focused almost exclusively on African Americans. There is a critical need to assess the attitudes of other racial and ethnic minorities. However, preliminary research suggests that other racial and ethnic minorities are also more distrustful of the health-care system than are white Americans. One study that assessed the attitudes of African American and Hispanic women regarding their willingness to undergo breast cancer screening revealed racial differences. It found that Hispanic and African American women were less likely to perceive the testing as beneficial, and that Hispanic women were the most opposed to screening before adjustment for other sociodemographic factors. The lower levels of trust of the African American and Hispanic women were also associated with less adherence to recommended breast screening protocols, suggesting that a lack of trust may be a barrier to racial and ethnic minorities seeking preventive care.[25]

Other studies suggest the existence of lower levels of trust in Asian, Hispanic, and Native American communities. Research has demonstrated that Hispanics are less willing to donate organs than are whites.[26] Culturally sensitive organ recruitment programs could play a role in increasing organ donation from minority communities. For example, a study conducted on Native American reservations revealed that Native Americans were more likely to donate if asked by a health care worker from their own culture.[27] Native Americans have also expressed distrust of genetic research. Other studies have demonstrated that Asian Americans are less likely than white Americans to be satisfied with their care and less likely to have trust in their physician.[28,29] Ngo-Metzger et al found that rates of dissatisfaction and loss of trust were higher in Asian Americans who thought that their physicians did not listen to them or did not understand their backgrounds or values.[28] These findings underscore the importance of cross-cultural education and communication skills in promoting trust in clinical settings.

Research has also indicated that it is important to take both race and gender into consideration to obtain a fuller understanding of issues of trust and racial and ethnic minorities. Doescher et al found racial and ethnic disparities in perceptions of physician style and trust.[14] Both African American and Hispanic patients reported less positive perceptions of physicians than did white patients; the differences, however, were most pronounced in African American and Hispanic men. In a telephone survey that examined the attitudes of 399 Baltimore residents, Boulware et al found racial and gender differences in willingness to donate blood and cadaveric organs.[20] African American (41%) and white (59%) women were less likely to be willing to donate blood than African American (66%) and white (86%) men. In addition, a majority of the white respondents had agreed to be cadaveric organ donors, whereas only a minority of the African American respondents had. Sixty-five percent of the white men surveyed had signed up to be organ donors, as had 60% of the white women. In contrast 38% of the African American women surveyed had signed up to be organ donors and only 19% of the African American men had. Mistrust of hospitals and concerns about hospital discrimination explained most of the differences in willingness to donate blood, whereas religious beliefs and spirituality explained most of the differences observed in willingness to donate organs among the four groups.

▶ WHY THE DISTRUST?

The reasons underlying the erosion of trust of the general public toward medicine also affect the attitudes of racial and ethnic minorities; however, given their lower levels of trust, additional causes must be considered. A complex interplay of social, political, cultural, and historical factors influence the expectations, beliefs, attitudes, and behaviors that patients bring to the health-care system.

Historical examination helps shed light on the attitudes of racial and ethnic minorities toward medical care and medical research. The Tuskegee Syphilis Study, the 40-year US government study (1932–1972) in which 399 black men from Macon County, Alabama, were deliberately denied effective treatment for syphilis in order to document the natural history of the disease is frequently cited as the primary source of distrust, particularly among African Americans. However in an article on the history of African American attitudes toward medical research, Gamble has noted that the distrust predated public revelations of the Tuskegee Syphilis Study and that African Americans' attitudes toward medical care and research are far more complex than can be attributed to one historical event.[30] They are also rooted in other historical experiences, such as slavery and legalized segregation, as well as contemporary racial discrimination.

Moreover, empirical research about the influence of the Tuskegee Syphilis Study is equivocal. A 1997 telephone survey of 218 African Americans and 203 white Americans from Jefferson County, Alabama, found that 52% of the African Americans and 46% of the whites knew about the Study. Twenty-two percent of the African Americans stated that the Study made them less willing to participate in a research study, compared with 10% of white respondents.[31] In contrast, a 2000 study found that awareness of the Tuskegee Syphilis Study did not influence an individual's willingness to participate in a clinical trial.[32] The researchers based their findings on ten focus groups conducted with 103 African Americans also from Alabama. A 2002 survey of 91 African Americans and 88 white Americans from Detroit also found racial differences in knowledge about the Tuskegee Syphilis Study.[33] Eighty-one percent of African Americans and 28% of whites had knowledge of the Study. This research revealed that white respondents were more likely than African American respondents to be willing to participate in medical research and that African Americans were less likely to believe that all racial and ethnic groups shared the risks and burdens of medical research. The researchers, however, found that knowledge of the Tuskegee Syphilis Study alone did not influence the willingness of an individual to participate in a research study. Furthermore, although many African Americans know about the Tuskegee Syphilis Study, many hold inaccurate views about it. For example, a persistent myth about the study is that the men were injected with syphilis. Nonetheless the Study is part of the collective memory of many African Americans and continues to exert a profound impact on mind-sets of many African Americans because it has become a symbol of their mistreatment by both the federal government and the medical profession.[30,34-36]

The histories of other racial and ethnic minorities also help further our understanding of the foundations of distrust. US immigration policies have influenced the attitudes of Latinos toward medical care. In 1994, California voters approved Proposition 187, which denied undocumented immigrants (or those suspected of being so) access to state services, including health care and public education. The referendum never went into effect because it was declared unconstitutional at the federal district court level and Governor Gray Davis decided not to appeal this decision. Despite the failure of Proposition 187, undocumented immigrants in California and in other locations often view health-care workers as agents of immigration authorities and therefore are often reluctant to access health-care services.[37]

The experiences of Latina women as victims of reproductive abuse have also contributed to attitudes of distrust. For example, in a study conducted in 1969 at a family planning clinic in Austin, Texas, poor mostly Chicana women received what they believed to be contraceptives. However 76 patients, without their knowledge, received placebos. Those who became pregnant were not provided with abortion services even after they requested them.[38] In addition, there is evidence of high rates of sterilization of Puerto Rican women, both in New York City and in Puerto Rico; and of Chicanas in California and in the Southwest.[39] The International Planned Parenthood Federation and the Puerto Rican government waged a sterilization campaign on the island that proved so successful that by 1968, more than one third of women of childbearing age on the island had been sterilized, the highest percentage in the world at the time.[40] Puerto Rican women were used extensively during the 1950s as research subjects in early clinical trials of birth control pills, intrauterine devices, and contraceptive foam.[39]

Research abuses have also occurred in Native American communities. A sterilization effort on Indian reservations during the 1970s left more than 25% of Native American women sterile. Between 1973 and 1976, physicians at four Indian Health Service hospitals sterilized more than 3000 women without obtaining adequate consent.[40] The distrust of Native Americans toward medical institutions must be understood in the context of the abrogation of treaty rights, the desecration of sacred burial grounds, and the history of off-reservation boarding schools.[41]

Notwithstanding the importance of these historical events, the most critical factor in understanding the attitudes of minorities toward medical providers and institutions is the continuing discrimination and unequal treatment of racial and ethnic minorities in today's society. An ever-growing body of research has definitively demonstrated racial and ethnic disparities in access to care and quality of care. To offer just a few examples, relative to whites, African Americans—and in some cases Hispanics—are less likely to receive appropriate cardiac procedures; less likely to receive hemodialysis and kidney transplantation; less likely to receive state-of-the art care for human immunodeficiency virus (HIV) infection and acquired immunodeficiency syndrome (AIDS); and more likely to receive lower quality preventive services even when variations such as insurance status, income, age, and coexisting condition are taken into account.[42–44] In addition, trust is a social contract that builds over time, and a lack of health insurance negatively affects the continuity of care. Racial and ethnic minorities are significantly less likely than white Americans to have health insurance. In 2002, approximately 32% of Latinos were uninsured. In comparison, 20% of African Americans, 18% of Asian Americans, and 12% of white Americans did not have health insurance.[45]

This research confirms the beliefs of members of minority groups that their race or ethnicity may determine the quality of their health care. Distrust, it seems, may result from experientially based expectations for care. A 1999 study commissioned by the Kaiser Family Foundation found that 67% of the African Americans surveyed stated that they were very or somewhat concerned that they or a family member would be treated unfairly in the future when they sought medical care because of their race or ethnicity.[46] Fifty-eight percent of the Latinos polled were very or somewhat concerned that they or a family member would be treated unfairly when they sought health care. In contrast, only 24% of whites in the survey stated that they were very or somewhat concerned that they or a family member would be treated unfairly because of their race or ethnicity. A 2002 Kaiser Family Foundation survey revealed that minority physicians also believe that racial and ethnic minorities receive poorer health care than do white Americans.[47] This survey found that 77% of African American physicians, 52% of Latino physicians, 33% Asian physicians, and 25% of white physicians said that the health-care system very or somewhat often treated people unfairly based on their race and ethnicity. To be sure, individuals who have experienced racism or perceive racism in the health-care system are less likely to place trust in the system.

▶ STEPS TOWARD A TRUSTWORTHY HEALTH-CARE SYSTEM

Crawley offers an important corrective to the distrust literature.[48] She notes that most of the research on trust and minority communities has focused on the attitudes of these populations toward providers and health-care institutions. Crawley criticizes such an approach as inadvertently promoting stereotypes that minority Americans are inherently mistrustful. Such stereotyping, she argues, might convince researchers to curtail their efforts to recruit minorities into clinical trials or lead clinicians to omit full explanations of treatment options for minority patients because of a belief that they would be nonadherent to therapeutic recommendations.

Crawley views distrust as a breach of trust and calls for a paradigm shift that focuses on trustworthiness rather than on distrust. Such a shift puts the onus on health-care professionals and health-care institutions to address the problem of trust. It encourages them to look within their own environments and institutions for the sources of untrustworthiness. Her work prompts the critical question, "What have health-care professionals and health-care institutions done to demonstrate that they deserve the trust of racial and ethnic minorities?"

There are several steps that health-care professionals and health-care institutions can take to create a trustworthy health-care system for racial and ethnic minorities. Initiatives that help staff and institutions to provide care in a culturally competent fashion need to be advanced and supported. Cultural competence education can help providers better understand the histories, culture, experiences, preferences, and health behaviors of their minority patients. Increasing physicians' knowledge of the African American experience, including the Tuskegee Syphilis Study and the history of racism in this country, would help them better understand the perceptions of some of their African American patients. Cultural competence could also help health-care professionals bridge cultural divides by providing them with a better understanding of a racial or ethnic minority group's views of symptoms and illness. For example, knowledge of the health behaviors of Asian populations could help providers see that distrust of the Western health-care system and patients' perceptions that Western practitioners are critical of Asian health beliefs can manifest as lack of adherence, ranging from refusal to follow treatment recommendations to reluctance to consult Western physicians.[49] But cultural competence must go beyond the creation of training programs; it must become part of the institutional fabric of the US health-care system. The February 2000 decision of the Liaison Committee on Medical Education, the body responsible for accrediting medical schools, to mandate that cultural competence be a criterion for medical school accreditation is an example of an important step in the institutionalization of cultural competence.

Research has demonstrated that health-care professionals need good communication skills to facilitate the development of trusting relationships with patients. Thus, it is important that health-care professionals have training that advances communication skills emphasizing honesty, respect, and inclusiveness. To promote the importance of good communication skills for quality health care, it may be necessary to have the assessment of such skills as a requirement of professional certification.

Studies have also shown that language barriers can adversely affect the development of trusting relationships with racial and ethnic minorities. Health-care institutions should create programs that address the needs of their patients with limited English proficiency (LEP), especially in light of the nation's changing demographic shifts. According to data from the National Health Law Program, 15 states have had a greater than 100% LEP growth between 1990, and 2000. Under Title VI of the Civil Rights Act and its implementing regulations, health-care providers who receive federal funds have a legal obligation to ensure that people with LEP have meaningful access to health services. Failure to do so would constitute discrimination based on national origin. However, many health-care providers and institutions have opposed the implementation of Title VI because they view it as an unfunded mandate. In addition, many providers do not know the expectations of Title VI and how to implement this federal mandate. Overcoming language barriers is critical to the development of trust. Thus, it is important that health-care institutions and providers develop efficient and cost-effective practices that implement Title VI.

Health-care providers and institutions can also improve the levels of trust of minority patients by supporting efforts to diversify the health-care professions and to eliminate racial and ethnic disparities in health care. Research has demonstrated that racial and ethnic concordance between patient and provider was associated with more positive satisfaction with the care received. Patients believed that these visits were more participatory, supportive, and less discriminatory—in other words, more trustworthy. At a time when affirmative action and diversity initiatives are increasingly under attack, it is important that health-care providers and institutions advocate for the continuation of diversity programs and make the case that such programs are critical for the provision of quality health care. Likewise, it is important that health-care providers and health-care institutions be visible supporters of efforts to eliminate racial and ethnic disparities in health care. Such advocacy would demonstrate to racial and ethnic minority patients that health-care providers and health-care institutions acknowledge the disparate treatment that they may receive in the health-care system and are prepared to address the problem.

Research into understanding the role of trust in improving the quality of care is in its early stages of development, especially with regard to minority populations. More studies need to be done to develop validated measurement instruments and to better elucidate the mechanisms of the ways in which trust influences health care. Much of the research on trust in minority populations has focused on African Americans, resulting in a significant research gap with respect to other minority populations. In addition, most of the research has concentrated on the role of physicians in influencing trust; more work is needed to understand the role of other health-care professionals.

Another critical step in the development of a trustworthy health-care system for minority populations is for health-care providers and health-care institutions to provide mechanisms for community consultation, evaluation, and collaboration. They must develop strong relationships with members of minority communities so that community members can assist them in determining sources of distrust and activities to address and overcome them. For example, researchers may think that the source of distrust is the Tuskegee Syphilis Study when it may in fact be a local or institutional breach of trust. By consulting members of minority communities, health-care providers and health-care institutions clearly demonstrate that they respect the needs, thoughts, and experiences of racial and ethnic minorities and understand that trust is something that should be earned, not assumed.

On May 16, 1997, President Bill Clinton apologized for the Tuskegee Syphilis Study in a White House ceremony. The legacy of distrust that has become associated with the Syphilis Study prompted the campaign for the apology. Commenting on the need for the apology, Dr David Satcher, then Surgeon General and Assistant Secretary for Health and Human Services remarked, "The distrust is hurting us. I think we've got to really focus on it."[50] Those words still hold today.

► Case Study

Mrs Elizabeth Jones is a 79-year-old black woman with a history of high blood pressure and diabetes. A widow, she is a retired high school principal who is very active in her church and volunteers in the Foster Grandparent program. One evening she develops paralysis on the left side of her body and her family rushes her to the local hospital, where she is diagnosed with a stroke and is admitted to the hospital's intensive care unit in stable condition. She is conscious but has difficulty speaking and cannot move her left arm or leg. The next day, she is visited by the neurology team, which includes the attending physician, chief resident, junior resident, and two medical students. All members of the team are white and none has ever met Mrs Jones. Dr Charles, the attending physician, greets her, "Hello Elizabeth. How are you doing today?" During his visit with Mrs Jones, Dr Charles does not make eye contact with her or her son who is in the room. He talks about her medical condition with the other members of the team as if the family were not there. He approaches the issue of end-of-life care. He asks her if she would want her heart restarted if it stopped. He also asks her whether she would want life support systems withheld if her condition were to drastically worsen. She says that she does not know. "Well we need to have these things on your chart as soon as possible," the attending replies. At this point the son confronts the physician because of the disrespectful manner in which his mother has been treated. "First of all, her name is Mrs Jones, not Elizabeth. You are asking these questions about withholding treatment because she is an elderly black woman. I am sure that you do not ask white patients these questions. I know that black patients receive different care than white patients. You think that because she is black that she is poor and cannot pay for her treatment. That is why you are asking these questions. She does have insurance." As he leaves the room, Dr Charles responds, "Black and white patients receive the same care. This is not a racial issue."

Later that afternoon, Mrs Jones's primary physician, Dr Ruggere, who is also white, comes to visit her. She has been his patient for more than 10 years. "Hello, Mrs Jones. Hello Mr. Jones," he says as he sits down on her bed. Holding her hand, he discusses her medical condition and her fears. He too approaches the issue of end-of-life care. "For several years we have discussed what you would want done if you became critically ill and could not make decisions for yourself. I know that you have also discussed this with Reverend Morris. I know that this is a difficult discussion for you, but we need to move toward making some decisions." The son again raises his concerns about the differences between the treatment of black and white patients. Dr Ruggere asks why he thinks this. The son explains that black lives are not often

valued as much as white lives. "The Tuskegee Syphilis Study showed that. I have also read some newspaper articles about recent medical research that confirms that black patients are treated differently than white patients." "Yes, I know about the Syphilis Study and am familiar with those recent medical studies. I understand your concerns," Dr Ruggere responds. He reassures Mr Jones that his mother, along with the family, not physicians, would be making the decisions. Mrs Jones says that she is afraid to have this discussion without other family members being present. "I understand," Dr Ruggere replies. "Why don't we call your daughter and other son, and perhaps Reverend Morris and I can meet with them later." Mrs. Jones's son thanks the physician and agrees to set up a family meeting.

▶ SUMMARY AND RECOMMENDATIONS

Trust is the cornerstone of the provider–patient relationship and the foundation for quality health-care delivery and outcomes. It is also an element of constructive relationships between investigators and participants in biomedical research. Caring and comfort, technical competence, and good communication skills have been identified as physician behaviors that engender trust.

Research has documented that racial and ethnic minorities have lower levels of trust in medical providers and in medical institutions than do white Americans. Distrust can adversely affect health outcomes and contribute to racial and ethnic disparities in health and health care. It leads to decreased patient satisfaction, low enrollment in clinical trials, greater reluctance to seek medical care, poorer patient adherence to treatment recommendations, and increased unwillingness to donate organs. Race concordance between patient and physician is positively correlated with higher perceptions of quality of care, communications, patient satisfaction, and participatory decision making.

▶ **TABLE 25–1.** Summary of Recommendations

- Initiatives that help health-care professionals and institutions to provide culturally competent care should be advanced and supported
- Health-care professionals need training to develop communication skills that emphasize honesty, respect, and inclusiveness
- Efficient and cost-effective measures that implement Title VI of the Civil Rights Act should be developed to serve racial and ethnic minorities with limited English proficiency
- Health-care providers and institutions must become visible advocates of efforts to increase the diversity of the health-care profession and to eliminate racial and ethnic disparities in health
- More research must be conducted to better understand the role of trust in improving the quality of care for minority patients; this research must include all minority populations
- Health-care providers and institutions need to have strong relationships with the communities that they serve. Mechanisms for community consultation, evaluation, and collaboration must be developed

Trustworthiness, rather than distrust, may be a more useful conceptual framework to discuss the relationship of minority populations to the health-care system. It shifts the onus to health-care professionals and health-care institutions to address the problem of trust. Health-care professionals and health-care institutions can initiate several activities to create a trustworthy health-care system for racial and ethnic minorities. Recommendations aimed at achieving this goal are summarized in Table 25–1.

Most of the research on issues of trust in minority communities has focused almost exclusively on African Americans. There is a critical need to assess the attitudes of other racial and ethnic minorities. Preliminary research suggests that other racial and ethnic minorities are also more distrustful of the health-care system than are white Americans.

Race and gender play roles in the development of trust. African American and Hispanic men report less positive perceptions of physicians. The erosion of trust in minority communities is a complex interplay of social, political, cultural, and historical factors. Empirical research on the impact of the Tuskegee Syphilis Study is equivocal.

▶ REFERENCES

1. Mechanic D. Changing medical organization and the erosion of trust. *Milbank Q* 1996;74(2):171–189.
2. Ahern MM, Hendryx MS. Social capital and trust in providers. *Soc Sci Med* 2003;57(7):1195–1203.
3. Balint J, Shelton W. Regaining the initiative. Forging a new model of the patient–physician relationship. *JAMA* 1996;275(11):887–891.
4. LaVeist TA, Nickerson KJ, Bowie JV. Attitudes about racism, medical mistrust, and satisfaction with care among African American and white cardiac patients. *Med Care Res Rev* 2000;57(suppl 1):146–161.
5. Rotter JB. A new scale for the measurement of interpersonal trust. *J Pers* 1967;35(4):651–665.
6. Mechanic D, Schlesinger M. The impact of managed care on patients' trust in medical care and their physicians. *JAMA* 1996;275(21):1693–1697.
7. Goold SD. Trust, distrust and trustworthiness. *J Gen Intern Med* 2002;17(1):79–81.
8. Goold SD. Trust and the ethics of health care institutions. *Hastings Cent Rep* 2001;31(6):26–33.
9. Pederson LA. Racial differences in trust: Reaping what we have sown? *Med Care* 2002;40:81–84.
10. Kao AC, Green DC, Davis NA, et al. Patients' trust in their physicians: Effects of choice, continuity, and payment method. *J Gen Intern Med* 1998;13(10):681–686.
11. Safran DG, Taira DA, Rogers WH, et al. Linking primary care performance to outcomes of care. *J Fam Pract* 1998;47(3):213–220.
12. Thom DH, The Stamford Trust Study Physicians. Physician behaviors that predict patient trust. *J Fam Prac* 2001;50:323–328.

13. Boulware LE, Cooper LA, Ratner LE, et al. Race and trust in the health care system. *Public Health Rep* 2003;118:358–365.

14. Doescher MP, Saver BG, Franks P, et al. Racial and ethnic disparities in perceptions of physician style and trust. *Arch Fam Med* 2000;9(10):1156–1163.

15. Ayanian JZ, Cleary PD, Weissman JS, et al. The effect of patients' preferences on racial differences in access to renal transplantation. *N Engl J Med* 1999;341(22):1661–1669.

16. Cooper-Patrick L, Gallo JJ, Gonzales JJ, et al. Race, gender, and partnership in the patient–physician relationship. *JAMA* 1999;282(6):583–589.

17. LaVeist TA, Nuru-Jeter A. Is doctor–patient race concordance associated with greater satisfaction with care? *J Health Soc Behav* 2002;43(3):296–306.

18. Cooper LA, Roter DL, Johnson RL, et al. Patient-centered communication, ratings of care, and concordance of patient and physician race. *Ann Intern Med* 2003;139:907–915.

19. Saha S, Komaromy M, Koepsell TD, et al. Patient–physician racial concordance and the perceived quality and use of health care. *Arch Intern Med* 1999;159(9):997–1004.

20. Boulware LB, Ratner LE, Cooper LA, et al. Understanding disparities in donor behavior: Race and gender differences in willingness to donate blood and cadaveric organs. *Med Care* 2002;40:85–95.

21. Siminoff LA, Arnold R. Increasing organ donation in the African-American community: Altruism in the face of an untrustworthy system. *Ann Intern Med* 1999;130(7):607–609.

22. Kass NE, Sugarman J, Faden R, et al. Trust, the fragile foundation of contemporary biomedical research. *Hastings Cent Rep* 1996;26(5):25–29.

23. Corbie-Smith G, Thomas SB, St George DM. Distrust, race, and research. *Arch Intern Med* 2002;162(21):2458–2463.

24. Corbie-Smith G, Thomas SB, Williams MV, et al. Attitudes and beliefs of African Americans toward participation in medical research. *J Gen Intern Med* 1999;14(9):537–546.

25. Thom DH, Kravitz RL, Bell RA, et al. Patient trust in the physician: Relationship to patient requests. *Fam Pract* 2002;19:476–483.

26. McNamara P, Guadagnoli E, Evanisko MJ, et al. Correlates of support for organ donation among three ethnic groups. *Clin Transplant* 1999;13(1 pt 1):45–50.

27. Danielson BL, LaPree AJ, Odland MD, et al. Attitudes and beliefs concerning organ donation among Native Americans in the upper Midwest. *J Transplant Coord* 1998;8:153–156.

28. Ngo-Metzger Q, Legedza AT, Phillips RS. Asian Americans' report of their health care experiences: Results of a national survey. *J Gen Intern Med* 2004;19:111–119.

29. Taira DA, Safran DG, Seto TB, et al. Asian-American patient ratings of physician primary care performance. *J Gen Intern Med* 1997;12(4):237–242.

30. Gamble VN. Under the shadow of Tuskegee: African Americans and health care. *Am J Public Health* 1997;87(11):1773–1778.

31. Green BL, Masisiak R, Britt M, et al. Participation in health education, health promotion, and health research by African Americans; Effects of Tuskegee syphilis experiment. *J Health Educ* 1997;28:196–201.

32. Fouad MN, Partridge E, Green BL, et al. Minority recruitment in clinical trials: A conference at Tuskegee, researchers and the community. *Ann Epidemiol* 2000;10(8 suppl):S35–40.

33. Shavers VL, Lynch CF, Burmeister LF. Racial differences in factors that influence the willingness to participate in medical research studies. *Ann Epidemiol* 2002;12(4):248–256.

34. Freimuth VS, Quinn SC, Thomas SB, et al. African Americans' views on research and the Tuskegee Syphilis Study. *Soc Sci Med* 2001;52(5):797–808.

35. Dula A. African American suspicion of the health-care system is justified: What do we do about it? *Camb Q Health Ethics* 1994;3(3):347–357.

36. Corbie-Smith G. The continuing legacy of the Tuskegee Syphilis Study: Considerations for clinical investigation. *Am J Med Sci* 1999;317(1):5–8.

37. Canlas LG. Issues of health care mistrust in East Harlem. *Mt Sinai J Med* 1999;66(4):257–258.

38. Veatch RM. "Experimental" pregnancy: The ethical complexities of experimentation with oral contraceptives. *Hastings Cent Rep* 1971;0(1):2–3.

39. Zambrana R. Inclusion of Latino women in clinical and research studies: Scientific suggestions for assuring legal and ethical integrity. In: Mastroianni AC, Federman D, eds. *Women and Health Research: Ethical and Legal Issues of Including Women in Clinical Studies.* Washington, DC: National Academy Press; 1994;232–240.

40. Roberts D. *Killing the Black Body: Race, Reproduction, and the Meaning of Liberty.* New York, NY: Pantheon; 1997.

41. Lex B, Norris J. Health status of American Indian

and Alaska Native Women. In Mastroianni AC, Federman D, eds. *Women and Health Research: Ethical and Legal Issues of Including Women in Clinical Studies.* Washington, DC: National Academy Press; 1994;192–215.

42. Mayberry RM, Mili F, Ofili E. Racial and ethnic differences in access to medical care. *Med Care Res Rev* 2000;57(suppl 1):108–145.

43. Smedley BD, Stith AY, Nelson AR, eds. *Unequal Treatment: Confronting Racial and Ethnic Disparities in Health Care.* Washington, DC: National Academy Press; 2003.

44. Physicians for Human Rights. *The Right to Equal Treatment: An Action Plan to End Racial and Ethnic Disparities in Clinical Diagnosis and Treatment in the United States.* Boston, Mass: Physicians for Human Rights; 2003.

45. Alliance for Health Reform. Closing the gap: Racial and ethnic disparities in healthcare. *J Natl Med Assoc* 2004;96:436–440.

46. Henry J Kaiser Family Foundation. *Race, Ethnicity & Medical Care: A Survey of Public Perceptions and Experiences.* Menlo Park, Calif: Henry J Kaiser Family Foundation; 1999.

47. Henry J Kaiser Family Foundation. *National Survey of Physicians: Part 1: Doctors on Disparities in Medical Care.* Menlo Park, Calif: Henry J Kaiser Family Foundation; 2002.

48. Crawley LM. African-American participation in clinical trials: Situating trust and trustworthiness. *J Natl Med Assoc* 2001;93(12 suppl):14S–17S.

49. Sung CL. Asian patients' distrust of western medical care: One perspective. *Mt Sinai J Med* 1999;66 (4):259–261.

50. Trafford A. The ghost of Tuskegee. *The Washington Post* 1997; 6 May:A19.

CHAPTER 26

Participation of Minorities in Research and Clinical Trials

DAVID GRANDISON, MD, PhD

▶ **INTRODUCTION**

Elements within the clinical research and health-care communities that led to the US Public Health Service Study of untreated syphilis in African American men at Tuskegee Institute[1] may persist today. Widespread awareness of this infamous study constitutes a continuing barrier to African American and other minority participation in clinical research. These elements may also contribute to the significant health disparities between African Americans and other minorities, on the one hand, and majority group members on the other. Proactively addressing these elements is key to increasing African Americans' and other minorities' participation in clinical research, improving public health, and reducing health disparities.

▶ **THE SHADOW OF TUSKEGEE**

The US Public Health Service Syphilis Study at Tuskegee depicts a dark shadow of racism, medical arrogance, scientific bureaucracy, and a disregard for the value of human subjects participating in clinical research. The US Public Health Service Tuskegee Syphilis Study has often been described as the pivotal reason African Americans distrust clinical researchers and the health-care system in general. An article by Gamble[2] entitled "Under the Shadow of Tuskegee: African Americans and Health Care," in contrast, strongly suggested that the elements of distrust, suspicion, and fear of clinical researchers and the health-care system predate the Tuskegee Study. Gamble stated, "An examination of the syphilis study within a broader historical and social context makes it plain that several factors have influenced, and continue to influence, African Americans' attitudes toward the biomedical community." She described the exploitation and abuse of blacks by researchers and the health-care system during slavery and after the US Civil War, and suggested these are important factors contributing to the attitude of mistrust many African Americans have toward participating in clinical research. Fear of exploitation, abuse, racism, and distrust played a role in the establishment of so-called black hospitals. Yet black hospitals were not a protection against blacks being exploited by clinical researchers and the health-care system: The US Public Health Service Study of untreated syphilis in 400 black men was conducted in the "for blacks" veteran hospital in Tuskegee,

Alabama. Furthermore, black health-care professionals, with or without their understanding of the study's mistreatment of its subjects, participated in the experiment.

The powerful legacy of the US Public Health Syphilis Study endures, in part, because the racism and disrespect for black lives that allowed it reflect black people's contemporary experiences with the medical profession.[3] In addition to Gamble, numerous researchers argue this study is the most important reason that African Americans distrust clinical research and the health-care system.

The imprinting of this study on the minds of black people does not fully explain the low numbers of blacks participating in clinical research. Corbie-Smith et al[4] studied reasons for low participation in clinical trials among African Americans to identify and conceptualize barriers and facilitators to participation in clinical research. The study also examined attitudes and beliefs about the informed consent process, knowledge about the US Public Health Syphilis Study, and the perceived benefits and risks of participation in clinical research. African American participants described distrust of the medical community as a prominent barrier to participation in clinical research. Study participants also described real and perceived examples of exploitation to support their distrust of researchers. Corbie-Smith noted that distrust of clinical research is not unique to African Americans; it has been observed among all races after recently confronting health problems allegedly arising from unethical researcher conduct.

▶ FACTORS INFLUENCING MINORITY PARTICIPATION

Shavers et al[5] studied factors that influence African Americans' willingness to participate in medical research studies. According to the study, approximately 50% of study participants indicated there were conditions under which they would participate in clinical research, particularly if it would help a friend or relative or if it would be of direct benefit to the participant. Although knowledge of the US Public Health Service Syphilis Study was associated significantly with the unwillingness to participate in clinical research, distrust of clinical researchers was also likely exacerbated by US social history. In a separate paper, Shavers et al[6] examined racial differences in the prevalence of sociocultural barriers as a possible explanation for the underrepresentation of African Americans in clinical research. The study showed that the differences in the willingness to participate were primarily due to the relatively lower level of trust among African Americans for the clinical researcher. African Americans were also less willing to participate in clinical research if they attributed high importance to the race of the physician when seeking medical care, and if they knew about the US Public Health Service Syphilis Study.

Several factors may underlie the underrepresentation of African Americans and other minorities in clinical research. Minorities may lack awareness about clinical research studies[7] and may fear being used as "guinea pigs." Economic barriers may contribute to fewer minorities participating in clinical research, especially if they are required to pay for research-related expenses such as hospitalization, child care, or transportation.[8] Minority physicians' reluctance to refer minority patients also may limit their participation in clinical research.[9] Jean et al[10] commented that it is important to avoid picking the most affluent to participate in studies, so that results will be generalizable to the poor and underserved. Clinical trials with eligibility requirements based on educational status, material goods, or transportation may create barriers to participation by ethnic minorities as well as poor and underserved populations. Study sponsors may sometimes inadvertently discourage study participation by diverse subjects in an effort to increase the likelihood of protocol compliance.[11] Some minorities may also misinterpret the informed consent procedure and believe that it serves as a liability waiver for researchers. Along with the preceding barriers that reduce participation, minorities may avoid participation for other reasons, such as a fatalistic attitude about a particular disease or concerns about the racial composition of the research staff, or both.[9]

Freimuth et al[12] evaluated barriers to clinical research participation and the impact of past abuses of human subjects through clinical research. They conducted focus groups with African Americans in Los Angeles; Chicago; Washington, DC; and Atlanta. The purpose of the study was to understand attitudes toward research among African Americans, to assess knowledge of and beliefs about the Tuskegee Syphilis Study, and to identify strategies to overcome barriers to participation in clinical research. The study found that accurate knowledge about research was limited, lack of understanding and trust of informed consent procedures was problematic, and distrust of researchers posed a substantial barrier to recruitment. The study also found that, in general, African American participants believed research is important, but they clearly distinguished between types of research in which they would be willing to personally participate. Solutions recommended by the authors to improve minority participation in research included improving communication between referring physician and research subjects, developing culturally relevant educational materials, increasing minority outreach, and increasing involvement of the referring physician.

▶ CURRENT STATUS OF MINORITY PARTICIPATION IN CLINICAL RESEARCH

Lower minority participation in clinical research is a concern for both research and public health reasons. Without adequate minority enrollment in clinical trials, investigators cannot learn about differences in clinical responses among racial and ethnic minority groups or ensure the generalizability of clinical study results. Reasons for continued underrepresentation of African Americans and other minorities in clinical research and clinical trials must be addressed to enhance public health and to reduce health disparities.

The experiences of most African Americans and other minorities have been shaped by the influence of their race or skin color through segregation, civil rights validation, and racism. Disparities in health and health care strongly suggest that issues of race persist in the 21st century as remnants of slavery. Byrd[13] stated that racism is at least partly responsible for the fact that since arriving as slaves, African Americans have had the worst health care, the worst health status, and the worst health outcomes of any racial or ethnic group in the United States.

Racial and ethnic minority populations are among the fastest growing segments of all US communities, yet these populations have poorer health and remain medically underserved. African Americans and other underserved minorities remain behind the overall US population on virtually all health status indicators,[14] underscoring the importance of continued focus on clinical research to help reduce and eliminate the burden of health disparities among racial and ethnic minorities. *Healthy People 2010* noted that the 20th century saw remarkable and impressive improvements, with a significant decrease in infant mortality and a significant increase in life expectancy.[15] *Healthy People 2010* builds on the premise of 20 years of improvement in quality and healthy life, which began with the first set of health objectives published in 1979.[16] However, despite impressive improvement in quality and years of healthy life, a significant decrease in infant mortality rate, and a significant increase in life expectancy, on average, African Americans, Native Americans, and Alaska Natives still have the highest overall rates of death and infant mortality. A report on cancer clinical trials resources for Native Americans indicates that historically, Native Americans have been overresearched, yet outcomes have been underreported. As a result, Native American communities initially react to research and researchers with anger when no information is found as to how or why cancer and other diseases act differently in Native Americans.

Increasing minority participation is an important avenue to reducing health disparities. The relative absence of African Americans and ethnic minority participation in clinical research has received considerable attention due to recent government mandates for their inclusion in all human subject research. Inclusion of minorities in clinical research became a federal legal requirement in 1993. The National Institutes of Health Revitalization Act of 1993 deemed it imperative that research involving human subjects obtain information about both women and men, and from diverse ethnic and racial groups. The Food and Drug Administration (FDA) also mandates inclusion of minorities in clinical drug trials. The FDA's 1988 guidelines for the format and content of the clinical and statistical sections of new drug applications emphasize the importance of including analysis of demographic subset data in the application. The Food and Drug Modernization Act of 1997 also prompted the FDA to examine issues related to the inclusion of racial and ethnic groups in clinical drug trials.[17] Despite these government mandates to include special population groups such as minorities and women in clinical research, recruitment and retention of minorities in clinical research continue to represent major challenges for clinical researchers.

► CANCER RESEARCH

Overall patient participation rates in cancer clinical trials range from 3% to 20%; these rates are especially low in cancer clinical trials involving minority populations.[18] Cancer remains a major health threat to and is a leading killer of African Americans, second only to heart disease. Overall incidence and mortality rates for cancer among African Americans are higher than those for whites, but African Americans are still significantly underrepresented in clinical research aimed at finding treatment for such diseases. The difficulty of recruiting adequate numbers

of minority subjects is illustrated by analysis of data from National Cancer Institute (NCI)–sponsored nonsurgical treatment trials for four types of cancer. From 1996 through 2002, 75,215 patients were enrolled in NCI cooperative trials for breast, lung, colon, and prostate cancers. Approximately 9.2% of trial participants were black, 3.1% were Hispanic, 1.7% were Asian or Pacific Islander, and 0.3% were American Indian or Native Alaskan; 86% were white. Murphy et al[19] noted that although the total number of trial participants increased during the study period, representation of racial and ethnic minorities decreased. The authors suggested that several barriers might exist among minority groups, impeding their enrollment into clinical trials. These include past and ongoing patterns of discrimination, resulting in decreased trust in the health-care system among minority patients. Another barrier is that minorities are more likely to be guarded in statements about or to conceal their concerns about exploitation, the risks of experimental treatment, and motivations of researchers.

Cancer researchers from the Eastern Cooperative Oncology Group (ECOG)[20] conducted a study to identify potential barriers and solutions to African American enrollment in clinical trials. ECOG designed a survey to solicit the insight of African American physicians in the National Medical Association (NMA) about ways to increase minority participation in ECOG clinical trials. Seventy percent of NMA physicians cited mistrust of the research centers, fear of losing patients, and lack of respect from ECOG investigators as the most important barriers to referring minority cancer patients to participate in ECOG clinical trials.

Tejeda et al[21] evaluated the inclusion of African Americans, Hispanics, and non-Hispanic whites in NCI-sponsored trials from 1991 to 1994. They demonstrated that NCI clinical trials were, as a whole, racially and ethnically representative of the US population, suggesting there was equal access to NCI clinical trials. However, even though whites experience higher incidence rates, African American women experience higher death rates from breast cancer than any other racial or ethnic group. African Americans are 30% more likely to die from cancer than white Americans and have the highest age-adjusted incidence and mortality rates for several types of cancers. African American men have the highest prostate cancer incidence rate in the United States and a death rate for prostate cancer more than twice that of any other racial or ethnic group. This has not, however, translated into increased enrollment into clinical trails. Even though African American men were more receptive to prostate cancer clinical trials, they still distrusted the medical establishment and were fearful of being used as "guinea pigs" in clinical research.[22] In 1990, in response to low numbers of minorities participating in clinical trials, NCI established the Minority-Based Community Clinical Oncology Program (MB-CCOP).

▶ HEART FAILURE RESEARCH

According to one analysis[23] of multiple research protocols for congestive heart failure therapies, although racial and ethnic minorities comprise 30% of heart failure patients, research protocols for congestive heart failure enrolled primarily nonminority participants, with only 15% of patients in these studies representing racial or ethnic minorities. Not including these population groups, especially African Americans, in clinical trials for heart failure is of critical importance because clinical data suggest congestive heart failure is a unique malady in African Americans. According to Yancy,[24] heart failure in African Americans usually has a more troubling prognosis and potential variances in response to current medical therapies. The consequence of underrepresenting minority populations in congestive heart failure research is to neglect the population that bears the greatest burden of this disease and to increase the cost of health disparities. A review of randomized controlled heart failure clinical trials by Heiat et al[23] concluded that

these studies focused on a relatively small segment of the heart failure population, with sparse representation of minority women and the elderly.

▶ HIV/AIDS AND OTHER CHRONIC DISEASE RESEARCH

At a 1998 conference entitled "Diverse Perspectives of Clinical Trials," sponsored by the FDA, Brawley[25] reported on two MB-CCOP studies to show the extent to which minorities participate in cancer research. In the first, 7809 newly diagnosed cancer patients were enrolled, with similar rates for whites, Hispanics, and African Americans. In the second, of 820 patients eligible for enrollment, 62% of whites, 70% of Hispanics, and 61% of African American patients enrolled. Brawley suggested that these data demonstrate that hospitals that have good relationships with their communities can enroll Hispanic and African American subjects at a rate similar to that for whites. He noted that although NCI cooperative studies enroll large numbers of minority patients in treatment trials, they are unable to achieve similar success in prevention trials. He suggested that one possible reason for the difference is that prevention trials generally attract individuals who are more highly educated and economically secure.

To improve Native Americans' participation in clinical research, NCI established two Native American cancer control research networks. The purpose of the networks is to develop and promote a cadre of cancer prevention and control scientists to conduct culturally sensitive research among Native American populations. The primary objective of the research is to reduce morbidity and mortality from cancer.

The low numbers of Native Americans participating in clinical trials is illustrated by a 1992 breast cancer prevention trial sponsored by the National Surgical Adjuvant Breast and Bowel Project (NSABP). Of the 13,388 women enrolled in the study, only 34 were Native Americans, and only 27 completed the study.

A primary reason for nonparticipation by Native Americans in clinical trials is reported to be lack of information and limited opportunities to learn about clinical research and clinical trials. To improve enrollment and communication, when NSABP began the study of tamoxifen and raloxifene (STAR) breast cancer prevention trial, it established a relationship with the Native American community by hiring Native American coordinators and developing culturally specific educational materials.[26]

Stone et al[7] observed that the incidence of HIV infection was six times higher in African Americans and two times higher in Latinos than in whites but observed that women and patients of color were significantly less likely than whites to have participated in an AIDS clinical trial. King[11] also observed that pharmaceutical companies, in an effort to obtain licensing approval, may deliberately avoid recruiting marginalized populations, especially minority groups, substance abusers, and homeless persons to clinical trials because they believe poor compliance is common among these groups of research subjects.

Gifford et al[27] reported that 14% of adults receiving HIV treatment in the United States participated in a clinical trial between 1996 and 1998. They indicated that factors associated with participation in a clinical trial of HIV treatment included non-Hispanic white race, male sex, a history of homosexual contact, education beyond the high school level, annual income greater than $25,000, private fee-for-service health insurance, and residence within 1 mile of a center participating in such a trial. Much of the improvement in outcome for patients with HIV infection resulted from widespread use, after 1996, of highly active antiretroviral therapy (HAART). Ninety percent of HIV-infected patients with private insurance, and 79% of patients without insurance, had received such therapy through clinical trials. Gifford et al further demonstrated that black race and Hispanic or "other" ethnicity negatively influenced access to clinical trials.

It is important to increase the participation of African Americans and Hispanics in clinical trials to identify effective prevention and treatment strategies for cancer, diabetes, hypertension, obesity, HIV/AIDS, and other chronic diseases that disproportionately affect minority communities. Issues related to race and ethnicity may affect disease severity, progression, and response to therapy. Svensson's[8] review of African American representation in clinical trials observed that of 13 studies examining the efficacy and safety of antihypertensive drugs, only 8 enrolled at least one African American subject and in only one study was there an attempt to identify race-based differences in antihypertensive response to the investigational drug.

► THERAPEUTIC CLINICAL TRIALS

Britton et al[28] observed that although randomized controlled trials are considered the gold standard in terms of evaluating the effectiveness of therapeutic interventions, such trials are susceptible to challenges to their external validity if those participating are unrepresentative of the reference population for whom the therapy is intended. They conclude that narrow inclusion criteria for clinical trials may increase precision and reduce the number of subjects lost to follow-up, but an important disadvantage is uncertainty about extrapolation of trial results to all groups that might benefit from the therapy.

Corbie-Smith et al[4] examined the question of whether inclusion of minority participation in therapeutic clinical trials translated into reporting of trial results, so that the findings from clinical research could provide evidence to motivate changes in clinical practice addressing issues of disparities. They reviewed 253 clinical trial results from 1989 to 2000 published in three major internal medicine journals: *Annals of Internal Medicine, Journal of the American Medical Association,* and the *New England Journal of Medicine.* Their review showed the analysis of clinical results by race and ethnicity was reported in only two trials and by gender in only three. In diseases for which there are known racial and ethnic disparities, many clinical trials did not report race and ethnicity of study participants, and almost none reported results by race and ethnicity. The authors concluded, "Although federal initiatives mandate inclusion of minority groups in research, that conclusion has not translated to reporting of results that might guide therapeutic decisions."[28]

Evelyn et al[29] conducted a retrospective analysis of FDA medical officers' reviews of therapeutic clinical trial protocols and product labeling for 185 new molecular entities approved by the Center for Drug Evaluation Research between 1975 and 1999. The review was conducted to evaluate the extent to which racial and ethnic groups participated in clinical trials of newly approved drugs and the extent to which sponsors presented race-related information in the labeling approved for those products. The study showed that blacks were included in these clinical trials more frequently than other minorities, but that their participation declined from 12% to 6% from 1995 to 1999. Hispanic representation in these clinical trials was far below their representation in the US population. Product labeling for only 84 of 185 of the products (45%) contained some statement about race; however, in only 15 of 185 (8%) were the differences related to race described. It should be noted that 50% of the drug effects described in association with race or ethnicity were pharmacokinetic, 39% related to efficacy, and 11% related to safety. Also of note is that only one, of the 185 products reviewed, recommended changes in dosage based on racial effects.

▶ IMPORTANCE OF MINORITY INCLUSION

Improving minority participation in clinical research is a concern both for research and public health reasons. Without adequate minority enrollment in clinical trials, investigators cannot learn about potential differences in clinical responses among racial and ethnic minority groups or ensure the generalizability of clinical study results. Reasons for continued underrepresentation of African Americans, Hispanics, Native Americans, and other minorities in clinical research and clinical trials must be addressed for the good of public health, to reduce health disparities, and to reduce the cost of health care. It is important to develop effective strategies to increase racial and ethnic minority participation in clinical trials to identify effective prevention and treatment strategies for cancer, diabetes, hypertension, obesity, HIV/AIDS, and other chronic diseases that disproportionately affect minority communities. This is especially true since genetic studies[30] strongly suggest that issues related to race and ethnicity may influence disease severity, progression, and response to therapy.

Use of new treatments or drugs should be based on the results of adequate and well-controlled clinical trials and include subjects reflecting the range of patients expected to benefit from treatment or drugs. When minorities are underrepresented in clinical trials, there is often inadequate information upon which to assess the efficacy and safety of new drugs for use with members of minority groups.

The opportunity to participate in clinical research carries both potential risks and benefits. Potential benefits include access to state-of-the-art care and improved disease monitoring. To the extent to which clinical research participation provides benefits to participants, noninclusion of ethnic minorities denies them the chance to benefit.

Fairness demands equal opportunity for enrollment of minorities in clinical trials whenever clinically appropriate. However, to rebuild trust and confidence among minority populations and thereby increase their participation in clinical research will require substantial time and effort on the part of the clinical research and health-care communities. Historical abuses and current inequities at the hands of the clinical research and health-care communities help validate reasons for the mistrust and suspicions African Americans, Hispanics, Native Americans, and other ethnic minorities hold toward clinical researchers. Clinical investigators who wish to engage minorities in research must take time to develop effective strategies for educating potential minority participants about the importance of clinical research and clinical trials. They must be willing to discuss the concerns of potential minority participants openly, provide opportunities to ask questions, and avoid reacting defensively when responding to expressions of mistrust, suspicion, and other barriers that deter racial and ethnic minorities from enrollment in clinical trials.

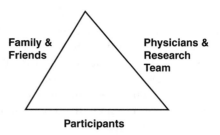

Figure 26–1. The recruitment triangle. *(Adapted from Gorelick PB, Harris Y, Burnett B, et al. The recruitment triangle: Reasons why African Americans enroll, refuse to enroll, or voluntarily withdraw from a clinical trial. An interim report from the African American Antiplatelet Stroke Prevention Study [AAASPS]. J Natl Med Assoc 1998;90(3): 141–145.)*

▶ PROVIDER ATTITUDES

King[11] acknowledged that beliefs, behavior, attitudes, perceptions, and expectations influence both patients and physicians, and that these factors may affect the patient–physician relationship. King further suggested that health-care providers, much like the rest of society, harbor prejudicial attitudes toward minority groups. Patients often respond to perceived attitudes with mistrust of the physician and the research staff, and reluctance to comply with treatment. Such patients would probably not choose to volunteer as participants in clinical research. Recognizing these attitudes and beliefs and improving communications between the minority subjects, the clinical investigator, and the referring health-care professional is key to reducing these barriers and building a trusting and supportive research environment for the minority subject.

▶ BUILDING TRUST

Shavers et al,[5] in evaluating factors that influence African Americans' willingness to participate in medical research studies, indicated that suspicion resulting from racial discrimination is a major contributor to the distrust that impedes African Americans' participation in clinical research. Building trust with African Americans depends on reducing repeated occurrences of the conditions and experiences that cause distrust. The authors suggested that researchers establish relationships built on mutual respect with the minority community. Researchers must provide frank and thorough explanations to the minority community for conducting clinical studies, commit to ethical research conduct, and describe provisions made to protect human subjects. Fouad et al[31] recognized the importance of early community involvement in planning the recruitment of minorities into clinical studies. Not involving trusted community representatives in planning for clinical research might result in mistrust and alienation in minority communities.

Creation of clinical research advisory committees (CRACs) with representation from a cross-section of the minority community is one method to engage the community in clinical research. The CRAC could become a vital tool to help researchers interact with the minority community to educate, train, and exchange information. Such committees can also assist the research community in dispelling suspicion and earning the trust needed to face future challenges and opportunities of clinical research.

▶ **TABLE 26–1.** Summary of Recommendations for Increasing Participation of Minorities in Clinical Research

- Reduce perceptions of racism and discrimination among members of the research team
- Build a trusting relationship between the subject and the research team
- Overcome inherent mistrust in the researcher and the research team
- Reduce subjects' fears of exploitation and abuse by the researcher
- Develop a culturally sensitive research team
- Address financial concerns about participation in clinical research, such as the cost of child care, elder care, transportation, and time conflicts with work
- Educate subjects about the risk of participation in clinical research
- Improve communication skills of the research team
- Address language barriers
- Refer subjects with other health-care or social needs to appropriate resources
- Engage community representatives in planning the research agenda
- Involve churches and other community organizations

▶ **SUMMARY AND RECOMMENDATIONS**

Plans for overcoming barriers to increasing participation of minorities in clinical research should include the strategies outlined in Table 26–1. Gorelick et al[32] suggested that organizers of clinical trials be aware of the "recruitment triangle" in soliciting subjects' participation in clinical trials. Understanding the respective roles of the potential subject, key family members or friends, and the primary physician, and their influence on the decision-making process facilitate the process of enrollment into trials (Fig. 26–1).

Clinical research stands on the threshold of new explorations into the biology of disease, and opportunities for developing more precise,

efficacious, and safe therapies through genetics and pharmacogenomic research. The challenge for the research community is to partner with minority communities in developing effective strategies to eradicate suspicion and doubt, improve the efficiency of clinical research, and facilitate the transfer of new therapies from bench to bedside. These must be balanced against potential harm to subjects and minority communities. The challenge for the minority community is for more minority physicians, research investigators, and health-care professionals to assist in educating their communities about the benefits of clinical research and the promise it holds for eventually eliminating health disparities among millions of Americans of racially and ethnically diverse heritage.

▶ **REFERENCES**

1. Revery S. *Tuskegee's Truths*. Chapel Hill, NC: University of North Carolina Press; 2000.
2. Gamble VN. Under the shadow of Tuskegee: African Americans and health care. *Am J Public Health* 1997;87(11):1773–1778.
3. Brawley OW. The study of untreated syphilis in the Negro male. *Int J Radiat Oncol Biol Phys* 1998;40(1):5–8.
4. Corbie-Smith G, Thomas SB, Williams MV, et al. Attitudes and beliefs of African Americans toward participation in medical research. *J Gen Intern Med* 1999;14(9):537–546.
5. Shavers VL, Lynch CF, Burmeister LF. Factors that influence African-Americans' willingness to participate in medical research studies. *Cancer* 2001;91(1 suppl):233–236.
6. Shavers VL, Lynch CF, Burmeister LF. Racial differences in factors that influence the willingness to participate in medical research studies. *Ann Epidemiol* 2002;12(4):248–256.
7. Stone VE, Mauch MY, Steger K, et al. Race, gender, drug use, and participation in AIDS clinical trials. Lessons from a municipal hospital cohort. *J Gen Intern Med* 1997;12(3):150–157.
8. Svensson CK. Representation of American blacks in clinical trials of new drugs. *JAMA* 1989;261(2):263–265.

9. El-Sadr W, Capps L. The challenge of minority recruitment in clinical trials for AIDS. *JAMA* 1992;267(7):954–957.

10. Jean S, Richter KP, Ahluwalia JS, et al. Reasons for ineligibility for a randomized clinical trial. *J Health Care Poor Underserved* 2003;14(3):324–330.

11. King TE Jr. Racial disparities in clinical trials. *N Engl J Med* 2002;346(18):1400–1402.

12. Freimuth VS, Quinn SC, Thomas SB, et al. African Americans' views on research and the Tuskegee Syphilis Study. *Soc Sci Med* 2001;52(5):797–808.

13. Byrd WM, Clayton LA. Race, medicine, and health care in the United States: A historical survey. *J Natl Med Assoc* 2001;93(3 suppl):11S–34S.

14. Levine RS, Foster JE, Fullilove RE, et al. Black–white inequalities in mortality and life expectancy, 1933–1999: Implications for Healthy People 2010. *Public Health Rep* 2001;116(5):474–483.

15. US Dept of Health and Human Services. *Healthy People 2010: Understanding and Improving Health,* 2nd ed. Washington, DC: US Government Printing Office; 2000. Available at: http://www.health.gov/healthypeople/.

16. US Public Health Service, Office of the Surgeon General. *Healthy People: The Surgeon General's Report on Health Promotion and Disease Prevention.* Washington, DC: US Government Print Office; 1979. DHEW Publication No. (PHS) 79-55071.

17. Food and Drug Administration Modernization Act of 1997, Pub L No. 105-115, November 21, 1997.

18. Giuliano AR, Mokuau N, Hughes C, et al. Participation of minorities in cancer research: The influence of structural, cultural, and linguistic factors. *Ann Epidemiol* 2000;10(8 suppl):S22–34.

19. Murthy VH, Krumholz HM, Gross CP. Participation in cancer clinical trials: Race-, sex-, and age-based disparities. *JAMA* 2004;291(22):2720–2726.

20. McCaskill-Stevens W, Pinto H, Marcus AC, et al. Recruiting minority cancer patients into cancer clinical trials: A pilot project involving the Eastern Cooperative Oncology Group and the National Medical Association. *J Clin Oncol* 1999;17(3):1029–1039.

21. Tejeda HA, Green SB, Trimble EL, et al. Representation of African-Americans, Hispanics, and whites in National Cancer Institute cancer treatment trials. *J Natl Cancer Inst* 1996;88(12):812–816.

22. Robinson SB, Ashley M, Haynes MA. Attitudes of African-Americans regarding prostate cancer clinical trials. *J Community Health* 1996;21(2):77–87.

23. Heiat A, Gross CP, Krumholz HM. Representation of the elderly, women, and minorities in heart failure clinical trials. *Arch Intern Med* 2002;162(15):1682–1688.

24. Yancy CW. The role of race in heart failure therapy. *Curr Cardiol Rep* 2002;4(3):218–225.

25. Brawley OW. *Diverse Perspectives of Clinical Trials, in U.S. Food and Drug Administration: Deadly Diseases and People of Color: Are Clinical Trials an Option?* Available at: http://www.fda.gov/oashi/patrep/perspectives.html.

26. Boesch M. Developing cancer clinical trial resources for Native Americans. *Cancer Practice* 2002;10(5):263–264.

27. Gifford AL, Cunningham WE, Heslin KC, et al. Participation in research and access to experimental treatments by HIV-infected patients. *N Engl J Med* 2002;346(18):1373–1382.

28. Britton A, McKee M, Black N, et al. Threats to applicability of randomised trials: Exclusions and selective participation. *J Health Serv Res Policy* 1999;4(2):112–121.

29. Evelyn B, Toigo T, Banks D, et al. Participation of racial/ethnic groups in clinical trials and race-related labeling: A review of new molecular entities approved 1995–1999. *J Natl Med Assoc* 2001;93(12 suppl):18S–24S.

30. Comuzzie AG. The emerging pattern of the genetic contribution to human obesity. *Best Pract Res Clin Endocrinol Metab* 2002;16(4):611–621.

31. Fouad MN, Partridge E, Wynn T, et al. Statewide Tuskegee Alliance for clinical trials. A community coalition to enhance minority participation in medical research. *Cancer* 2001;91(1 suppl):237–241.

32. Gorelick PB, Harris Y, Burnett B, et al. The recruitment triangle: Reasons why African Americans enroll, refuse to enroll, or voluntarily withdraw from a clinical trial. An interim report from the African American Antiplatelet Stroke Prevention Study (AAASPS). *J Natl Med Assoc* 1998;90(3):141–145.

CHAPTER 27

Disparities in Patient Safety

HARVEY J. MURFF, MD, MPH
DANIEL J. FRANCE, PhD, MPH
ROBERT S. DITTUS, MD, MPH

▶ INTRODUCTION

A 32-year-old Hispanic woman presents to a community hospital emergency department (ED) complaining of abdominal pain. Although she can speak some English, she is more comfortable using Spanish as her primary language. The ED provider interviews the patient with the help of a nonclinical hospital employee who has some Spanish-language skills. Based on the patient's history, physical examination, and a urinalysis, the provider determines that the woman has a urinary tract infection and prescribes sulfamethoxazole-trimethoprim, a common antibiotic. The patient goes home and begins taking the medication.

Within hours, she develops a diffuse rash, facial swelling, chest pain, and wheezing, and becomes acutely short of breath. Her family calls emergency services. The woman is diagnosed as having an anaphylactic reaction, and the paramedics initiate emergency treatment in the field. After she is stabilized, the woman is transported to the emergency department of another hospital for further evaluation. A provider, fluent in Spanish, learns that the patient has had a prior severe allergic reaction to sulfa-containing drugs and has a known allergy to these medications. The provider documents this allergic reaction within the patient's medical record at this hospital. The patient makes a complete recovery and goes home the following morning.

Recent data have suggested that the frequency of serious injuries and even death secondary to medical errors is strikingly high. These observations have catalyzed research devoted to patient safety. Data are beginning to describe adverse events (injuries due to medical management and not a patient's underlying disease process), why they occur, and opportunities for their prevention. Because disparities in health-care access and quality of care are known to permeate the health-care system, subgroups of patients may be at higher risk for medical adverse events. This chapter reviews the current evidence that serves as the foundation for patient safety research, describes the fundamental reasons that safety problems exist in health care, and reviews the evidence regarding health disparities and patient safety.

Much debate exists regarding the types of problems that represent a safety lapse. Although some definitions include episodes in which an individual received an unnecessary test (overuse error) or did not receive a necessary test (underuse error) as clear examples of patient safety problems,[1] this chapter focuses on occurrences in which patients experience injuries specifically related to their medical management. An example of this type of problem would be the individual who inadvertently received a 10-fold overdose of a narcotic medication that resulted in oversedation and respiratory distress.

▶ THE PROBLEM OF PATIENT SAFETY

Public attention has recently been focused on patient safety due to two recent Institute of Medicine (IOM) reports; however, data existed long before these reports were published detailing some of the problems with patient safety. One of the earliest studies to evaluate negligent iatrogenic injury in the United States was the California Medical Insurance Feasibility Study.[2] This study, initially published in 1974, involved a review of more than 20,000 medical records. Seeking any evidence of iatrogenic injury, it identified 4.65 injuries occurring to medical patients for every 100 hospitalizations. Of these injuries, 17% involved some form of medical negligence. Despite these early observations that a problem existed in the delivery of safe care to the American public, there was little public or professional response to these data.

In the mid-1980s, the Harvard Medical Practice Study[3,4] included a medical chart review of more than 30,000 patients admitted to one of 51 acute care hospitals in New York State. Adverse events occurred in 3.7% of hospital admissions, with 69% of injuries being caused by human error. Common causes of adverse events included surgical procedure complications, adverse drug events, and hospital-acquired infections. Subsequent studies examined why iatrogenic injuries were so common and the root causes of these errors. Seminal articles by Leape et al[5] began to call attention to possible "system failures" within the US health-care system that facilitated human error and adverse events.

Further work at Harvard[6] and Latter-Day Saints Hospital in Utah[7] demonstrated that advances in hospital information systems could reduce the rates of many types of adverse events. Despite evidence to support the benefits of information technology in reducing medication errors, the adoption of such systems remains slow. A large, chart review-based study further supports the findings of its predecessors. The Colorado and Utah Study[8] repeated the same methodology as the Harvard Medical Practice Study and found that 2.9% of hospitalizations were associated with an iatrogenic injury. In this study, 6.6% of adverse events resulted in the patient's death, and approximately 30% of the adverse events were due to negligence.

Despite several large American studies, and an equally substantial Australian study,[9] little public or professional attention was focused on patient safety until very recently. In 2000, the medical community was shocked by the release of the IOM's landmark report, *To Err is Human: Building a Safer Healthcare System.*[10] This report estimated that 44,000 to 98,000 Americans die each year because of medical errors, with over one million patients being injured.[11] Following these reports, a flood of media attention and increased governmental funding support helped produce the field of patient safety research. The Agency for Healthcare Research and Quality made improving patient safety one of its top priorities and set aside over $55 million to study medical errors. Industry groups also became involved. A notable example is the Leapfrog Group, a consortium of over 150 different private and public organizations, which as a whole represent approximately 34 million individuals within the United States. The goal of the Leapfrog Group are to use its market power to force hospitals to adopt safe practices, and several hospital systems have adopted its recommendations.

Patient safety has emerged as a new area of emphasis with public, private, and governmental support. The safety problems that Americans face when interfacing with their health-care system are sobering, but much effort is being focused at improving these problems. Little evidence exists that has specifically evaluated whether certain groups of people experience a disproportionate share of adverse events. This remains an important yet largely unexplored question. A review of the existing evidence regarding this question appears later in this chapter. Next, however, we summarize the mechanisms behind medical errors and why patients are often at risk.

▶ A SYSTEMS APPROACH TO PATIENT SAFETY

In 2001, the IOM released *Crossing the Quality Chasm* as a follow-up to its sobering report on health-care safety, *To Err is Human: Building a Safer Health System. Crossing the Quality Chasm* expanded the IOM's field of view to include the full dimensionality of health-care quality.[12] The report provides a diagnostic assessment of the current health-care system and offers a roadmap for change and improvement across six specific dimensions of care (Table 27–1).

In the report, the IOM provides evidence that improvements in the quality of the US health-care delivery system are being far outpaced by advances in clinical knowledge and technological innovation. The IOM asserted that high-quality care will not be achieved by further stressing the current system of health care. Instead, health care must adopt a systems approach to improvement, in view of the fact that

▶ **TABLE 27–1**. Institute of Medicine's Six Dimensions of Care

- Safety
- Effectiveness
- Patient-centeredness
- Timeliness
- Efficiency
- Equity

systems must be designed or redesigned to provide high-quality care.

The systems approach to improvement shifts the focus from the actions of individual care providers to the multiple factors that influence provider behavior and, ultimately, patient outcomes.[5] The systems model is a product of industrial and systems engineering and has been studied extensively in other high-risk industries such as aviation and nuclear power. Exploring systems thinking in the context of risk and safety will provide important insights into the potential sources of health disparities in safety and across all dimensions of care. Limited research has been published to date on disparities in patient safety, but this may reflect limitations in the models or frameworks used to pursue such inquiry. Investigators are now beginning to use systems theory to study and understand how factors extending far beyond the bedside may contribute to adverse events or conditions that lead to harm. A systems model provides a means to study the relationship among patient safety and its many interrelated factors, including human, system, cultural, and societal factors.

Human Error

James Reason's (1990) classical definition of human error is "the failure of a planned action to be completed as intended or the use of a wrong plan to achieve an aim."[13] Errors in medicine are generally defined in terms of an act or action made by a care provider that affects the patient.[14] The theory of cognition states that there are three basic mechanisms of thought that lead to action: skills-based, rules-based, and knowledge-based cognitive processes.[15] These processes span the range from unconscious to conscious thought processes.

Skills-based processes are automatic actions that require virtually no thought to perform. These processes require an individual to follow a set of instructions but not necessarily understand the reasoning behind them. Rule-based processes require individuals to match context to problem. Rules are generally in the "if X then Y" form and can be based on past experience or explicit instructions. Knowledge-based processing is a highly conscious process and involves analytic thought—processing and analyzing subjective knowledge.

When cognitive processes break down, human error results in the form of slips, lapses, and mistakes. Slips are errors of action that result when there is poor execution of a good or appropriate plan. Lapses are internal events that generally involve memory failures. Mistakes are errors of intention, such that bad plans are executed flawlessly. Reason proposed that human error, in any of its forms, occurs as active failures at the sharp end (ie, bedside) or as latent failures at the blunt end (ie, far removed from the patient or even the clinical setting). Regardless of where these errors occur, they all describe acts or behaviors.[14]

As documented in *To Err is Human,* health care has historically overemphasized the role of human actions in the error equation. As a result of focusing on deficiencies in the performance of its workforce, health care propagated a culture of blame and shame rather than system-based learning and improvement. The people-focused approach only created mistrust and fear of retribution in the workforce, limiting health-care provider involvement and participation in safety improvement efforts.[5] Safety interventions implemented during this era focused primarily on retraining poorly performing staff and rewriting policies and procedures to fix points of failure. Today's systems-focused framework for patient safety shifts the focus from errors and the humans who commit them to the conditions and factors that create unsafe conditions—for both health-care providers and patients.

Human Behavior and Performance Shaping Factors

Human behavior is typically defined as the interaction of person and environment.[14] Lewin[16] defined behavior as a function of a person not in isolation, but of a person in continuous interaction with the environment. This definition provides important insight into understanding human error and provides a foundation for systems thinking. As Bogner states in her book, *Misadventures in Health Care,*[14] the definition acknowledges that although humans are naturally error-prone, their performance is influenced by their interactions with many complex and dynamic factors.

In the early 1980s, human factors engineers, cognitive psychologists, and safety scientists began to transition away from studying errors and accidents in industry to studying the multitude of factors that shape or influence human behavior and performance. The major motivation for this transition in research focus was the realization that error and accident analyses are retrospective approaches that require the accumulation of accidents, tragedies, and catastrophes to prevent future mishaps. Studying these factors, coined *performance shaping factors,* became appealing to researchers because it provided a means to conduct prospective safety analyses. Performance shaping factors are the conditions or factors that influence provider behavior for the positive or negative. In the case of human error, performance shaping factors work against the good intentions of the care provider in a manner that impairs performance and ultimately compromises patient safety. The general categories of performance shaping factors are[17–19] individual factors (ie, experience, training, physiologic or psychological state), task-related factors (ie, workload, vigilance), equipment and tools (ie, technology and user interfaces), interpersonal factors (ie, teamwork), care environment factors (ie, facility layout, cleanliness), and organizational or cultural factors (ie, work schedules or work policies). The idea of performance shaping factors caught the interest of patient safety researchers, especially in anesthesiology, about a decade after their emergence in reliability and safety engineering.[20–22] Soon after, performance shaping factors became an important building block in the development of systems theory in health care.

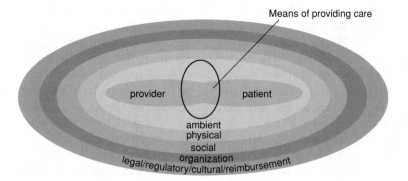

Figure 27–1. The systems approach model of error. (The artichoke model)

Systems Approach Models of Error

James Reason divided the human contributions to the breakdown of complex systems into two categories: active failures and latent failures.[17] These failures differ based on who initiated them and how long they take to have an adverse effect. People working at the sharp end (ie, bedside) of the health-care system commit active failures, and the impact of these failures is usually felt immediately. People working at the blunt end of the system (ie, upper echelons of administration) commit latent errors, and the effects of these failures may take years to be realized. Latent errors are often flaws in system planning, design, structure, maintenance, or training, and they are often only apparent when they are triggered by active failures to penetrate or bypass system defenses and safeguards. These errors most directly correlate with the concept of performance shaping factors. Reason asserts that latent failures are inevitable and are inadvertently designed into all systems. However, they can be diagnosed and removed before they cause errors and adverse outcomes.

Health care is a dynamic process, and its delivery requires the interaction of three primary components: (1) the provider, (2) the means of providing care, and (3) the patient. These components are interrelated and interdependent, so changes in one often affect the others. For example, the health of the care provider, physical or mental, may affect how that provider performs in using a medical technology on a patient. Similarly, a surgical device of poor ergonomic design may adversely affect a surgeon's performance in using that device on a patient, resulting in patient injury. Finally, a physical condition of a patient, perhaps morbid obesity, may cause changes in standard clinical procedures that inadvertently lead to error and patient injury. This systems view of health-care delivery muddies the simplified view that health-care providers are the sole cause and source of errors in medicine.

Bogner extends the systems model by suggesting that the three components of health-care delivery—provider, means for providing care, and patient—form a subsystem of the larger basic care-providing system.[23] Surrounding the core subsystem of care delivery are five systems or categories of interrelated factors that define the context of care. These systems that encircle the care delivery subsystem are ambient conditions, physical environment, social environment, organizational factors, and the overarching legal-regulatory-reimbursement-national culture factors.

The model (see Fig. 27-1) suggests that far-reaching forces at the social, organizational, or national level contribute directly or indirectly to the cognitive slips, lapses, and mistakes that translate into error or even nonequitable care at the bedside. The model proposes that a ripple effect results whenever any shell or leaf is perturbed. However, in this model ripples always emanate inward toward the health-care delivery subsystem that lies at the center. So changes in any system affect all systems within its circumference. Changes in the outermost level, the legal-regulatory–reimbursement-cultural level, have the most profound impact on the basic care-providing system. For example, state and national laws protecting adverse event reporting from legal discovery improve the safety climate and culture (ie, blame-free) of an organization. A safe organizational culture will increase provider participation in incident reporting and safety improvement. The model supports the notion that errors and disparities in health care are created and propagated by failures in the health-care system in addition to failures resulting from individual provider behaviors.

Implications for Future Research

Systems models of error provide a framework for considering and evaluating disparities in health-care quality and safety. The framework requires one to consider not only the act of health care, but also its context. Disparities result when social, cultural, regulatory, political, or other factors knock the health-care system out of balance. Equity in each and every level of the system must be achieved and maintained to restore this equilibrium. Future research should focus on the barriers that exist or develop at the interfaces of the health-care subsystems.

▶ DISPARITIES IN PATIENT SAFETY

Patient safety is an important element of overall health-care quality. Errors of commission, such as a failure to diagnose or an inappropriate delay in diagnosis, and errors of omission, such as failure to meet a recommended level of care (eg, inappropriate monitoring of glucose control in a diabetic patient), arguably produce unsafe medical conditions. Much data exist documenting disparities in time to medical diagnoses and adherence to treatment guidelines between ethnic

and racial groups. As previously noted, much of these data are reviewed within the disease-specific context of other chapters of this text. For the purposes of this chapter, we focus specifically on injuries resulting from medical care.

Few groups have made the examination of health-care disparities associated with patient safety a priority of their research agenda. This lack of focus on disparities may be a result of the current conceptual frameworks that point to health-care systems, rather than individual providers, as the cause of most medical errors and the major opportunities for improvement. Such systems do not have as obvious a capacity for discrimination as individual providers. However, much data exist that suggest that patients of different cultures have very different interactions with the medical system that could result in safety disparities.[24,25]

System attributes such as good communication and participatory decision making differ among cultural groups.[26,27] Discontinuity with a health-care provider is more common among African Americans and Hispanics than whites. Access to a regular provider is less common.[28,29] Rates of satisfaction with providers are typically lower in nonwhites.[25,30] As a result, levels of trust between a provider and patient are lower, particularly in situations in which there is racial disconcordance between provider and patient.[26,31]

Good communication, available access, and continuous care are all important system properties that if disrupted could potentially result in medical injury. Although there is little direct evidence to indicate whether certain racial or ethnic groups experience a disproportionate share of medical errors, there is mounting indirect evidence to suggest this possibility.

Rates of Adverse Events Among Ethnic and Racial Groups

Adverse events can be identified by several methods. The most frequently employed is thorough third-party chart review. This method typically involves chart prescreening, by either electronic or manual means, followed by physician review. Alternatives have included prompted physician reporting, direct observation of clinical care, and patient interviews.

Three studies employing chart review have been conducted from which data can be derived regarding adverse event rates in minority groups. The largest study to date involved data collected as part of the Harvard Medical Practice Study. Burstin et al evaluated over 30,000 hospital admissions occurring in 51 New York state hospitals in 1984.[32] Adverse events were identified in 1278 admissions and negligent adverse events in 306 admissions. Race data were obtained from the New York Statewide Planning and Research Cooperative System database and coded as either "white" or "black." On univariate analysis, black patients had an adverse event rate of 5.4% compared with 4.0% for white patients—a difference that was not statistically significant. Black patients were more likely to have an adverse event due to negligence when compared with white patients (36% versus 23.6%, P value <0.05). However, after adjusting for patient age, diagnostic-related risk, income, and insurance payer status, black race was not associated with an increased risk for adverse events or negligent adverse events (odds ratio 1.13, 95% confidence interval [CI] 0.84 to 1.51 and 1.48, 95% CI 0.80 to 2.75, respectively). In this study only insurance status was associated with increased risk for having an adverse event, with uninsured patients having an odds ratio of 2.35 (95% CI 1.40 to 3.95) of having an adverse event when compared with individuals with health insurance.

The remaining studies focused only on adverse drug events as the outcome measured. Adverse drug events are medical injuries that result from medication use. Adverse drug events can result from several different mechanisms, including ordering errors, such as ordering the wrong drug for a patient; administration errors, such as giving an incorrect drug dose; or problems in monitoring, such as failing to detect a serious drug-to-drug interaction.

Bates et al, in 1999, conducted a nested case-control study of 2240 hospitalized adults admitted to two large tertiary care hospitals in Boston, Massachusetts.[33] Adverse drug events were first identified by either hospital nurses or pharmacists or by a research nurse who visited the study wards twice daily. Potential incidents were then referred for physician review. Adverse drug events were found in 139 patients (6% of all admissions). Patient race was reported as white versus nonwhite. Within the entire cohort, 25% of patients were classified as nonwhite. In the 139 patients who experienced an adverse event, 24% were nonwhite. In a further, subgroup analysis of preventable adverse drug events (medication injuries due to human error), 31% of individuals who experienced a preventable adverse drug event were classified as nonwhite. Although in this study nonwhites tended to experience higher rates of preventable adverse events than whites, the difference was not statistically significant and the overall number of preventable adverse events was quite small (N = 42).

A second study from the same group evaluated adverse drug events occurring in nonhospitalized adults.[34] This study relied on a computerized monitor to detect potential adverse drug events, which were then confirmed by manual physician review. This study involved ambulatory records for 15,665 patients. Within this cohort, 2077 (13%) individuals were reported as black, 781 (5%) as Hispanic, 155 (1%) as Asian, and 5475 (35%) as "other." The investigators manually reviewed a random sample of all the electronically identified charts. One hundred and twenty-one adverse drug events occurring in 97 patients were identified. Based on these findings the investigators estimated that 864 adverse drug events, or 5.5 per every 100 patients, occurred within the entire cohort. Within this group of 97 patients experiencing an adverse drug event, 18% were reported as black, 6% as Hispanic, 1% as Asian, and 16% as "other." Thus, whereas 13% of the entire cohort was identified as African American, 18% of individuals experiencing an adverse drug event were black; however, this difference was not statistically significant and might thus be due to chance alone.

Chart review is not the only method of detecting adverse events. In a study conducted by O'Neil et al, the investigators compared prompted physician reporting with manual chart review to identify adverse events.[35] The study was conducted on the medical service of the Brigham and Women's Hospital in Boston and involved 3141 hospitalized patients. Seventeen percent (527) of the study cohort were identified as black, 6% (178) as Hispanic, 1% (32) as Asian, and 0.2% (7) as "other." This study is notable in that although prompted physician review identified an equivalent number of patients experiencing adverse events when compared with manual review (89 versus 85), these two methods of adverse event detection overlapped in only 41 patients. Of the 44 adverse events identified by chart review alone, 7% occurred in black patients and 11% in individuals reported as "other." In the 48 adverse events identified through prompted physician review but not seen on chart review, 19% occurred in black patients and 2% occurred in "other." Although there was no statistically significant difference in adverse event rates among racial or ethnic groups, this finding suggests a potential limitation of chart review in determining race-specific rates of adverse events. Interestingly, physician reporting identified almost twice as many preventable adverse events (ie, those due to a human error) as the chart review methodology.

Direct observation has also been employed to detect adverse events in hospitalized medical patients. In a study conducted by Andrews et al,[36] trained ethnographers attended medical work rounds and nursing shift changes and recorded adverse events mentioned in the course of these communications. Of the 1047 patients followed in the study, 18% experienced at least one serious adverse event. This rate is substantially higher than rates extrapolated from chart review and again suggests limitations to the chart review methodology. Within this cohort of patients, 47.3% of patients were identified as nonwhite, while 49% of patients experiencing an adverse event were identified as nonwhite. Another observational study relied on attending physicians on a general medicine service to detect and report medical errors committed by the housestaff.[37] Five hundred and twenty-eight patients were evaluated. Twelve percent of individuals with no errors occurring during their care were African American, 4% were Hispanic, and 0.8%, Asian. Of the 22 patients with an adverse event, none were African American or Asian American, and 5% were Hispanic. In the 33 patients who experienced near-misses (a medical error occurred but no injury resulted), 21% were African American, 3%, Hispanic, and 3%, Asian American.

Few studies have identified adverse events based on patient observations. A study conducted in four adult primary care practices in Boston surveyed 1202 outpatients immediately after a clinic visit.[38] Reports of adverse drug events were reviewed by two physicians to confirm whether in fact an adverse drug event had occurred. Of the 661 respondents, 11% (74) identified themselves as African American and 7% as "other." Of the 162 patients who identified an adverse drug event, 11% were black and 6%, "other, nonwhite."

In general, no studies have found a statistically significant difference in rates of adverse events, although some have noted higher frequencies in African Americans. Because adverse events typically occur in about 3% to 6% of admissions, studies must review potentially thousands of charts to accumulate a sufficient number of adverse events for study. Furthermore, to conduct a subgroup analysis based on race requires even further division of the overall numbers. Because of the overall size of the Harvard Medical Practice Study, it is unlikely that the lack of association between patient race and medical injuries represents a false-negative result. These results, however, could still underestimate an effect if they rely on chart review if, in fact, this method of adverse event detection underestimated medical injuries to African American groups.

▶ **TABLE 27-2.** Summary of Major Findings Regarding Disparities in Patient Safety

- Over one million patients are injured each year as a result of errors with their medical care.
- Although humans are naturally error-prone, their performance is influenced by their interactions with many complex and dynamic factors.
- The systems models of human error suggest that social, cultural, regulatory, and political factors can contribute to the overall safety of a health-care system, thus providing a strong rationale why patient safety disparities might exist.
- Little evidence exists that has specifically evaluated whether certain groups of people experience a disproportionate share of adverse events.
- Although in some studies the frequencies of adverse events were higher in minority groups, these findings were neither consistent nor statistically significant.
- As a patient safety research agenda continues to emerge, studies need to be conducted to specifically address these questions.

▶ **TABLE 27-3.** Recommendations for National Priorities to Ameliorate Disparities in Patient Safety

- Governmental and nongovernmental bodies must continue to place a high priority on funding research related to improving patient safety, because medical injuries are strikingly prevalent in the United States population.
- As a national patient safety research agenda continues to evolve, specific emphasis needs to be directed at addressing whether disparities in rates of patient injuries exist, whether certain groups are more likely to experience certain types of injuries, and whether different adverse event detection methods more accurately identify adverse events in certain patient groups.
- Although the Harvard Medical Practice Study did not find an association between patient race and adverse event risk, these findings should be confirmed in other large epidemiologic studies; a few large epidemiologic studies exist, which could reanalyze previously collected data to evaluate whether patient race might be a risk factor for adverse events.
- Future studies of patient safety should consider evaluating how patient ethnicity and race might influence the effectiveness of patient safety interventions.

Race As a Predictor of Adverse Events

Few studies have evaluated race as a potential predictor of adverse events. In fact, much of the literature regarding predictors for adverse events has resulted from case-control studies, which have used race as a matching variable. In view of this, one cannot determine just what effect race might have on the probability of experiencing an adverse event. One study that was designed to evaluate this question looked at the rates of inappropriate prescribing of medications to elderly individuals.[39] Using the 1997 National Ambulatory Medical Care Survey, the investigators determined that inappropriate medications were being prescribed in frequencies per visit of 10.3% for whites, 9.7% for blacks, and 1.9% for other minorities. Al-

though these data would suggest that minority elderly patients are not at increased risk of being prescribed inappropriate medications, African Americans were more likely to be prescribed four or more prescriptions per visit than whites (22.7% versus 17%). Number of prescriptions remains the only consistently demonstrated patient risk factor for the occurrence of an adverse drug event. A second study asking this same question found elderly nonwhites no more likely to receive inappropriate medications than elderly whites.[40]

Although no data exist that demonstrate higher rates of adverse events in minorities than in nonminorities, some data suggest that not speaking English is a risk factor for medical errors. In a study involving a pediatric outpatient population, errors were frequently found because of language translation.[41] The investigators noted a mean of 31 errors per encounter. Of these interpretation errors, almost two thirds had potentially significant clinical consequences. Ad hoc translators (those who were not professional translators employed by the study institution) were much more likely to make a clinically significant error in translation than professional translators.

▶ SUMMARY AND RECOMMENDATIONS

As a field for basic and applied scholarship, patient safety has emerged as a response to unacceptably high rates of medical errors. Much of the knowledge regarding why errors are so prevalent in medicine springs from work performed in other industries, such as aviation or nuclear power. Little research has been conducted to evaluate whether specific groups of people experience a disproportionate share of adverse events. However, emerging evidence suggests that this could be a possibility. Injuries from medical care exact a substantial toll in the United States in patient morbidity and mortality as well as in financially overburdening an already expensive health-care system. Further study is needed to identify subpopulations at higher risk for medical errors and to improve patient safety among all individuals receiving health care. Summaries of the findings and recommendations discussed in this chapter appear in Tables 27–2 and 27–3.

▶ REFERENCES

1. Chassin MR. Is health care ready for Six Sigma quality? *Milbank Q* 1998;76(4):565–591,10.
2. Mills DH. Medical insurance feasibility study. A technical summary. *West J Med* 1978;128(4):360–365.
3. Brennan TA, Leape LL, Laird NM, et al. Incidence of adverse events and negligence in hospitalized patients: Results of the Harvard Medical Practice Study I. 1991. *Qual Saf Health Care* 2004;13(2):145–151; discussion 51–52.
4. Leape LL, Brennan TA, Laird N, et al. The nature of adverse events in hospitalized patients. Results of the Harvard Medical Practice Study II. *N Engl J Med* 1991;324(6):377–384.
5. Leape LL. Error in medicine. *JAMA* 1994;272(23):1851–1857.
6. Bates DW, Leape LL, Cullen DJ, et al. Effect of computerized physician order entry and a team intervention on prevention of serious medication errors. *JAMA* 1998;280(15):1311–1316.
7. Classen DC, Pestotnik SL, Evans RS, et al. Computerized surveillance of adverse drug events in hospital patients. *JAMA* 1991;266(20):2847–2851.
8. Thomas EJ, Studdert DM, Burstin HR, et al. Incidence and types of adverse events and negligent care in Utah and Colorado. *Med Care* 2000;38(3):261–271.
9. Wilson RM, Runciman WB, Gibberd RW, et al. Quality in Australian Health Care Study. *Med J Aust* 1996;164(12):754.
10. Kohn LT, Corrigan JM, Donaldson MS, eds. *To Err is Human: Building a Safer Healthcare System.* Washington, DC: National Academy Press; 2000.
11. Weingart SN, Wilson RM, Gibberd RW, et al. Epidemiology of medical error. *BMJ* 2000;320(7237):774–777.
12. Corrigan JM, Kohn LT, Donaldson MS, et al. *Crossing the Quality Chasm: A New Health System for the 21st Century.* Washington, DC: National Academy Press; 2001.
13. Reason J. Human error: Models and management. *West J Med* 2000;172(6):393-396.
14. Bogner MS. *Misadventures in Health Care: Inside Stories.* London, England: Lawrence Erlbaum Associates; 2004.
15. Rasmussen J. The role of error in organizing behaviour. 1990. *Qual Saf Health Care* 2003;12(5):377–383; discussion 83–85.
16. Lewin B. *Principles of Topological Psychology.* New York, NY: McGraw-Hill; 1966.
17. Reason JT. *Human Error.* New York, NY: Cambridge University Press; 1990.
18. Sargent TO, Blum RB. Predicting and controlling variable performance shaping factors. *Trans Am Nuclear Soc* 1980;34:693–694.

19. Embrey D. Incorporating performance shaping factors into the assessment of human reliability. *Trans Am Nuclear Soc* 1980;34:162–163.
20. Gaba DM. Human error in anesthetic mishaps. *Int Anesthesiol Clin* 1989;27(3):137–147.
21. Howard SK, Gaba DM, Fish KJ, et al. Anesthesia crisis resource management training: Teaching anesthesiologists to handle critical incidents. *Aviat Space Environ Med* 1992;63(9):763–770.
22. Weinger MB, Slagle J. Human factors research in anesthesia patient safety. *Proc AMIA Symp* 2001: 756–760.
23. Bogner MS. Error: It's what, not who. *TraumaCare* 2000;8(2):82–84.
24. Shi L. Experience of primary care by racial and ethnic groups in the United States. *Med Care* 1999;37(10):1068–1077.
25. Murray-Garcia JL, Selby JV, Schmittdiel J, et al. Racial and ethnic differences in a patient survey: Patients' values, ratings, and reports regarding physician primary care performance in a large health maintenance organization. *Med Care* 2000; 38(3):300–310.
26. Cooper-Patrick L, Gallo JJ, Gonzales JJ, et al. Race, gender, and partnership in the patient–physician relationship. *JAMA* 1999;282(6):583–589.
27. Quill TE. Recognizing and adjusting to barriers in doctor–patient communication. *Ann Intern Med* 1989;111(1):51–57.
28. Blendon RJ, Aiken LH, Freeman HE, et al. Access to medical care for black and white Americans. A matter of continuing concern. *JAMA* 1989;261(2):278–281.
29. Fichtenbaum R, Gyimah-Brempong K. The effects of race on the use of physician's services. *Int J Health Serv* 1997;27(1):139–156.
30. Hulka BS, Kupper LL, Daly MB, et al. Correlates of satisfaction and dissatisfaction with medical care: A community perspective. *Med Care* 1975;13(8):648–658.
31. Doescher MP, Saver BG, Franks P, et al. Racial and ethnic disparities in perceptions of physician style and trust. *Arch Fam Med* 2000;9(10):1156–1163.
32. Burstin HR, Lipsitz SR, Brennan TA. Socioeconomic status and risk for substandard medical care. *JAMA* 1992;268(17):2383–2387.
33. Bates DW, Miller EB, Cullen DJ, et al. Patient risk factors for adverse drug events in hospitalized patients. ADE Prevention Study Group. *Arch Intern Med* 1999;159(21):2553–2560.
34. Honigman B, Lee J, Rothschild J, et al. Using computerized data to identify adverse drug events in outpatients. *J Am Med Inform Assoc* 2001;8(3):254–266.
35. O'Neil AC, Petersen LA, Cook EF, et al. Physician reporting compared with medical-record review to identify adverse medical events. *Ann Intern Med* 1993;119(5):370–376.
36. Andrews LB, Stocking C, Krizek T, et al. An alternative strategy for studying adverse events in medical care. *Lancet* 1997;349(9048):309–313.
37. Chaudhry SI, Olofinboba KA, Krumholz HM. Detection of errors by attending physicians on a general medicine service. *J Gen Intern Med* 2003;18(8):595–600.
38. Gandhi TK, Weingart SN, Borus J, et al. Adverse drug events in ambulatory care. *N Engl J Med* 2003;348(16):1556–1564.
39. Huang B, Bachmann KA, He X, et al. Inappropriate prescriptions for the aging population of the United States: An analysis of the National Ambulatory Medical Care Survey, 1997. *Pharmacoepidemiol Drug Saf* 2002;11(2):127–134.
40. Goulding MR. Inappropriate medication prescribing for elderly ambulatory care patients. *Arch Intern Med* 2004;164(3):305–312.
41. Flores G, Laws MB, Mayo SJ, et al. Errors in medical interpretation and their potential clinical consequences in pediatric encounters. *Pediatrics* 2003;111(1):6–14.

CHAPTER 28

Health-Care Disparities in Medical Genetics

G. Bradley Schaefer, MD, FAAP, FACMG

Georgia M. Dunston, PhD

► INTRODUCTION

Human genetics refers to the research and clinical practice of genetics as it relates to human beings. This is distinct from medical and clinical genetics, which is a subset of human genetics. Medical and clinical genetics is the application of human genetic research and information to health care. The terms *medical genetics* and *clinical genetics* are essentially the same, and for the purposes of this chapter, the term *medical genetics* will be used.

The effect of critical factors such as socioeconomic status, education, and ancestry on health-care disparities has been discussed elsewhere in this book. These issues clearly interface with human genetics and are woven throughout this chapter. This chapter focuses on issues specific to medical genetics and their direct effects on health care disparity.

Until recently, the traditional role of genetics in medicine was limited to the study of uncommon unifactorial conditions (eg, chromosomal and single gene disorders). However, advances in medical genetics have shown that the traditional constructs of Oslerian medicine, which emphasize external, identifiable, and single factor causes, are incomplete and insufficient for the explanation of most human medical conditions.[1] Fueled by information from the Human Genome Project and the development of a wide variety of novel tools and techniques, it is now possible to clinically apply an understanding of complexly inherited traits. The veritable explosion of genetic information has resulted in the evolving scope of medical genetics and its incorporation into all aspects of clinical practice and health-care education. Today, all health-care providers must have a basic understanding of medical genetics. In most, if not all, centers for health-care education, the curricula of disciplines as diverse as medicine, nursing, dentistry, pharmacy, and the allied health services include instruction in this discipline. This will continue for many decades.

Historically, there has been a natural alliance between medical genetics and public health, and this has been evidenced by multiple collaborative projects at the regional, state, and federal level. As the practice of medical genetics has evolved, so has its integration with public health policies and procedures. This includes such efforts as the establishment of regional genetic networks through the Genetics Services branch of the Health Resources and Services Administration (HRSA), public policy and practice for newborn and other population screening, and the funding of the Human Genome Project.

The Human Genome Project bears special mention. This project was an international collaborative that officially began in 1990 and was the single most ambitious scientific endeavor ever undertaken. The overriding theme of the project was to decode the entire sequence of the human genetic blueprint. Specific goals were to:

1. Identify all genes in human DNA.
2. Determine the sequence of 3 million base pairs of nucleotides in the human genome.
3. Store the collected information in electronic databases.
4. Improve the tools for data analysis.
5. Transfer related technologies.
6. Address the ethical, legal, and social implications (ELSI) of this rapidly evolving information database.

Cumulative information for the identified genes and gene sequences was published simultaneously in the journals *Science* and *Nature* in 2001.[2,3] The Human Genome Project was formally completed in 2003. Driven by a competitive effort from the private sector, this government project finished ahead of schedule and under budget.

As expected, the completion of the project has provided an overwhelming amount of powerful information. One of the first practical pieces of information generated was a significant reduction in the number of estimated human genes. Prior to the Human Genome Project, it was estimated there were approximately 100,000 functioning human genes; with completion of the project, it is now estimated that 20,000 to 25,000 genes are all that are needed for human development and physiology.[4] Success in achieving the stated goals of the Human Genome Project has been reviewed and deemed a success in goals 3 through 5, with unimaginable amounts of information stored in databases, improved tools, and public access

allowing transfers of the related technologies. The success of the ELSI Project is more difficult to assess. Many questions have been raised, yet to date, few clear answers to the questions posed have emerged. However, this is not to minimize the importance of the ELSI Project. It is of prime importance that the project was designed with consideration of these issues in mind from the start.

Although all human genes have been "identified," it is not yet known what many of them do or how they relate to human disorders. Currently, there are approximately 600 to 700 genetic tests[5] that target specific genetic disorders, well short of the tens of thousands of genes hypothesized to affect human health. Much work in this area remains to be done over the next 20 to 25 years. Impetus and momentum from the Human Genome Project will continue; its findings will be at the center of human medical research for decades to come.

This chapter is organized to reflect the multiple levels at which genetics can interface with the occurrence of human health disparities. Most directly, one would think about genetic changes directly producing health-care inequities as they affect the health of the individual. However, the question is more complex and includes issues of access to services, access to information, and the possibilities of genetic discrimination at all levels. In the context of the other chapters in this book, it should be noted that any human disease—genetic or not—can produce health-care disparities. It is important to consider how medical genetics differs from other medical services. There are overlaps, as far as access and information, but there are many potentially unique aspects, including issues such as predictive and presymptomatic testing.

Finally, it is not within the scope of this chapter to define specific genetic terms or to explain basic genetic concepts. An effort has been made to minimize the genetic jargon used in this chapter. Those desiring explanations and definitions of genetic terms can find them in a number of standard genetics textbooks.[6–8]

▶ MODERN MEDICAL GENETICS

For the majority of the history of the practice of medical genetics, emphasis has been placed on rare yet easily noticeable genetic conditions. By and large, these conditions have been disorders of major gene influence (single-gene disorders such as sickle cell anemia) or readily observable chromosome disorders such as Down syndrome (trisomy 21). The observation and description of these disorders led to a misconception that genetic mutations represent rare events. Recent insights into genetic influence on almost all human medical conditions have led to the important insight that mutations are, in fact, common events that occur in humans throughout the life cycle.

As understanding of medical genetics has advanced, the rare conditions that were originally described have come to represent almost the exception to the rule rather than the mainstay of medical genetic understanding. Sickle cell anemia remains one of the few conditions that is largely straightforward from a genetic standpoint in that it represents a genetically homogenous condition with a single gene influence producing most of the understandable clinical manifestations of this condition.

In contrast, in the daily practice of medicine, most conditions show a more complex relationship of genetic and environmental influences. From the mid-1970s through 1980s, the concept of multifactorial inheritance moved to the forefront. Multifactorial inheritance was envisioned as a continuum of genetic and environmental influences that was disease specific. Multifactorial inheritance is invoked when the following conditions are met:

- Genetic variability exists, yet no clear mode of inheritance can be identified.
- Family studies indicate an increased risk for near relatives to be affected.
- Complicated pathophysiologic and morphogenic processes are involved.
- Expression of the condition requires both biologic influences and environmental factors.

Given this definition, it is clear that most, if not all, of the more common human diseases (diabetes, atherosclerosis, hypertension, allergies, etc) exhibit a pattern of multifactorial inheritance.[9] Multifactorial conditions are envisioned as the cumulative product of so-called liabilities that increase the probability of the disease within a range of favorable to unfavorable environmental factors and from protective to predisposing genetic factors. Multifactorial conditions are expressed when the cumulative contributions of all genetic and environmental liabilities exceed a theorized biologic threshold. The threshold is the point at which the capacity of the organism to defend against this liability is overcome. The relationship of genetics to human disease in multifactorial disorders is characterized by:

- A relationship of the recurrence risk to the population frequency.
- A nonlinear decrease in the frequency with increasing distance of relationship.
- An increased risk with number of affected individuals.
- An increased risk with increased severity.
- An increased risk that the persons of rare genes are affected.

For many conditions today, the multifactorial model of inheritance is still the only model that can be applied. Thus, genetic counseling and recurrence risk information are still based on population (empirical) data. Although this can be helpful for families, it is inherently limited information.

Over the past two decades, great insight has been gained into the understanding of complexly inherited traits. Other models of inheritance have emerged that are, in fact, refinements of the multifactorial model. It is important to note that these different models may not be mutually exclusive, with considerable overlap among them for any given disorder.

One example of these models is *polygenic inheritance*. This refers to the additive contribution of a small number of genes to a quantitative trait. Polygenic inheritance is the best explanation for human quantitative traits such as height, weight, and intelligence. Another example is *multilocus inheritance,* which refers to the sequential accumulation of mutations in certain pathologic process and appears to be the best model for the pathogenesis of human cancers. The term *multiprocess disorders* refers to multiple, complex physiologic conditions that contribute to a particular disorder. Within each process, there are multiple genes that may influence the pathophysiology of process. An excellent example of multiprocess involvement would be that of type 2 (insulin-resistant) diabetes.

With rare exceptions, such as sickle cell anemia, human conditions show some degree of genetic heterogeneity. In other words, more than one locus (gene) can cause a specific well-defined disorder. Some conditions show marked genetic heterogeneity. For instance, at least 25 loci that are causally related to the spinocerebellar ataxias (slowly degenerative disorders of the cerebellum and brainstem) have now been described, but 10% of families with this condition still cannot be explained by any of the identified loci.[10]

One of the most exciting advances in understanding genetic and environmental interactions has been the concept of *genetic susceptibility.* Buehler et al[11] were the first to describe a molecular susceptibility to a known environmental influence in 1986. They described the biochemical and genetic basis for susceptibility to Fetal Dilantin Syndrome, birth defects induced in an infant if the mother takes the medication hydantoin. Subsequently, there was an explosion of information related to genetic susceptibility. Recent studies have shown that assumed environmental influences such as outcomes in head trauma show differential susceptibilities based on genetic polymorphisms. In this event, polymorphisms in the apolipoprotein E gene, the same gene that is hypothesized to produce susceptibility to the occurrence of Alzheimer disease, predict with a high degree of accuracy those who are likely to have a poorer outcome of head trauma than those with different polymorphisms.[12]

Another feature of modern medical genetics has been the recognition of so-called atypical inheritance patterns. All the presumed basic rules of human genetics have been shown to have exceptions. Currently described mechanisms of atypical inheritance include a variety of inheritance patterns such as genomic imprinting, uniparental disomy, mosaicism, genetic anticipation, expanding trinucleotide repeats, transposable elements, mitochondrial inheritance, triallelic inheritance, and digenic inheritance. Although beyond the scope of this discussion, it is important to note the existence of these atypical inheritance patterns and to recognize that these concepts are not just theoretical but have direct clinical applications in the day-to-day practice of medical genetics. Further, it is essential that this highly complex information be relayed to the patient in some understandable context.

In this vein, genetic counselors remain essential to delivery of inheritable disease information. Genetic counselors are sophisticated in their knowledge of genetic disorders and specifically trained to explain complex concepts to individuals of varying backgrounds. For example, if a child is diagnosed as having fragile X syndrome, an X-linked form of mental retardation, final genetic testing will confirm the cause of this condition. The information that must be imparted to the family is that "Your child has an X-linked semidominant disorder that shows genetic anticipation due to an expanding trinucleotide repeat of the *FMR1* gene"—concepts that are not readily understood by the population in general. In the example of fragile X syndrome, parental carriers of this condition may have partial effects, including disorders of cognition and behavior, that further complicate a provider's ability to deliver this information accurately and in a useable manner to the family. In addition to delivering this information in an understandable manner, the provider must also deliver it in a culturally and linguistically appropriate way.

Recent passage of the Health Insurance Portability and Accountability Act of 1996

(HIPAA) has had multiple effects on the provision of medical care. One issue that has not been completely sorted out is what effect this will have on the practice of medical genetics.[13] Specifically, will attempts to protect the patient's privacy impede the flow of genetic information? One simple example that has been mentioned is whether the placement of family history information into the chart of the proband (the patient who is being treated) is a violation of privacy guidelines for other affected family members.

► ACCESS

Disparities in Access to Clinical Genetic Services

An overriding inequity in medical genetics is lack of access to clinical genetic services for large numbers of individuals. There are multiple reasons for the limited access to services, including the relative newness of the field, lack of public and professional awareness of the field and what it can offer, small numbers of providers, unequal distribution of existing providers, and fiscal realities of medical genetics as a reimbursable service.

Medical genetics is a relatively new specialty, dating from the early 1970s. As such, the number of providers is significantly limited. In addition, providers are typically located in tertiary care centers. Other access issues include problems with geographic distribution, particularly in larger, less-populated states. In the upper Midwest, for example, there are large areas in which patients may be 300 miles or more from the closest genetic health-care professional. States such as North and South Dakota, Wyoming, and Kansas may have less than one full-time equivalent of professional time committed to clinical genetic services for the entire state. The paucity of health-care providers in medical genetics is compounded by the fact that there is little expectation of improving the shortage in the near future because relatively few individuals are currently receiving training in medical genetics specialties. In 2004, a total of 61 medical geneticists were training in 47 programs for all of North America.[14]

Contributing to the paucity of health-care providers in this field is the fact that human genetic services typically are viewed in university settings as money-losing services. Therefore, many academic institutions are reducing or eliminating health-care professionals in the area of genetics. There are also few, if any, private practice opportunities in the field of medical genetics. Many insurance providers have specific clauses denying genetic testing and services, based on the position that these are experimental or nonmedical services. Within medicine, one of the significant problems of inadequate reimbursement for medical genetic services is related to the fact that clinical genetics was only recently (in 1991) recognized by the American Medical Association. Without ICD-9 and CPT codes to provide the necessary vehicle for reimbursement of services, such as genetic counseling and obtaining pedigrees, clinical geneticists cannot be reimbursed for the services they provide, again contributing to the lack of financial incentives for employing these specialists.

Another significant access barrier to genetic services relates to the high cost of new technology. New clinical genetic tests become available on a daily basis. Many of them, however, cost literally thousands of dollars. In addition, many are offered at only a few internationally scattered laboratories. The complexities of international law and policy often impede the process of having a specific test performed if the sole laboratory offering the test is outside of the country. State boundaries also create major impediments to patients accessing these tests— particularly those dependent on Medicaid and Medicare funding for their health care. Many, if not most, of these laboratories are unwilling to accept entitlement payments from outside their own state. A patient with Medicaid or Medicare coverage who has a rare genetic condition may be unable to obtain specific indicated testing if the test is not performed in a laboratory located within his or her home state. The high cost of technology has an even greater impact on new treatments. Innovative therapies for several genetic disorders have been developed,[15] but the cost of these sometimes approaches several hundred thousand dollars per year for the administration of a single medication.

Access to Clinical Genetic Information

Access to information empowers people to take charge of their health. Distribution of medical information is an issue for all medical specialties, but particularly for medical genetics and public health. The newness of the field and the complexities of its underlying basic science have created an intimidating image. This has resulted in information barriers for both health-care professionals and laypersons, as highlighted by the saga of folic acid and its role in the prevention of birth defects.

Over the past decade, a large body of literature has developed that clearly documents the effects of folic acid in the prevention of birth defects. Taking a vitamin supplement containing 0.4–4.0 mg of folic acid prior to and during pregnancy lowers the risk of birth defects, including spina bifida, cleft lip or cleft palate, congenital heart defects, limb anomalies, and pyloric stenosis, by as much as 70%.[16] Folic acid is part of the B vitamin complex; it is relatively inexpensive and has no significant side effects or toxicity. Women of childbearing age can do something as simple as take a cheap, safe vitamin supplement and significantly reduce the risk of birth defects in their children. The greatest benefit of folic acid is achieved if it is started 2 to 3 months before conception. Despite this information, it is significant that only 30% to 40% of women of childbearing age in the United States currently take the recommended dietary supplement of folic acid.[17] In addition, recent surveys suggest that only 60% to 75% of women have even "heard of" this information, despite several large national campaigns to increase folic acid awareness.[18] These data highlight the importance of access to information and the risks

when such information is not universally accessible.

As noted earlier, the rate of change in genetic information is staggering. One of the stated goals of the Human Genome Project was to make the information generated from the project available to the professional and lay public via electronic databases. This has led to development of sophisticated databases that are Internet-accessible and consistently updated. Table 28–1 provides a list of URLs to medical genetic information that was active at the time of publication; note that many websites change host sites quickly. Despite the fact this information is web-based and available at no charge, another disparity arises from the fact that not all persons have Internet access. Recent surveys suggest that only 60% of Americans have ready Internet access and approximately 80% "use it occasionally."[19] Socioeconomic factors play strongly into the discrepancy of access to Internet service. An additional factor complicating the presence of genetic information on the Internet is the lack of standards for information posted. Unfortunately, much misinformation about medical genetics resides on the Internet, and patients are often misled by claims for unproven therapies that promise miraculous results. This can lead to participation in misrepresented clinical "trials" as well as mistrust of health-care professionals who adhere to evidence-based therapies and standards.

▶ POPULATIONS

Race and Ethnicity

There are few issues that are more emotionally charged in the application of basic genetic science than the biology of race and ethnicity. As thoughtful consideration has been given to this topic, several consistent themes have emerged. The concepts of race and ethnicity are contextual and politically and socially defined terms. As information about the inherent genetic basis of humankind continues to accumulate, it has become clear that the concepts of race and

▶ **TABLE 28–1.** Selected URLs for Reference in Medical Genetics

Source	Website
American Academy of Pediatrics, Committee on Genetics	*http://www.aap.org/visit/cmte18.htm*
American College of Medical Genetics	*http://www.acmg.net/*
GDB Human Genome Database	*http://www.gdb.org/*
Gene Tests	*http://www.genetests.org/*
Genetic Alliance	*http://www.geneticalliance.org/*
Genetics Education Center, University of Kansas Medical Center	*http://www.kumc.edu/gec/*
Human Genome Project	*http://www.ornl.gov/sci/techresources/Human_Genome/home.shtml*
National Center for Biotechnology Information	*http://www.ncbi.nlm.nih.gov/*
Online McKusick's Inheritance in Man (OMIM)	*http://www3.ncbi.nlm.nih.gov/entrez/query.fcgi?db=OMIM*
World of Genetic Societies	*http://genetics.faseb.org/*

ethnicity are often misleading and insufficient to accurately study human variability. When viewed at the molecular level, populations originally defined by race or ethnic parameters have been shown to be less distinct than originally thought. A more practical understanding is that population clusters should be identified by genotype analysis, which is more informative and biologically valid than identification by race or ethnicity.[20] This hypothesis has been corroborated by experience in the realm of newborn screening.

Newborn screening for genetic and metabolic disorders has been practiced for decades and has produced the largest body of information on how to effectively conduct population screening efforts. As newborn screening programs have expanded the list of disorders screened for in the past 10 to 15 years, the question of selective population screening has arisen in areas such as hemoglobinopathies and cystic fibrosis. Screening for hemoglobinopathies only in individuals of African, Mediterranean, and Southeast Asian descent and for cystic fibrosis in Northern European populations, would be "cost effective" given the relatively high frequency of these disorders in the respective populations. However, problems with self-reporting and identification of ethnicity discrimination

and stigmatization have shown that selective screening does not translate into reasonable clinical efforts. Experience has shown that race and ethnicity have little relationship to much of the new genetic information. Because selected population screening for hemoglobinopathies has been abandoned, significant numbers of hemoglobinopathies have been identified in the "non–high-risk" populations.

Much emphasis has been given to the development of haplotype maps. Haplotype maps are "sizable regions over which there is little evidence for historical recombination and within which only a few common haplotypes exist."[21] In nonscientific terms, haplotypes have been called "DNA neighborhood blocks." These maps are the underpinning of recent powerful strategies for finding genes that contribute to complex traits. In October 2002, the International Human Haplotype Map Project Consortium was initiated to programmatically construct comprehensive haplotype maps to facilitate comprehensive disease association studies.[22] These maps are based on the concept that variation is not randomly distributed and that differences will be identifiable in select populations. For these maps to be effective and provide information that translates into human medical practice, it is imperative that "the basic information of types, frequencies and distribution of the polymorphisms in all human populations is ascertained."[23] The goal is that this information should be collated for all populations, giving all the same hope of medical benefits from genetic discoveries.

Another influence of race and ethnicity in clinical genetics is in the area of differential responses to therapy. Recent reports have documented differences in response between specific racial and ethnic groups to specific medications, raising the prospect of using genotypic information to create customized medicines. However, it has quickly become apparent that race is likely to have little to no direct influence on response to medication; this type of "tailored" pharmacology must, of necessity, be based at the individual level.[24]

Mounting evidence in the medical literature, reason, and experience are demonstrating that the concepts of race and ethnicity as identifiers of homogenous populations are inadequate. Despite this, the current practice of medical genetics still relies on standards of care that are related to conditions that occur in defined high-risk populations based on ancestry. Current practitioners would be legally liable if they did not offer carrier screening for Tay-Sachs disease to couples of Ashkenazi (Eastern European) Jewish descent in anticipation of childbearing. Table 28–2 lists eight specific genetic disorders that are screened for in commercially available "Ashkenazi Jewish Panels" because these disorders are known to occur at a significantly higher rate in this population. It is acceptable

▶ **TABLE 28–2.** Commonly Offered Tests in the "Ashkenazi Jewish Panel"

Bloom syndrome
Canavan disease
Familial dysautonomia
Fanconi anemia
Gaucher disease
Mucolipidosis type IV
Niemann-Pick disease
Tay-Sachs disease

▶ **TABLE 28–3.** High-Risk Groups for Specific Genetic Conditions (Based on Ancestry)

Ancestry	Condition
African	Sickle cell disease
French Canadian	Tay-Sachs disease
Mediterranean	Hemoglobinopathies
Native Alaskan	Congenital adrenal hyperplasia
Northern European	Cystic fibrosis

to offer screening to this population and in this case, targeted population screening is not perceived as negative by the patient group. Within the Ashkenazi community, Tay-Sachs screening is typically considered desirable and beneficial and community initiatives to increase awareness and utilization of genetic screening are routine events. Table 28–3 provides additional examples of known associations between populations defined by ancestry and specific genetic disorders that occur with increased frequency within them. These associations are well recognized and medically important in the care of individuals from these population groups.

Finally, the potential for racial stigmatization of any racial or ethnic group remains a significant concern. The stereotypic association of fetal alcohol syndrome with Native American populations serves as a prime example. Few reliable epidemiologic studies exist to quantify whether an association exists, yet this is assumed to be the case in most health-care and lay communities. The assumption ignores the reality that the designation "Native American" does not identify a homogenous population. As a group, people who self-identify as Native Americans represent an extremely heterogeneous group of individuals. Striking differences exist among tribes in relationship to use of alcohol, and many Native American tribes actually have significantly lower alcohol use rates than those of the general population. In addition, notable tribal and presumably genetic differences exist in the teratogenic response to alcohol. Given the same amount of alcohol exposure, there are differences in the degree of effect. In light of these facts, it is not surprising that the incidence of fetal alcohol syndrome varies greatly among Native American tribes;[25] a fact that is seldom acknowledged by providers of health care to this group.

Definition of Disease

A well-established medical aphorism holds that "the patient defines his or her own 'dis' 'ease',"[26] and it should not be surprising that different populations perceive disease in markedly divergent ways. What may be considered disease in one group may not be viewed as such in another.

Nobles[27] noted that African philosophy places emphasis on past and present, rather than on the future. As a result, the predictive and probablistic nature of genetics might not carry the same weight and value within this population. Likewise, participation of Native American women in cancer screening programs has been historically low as a result of complex cultural values and beliefs. One difference is in the perception of potential outcomes of cancer treatments and, within the Native American community, a more fatalistic view of the possibility of a cure for cancer.[28] More favorable responses to potential interventions have been obtained with the use of culturally acceptable modes of communication such as "Talking Circles."[29] Thus, any attempt at successful genetic screening initiatives among Native American women with heritable breast and ovarian cancer must incorporate the knowledge of values and beliefs and the most effective methods of communication.

▶ ISSUES IN MEDICAL GENETICS

Genetic Conditions As Contributors to Health-Care Disparities

Multiple Congenital Anomalies
Children born with multiple birth defects represent a particularly complex set of problems for health-care providers. The problem of basic access to health care is compounded by the high number of medical comorbidities and the need for coordinated case management. These children require access to multiple specialists, who often practice at different medical centers. It is common for one child with a complex disorder to require the care of 10 to 15 different pediatric subspecialists. Over the past 20 years, interdisciplinary care has evolved as part of the solution to such problems, but interdisciplinary clinics have significant access limitations. There are relatively few of them, and most are in tertiary or quaternary care settings and thus geographically distant from much of the population. Even when they have adequate insurance, parents of a medically fragile child may find access problems to be practically and emotionally overwhelming.

Cognitive Deficits
Many genetic conditions also have a major effect on cognition, which can be manifested as mental retardation, developmental delays, learning disabilities, or a combination of these effects. Individuals with cognitive delays obviously may have significant problems with health-care access based on their own cognitive limitations. There may also be disparities in provision of care to individuals with these problems. Federal programs often are helpful to individuals up to the age of 21 years; however, there is a tremendous discrepancy in access to services for cognitive delays and other genetic conditions for individuals once they reach adulthood.

From a public health perspective, understanding the genetic basis of behavior holds the greatest potential for preventing disease and correcting disparities. For example, evidence of the genetic basis of addictions has recently come to light.[30] Specific polymorphisms in dopamine and nicotinic receptors have been shown to be significant predictors of nicotine addiction and varying responses to cessation treatment programs.[30–32] In fact, these associations have been so highly correlated that personalized therapy trials are underway.[33] Early information from these trials has led to optimism that "with advances in molecular biology and genomics technology, individualized tailoring of smoking cessation therapy to genotype is within our grasp."[34]

As the understanding of such concepts increases, however, so does the level of complexity. Polymorphisms in these same genes (*DRD2A1* and *CYP2B6*) have relationships to other comorbid phenomena, such as alcohol use and food intake associated with smoking behavior.[30,35] Likewise, in the multifactorial model of complex traits, the effects of socioeconomic and other environmental factors cannot be ignored and have been shown to interact directly with the genetic background.[36]

Neurobehavioral Disorders

Medical care for many individuals with genetic conditions is complicated by the issue of "dual diagnosis." Many genetic conditions have the comorbid occurrence of behavioral or psychiatric conditions such as the autism spectrum disorders, with its associated problems of socialization and communication; attention deficit/hyperactivity disorder (ADHD); or major psychiatric conditions, such as schizophrenia and bipolar disorder. The presence of an associated behavioral disorder greatly complicates all aspects of health-care delivery for these individuals because of the extremely low number of providers experienced in the "dual diagnosis" arena.

Genetic Discrimination

Genetic discrimination, a term that has only recently been added to the working health-care vocabulary, is a major concern to the public. By far the single most common reason people decline services for genetic evaluation or testing is the spectre of genetic discrimination.[37] The question among these individuals is, "Will/can my personal genetic information be used in a detrimental manner, rather than for my benefit?" Surveys regarding concerns about the influence of genetic information on insurance and employment showed that 75% to 80% of respondents surveyed do not want their insurance provider or their employer to have access to genetic information.[38]

Concern over genetic discrimination is great, but the question remains as to how serious the problem really is. According to the Council of Responsible Genetics,[39] over 500 cases have been reported in which insurance or employment was lost, based on genetic discrimination. Although 500 cases may not sound like many in the overall context of the number of services provided, there is fear that this represents the "tip of the iceberg." One of the authors (GBS) served on the Nebraska Commission on Human Genetic Technology, which performed a formal survey of the entire state of Nebraska. The commission found that only a handful of legitimate complaints had been registered with the state based on genetic discrimination over the previous 2 years.

Government has addressed these issues through a variety of efforts designed to protect the public from genetic discrimination. Currently, 41 states have enacted legislation related to genetic discrimination in health insurance, and 31 have laws for protection from genetic discrimination in the workplace. Comprehensive national legislation introduced by former President Clinton would have banned health plans from discriminating based on genetic information, but was not enacted by Congress. In February 2000, President Clinton issued an executive order that prohibited the federal government from obtaining genetic information in employment practices.

Participation in Genetic Research

Another emotionally charged topic is the area of genetic research and the disparities it may produce in health care.[40] Subject participation in genetic research is a double-edged sword. From one point of view, limited group participation in genetic research could lead to discoveries that might benefit the health of the group as a whole.

Alternatively, the potential for exploitation and stigmatization of individuals who participate remains a substantial issue. The solution requires formal assurances and safeguards to ensure that the ultimate goal of the research is the improvement of community health and well-being. Research should focus primarily on identifying the genetic and environmental components of disease, thus facilitating early detection, effective treatment, and ultimately prevention.[23] Caution is also needed so that overemphasis on genetics as a major etiologic factor in health-care disparities does not allow researchers to overlook other contributing factors to disparities that may be equally or more important. Failure to do so may reinforce racial stereotyping.[41]

Within the realm of genetic research on humans, the issues of informed consent, privacy, and confidentiality are paramount. The question yet to be answered is whether or not these issues are practically different for genetic conditions and have implications extending beyond the patient to the family.

It is also important that genetic research not be promoted with unrealistic expectations. There is a large chasm between identifying etiology and developing effective therapy. For example, although the etiology of Down syndrome (trisomy 21) has been known since 1959, there have yet to be major advances in the overall therapy for affected individuals.

Lastly, concerns over safety with gene therapy have been magnified as a result of the deaths of individuals participating in gene therapy studies. As a result, the pace at which genetic therapy research is proceeding has significantly slowed, but this is an important and necessary precaution.

Prevention

The goal of health-care professionals is the prevention of human disease and suffering, and nowhere has this been more apparent than in the area of genetic disorders. However, one of the major impediments has been the association in the public mind between prevention of genetic disorders and pregnancy termination. The issue of pregnancy termination is one of the most controversial in American society, and it is critical that public education efforts specifically emphasize that prevention of genetic conditions and birth defects is not tied completely to pregnancy termination. As previously noted, primary prevention such as the use of folic acid to prevent birth defects is a reality. Likewise, educational efforts to reduce fetal alcohol syndrome and other alcohol-related birth defects are educational issues, not moral or ethical ones. Prenatal diagnosis to identify birth defects such as neural tube defects may have benefits beyond the ability to consider pregnancy termination. Children identified with neural tube defects in the womb can be delivered prospectively, by elective Cesarian section, prior to the onset of labor. If this is accomplished, outcomes such as functional bowel and bladder control and ambulation are significantly improved.[42]

To implement prevention effectively, genetic literacy must improve, not only among the lay public, but also among health professionals. Genetic literacy is defined as the knowledge of risks, benefits, limitations, and implications of medical genetic services. Many current providers received medical training before the introduction of medical genetics into the educational curricula or practice of medicine.

▶ SUMMARY AND RECOMMENDATIONS

This chapter highlights the complex interface between medical genetics and health-care disparities. Several consistent themes emerge.

- The knowledge base for genetic information will continue to increase at an exponential rate.

▶ **TABLE 28–4.** Summary of Recommendations to Reduce Health-Care Disparities in Genetics

Genetic Services
- An overall increase in medical genetic services is needed to decrease disparity.
- Current strategies include outreach clinics to geographically disparate regions; Internet technology is increasing the use of telemedicine to deliver services to tertiary and quaternary providers at major medical centers to rural areas.
- There must be greater emphasis on interdisciplinary care and improved reimbursement for so-called nontraditional services provided by medical genetics counselors.

Education
- There is a need for ongoing education of health-care providers and the public; both groups must greatly improve their genetic literacy, and this information must be provided in a culturally and linguistically appropriate way.

Policy
- Major legislative and public health policies should be implemented, including Medicaid and Medicare policies that allow for reimbursement across state lines, particularly for unique testing.
- Legislation must be continuous and dynamically changing to protect against genetic discrimination.

Training of Health-Care Professionals
- A greater emphasis must be placed on training to increase the overall number of professionals and specialists in the field of medical genetics.
- Proactive efforts to recruit minority and underrepresented groups into these training programs must be made.

- The fund of knowledge for the basic science of genetics will continue to grow faster than related public policy or legislation.
- Genetics will be at the heart of clinical medicine and medical research for the next several decades

Strategies for reducing disparities pose considerable difficulties and implementing them will be a challenge. Recommendations for reducing health-care disparities in the area of genetics are summarized in Table 28–4.

▶ **REFERENCES**

1. Huddle TS, Centor R, Heudebert GR. American internal medicine in the 21st century: Can an Oslerian generalism survive? *J Gen Intern Med* 2003;18(9):764–767.
2. Venter JC, Adams MD, Myers EW, et al. The sequence of the human genome. *Science* 2001; 291(5507):1304–1305.
3. Lander ES, Linton LM, Birren B, et al. Initial sequencing and analysis of the human genome. *Nature* 2001;409(6822):860–921.
4. International Human Genome Sequencing Consortium: Finishing the euchromatic sequence of the human genome. *Nature* 2004;431(7011):931–945.
5. GeneTests. Copyright 1993–2004, University of Washington, Seattle, Wash: 2004. Available at: http://www.genetests.org/.
6. Nusbaum RL, McInnes RR, Willard HF. *Thompson and Thompson Genetics in Medicine*, 6th ed, rev reprint. Philadelphia, Pa: Saunders; 2004.
7. Pritchard PJ, Korf BR. *Medical Genetics at a Glance.* Oxford, England: Blackwell Science; 2003.
8. Pasternak JJ. *An Introduction to Human Molecular Genetics.* Bethesda, Md: Fitzgerald Science; 1999.
9. Glazier AM, Nadeau JH, Aitman TJ. Finding genes that underlie complex traits. *Science* 2002;298(5602):2345–2349.
10. Stevanin G, Bouslam N, Thobois S, et al. Spinocerebellar ataxia with sensory neuropathy

(SCA25) maps to chromosome 2p. *Ann Neurol* 2004;55(1):97–104.

11. Buehler BA, Delimont D, van Waes M, et al. Prenatal prediction of risk of the fetal hydantoin syndrome. *N Engl J Med* 1990;322(22):1567–1572.

12. Teasdale GM, Nicoll JA, Murray G, et al. Association of apolipoprotein E polymorphism with outcome after head injury. *Lancet* 1997;350(9084):1069–1071.

13. Cole LJ, Fleisher LD. Update on HIPAA privacy: Are you ready? *Genet Med* 2003;5(3):183–186.

14. American Board of Medical Genetics. Available at: http://genetics.faseb.org/genetics/abmg/about.htm.

15. Human Genome Project: Gene Therapy. 2004. Available at: http://genome.rtc.riken.go.jp/hgmis/medicine/genetherapy.html.

16. Botto LD, Olney RS, Erickson JD. Vitamin supplements and the risk for congenital anomalies other than neural tube defects. *Am J Med Genet* 2004;125C(1):12–21.

17. Centers for Disease Control and Prevention. Use of vitamins containing folic acid among women of childbearing age—United States. *MMWR Morb Mortal Wkly Rep* 2004;53(36):847–850.

18. Neill AM. The "Folic Acid Campaign": Has the message got through? A questionnaire study. *J Obstet Gynaecol* 1999;19(1):22–25.

19. Fox S, Fallows D. *Internet Health Resources.* Washington, DC: Pew Internet and American Life Project; 2004. Available at: http://www.pewinternet.org/reports/pdfs/PIP_Health_Report_July_2003.pdf.

20. Wilson JF, Weale ME, Smith AC, et al. Population genetic structure of variable drug response. *Nat Genet* 2001;29(3):265–269.

21. Gabriel SB, Schaffner SF, Nguyen H, et al. The structure of haplotype blocks in the human genome. *Science* 2002;296(5576):2225–2229.

22. Cardon LR, Abecasis GR. Using haplotype blocks to map human complex trait loci. *Trends Gene* 2003;19(3):135–140.

23. Dunston GM, Royal CDM. The human genome: Implications for the health of African Americans. In: Livingston IC, ed. *The Prager Handbook of Black American Health: Policies and Issues Behind Disparities in Health,* 2nd ed, Vol 2. Westport, Conn: Greenwood Publishing Group; 2004:758–768.

24. Smart A, Martin P, Parker M. Tailored medicine: Whom will it fit? The ethics of patient and disease stratification. *Bioethic* 2004;18(4):322–342.

25. Schaefer GB, unpublished data, 2004.

26. Deckert G, Medical school orientation, Oklahoma University School of Medicine; August 1978.

27. Nobles WW. African philosophy. Foundations for black psychology. In: Jones RL, ed. *Black Psychology.* Berkley, Calif: Cobb and Henry; 1991:47–63.

28. Burhansstipanov L, Bemis LT, Dignam MB. Native American cancer education: Genetic and cultural issues. *J Cancer Educ* 2001;16(3):142–145.

29. Hodge FS, Fredericks L, Rodriguez B. American Indian women's talking circle. A cervical cancer screening and prevention project. *Cancer* 1996;78(7 suppl):1592–1597.

30. Miksys S, Lerman C, Shields PG, et al. Smoking, alcoholism and genetic polymorphisms alter CYP2B6 levels in human brain. *Neuropharmacology* 2003;45(1):122–132.

31. Sabol SZ, Nelson ML, Fisher C, et al. A genetic association for cigarette smoking behavior. *Health Psychol* 1999;18(1):7–13.

32. Williams JM, Ziedonis D. Addressing tobacco among individuals with a mental illness or an addiction. *Addict Behav* 2004;29(6):1067–1083.

33. Walton R, Johnstone E, Munafo M, et al. Genetic clues to the molecular basis of tobacco addiction and progress towards personalized therapy. *Trends Mol Med* 2001;7(2):70–76.

34. Lerman C, Niaura R. Applying genetic approaches to the treatment of nicotine dependence. *Oncogene* 2002;21(48):7412–7420.

35. Epstein LH, Wright SM, Paluch RA, et al. Relation between food reinforcement and dopamine genotypes and its effect on food intake in smokers. *Am J Clin Nutr* 2004;80(1):82–88.

36. Broms U, Silventoinen K, Lahelma E, et al. Smoking cessation by socioeconomic status and marital status: The contribution of smoking behavior and family background. *Nicotine Tob Res* 2004;6(3):447–455.

37. Watson MS, Greene CL. Points to consider in preventing unfair discrimination based on genetic disease risk: A position statement of the American College of Medical Genetics. *Genet Med* 2001;3(6):436–437.

38. Employer-Employee Relations Subcommittee of House Education and the Workforce Committee hearing on "Genetic Non-Discrimination:

Examining the Implications for Workers and Employers"; 2004. Available at: http://tools-content.labvelocity.com/pdfs/4/63954.pdf.

39. Council on Responsible Genetics; 2004. Available at: http://www.gene-watch.org/problems/privacy.html.

40. Bates BR, Lynch JA, Bevan JL, et al. Warranted concerns, warranted outlooks: A focus group study of public understandings of genetic research. *Soc Sci Med* 2005;60:331–344.

41. Sankar P, Cho MK, Condit CM, et al. Genetic research and health care disparities. *JAMA* 2004;291:2985–2989.

42. Hanna DL, Fisher M, Schaefer GB. Update on cerebral palsy. Part II—Early identification and intervention. *Neb Med J* 1995;80(7):176–177.

CHAPTER 29

Community Health Centers

Margaret K. Hargreaves, PhD

Carolyne W. Arnold, ScD

William J. Blot, PhD

▶ INTRODUCTION

This chapter reviews the historical development of community health centers (CHCs) in the United States, their provision of basic health services to uninsured and poor in both urban and rural areas, and their promise in population-based health research. Originating in the neighborhood health center concept of the 1960s, CHCs today provide health and social services to more than 14 million individuals, nearly two thirds of whom belong to minority groups. CHCs also play a role in decreasing health disparities by becoming a nidus for health disparities research.

Special attention is paid to the Southern Community Cohort Study (SCCS), an ongoing investigation into the higher rates of incidence and mortality from most forms of cancer among African Americans. Recruitment into the SCCS is now taking place at CHCs across the South. The study serves as an example of collaborative CHC-based research into determinants of health disparities and indicates the potential for CHC-led involvement in the development of

community-supported measures aimed at disease prevention.

▶ FEDERALLY QUALIFIED HEALTH CENTERS SYSTEM

The federally qualified health centers (FQHC) system is perhaps the single most significant component of the health-care delivery system designed to correct health disparities. The FQHC system targets a range of vulnerable populations such as the elderly, children, the poor, the uninsured, the homeless, migrant laborers, and individuals living with human immunodeficiency virus (HIV) and acquired immunodeficiency syndrome (AIDS). The cornerstones of the system are CHCs. CHCs are operated by a variety of nonprofit organizations, local health departments, health and hospital departments, religious or faith-based organizations, medical schools, and other local government entities. Costs are covered through a variety of sources: private insurance, Medicare, Medicaid, children's health programs, sliding fee scales based on the patient's family income and size, foundation or corporate grants, government contracts, and other funds.[1,2]

Supported by 1RO1-CA91408-03; P20-MD000516-02; U54 CA91408-03; and P60 DK 20593-25.

Origin and Evolution of Community Health Centers

Contemporary CHCs represent an enduring legacy of the War on Poverty, the surviving heirs of the neighborhood health center (NHC) movement of the 1960s and early 1970s. Responding to the imperative to eradicate poverty and recognizing the reinforcing, self-perpetuating cycle of poverty on health, on March 16, 1964, President Lyndon B. Johnson, in a special message to Congress, introduced a program that came to be known as the War on Poverty. Shortly thereafter, Congress passed Public Law 88-452, the Economic Opportunity Act. Its declaration of purpose established public policy in relation to the elimination of poverty. The Act, divided into seven titles, was to provide employment and training opportunities for the poor and to provide community-developed, consumer-directed self-help programs through community action programs that aimed at the "maximum feasible participation of members of the community."[3]

One of the most far-reaching and unique features of CHCs has been the staunch involvement of community residents in the planning, development, and governance of health centers. The concepts of "community-developed," "consumer-directed," "maximum feasible participation" gave voice to community residents in decision making in community organizations. It opened new sources of psychological, financial, and political power as the poor found themselves having a say in, and in some instances even controlling, the programs and institutions that affect their lives.[3,4]

Originally, the Act did not concern itself with the development of a health services delivery system. Its intent was to establish social service programs that would enhance the productive ability of the poor and facilitate their transition from welfare to work. However, physicians H. Jack Geiger and Count Gibson, who were on the faculty of Tufts Medical School, saw the inextricable tie between the productive ability of the poor and their health status. They sought funding to establish a demonstration project,

Clinic 8S, in which the social conditions affecting health would be addressed.[3]

Viewing medical services as one vital component of the broader context of health and social well-being was a novel idea at the time. Although the Economic Opportunity Act was essentially an antipoverty program of services, Geiger and Gibson made a persuasive case that medical services were merely another social service. The Office of Equal Opportunity (OEO) agreed, believing the provision of both health care and job opportunities to neighborhood residents were important, and money was made available to demonstrate this new model of health-care delivery. Thus, OEO's involvement in health-care delivery and the development of the NHCs was born.

In 1965, Geiger and Gibson established the first NHC in the United States in Columbia Point, an isolated, largely black, low-income housing project in Boston.[3,4] Having worked in the civil rights movement in the early 1960s, Geiger and Gibson were also acutely aware of the special problems of rural poverty and the lack of health services in rural areas. Working with local residents in Mound Bayou, Mississippi, they established the Delta Health Center, the first rural health center in the country. A confluence of health and social legislation, including the enactment of Medicare and Medicaid legislation, also occurred in the same year as the initiation of NHCs.

Community Health Center Growth, Change, and Adaptation

NHCs were designed to meet the health and social needs of the poor and the at-risk. Their development filled a chasm in the infrastructure of the health-care system and addressed health disparities in minority populations. By the early 1970s, the OEO-NHC program was at its peak, with an estimated 200 NHCs nationwide. In the mid-1970s, the program was renamed the Community Health Center Program, and its scope was narrowed to concentrate on the delivery of medical care, with less emphasis on the social roles of NHCs. CHCs were encouraged to expand their services to the nonpoor.[1] By the early 1980s, the number of CHCs grew to approximately 800,[5] and today there are more than 1000 FQHCs and 3500 health center delivery sites in rural and urban settings, serving more than 14 million people.[6]

The goal of NHCs and subsequently CHCs was to provide comprehensive ambulatory services—preventive and rehabilitative as well as curative—to the poor living in inner cities and rural areas, services that were to be delivered sensitively, to be affordable and of high quality, and to intervene in the cycle of poverty. Although each center reflected its own community, they shared common characteristics. For example, in urban areas, they provided access and care to medically underserved, inner-city minority groups. In rural areas, CHCs more often served poor populations of mixed racial composition.[7] They used physicians, nurses, social workers, and community health workers in multidisciplinary team practice. Community health workers—indigenous neighborhood residents—were a new type of health worker that combined basic nursing with social service and outreach skills. In fact, CHCs pioneered in the training and employment of nurse practitioners and physician assistants.

Over the years, as with most organizations, political, policy, and priority shifts necessitated that CHCs adapt to the changing political, social, and economic conditions and take on new roles. By the early 1980s, CHCs focused on urban and rural medically underserved populations, and later in the decade, the strategies for the CHC program expanded to serve only high-need areas, work closely with state governments and medical societies, support only well-managed projects, promote self-sufficiency in projects, and help projects adapt to changing conditions.

In the 1990s, the age of managed care, some CHCs became affiliated with health maintenance organizations (HMOs) and other managed care forms. In 2002, President George W. Bush announced the Health Center Initiative. Over 5 years, the initiative proposed to add 1200 new facilities, eventually doubling the numbers of patients served.[8]

▶ COMMUNITY HEALTH CENTERS AND THE TREATMENT OF MINORITIES

Population Served

CHCs are now positioned to target medically underserved individuals and families throughout the United States. The target populations include 42 million uninsured Americans, 62 million rural Americans, and 78 million racial and ethnic minorities.[8] Of the more than 14 million people now served, 36% are white and 64% belong to minority groups. Of the total, 35% are Hispanic; 25%, African American; 4%, Asian and Pacific Islander; and 1%, American Indian and Alaska Native,[9] although the percentages vary considerably by area of the country, with much higher percentages of African American participants in the South. Nearly one third of patients served have limited English proficiency.[6] Almost 40% of these patients are uninsured; the remainder have Medicaid (36%), Medicare (7%), private (15%), or other public sources (3%) of insurance. The incomes of almost 70% are at the federal poverty level and below.[6]

Services Provided

CHCs serve a high-risk, low-income population that is expected to grow over the coming years. By virtue of their mission, CHCs must meet five unique requirements to be funded.[9] They must:

1. Be located in high need areas;
2. Provide comprehensive services;
3. Be open to all, regardless of income and insurance status;
4. Be governed by community boards; and
5. Follow rigorous administrative, clinical, and financial operational methods.

Services provided include not only primary and preventive health care, obstetric and gynecologic care, dental services, mental health and substance abuse services; radiologic and laboratory services, pharmacy, hearing and vision screening, and blood tests, but also supportive or so-called enabling services. These include case management, health education, parenting education, nutrition education, outreach, interpretation or translational services, transportation, and home visits,[10] which enable clients to achieve health-care goals. New roles assumed by CHCs, such as participation in Health Disparities Collaboratives (discussed later), contribute to that achievement.

Impact on Health Disparities

With such activities, there is growing recognition that CHCs are contributing to a decrease in health disparities. Recent analyses conducted by the National Association of Community Health Centers indicate that CHCs are contributing to quality health care that is satisfying to its clients[11]—clients who are also experiencing decreases in health disparities beyond those experienced by the general population. CHCs increase access to care and have been reported to reduce disparities in access to mammograms, and to decrease racial and ethnic differences in infant mortality rates, early prenatal care, tuberculosis, diabetes, and overall mortality.[12–13] According to Tommy Thompson, Secretary for Health and Human Services, "CHCs are the most effective tools to reduce health disparities."[14]

► COMMUNITY HEALTH CENTERS AND HEALTH DISPARITIES RESEARCH

Community Health Centers As Population-Based Centers for Health Research

The CHC network provides basic health services to a segment of US society, namely the poor and uninsured, that is often underrepresented in health research. Although the centers' primary functions relate to health care, CHCs can also engage in the conduct of research to evaluate the causes and prevention of chronic and acute illnesses. In some ways CHCs can serve as ideal laboratories for population-based research because they provide unique access to underserved populations; have earned the trust, respect, and appreciation of the populations served; and have or can arrange for the infrastructure and professional staffing needed for epidemiologic, behavioral, clinical, and other health studies.

The initiation of such research was in part stimulated by the Health Disparities Collaboratives, a national initiative for CHCs developed by the Bureau of Primary Health Care, Health Resources and Services Administration, and Department of Health and Human Services in 1999 to improve health outcomes for chronic conditions among the medically vulnerable.[10] The initiative is structured around the chronic care model, defined as a "population-based module that relies on knowing which patients need care, assuring that they receive knowledge-based care, and actively aiding them to participate in their own care."[15,16] Conditions addressed include diabetes, cardiovascular disease, cancer, asthma, depression, HIV, and prevention. The initiative is also based on the Plan-Do-Study-Act cycles from the continuous quality improvement field.[17] There were major challenges to implementing the collaborative, including need for more time and resources, difficulty developing computerized patient registries, team and staff turnover, and need for more administrative support.[17]

Southern Community Cohort Study

Our recent experience with CHCs as sites for health research arises from the conduct of the Southern Community Cohort Study (SCCS). The SCCS is a National Institutes of Health–funded epidemiologic investigation into the determinants of disparities in cancer incidence and mortality.[18] Plans call for a total of nearly 100,000 individuals, aged 40 to 79, to be recruited into the cohort over a 5-year span. More than two thirds of the participants will be African American, and more than half will be recruited from CHCs located in the states of Mississippi, Alabama, Georgia, Florida, South Carolina, Tennessee, and Kentucky, with possible future expansion to a broader geographic area.

The goals of the SCCS are to better understand the causes of cancer and other common illnesses so that measures aimed at disease prevention can be developed. In particular, the study aims to discover what underlies the disparities in cancer risk, including why people living in the Southeast experience higher rates of several types of cancer and why African Americans experience a disproportionate burden of cancer and other chronic diseases. As a cohort study, the SCCS will be able to evaluate, in addition to cancer, various potential risk factors for and determinants of the elevated risks of heart disease, hypertension and stroke, renal disease, diabetes, and other chronic illnesses among African Americans.

As noted elsewhere in this monograph, cancer mortality rates tend to be elevated among African Americans. Figure 29–1 illustrates the nearly 50% higher total cancer death rate among black men versus white men, with a similar but somewhat smaller disparity for women.[19] As seen in Figures 29–2 and 29–3, most individual cancers demonstrate the mortality disadvantage.[19] The higher mortality rates among African Americans tend to arise from a higher incidence of cancer, compounded by a poorer rate of survival once the cancer is diagnosed.[20]

The SCCS will study various potential contributors to the cancer differentials, including:

- Use of various tobacco products
- Diet (food groups, foods, macronutrients, micronutrients)
- Physical activity
- Personal and family medical history
- Over-the-counter and prescription medications
- Access to health care and barriers to health-care services

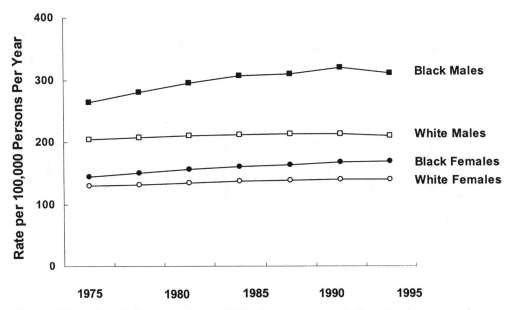

Figure 29–1. Trends in age-adjusted US total cancer mortality rates by sex and race. (Adapted by Blot from Ref. 19.)

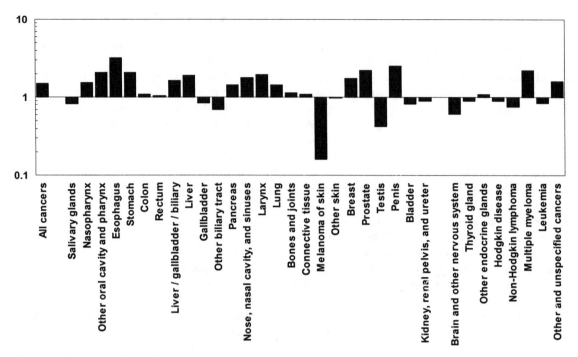

Figure 29–2. Ratios of national age-adjusted mortality rates for specific cancers among African American and white men, 1970 through 1994. (From Ref. 19.)

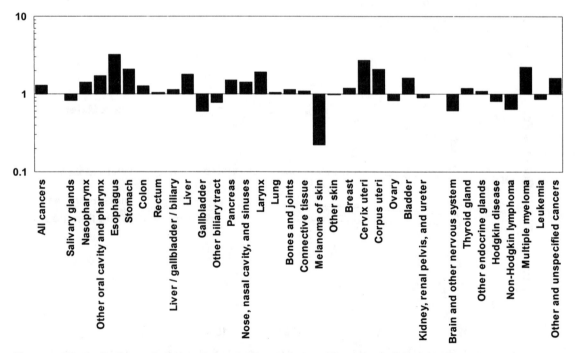

Figure 29–3. Ratios of national age-adjusted mortality rates for specific cancers among African American and white women, 1970 through 1994. (From Ref. 19.)

- Reproductive patterns
- Body size and obesity
- Occupational exposures
- Stress, depression, and social support
- Hormones
- Genetic predispositions

As of early 2004, more than 25,000 participants, including over 20,000 African Americans, have been recruited from CHCs throughout the South. At enrollment, comprehensive interview data, as well as blood and mouth cell samples, are collected from participants. Over the years, the cohort members will be periodically recontacted for follow-up information about changes in behaviors. The cohort rosters also will be linked with the National Death Index and with state cancer registries to identify deaths and incident cancers. Eventually, the interview data and frozen biologic specimens will be used to perform analyses assessing disease risk factors, including the interaction between endogenous susceptibility traits and exogenous environmental exposures.

CHC involvement has been critical in the planning, operation, and success of the SCCS. The NIH grant has thus far enabled funding to 25 CHCs in areas shown in Figure 29–4, with plans to more than double this number and expand into North Carolina, Virginia, West Virginia, Arkansas and Louisiana.

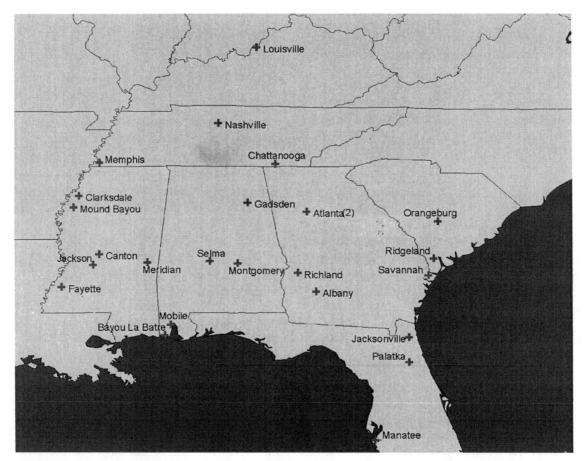

Figure 29–4. Initial community health centers in the Southern Community Cohort Study (SCCS).

The SCCS and CHCs are natural partners because both share a common goal of promoting and protecting the health of populations that traditionally have had limited resources. CHCs bring together the exact populations (poor, minority, and rural) that have been greatly underrepresented in medical research. Furthermore, the trusting environment in which to conduct health studies offered by the CHCs is important to counteract the mistrust sometimes directed toward researchers.

During the course of the SCCS, successful enrollment at the CHCs has been enhanced by having the support of the center's administration and health professionals. This has been achieved in simple ways that have key effects, such as the CHC preparing a letter of support for the study that can be shown to clinic patients, providing space for the interview and for displaying SCCS posters and brochures, and having staff who are knowledgeable about the study, its goals, and its importance.

CHCs have provided a fertile setting for recruitment. The SCCS clinic interviewers approach age-appropriate visitors to the center, introduce themselves, and provide information about the study. After obtaining informed consent from participants, the interviewers administer a specially designed computer-assisted interview that takes about 1 hour. The study takes advantage of existing CHC facilities for blood collection, with interviewers coordinating with CHC phlebotomists for blood sampling or collecting mouth rinse samples themselves. The biosamples are then sent via overnight delivery to Vanderbilt University Medical Center for long-term storage and later bioassay.

Table 29–1 shows selected characteristics of the initial participants in the SCCS. The educational level of these adults, aged 40 to 79 years, is low: approximately one third have a high school diploma, one third have lesser schooling, and the remaining third have greater schooling. Income is also low (median: approximately $14,000 annually). Participants tend to have a high prevalence of obesity and diabetes and a current smoking rate that is nearly double

▶ **TABLE 29-1.** Characteristics of Initial SCCS Participants

Indicator	Level
Median education	12 years
Median income	$ 14,000
Percent obese (BMI ≥ 30)	44%
Percent diabetes	21%
Percent parental history of cancer	33%
Percent female ever had mammogram	83%
Percent male ever had PSA screening	43%
Median time of last visit to dentist	51 months
Percent current smoker	45%

BMI = body mass index; PSA = prostate-specific antigen.

the national average. Hence, the population under study is at high risk for several chronic illnesses. Communication with the cohort participants about poor health behaviors (such as smoking) is under way, and selected targeted interventions are planned.

The CHC network has provided an ideal base for epidemiologic research on cancer and other common illnesses disproportionately afflicting African American and low-income populations. This model is suitable for expansion to other etiologic and preventive research endeavors.

Community Health Centers and Intervention Approaches

The Health Disparities Collaboratives and the SCCS are, respectively, excellent general and specific initiatives for the CHCs. The former tends to strengthen the service approach advocated by CHCs, and the latter, the research infrastructure, particularly with respect to etiologic studies. There is also room to test intervention approaches based on accepted behavioral models. The collaboratives demonstrate that many CHCs can be brought together to accomplish mutual objectives relating to diseases that occur with great frequency in these centers. The SCCS has demonstrated that the CHCs can participate in epidemiologic research. This experience and those of the collaboratives can be replicated to test true experimental designs. The CHC provides an excellent environment for the conduct of low-risk clinical trials and the community-based approach that is advocated as the best approach to a low-literacy, high-risk population. Many CHCs have demonstrated they can coordinate several projects at once; many are conducting several collaboratives simultaneously,[21] while others may be lead[22] or collaborating[23] institutions on large-scale REACH 2010 population-based projects.

The literature offers few examples of projects and programs designed to determine barriers to behavioral change or to test behavior change models for the population targeted by the CHCs. Nevertheless, CHCs offer enormous potential to help carry out research and establish the scientific basis for interventions to reduce health risks among all segments of the US population, especially those most in need. With the increased number of centers projected as a result of the new congressional initiatives, CHC-based research will assume even greater importance.

▶ SUMMARY AND RECOMMENDATIONS

Table 29–2 summarizes key points outlined in this chapter. Recommendations to ameliorate current disparities are provided in Table 29–3.

▶ **TABLE 29–2**. Summary of Major Findings Regarding Community Health Centers (CHCs)

- CHCs have evolved to provide basic health services to the uninsured and underserved in the United States
- Since the 1960s, CHCs have expanded in size and scope and now operate in over 3500 delivery sites nationwide
- Many CHCs provide services mainly to minorities, especially African Americans
- CHCs can serve as population-based centers for health research in populations often underrepresented in previous studies
- The Southern Community Cohort Study (SCCS) is a federally funded research project, now ongoing in CHCs throughout the South, to assess reasons for disparities in cancer and other diseases
- To date over 30,000 participants have been enrolled in the SCCS, providing a low-income cohort to be followed for future health outcomes
- CHCs may provide optimal settings for various research activities, including interventions to reduce the burden of cancer and other diseases in high-risk groups

▶ **TABLE 29–3**. Summary of Recommendations for National Interventions to Ameliorate Current Disparities

- The 5-year initiative to double the number of CHCs should be expedited because of the great need for health services among its client populations
- CHC participation should be encouraged in population and behavior research that has potential to decrease health disparities in the long term
- Appropriations for population, behavior, and intervention research initiatives should be increased to assess the determinants and means of reduction of health disparities
- Community-academic partnerships should be fostered to help develop Research Centers of Excellence where practical and effective methods for improving preventive and therapeutic health services can be initiated and evaluated

▶ **REFERENCES**

1. Federally Qualified Health Centers; 2002. Available at: http:www.ncsl.org/programs/health/fqhc.htm.
2. Sanchez EJ. Special centers offer health care to those in need. *Austin-American Statesman.* 2003.
3. Young D. *A Promise Kept: Boston's Neighborhood Health Centers.* Boston, Mass: Trustees of Health and Hospitals, City of Boston; 1982.
4. Geiger HJ. Community-oriented primary care: The legacy of Sidney Kark. *Am J Public Health* 1993;83(7):946–947.
5. Budget to Continue President's Initiative for the Uninsured: Efforts Include Health Centers, Tax Credits and Investments to Expand Access to Care; 2003. Available at: http://www.hhs.gov/news/press/2003pres/200302//.html.
6. Proser M. Quality and cost effective care at community health centers. Audioconference for National Conference of State Legislatures on Cost-Effectiveness and Health Outcomes of Community Health Centers. Washington, DC: National Association of Community Health Centers; 2004. Available at: http:// www.ncsl.org/programs.
7. Kovner AR. *Health Care Delivery in the United States.* New York, NY: Springer; 1995.
8. Duke EM. Remarks to the 8th Biennial Symposium on Minorities, the Medically Underserved, and Cancer. Washington, DC: Health Resources and Services Administration Press Office, US Dept of Health and Human Services; 2002. Available at: http://www.newsroom.hrsa.gov.
9. National Association of Community Health Centers: *Special Topics Issue Brief #2. The Role of Health Centers in Reducing Racial and Ethnic Health Disparities.* Washington, DC: NACHC; 2003.
10. National Association of Community Health Centers. *Health Centers' Role in Reducing Racial and Ethnic Health Disparities.* Washington, DC: NACHC; 2003.
11. Roby D, Rosenbaum S, Hawkins D. *Exploring Health Care Quality and Effectiveness at Federally-Funded Community Health Centers: Results from the Patient Experience Evaluation Report System (1993–2001).* Washington, DC: National Association of Community Health Centers; 2003.
12. Politzer RM, Yoon J, Shi L, et al. Inequality in America: The contribution of health centers in reducing and eliminating disparities in access to care. *Med Care Res Rev* 2001;58(2):234–248.
13. Shin P, Jones K, Rosenbaum S. *Reducing Racial and Ethnic Health Disparities: Estimating the Impact of High Health Center Penetration in Low-Income Communities.* Washington, DC: Center for Health Services Research and Policy, George Washington University; 2003.
14. Thompson T. Compassion and service: The importance of community health centers to America's health care future. Speech at the NACHC Policy and Issues Forum; Washington, DC; 2002. Available at: http://www.hhs.gov/news/2002/020320.html.
15. Health Disparities Collaboratives; 2004. Available at: http://www.healthdisparities.net/index.html.
16. Health Disparities Collaboratives: Models for Changing Practice; 2001. Available at: http://www.healthdisparities.net/about_models.html.
17. Chin MH, Cook S, Drum ML, et al. Improving diabetes care in Midwest community health centers with the health disparities collaborative. *Diabetes Care* 2004;27(1):2–8. Erratum in: *Diabetes Care* 2004;27(8):2099.
18. Southern Community Cohort Study; 2004. Available at: http://www.southerncommunitystudy.org.
19. Devesa S, Grauman D, Blot W, et al. *Atlas of Cancer Mortality in the United States 1950–94.* No. 99-4564. Washington, DC: National Institutes of Health; 1999.
20. Surveillance, Epidemiology and End Results (SEER) Program. SEER and Stat Database; 2003. Available at: http://www.seer.cancer.gov.
21. Barr MS. Baltimore medical system. Audioconference for National Conference of State Legislatures on Cost-Effectiveness and Health Outcomes of Community Health Centers. Washington, DC,: National Association of Community Health Centers; 2004. Available at: www.ncsl.org/programs.
22. Matthew Walker Community Health Center REACH; 2004. Available at: http://www.mwchc.org/REACH.htm.
23. Levy SR, Anderson EE, Issel LM, et al. Using multilevel, multisource needs assessment data for planning community interventions. *Health Promot Pract* 2004;5(1):59–68.

CHAPTER 30

Faith-Based Initiatives

GREGORY STRAYHORN, MD, MPH, PhD

► INTRODUCTION

Religious institutions in the United States have traditionally delivered social services to minority and socioeconomically disadvantaged groups. Many proponents argue that greater participation by faith-based groups in the health services arena has the potential to decrease health disparities among minority and socioeconomically disadvantaged populations.[1–4] Although available research fails to show that faith-based social services provide long-term, holistic service delivery solutions, evidence exists that faith-based organizations can provide short-term and effective health-promoting activities and interventions.[3,5] Although the majority of such research is focused on African Americans, findings concerning the potential impact of faith-based health interventions may also pertain to other groups.[5,6]

This chapter provides an overview of faith-based organizations' participation in social service and health activities that could have the potential to augment clinical and public health efforts to reduce health disparities. Among the topics discussed are the potential of faith-based organizations to address health issues through their role in their communities and their social service programs, the extent to which faith-based organizations participate in services that target their communities, the effectiveness of health-promoting programs, examples of health initiatives in faith-based organizations, government's role in supporting social outreach services of faith-based organizations, and methods to assist faith-based organizations in developing effective approaches to health-promoting programs.

► FAITH-BASED ORGANIZATIONS AND SOCIAL SERVICE

Health programs based in churches, synagogues, and other places of worship can potentially have a positive impact on people's health. African American faith-based organizations have deep historical roots in their communities and are closely linked to the cultural, social, and political environments of these communities. Sixty-one percent of African American adults attend religious services at least once a month, a rate that is substantially higher than that among whites (47%).[7] Compared with white congregations, African American congregations have a significantly higher rate of involvement in their communities' social and civil rights activities.[7] Churches have a similarly central role in Latino communities, particularly among less-acculturated, Spanish-speaking, poorly educated Hispanic women.[6,8]

Faith-based organizations already function as major channels of communication between their congregations and the larger community and could potentially be utilized for targeted health-promoting activities.[3,5] Many faith-based organizations provide social services independently and in collaboration with secular social agencies that target socioeconomically disadvantaged populations.[3,5,8–10] A focus on health promotion and the provision of appropriate health services might be a natural extension of these social services. Faith-based organizations, especially in African American communities, have a long history of sponsoring health promotion and education activities for their congregations and communities. Examples include screening for cancer, hypertension, diabetes, and high cholesterol; smoking cessation, physical activity, and nutritional health education and interventions; and coping with mental health problems in the family.[3,5,6,7,11–21]

Advocates of expanded faith-based social service delivery argue that faith-based groups are able to provide more effective social services than secular agencies because their religious character fosters the social and emotional reinforcement needed for effective social service programs. Empirical evidence for it is limited and mixed.[22]

Most faith-based organizations that provide social services target socioeconomically disadvantaged groups. Activities generally focus on food services, clothing, housing, substance abuse, and employment assistance. These are generally collaborative efforts with secular social service organizations.[22–24] Collaborations among health-care providers, secular social services agencies, and faith-based organizations could incorporate targeted health-care programs with the potential to improve the quality of life for vulnerable groups and congregants.

▶ LEVELS OF PARTICIPATION AND CHARACTERISTICS OF FAITH-BASED ORGANIZATIONS THAT PROVIDE SOCIAL AND HEALTH SERVICES

Although most churches provide some form of social outreach, few are engaged in intensive social service activities that require significant personnel or financial resources.[22–24] Churches with large congregations, substantial annual revenues, middle-class congregants, ministries that specifically focus on social outreach, more highly educated and full-time ministers, racially conscious African American ministers, and congregations and ministers with less conservative religious philosophies are more likely to provide social services. Recipients of most social services tend not to be members of the faith-based organizations' congregations but rather underserved and socioeconomically disadvantaged groups. Few provider congregations extend integration of these recipients into their regular religious activities. Services tend to focus on immediate and emergent needs such as housing, clothing, and food, rather than on long-term goals. Few programs provide "holistic, transformational services." Most faith-based organizations that provide social services do so in collaboration with secular social nonprofit and government agencies. More conservative and fundamentalist faith-based organizations are less willing to apply for or accept governmental support. It is noteworthy that black congregations are significantly more likely to provide some level of social services regardless of size, revenue, and urban, rural, or geographic location.[7–9,22–24] However, the degree of community involvement of African American churches has declined over time.[7]

The prevalence of faith-based organizations that provide specific health-oriented programs for their congregations or communities is unknown. Caldwell et al found that two thirds of African American churches provided outreach programs to meet family, health, and social services needs.[25] A recent systematic review of the literature found 386 articles that described health activities located in churches. In the articles reviewed, most programs targeted faith-based organizations' congregations or surrounding communities, African Americans and adults, and were categorized as faith-based (church initiated), faith-placed (initiated by health professionals or social agencies), or collaborative (jointly initiated).[5]

▶ EFFECTIVENESS OF FAITH-BASED, HEALTH-RELATED PROGRAMS

Information on outreach programs of faith-based organizations tends to be descriptive. Few empirical studies exist that measure program outcomes and evaluate their effectiveness. Faith-placed programs that are initiated by health professionals, who usually work at academic centers, are more likely to identify, measure, and evaluate outcomes. Chaves notes that the few systematic comparisons between religious and secular organizations doing similar work provide mixed results. For example, when religious nursing homes are compared with secular facilities, data suggest that the religious facilities may be more effective; whereas secular child-care centers have been found to provide higher quality care than religious alternatives. Compelling objective studies that support the effectiveness of faith-based organizations' social outreach programs do not exist.[22,23,24]

In Dehaven's systematic review of the faith-based literature from 1900 to 2000, only 28 out of 386 studies measured program outcomes or were designed to assess the programs' effectiveness. Most programs were described as faith-placed, tended to be clustered in certain geographic areas of the United States, and targeted the organizations' congregations and surrounding communities, African Americans, and adults. Thirteen studies provided process evaluations of health screening activities. The remaining 15 programs tested interventions and found statistically significant outcomes. The few studies that reported the results of faith-based and collaborative programs had similar findings. Thus, if properly designed and implemented, these studies suggest that regardless of whether programs are faith-based, faith-placed, or collaborative they can produce significant and positive health outcomes.[5]

▶ EXAMPLES OF HEALTH PROGRAMS IN FAITH-BASED ORGANIZATIONS

This section presents examples of outcome studies and case reports of the most frequent health initiatives of faith-based organizations. Examples of health initiatives include cancer screening; hypertension, diabetes, smoking cessation, physical activity, and nutritional health education and interventions; and mental health services.[5,11–21]

Mental Health

African Americans are less likely than whites to use mental health services, often reporting distrust of the mental health service system, the lack of available community mental health centers, misdiagnosis of psychiatric symptoms, and lack of resources to pay for treatment as factors that account for the underutilization of mental health services. African Americans tend to rely on an extended family network in times of need rather than seek help from outside organizations. The church is an important member of this extended kinship network.[19]

Concerns about mental health services provided by the clergy and faith-based organizations relate to incorrect diagnosis, failure to recognize the seriousness of psychiatric symptoms, and failure to refer for appropriate treatment. An ethical concern relates to the nontherapeutic relationships between clergy and congregants.[19]

Taylor et al published one of the most extensive literature reviews of mental health services in faith communities and provided by the clergy.[19] They focused primarily on the role of the clergy in the provision of mental health services in black churches. The literature suggests that clergy in general and especially African American clergy provide a significant amount of personal and family counseling in the form of socioemotional assistance or encouragement to increase church involvement. Thirty-nine percent of Americans consult their ministers for serious personal problems ranging from marital problems to substance or alcohol abuse, depression, teenage pregnancy, unemployment, and legal issues. Although half of the personal problems presented to ministers relate to marital issues, surveys of Hispanic groups indicate that ministers are consulted for a broad array of personal problems. Frequent church attendees, African Americans (especially women), and members of fundamentalist denominations are more likely to seek personal counsel from clergy, whereas Jews and infrequent church attendees tend to seek assistance for personal problems from psychiatrists or clinical psychologists.[19]

Clergy with more liberal theological philosophies and higher education are more apt to make referrals to community mental health agencies. Compared with white clergy, African American clergy are more likely to provide counseling to persons with mental health diagnoses and provide crisis intervention. Although African American clergy are more likely to recommend religious practices as a solution to mental health problems, when compared with white clergy, they have more connections with community mental health agencies and refer to professional mental services more frequently. The greater a church's ties are with community agencies, the more likely are African American clergy to refer to community mental health agencies.[19]

African American churches that provide mental health services demonstrate the following characteristics: large and middle-class congregations that provide a substantial pool of volunteers; access to internal and external funding sources through pledges, donations, and grants; facilities to accommodate health programs; and associations with community agencies in general; and full-time clergy.[19]

From the standpoint of congregants, Nooney and Woodrum found from a survey of church attendees that perceived positive social support is significantly correlated with low depression scores. Using data from the 1998 General Social Survey, which is a representative sample of all noninstitutionalized English-speaking persons 18 years of age or older, and through the use of path analysis, the authors found a direct relationship between churches' social support systems and mental health as measured by depression. Church attendance was not directly correlated with depression; however, attendance was directly and positively correlated with perceived social support. Although this study did not delineate the types of social support, the construct suggested a measure of instrumental (providing tangible assistance) and socioemotional support during difficult times. Although this study does not directly address the mental health outcomes of organized faith-based programs that provide direct mental health services or collaborate with community mental health agencies, it does suggest that congregants' mental health can be affected by social support systems within the church.[21]

To determine congregants' use of mental health support services that are located in churches, Pickett-Schenk examined a faith-placed mental health support program for church members who have family members with mental illnesses. Through collaboration with a large (6000-member) African American church in Chicago, members of a support group at a local mental health agency extended their support services to the church. With the permission of the church's health advisory board and backing of the minister, the support group was advertised to the entire congregation by ministers. Reading materials and information were disseminated at a booth during the church's annual health fair and at a 1-day mental health workshop in which mental health professionals were present to inform and recruit participants. A 1-year follow-up assessment of support group participants found high satisfaction, increased knowledge and understanding of mental illness and mental health service systems, and reported higher morale. The results of this study suggest that faith-placed mental health services that target families of the mentally ill can be effective.[20]

Taylor et al described the potential for faith-based organizations and community mental health or social work agencies to collaborate in developing effective mental health services in the African American community. They make the following recommendations:[19]

1. Engagement of the minister is pivotal.
2. Social service agencies should become familiar with churches' sociodemographic characteristics.
3. Agencies should educate churches and familiarize them with agency services.
4. Agency liaisons should be appointed to work directly with the churches. Gender may be an important consideration, depending on the gender of the ministers and the target of services.
5. Use a partnership or collaborative model.
6. Agency representatives should provide in-service training regarding the functions and resources of their agencies for the ministers and lay church members; similar in-services should be provided by either the minister, the church's health advisory board, or lay members to acquaint the agency liaison with the church's mission, resources, and goals regarding health promotion and education programs.[19]

Health Behavior Modification

Behavioral patterns contribute to health disparities within minority and socioeconomically disadvantaged groups. Health behaviors are directly linked to the prevention, diagnosis, and management of diseases such as diabetes, hypertension, and cancer that disproportionately affect African Americans and other minority groups. This section presents examples and outcomes of behavioral modification programs that were initiated in African American churches.

Dietary Behavior

As part of the *Healthy People 2010* initiative promulgated by former US Surgeon General David Satcher, increases in fruit and vegetable consumption became a national priority. As an example of a faith-placed intervention, Resnicow et al conducted a 1-year intervention that sought to increase fruit and vegetable consumption among congregants in 14 African American churches.[16] Participants were recruited and received pretest and posttest assessments as part of church-sponsored health fairs at baseline and the 1-year follow-up. Using an approach similar to that recommended earlier in the discussion of mental health initiatives, a liaison was hired by the investigators to assist in recruitment and retention of participants and the implementation of the health fairs. Church ministers assisted in the recruitment by encouraging congregants to participate.

Based on the number of members participating, incentives in the form of donations were awarded to each church. Churches were matched on socioeconomic status and size and randomly assigned to one of three conditions:

1. **Group 1.** Participants in this group (the control group) received standard nutrition education materials at baseline and culturally sensitive intervention materials at the 1-year posttest.
2. **Group 2.** This group received a culturally sensitive, multicomponent self-help intervention with one telephone cue call. The culturally sensitive materials consisted of a 23-minute video, entitled *Forgotten Miracles,* that used religious themes to motivate healthy eating, and an *Eat for Life* cookbook, with recipes submitted by congregants. The recipes contained at least a quarter serving of fruit or vegetables per portion and were low in fat. The cookbook also included information about the health benefits of fruits and vegetables, tips for shopping and storing them, and cooking techniques; printed educational materials from the National Cancer Institutes brochure (No. 95-3862); a food guide pyramid slide card (Positive Promotions, Brooklyn, NY); the Soul Food Pyramid (Hebni Consultants, Orlando, Fla); a quarterly newsletter (mailed to all participants); and several "cues" imprinted with the project

logo, the message "5-A-Day," (eg, refrigerator magnet, pen, scratch pad, pot holder, and erasable writing tablet). Two weeks after receiving the nutritional materials, participants received a cue call that encouraged them to use the materials.

3. **Group 3.** In addition to the nutritional materials received by groups 1 and 2, participants in group 3 received three counseling calls, at 3, 6, and 10 months after baseline. The calls incorporated motivational interviewing that focused on changing fruit and vegetable intake. Motivational interviewing is a psychotherapeutic approach developed for addictive behaviors; the approach helps participants work through their ambivalence about behavior change and allows counselors to tailor content and format of the encounter to match participants' readiness for change.[16]

Eighty-five percent of the initial sample was assessed at follow-up. Group 3 participants—who received motivational interviewing calls along with the culturally sensitive, multicomponent nutritional education materials—consumed significantly greater amounts of both fruits and vegetables as assessed by validated food frequency questionnaires than participants in groups 1 and 2, who received the self-help or nutrition educational materials. Groups 1 and 2 had similar fruit and vegetable consumption. For group 3, the net effect of the interventions was an approximate 1.1 servings per day increase in fruit and vegetable consumption.[16]

WEIGHT MANAGEMENT AND HYPERTENSION

Obesity is a risk factor for chronic diseases such as hypertension, type 2 diabetes mellitus, cancer, and osteoporosis, among others; it impedes their management and contributes significantly to morbidity. The Baltimore Church High Blood Pressure Program (CHBPP) offered a behaviorally oriented weight-control program to women who attended participating churches.

The program consisted of eight weekly 2-hour diet counseling and exercise sessions. This nonrandomized, pre- and postintervention program compared weight and systolic and diastolic blood pressure of the 184 African American and 3 Caucasian hypertensive women with mean age of 51 years who participated between 1984 and 1986. The effects of the 8-week intervention on blood pressure and weight for the 88 women taking antihypertensive medication were compared with that of 99 hypertensive women who were taking no medication. Significant within-person weight reduction was found in both the medication and nonmedication groups. The mean weight loss in both groups was 6 pounds. Almost 90% of women lost some weight. Of the 20 women who participated in the 6-month follow-up, 65% maintained or exceeded their weight loss at 8 weeks. The mean reduction in both systolic and diastolic blood pressure was greater in the medication group but declined significantly in both groups. Blood pressure reduction was significantly correlated with percent change in weight. This study suggests that church-based programs that target health behavior change and resultant improvements in health indices, such as weight and blood pressure, can occur and be sustained postintervention.[12]

A similar but more scientifically rigorous study was conducted in the 1990s in a collaboration between Baltimore churches and the Center for Health Promotion at the John Hopkins University School of Medicine. The study design and implementation was overseen by a steering committee consisting of the investigators and ministers of African American churches in Baltimore. In this 1-year follow-up, randomized, intention-to-treat trial, involving 16 African American churches, 529 women were assigned to one of three church-based nutrition and physical activity strategies: (1) a standard behavioral group intervention, (2) the standard intervention supplemented with spiritual strategies, and (3) a self-help control. The results from both active groups were similar and combined for analysis. Women in the intervention groups had significant weight reduction and decreases in waist circumference, systolic blood pressure, dietary energy, dietary total fat, and sodium intake. There were no significant changes in the self-help group. This study suggests that church-based interventions can significantly improve cardiovascular risk factor profiles in African American women.[17]

Cancer Screening

Breast cancer is the most frequently diagnosed cancer among women. Although the age-adjusted incidence rate of invasive breast cancer is lower in African American women compared with their white counterparts, the age-adjusted death rate is significantly higher. Mammography is the screening tool of choice for detecting breast cancer in early stages. However, significant disparities in mammography screening exist between minority women (Hispanic or Latino and African American) and white women. After age 65, the gap in mammography screening closes between Hispanic or Latino and white women and significantly narrows for African American women. However, based on disadvantaged socioeconomic status, using education and income as indicators, disparities in mammography screening increase dramatically.[26]

The literature includes several reports of faith-based programs designed to increase and sustain mammography screening adherence among minority and socioeconomically disadvantaged women. Duan et al conducted a 2-year trial in Los Angeles churches through the use of telephone counseling of female congregants. The investigators recruited 30 churches (8 predominately Latino, 12 African American, and 10 white) and randomized half, representing each minority group, to either peer telephone counseling or a control condition. Churches were matched on race and ethnicity or membership, size, resources, and denomination. A total of 1443 women aged 50 to 80 years of age were recruited through announcements by ministers during services, meetings, special events, open houses, recruitment events, and telephone contact. Peer counselors from the congregations of participating churches were hired and trained. The training was based on the health belief model, which advocates increasing awareness of vulnerability, cues to action, and individualized focus on decreasing perceived barriers to adherence. Women were provided with information on their risk of breast cancer and encouraged to ask their physicians for referral for mammography and information about convenient screening facilities. Counseling occurred annually by telephone. The primary outcome was annual mammography screening adherence status—undergoing at least one mammography during the previous 12 months.[6]

Of the original recruited cohort, 813 completed both the baseline and 1-year follow-up. The investigators concluded that "Peer telephone counseling in a faith-based setting maintained 7.5% more baseline-adherent participants than did the control condition" and was statistically significant.[6] This represented a 32% reduction in nonadherence in the maintenance group that received peer counseling. However, there was no significant difference between the peer telephone counseling and control groups for conversion to receive mammography screening. The findings were similar among the three racial and ethnic groups. Although the intervention did not affect conversion to mammography screening among nonadherent women, which is an important public goal for early diagnosis and treatment and the possible elimination of disparities in breast cancer survival, the study results did lend support for maintaining or improving screening adherence among women in faith-based organizations. In their discussions, the authors reviewed the challenges of implementing such an intervention in churches. These challenges included costs related to data collection and evaluation of the program's effectiveness, self-report of outcome data, and the lower than desired response rate. Additional challenges included the significant time required to build relationships with church partners, training and coordination of peer counselors, and the diversity of participants that affected recruitment and intervention implementation. They suggest that such partnerships should be viewed as long-term endeavors that could have payoffs beyond that of the study period.[6]

Hypertension

For African Americans, hypertension continues to be disproportionately prevalent, undertreated, and a significant cause of end-organ damage, morbidity, and related premature death. Many faith-based, faith-placed, and collaborative projects have demonstrated positive outcomes.

Smith and Merritt used the combination of an educational and social support model through the use of church-based nurses as an intervention to improve and sustain church members' knowledge, skills, and behaviors regarding hypertension control. The specific goals of the intervention were to (1) increase knowledge of hypertension and its management, (2) decrease and maintain sodium and cholesterol dietary intake, and (3) decrease and maintain blood pressure.[11] The project was conducted among a convenience sample of 17 urban churches, with congregation sizes ranging from 150 to 4000 members, predominately African American, representing two Catholic and 15 Protestant groups, and located in the Chicago metropolitan area. Two churches were participants in the American Heart Association of Metropolitan Chicago program.

The pretest–posttest, nonequivalent, no-control group design project consisted of two phases. Phase one involved the recruitment of nurses from church congregations to train and serve as hypertension health educators and to provide support to hypertensive participants. Ministers in participating churches recruited nurses from their congregations and also referred other health professionals to serve as health educators. Nurses and other health professionals who volunteered participated in three, 8-hour, in-service training sessions and received continuing education credits. Important components of the training included experiential activities, assessment of hypertensive

patients' educational needs, determination of how such programs should fit into the church's structure, program planning skills, identification of resources, skills to match learner's needs with educational methods and techniques, creation of an environment conducive to education, methods of evaluating individual and overall educational programs and specific strategies, specific content on trends, and issues in hypertension management. All health education trainees underwent a post-training assessment to determine their readiness for implementing the hypertension education program at their churches.

In phase two, groups of 5 to 20 hypertensive participants at each church, after providing consent, received a syllabus that described intervention goals and listed the course content and specific objectives. Each study member participated in eight 1-hour educational sessions. To standardize the curriculum, guides developed by the principal investigator were used. Blood pressures were obtained using a standardized method at each class, immediately after the intervention period, and again 3 months postintervention. All blood pressures were recorded in each participant's confidential record. Immediately after the intervention and again 3 months postintervention, data were collected face to face. The church health educators provided support and education to hypertensive participants during classes, through contacts outside of classes, during home visits, and by telephone. When available, family members were included in the support efforts. Sixty-four church health professionals were trained as health educators.[11]

Ninety-seven church members of the 17 churches met the inclusion criteria and were included in the project. Significant changes in general knowledge of hypertension and drug management was found among the hypertensive participants from baseline to immediate postintervention and from immediate postintervention to 3 months postintervention. Perception of social support remained stable throughout the three periods.[11]

Smoking Cessation

African Americans bear the greatest health burden from smoking. During the 1970s and 1980s, death rates from respiratory cancers in African Americans increased among women and men; these rates have declined during the 1990s among African American men and plateaued among African American women.[26] When compared with other racial and ethnic minorities, middle-aged African Americans are more likely to die of smoking-related diseases such as coronary heart disease, stroke, and lung cancer. The dramatic increase in smoking incidence among African American youth during the 1990s portends significant future increases in tobacco-related morbidity and mortality. Although African Americans report a higher desire to quit smoking, smoking cessation rates among African Americans are lower than those for Caucasians.[27] The disparity in smoking cessation rates is attributed to lack of access to health and smoking cessation programs (especially for rural African Americans) and the failure of cessation programs to incorporate the cultural norms of African American communities. Two studies that were implemented in African American churches to address these concerns are summarized below: one targeted rural and the other, urban, populations.[14,15]

Voorhees et al conducted a church-based smoking cessation intervention on readiness to quit that assessed the effect of an intensive, culturally relevant, spiritually based church intervention on smoking behavior stages versus a minimal self-help strategy. Given the paucity of work on Prochaska and Diclemente's stages of change model with African American populations and previous studies of smoking cessation that suggest smokers move through a series of changes toward readiness to quit when participating in smoking cessation programs, the investigators targeted their study to urban, church-going African Americans. Twenty-three African American churches were recruited from 23 contiguous census tracts in and around Baltimore. The churches selected were known to ministers on the study's steering committee and were

active in community and church-related social and health issues. Baseline and 1-year follow-up data for study participants were collected at church health fairs. To compare participants' quit rates with secular trends among the church-going population of their catchment area, investigators conducted a cross-sectional, random-digit dialing survey during the follow-up period. Churches were randomly assigned to the intervention or control condition.[14]

The intervention included from one to four pastoral sermons on smoking; testimony during church service from individuals going through the quit process; training of lay volunteers to serve as smoking cessation counselors; access to individual and group support, supplemented with spiritual audiotapes containing gospel music; a day-to-day scripturally guided stop-smoking booklet; and baseline and follow-up health fairs that evaluated cardiovascular risk status and smoking status. Participants assigned to the minimal self-help group received the same baseline health fair intervention with the same health status feedback and were given the American Lung Association pamphlet entitled, *Don't Let Your Dreams Go Up In Smoke, designed for African Americans*.[14]

Baseline and postintervention questions consisting of the Prochaska and Diclemente stages of change items and smoking status were the primary outcome variables. To validate quit status, exhaled carbon dioxide and saliva nicotine levels were collected from participants categorized as quitters at follow-up. Compared with the random-digit dialing survey respondents, both the intensive and minimal intervention groups had significantly higher quit rates. However, quit rates for the two intervention groups did not differ significantly. The two intervention groups had similar baseline stages of change scores, but differed significantly at follow-up in favor of the intensive intervention group. A significantly higher proportion of the minimal intervention group made no change or regressed to earlier stages. Positive progress was most pronounced among Baptists in the intensive intervention group. The authors suggest that "the spiritual nature of the intervention and the interaction of the belief structures of specific denominations make (the church) an ideal arena in which specific health promotion and disease prevention strategies can be applied."[14] They also point to the importance of having the church leadership involved at all levels of project development, implementation, evaluation, and interpretation of results.[14]

Schorling et al developed a church-based smoking cessation program in two rural Virginia counties with large populations of African Americans through the development of a community health coalition, the Alliance of Black Churches Health Project. The goal of the project was to use the churches in one county to design and develop a smoking cessation program that would extend to the community, while developing a similar community health coalition in a neighboring county whose citizens served as the control population. Each county health coalition was developed by church and community leaders. A coordinator was assigned to each county to identify local agencies and community leaders, assist with coalition board organization, conduct community health needs assessment, and develop community resource inventories. Community coalitions were composed of laypersons and ministers. The project was guided by the philosophy of community empowerment and sought to improve the community's ability to identify and deal with important health problems. Although the community coalition boards were encouraged to develop health-related community projects, both boards agreed to participate in the smoking cessation project, with one county serving as the control.[15]

Similar to the Voorhees study, the community coalition boards participated in the project design and planning. After determining that a random-digit dialing survey would not work in the two populations and recruitment of study participants through churches was not feasible in the rural communities, an in-person household survey was conducted with data collected by the University of Virginia's Center for Survey Research. The survey identified 3744 African Americans in the two counties, including 965 smokers. Six-hundred and fifty-two smokers completed the baseline survey, and 452 were resurveyed at 18 months postintervention. The respondents were classified based on their smoking status and stages of change at baseline and follow-up.[15]

The intervention program consisted of one-on-one counseling with self-help materials. The counselors were selected by their churches and received 8 hours of training that focused on specific recruitment and counseling skills. The training included guidelines for dealing with smokers at different levels of the stages of change model. Counselors were encouraged to discuss the program with their congregations at large. To extend the smoking cessation project to the community, a multichannel approach was developed that used both church and nonchurch avenues to deliver interventions. The control county chose hypertension as its health issue and implemented similar approaches. Although not significant, the smoking cessation rate of the intervention county exceeded that of the control county. Frequent church attendance was significantly associated with smoking cessation. The difference in stages of change from baseline to follow-up significantly favored the intervention county.[15]

Although the authors discuss several limitations of the study, they point to the success of developing health-related interventions for African American populations in rural areas through the development of church–community coalitions. Twelve months after the completion of the first health-related project, the coalitions in both counties continued their activities of providing health promotion programs to their communities. The authors suggest that this model can be replicated in other communities where there are limited health promotion, education, and support resources.[15]

The Voorhees and Schorling studies demonstrate that health education and promotion programs that target minority groups and their communities, especially African Americans, can be designed, planned, and implemented in churches or by community coalitions that include church leaders. Programs that appear to have the greatest potential endurance make church and community leaders and lay volunteers equal partners and help the leadership to develop skills for coalition building and assessment of community health needs and resources. Although urban churches with large, middle-class congregations are more likely to have health ministries or provide other social services, Schorling et al demonstrated that sustainable health promotion programs can be implemented in rural communities whose church congregations are small and not affluent.

One glaring problem with most of the programs reviewed is the absence of significant or any male participation. Given that African American men have worse health indices and shorter life expectancy than African American women, health promotion and education programs that target men must be designed, implemented, and evaluated for efficacy and effectiveness.

▶ ROLE OF GOVERNMENT IN FAITH-BASED SOCIAL SERVICES

In 1996, during the debate on welfare reform, legislation was passed at the national level that included a provision for "charitable choice." This legislation required states to include religious organizations as eligible contractees if states contracted with nonprofit agencies for social services. The legislation provoked debate among religious denominations regarding the separation of church and state and the potential intrusion of government on religious autonomy. Although the charitable choice initiative has been promoted by conservative sectarian groups and politicians, surveys of conservative religious denominations find that they are less likely to accept government funding for their social programs. On the other hand, despite being the most vocal critics of charitable choice, Catholic and liberal-to-moderate Protestant denominations are more likely to apply and ac-

cept government funding for social programs. African American congregations are most willing to accept government funding for their social services. This willingness is attributed to the role of the African American churches in providing social services and political guidance to their congregations and to African American ministers' higher participation in political issues.[8,9,23,24]

In contradiction to suppositions put forward by proponents of the charitable choice initiative, on their own, social service activities provided exclusively by churches tend to be limited to enterprises that are short term, emergency oriented, and less focused on relationship building. Minimal church volunteer participation and financial resources support such programs. More long-standing, holistic, relationship-building programs occur when faith-based organizations or congregations collaborate with secular or government agencies. African American congregations are more likely than their Caucasian counterparts to collaborate with secular organizations and accept government funding to support their social service activities.

Limited financial resources pose a major barrier to churches' ability to develop, implement, and sustain social programs, including health promotion and educational programs. Through funding from agencies that provide charitable choice and collaboration with secular and government agencies, the financial barriers to developing and sustaining programs that target health disparities could be substantially reduced. Agency expertise in providing social services, coupled with the churches' community relationships, could serve to create successful programs.[3,7,8]

▶ SUMMARY AND RECOMMENDATIONS

Faith-based organizations have the potential to become important participants in public health efforts to eliminate health disparities among minority and socioeconomically disadvantaged populations. Efforts to introduce health promotion and education programs as part of the social mission of churches show promise for their effectiveness to positively influence health behaviors and outcomes. However, these efforts are usually short term (1 to 2 years) and part of research studies, and few focus on male health.

Successful, holistic, long-term, relationship-building programs are usually collaborations among health professionals, usually from academic centers, local or regional church pastoral and lay leaders, community leaders, and secular agencies. Support of the clergy is pivotal, although lay church members are most likely to participate in the day-to-day activities. Such collaborations require the development of trust among collaborators and equal partnerships and participation in the design and implementation of programs. Agency collaborators must learn the sociodemographic characteristics of churches. This knowledge is important when determining the churches' capacity to participate in health-related projects. Agency collaborators should educate church leaders about agency services, resources, and expertise. Agency liaisons should be appointed who will maintain the link between the church and the agency. Education should be bidirectional; churches should educate agency collaborators on the influence of church beliefs and practices on personal and family experiences.[19]

Collaborations with academic health centers to test the feasibility or effectiveness of health promotion and educational programs in church-based and community settings requires similar attention to the development of trust and partnerships. Additionally, academic collaborators should assist church and community leaders with the development of skills to conduct congregational and community health needs assessments, identify resources to support and sustain programs, and empower them to eventually take control over the consequences that are important to the members and their broader

community. Such collaborations should assist churches and communities to develop organizational structures that ultimately lead to independence in addressing community health problems.[5,15,18,19,28]

Although faith-based health promotion and education programs show promise in the effort to eliminate health disparities, little work has been done to determine program effectiveness. Given the limited personnel, financial, and expert resources required to develop, implement, and sustain programs, it is important that programs be designed to affect the intended outcomes. Thus, evaluation procedures should be an integral part of program development but should not be financially and technically burdensome. To determine the feasibility and effectiveness of programs, both process and outcome evaluations are necessary. Dees and Garcia offer a total continuous quality improvement model—Plan, Do, Check, Act Cycle (PDCA)—that can be applicable for faith-based and community collaborative program evaluation.[29] This model incorporates needs assessment, program goal and objective development, program design and implementation, process and outcome evaluation, and program refinement and continuation. Social service agencies and academic health professionals can assist faith-based and community organizations to incorporate similar evaluation processes in their health promotion and education programs. This or a similar evaluation approach will be necessary to determine program feasibility and effectiveness and avoid applying resources to ineffective programs.

▶ REFERENCES

1. Hatch J, Derthick S. Empowering black churches for health promotion. *Health Values Achieving High Level Wellness.* 1992;15(5):3–9.
2. Chatters LM, Levin JS, Ellison CG. Public health and health education in faith communities. *Health Educ Behav* 1998;25:689–699.
3. Peterson J, Atwood JR, Yates B. Key elements for church-based health promotion programs:

Outcome-based literature review. *Public Health Nurs* 2002;19(6):401–411.

4. Foege WH, O'Connell U. *Healthy People 2000: A Role for American's Religious Communities*. Chicago, Ill: Park Ridge Center and Carter Center; 1990.

5. Dehaven MJ, Hunter IB, Wilder L, et al. Health programs in faith-based organizations: Are they effective? *Am J Public Health* 2004;94(6):1030–1036.

6. Duan N, Fox SA, Derose KP, Carson S. Maintaining mammography adherence through telephone counseling in a church-based trail. *Am J Public Health* 2000;90(9):1468–1471.

7. Chaves M, Higgins LM. Comparing the community involvement of black and white congregations. *J Sci Study Religion* 1992;31(4):425–440.

8. Ebaugh HR, Pipes PF. Immigrant congregations as social service providers: Are they safety-nets for welfare reform? In: Nesbitt P, ed. *Religion and Social Policy*. Walnut Creek, Calif: AltaMira; 2001.

9. Chaves M, Tsitsos W. Congregations and social services: What they do, how they do it, and with whom. *Nonprofit Voluntary Sector Q* 2001;30:376–380.

10. Ebaugh HR. Where's the religion? Distinguishing faith-based from secular social service agencies. *J Scientific Study Religion* 2003;42(3):411–416.

11. Program for African Americans with hypertension. *Ethn Health* 1997;2(3):243–253.

12. Kumanyika SK, Charleston JB. Lose weight and win: A church-based weight loss program for blood pressure control among black women. *Patient Educ Counseling* 1992;19(1):19–32.

13. Irwin C, Braithwaite R. A church-based diabetes education program for older, African-American women. *Am J Health Stud* 1997;13(1):1–7.

14. Voorhees CC, Stilman FA, Swank RT, et al. Heart, body, and soul: Impact of church based smoking cessation intervention on readiness to quit. *Prev Med* 1996;25:277–285.

15. Schorling JB, Roach J, Siegel M, et al. A trial of church-based smoking cessation interventions for rural African Americans. *Prev Med* 1997;26:92–101.

16. Resnicow K, Jackson A, Braithwaite R, et al. Healthy Body/Healthy Spirit: A church-based nutrition and physical activity intervention. *Health Educ Res* 2002;17(5):562–573.

17. Yanek LR. Project joy: Faith based cardiovascular health promotion for African American women. *Public Health Rep* 2001;116(1S):68–81.

18. Ammerman A. The PRAISE! project: A church-based nutrition intervention designed for cultural appropriateness, sustainability, and diffusion. *Health Promotion Pract* 1998;19:173–202.

19. Taylor RJ, Ellison CG, Chatters LM, et al. Mental health services in faith communities: The role of clergy in black churches. *Social Work* 2000;45(1):73–87.

20. Pickett-Schenk SA. Church-based support groups for African American families coping with mental illness: Outreach and outcomes. *Psychiatr Rehabil J* 2002;26(2):173–180.

21. Nooney J, Woodrum E. Religious coping and church-based social support as predictors of mental health outcomes: Testing a conceptual model. *J Sci Study Religion* 2002;41(2):359–368.

22. Chaves M. Going on faith: Six myths about faith-based initiatives. *Christian Century* 2001;118(25):20–24.

23. Chaves M. Religious congregations and welfare reform. *Society* 2001;38(2):21–29.

24. Chaves M. Congregations' social service activities. No. 6 in: *Charting Civil Society, A Series by the Center on Nonprofits and Philanthropy*. Washington, DC: Urban Institute; 1999.

25. Caldwell CH, Greene AD, Billingsley A. Family support programs in black churches: A new look at old functions. In: Kagan LS, Weisbourd B, eds. *Putting Family First*. New York, NY: Jossey-Bass; 1994:137–160.

26. National Cancer Institute, Surveillance Research. Available at: http://surveillance.cancer.gov/statistics/.

27. Satcher D. Tobacco use among racial/ethnic minorities. *A Report of the Surgeon General—Executive Summary*. Washington, DC: US Dept of Health and Human Services, Centers for Disease Control and Prevention; 1998. Available at: http://www.cdc.gov/tobacco/sgr/sgr_1998/index.htm.

28. La Verne R, Hatch J, Parrish T. The role of a historically black university and the black church in community-based health initiatives: The Project DIRECT Experience. *J Public Health Manag Pract* 2003;(suppl):S70–S73.

29. Dees JP, Garcia MA. Program planning: A total quality approach. *AAOHN J* 1995;43(5):239–244.

CHAPTER 31

Complementary and Alternative Medicine

Michael D. Floyd, md, msci*

► INTRODUCTION

Complementary and alternative therapies run the gamut from A to Z; by one count, there are at least 1800 different therapies and systems of care encompassing acupuncture through zootherapy.[1] Complementary and alternative medicine (CAM) has been defined as the field of health care outside Western allopathic medicine that includes treatments and health-care practices not taught in allopathic schools of medicine[2] and, until recently, not discussed in their curricula.[3] These treatments and practices are not used in US hospitals and are generally not reimbursed by medical insurance companies, although this has begun to change.[4] CAM therapies used alone are referred to as *alternative therapies;* when used in conjunction with conventional medicine, they are referred to as *complementary.*[5]

Edzard Ernst, one of the world's leading authorities, defined CAM as "diagnosis, treatment and/or prevention which complements mainstream medicine by contributing to a common whole, by satisfying a demand not met by ortho-

doxy or by diversifying the conceptual frameworks of medicine."[6] Ernst's definition provides insight into at least one reason for growing use of CAM: Consumer-patients cite a desire for a more holistic approach to treatment. Dissatisfaction with traditional medicine can also be a motive for using alternative therapies, although evidence shows most individuals use CAM therapies in conjunction with conventional medical services, not as a substitute for them.[7]

► POPULATION STUDIES

Use of alternative therapies increased markedly during the last decade of the 20th century. Prior to the 1990s, Western allopathic medicine was dismissive of CAM primarily because there was little scientific evidence to support the efficacy of many modalities. However, consumer use of and demand for CAM prompted mainstream medicine to take another look.

Although they are not the sole studies, Eisenberg's reports in 1993 and 1998 provide the baseline against which most subsequent change has been measured. Using a national random-digit dialing survey in 1991, Eisenberg et al estimated CAM usage at 33.8% among US adults, 425 million visits to CAM providers annually,

*The McGraw-Hill Companies acknowledge the substantial editorial contributions of Donna M. Frassetto and Nancy N. Woelfl in preparation of this chapter.

and expenditures of approximately $13.7 billion for CAM therapies.[2] By 1997, usage had increased to 42.1%, provider visits to 629 million, and expenditures, conservatively estimated, to $27 million.[8] Herbal and nutritional supplement use also rose dramatically to between $4 and $8 billion by 1999.[8] Demographically, typical alternative users were 25- to 45-year-old college graduates who paid cash for the services not covered by insurance. Types of therapy, which varied by user, included acupuncture, biofeedback, herbal remedies and nutritional supplements, massage, and meditation. Utilization studies suggested racial and ethnic minorities (African Americans, Hispanics, Asian Americans, and Native Americans) were as likely to use CAM therapies as Caucasians.[9]

Astin found the problems that brought patients to CAM practitioners were similar to those that brought them to allopathic physicians and that four specific health problems were highly predictive of CAM utilization: back problems, chronic pain, anxiety, and urinary tract problems.[9] Barrett observed that CAM users were people with health concerns trying to prevent or treat illness, noting that persons with chronic health problems were two to three times more likely to seek CAM therapies than their healthy counterparts.[4]

The most current national snapshot of CAM utilization comes from the 2002 US National Health Interview Survey (NHIS).[10] Conducted by the National Center for Health Statistics (NCHS), this survey collected data from 31,044 adults aged 18 years and older using computer-assisted personal interviews (CAPI). The Alternative Health/Complementary and Alternative Medicine supplemental questionnaire included questions on 19 CAM therapies, representing a cross-section of provider-based, self-administered, and spiritual therapies. The 10 provider-based therapies included in the questionnaire (and described in Appendix 31-A) were acupuncture, Ayurveda, biofeedback, chelation, chiropractic, energy healing (reiki), folk medicine, hypnosis, massage, and naturopathy; the 8 self-administered therapies (see Appendix 31-A) were herbal medicine, home-

opathy, megavitamin therapy, special diets, qi gong, tai chi, yoga, and relaxation techniques (meditation, guided imagery, progressive relaxation, deep-breathing exercises); and the spiritually based therapies were self-prayer, sacramental rites, prayer chains, and prayer by others.

Thirty-six percent of respondents aged 18 and over had used a CAM therapy other than prayer in the 12 months immediately preceding the 2002 NHIS survey. When the definition of CAM was expanded to include prayer for health reasons, 62% reported CAM use during this same period. Approximately 50% had used a CAM therapy other than prayer at least once during their lifetime; when the definition of CAM included prayer, lifetime use rose to 74.6%.

Of the 10 CAM therapies most commonly used within the 12 months preceding the 2002 NHIS survey, most were mind–body interventions. They included prayer for one's own health (43%), prayer by others for the respondent (24.4%), herbal therapies and natural products (18.9%), deep-breathing exercises (11.6%), participation in a prayer group for health restoration (9.6%), meditation (7.6%), chiropractic care (7.5%), yoga (5.1%), massage (5.0%), and diet-based therapies (3.5%).

Respondents indicated CAM was most often used to treat back pain or problems, head or chest colds, neck pain or problems, joint pain or stiffness, and anxiety or depression. Barnes observed this was not surprising given that approximately one quarter to one third of the adult population suffer from musculoskeletal disorders in any given year, yet many forms of chronic pain are not highly responsive to conventional medical treatment.[10]

Consistent with earlier reports, the 2002 NHIS found CAM usage was associated with gender, education, and health status[8,9,11-13] Women were more likely to use CAM than men; persons with higher educational attainment were more frequent users than the less educated; and those who had been hospitalized within the past year demonstrated greater frequency of use.

► UTILIZATION OF CAM THERAPIES BY MINORITIES

Several government studies describe disparities in allopathic health services to minority communities[14-21] that parallel the rapid increase in CAM usage. Historically African Americans, Native Americans, and Hispanics have used home remedies to lower healthcare costs. When viewed against census data on household income and poverty levels, the degree of utilization and types of alternative therapies used in racial and ethnic minority communities become both economic and health outcome issues. Research is ongoing, and it is not yet known whether use of alternative medicine in minority communities results from health disparities or causes them.

There is a growing body of evidence regarding use of CAM therapies by racial and ethnic minorities in the United States. This is due in large part to the efforts of the federal government to address disparities in health status among US citizens. In 1985, the US Department of Health and Human Services released the Report of the Secretary's Task Force on Black and Minority Health.[22] This landmark report acknowledged that blacks, Hispanics, Native Americans, and Asian Americans had failed to benefit equally from advances in medical science and documented the magnitude of the problem. The Institute of Medicine revisited health disparities in 2003 and concluded there was still a distressing lack of progress toward narrowing the gap in health status.[23] *Healthy People 2010* particularly targets health disparities in its plan of action.[21]

Consistent with its commitment to reducing and eliminating health disparities, the federal government created the Office of Alternative Medicine, which was later redesignated the National Center for Complementary and Alternative Medicine. It has also directed increased research funding toward this problem and holds federal agencies accountable for reliable, proactive data collection so that progress or lack thereof can be measured.

Struthers and Nichols[5] reviewed 26 research studies on use of CAM by ethnic and racial minorities. Fourteen studies explored diverse issues related to CAM use by racial and ethnic populations, including frequency of use, differences between majority and minority patterns of use, reasons for use, and predictive factors. Eight of the 14 studies demonstrated that racial and ethnic minorities use CAM; 6 found no significant differences in majority and minority use of alternative therapies. Seven of the studies dealt with use of CAM therapies for treatment of cancers and HIV among racial and ethnic minority populations. These studies highlighted the fact that many subjects were using CAM therapies prior to diagnosis of their illness. An additional 5 studies reviewed patterns of CAM use by specific ethnic and racial groups, particularly Hispanics. These studies confirmed use by the respective subject groups and explored reasons for seeking, using, or declining to use CAM. Overall, 19 of the 26 studies documented high CAM use among racial and ethnic minority populations, while 7 found no significant differences between minority and majority users of alternate therapies. Sample sizes of the studies reviewed ranged from less than 100 to more than 2000, but most were convenience samples, not representative national probability samples.

Among national surveys that examine use of CAM therapies by racial and ethnic minorities, Mackenzie et al[24] used data from the 1995 National Comparative Survey of Minority Health Care in an effort to identify predictors of CAM utilization among racial and ethnic minorities. These investigators examined the relationship among age, gender, ethnicity, education, income, insurance status, national origin, and utilization of five CAM therapies (acupuncture, chiropractic, herbal medicine, home remedies, and traditional healers). Louis Harris and Associates, Inc, a professional research organization, conducted the 25-minute telephone interview in six languages (English, Spanish, Mandarin, Cantonese, Korean, and Vietnamese). Among the 3789 potential respondents, minorities were oversampled. A 60% response rate was achieved, generating minority samples of sufficient size to generate statistically reliable results. Non-Hispanic whites represented 32% of the sample; non-Hispanic blacks, 31%; Asian Americans, 18%; Hispanics, 17%; and Native Americans, 2%.

Among respondents in this survey, 43.1% reported using one or more of the five CAM modalities in the 12 months preceding the survey. Ethnic groups demonstrated similar rates of use, with non-Hispanic whites reporting 43.5%; non-Hispanic blacks, 42.6%; Hispanics, 40.7%; Native Americans, 39.6%; and Asian Americans, 39%. These differences were not statistically significant. Consistent with earlier findings, female gender and educational attainment were predictive, along with health insurance status. Ethnicity did not predict CAM use; however, the investigators did observe preferences and patterns of use that were ethnically related. Asian Americans were 12 times more likely to use acupuncture than any other group. Asian and Native Americans were most likely to report use of an herbal remedy. Caucasians were the most frequent users of chiropractic, a therapy seldom selected by the other ethnic groups in this sampling.

Keith et al[25] used data from the 1996 Medical Expenditures Panel Survey to assess the effects of race and ethnicity on use of CAM in the United States. The Medical Expenditure Panel (MEP) Survey is a nationally representative survey of medical care use, expenditures, sources of payment, and insurance coverage conducted by Agency for Healthcare Research and Quality (AHRQ). It draws on subsets of NHIS respondents, with an oversampling of African Americans and Hispanics. Similar to the study by MacKenzie et al, this study sought to identify predictors of use for 11 provider-based therapies (acupuncture, biofeedback, herbal remedies, homeopathic therapy, hypnosis, massage therapy, meditation, nutritional advice, spiritual healing, traditional cultural medicine, and other therapies named by respondents). The effects of ethnicity, socioeconomic status, three health status and source-of-service indi-

cators, and five demographic variables were considered.

The investigators restricted analysis to 13,208 of the 23,230 respondents, focusing on adults younger than 65 years of age on the assumption they were wage earners who would have more disposable income to spend on alternative therapies not covered by health insurance.

Findings indicated that 6.5% of respondents had used some form of CAM therapy in the 12 months preceding the survey. Although this is considerably lower than estimates observed in other national surveys, it is consistent with findings of other MEP surveys. CAM use was highest among Asians (8.1%), followed by whites (7.1%), Hispanics (5%), and African Americans (3.2%). African Americans and Hispanics were less likely to use alternative therapies than whites. Asian Americans did not differ significantly in utilization from whites. Individuals who were dissatisfied with the availability of conventional health care and those who were in poor health but satisfied with their conventional provider were more likely to use complementary and alternative therapies. The investigators concluded that when Americans turn to CAM, it has more to do with being dissatisfied with the health-care system in general rather than their specific provider.

Ni et al[7] examined use of 12 different alternative therapies using data from the 1999 NHIS. An estimated 28.9% of US adults had used at least one therapy in the 12 months preceding the survey. The most commonly used therapies were spiritual healing or prayer (13.7%), herbal medicine (9.6%), and chiropractic manipulation (7.6%). The typical CAM user was a well-educated (16 years or more) non-Hispanic white woman between the ages of 35 and 54. Overall CAM use was higher for non-Hispanic whites (30.8%) than non-Hispanic blacks (24.1%) or Hispanics (19.9%). Although those who were insured demonstrated high use of CAM, the difference was not significant after controlling for age, gender, and education. Compared with nonusers, CAM users were more likely to use conventional medical services.

Graham et al[26] performed one of the most recent studies of CAM usage among racial and ethnic minorities using data from the 2002 NHIS. Data obtained using the 2002 Alternative Health/Complementary and Alternative Medicine supplement, described earlier, represent a significant improvement over previous CAM data because they represent more modalities in greater detail. Minorities were oversampled in an effort to produce statistically reliable sample sizes. Non-Hispanic blacks and Hispanics each account for approximately 12% of the total sample.

Use of 19 different CAM therapies during the 12 months preceding the survey as well at other times during the respondent's lifetime was explored. For therapies used in the 12 preceding months, detailed follow-up questions were asked about the health problem or condition being treated, reasons for choosing the therapy, whether the costs were covered by insurance, satisfaction with the treatment, and whether the respondent's conventional medical provider knew he or she was using the therapy.

Graham et al found use was common overall among the survey population, and correlates of use were consistent with previous studies. Female gender, educational attainment, higher income status, regional factors, and age were all associated with higher rates of CAM use. These factors are particularly descriptive of non-Hispanic white users. Respondents were also more likely to use CAM if they had visited a conventional health professional within the previous 6 months. Excluding prayer, the most frequently used therapies were herbal medicine, relaxation techniques, chiropractic, yoga, and massage.

CAM use was highest for non-Hispanic whites (36%), followed by Hispanics (27%), and non-Hispanic blacks (26%). After controlling for other sociodemographic factors, non-Hispanic black and Hispanic ethnicities were associated with less CAM use.

Graham et al also found preferences and patterns of use that were ethnically related. When the definition of CAM included prayer, blacks demonstrated highest use of prayer-based therapies (67%). They were less frequent users of somatically based therapies and rarely used chiropractic. When faced with what they perceived to be worsening health status, their use of CAM declined. African American use of CAM therapies was also influenced by health insurance status.

Hispanics, in contrast, showed strong association between self-perceived deterioration in health status and increased utilization of alternative therapies. More frequently than any other ethnic or racial group, Hispanics indicated they used CAM because conventional medical treatments were too expensive.

Even though national probability sampling of CAM utilization is now performed on a regular basis, it is still difficult to identify and profile the typical user of alternative therapies. Struthers, Mackenzie, and Graham[5,24,26] address the challenges of conducting research in this area. Mackenzie et al noted that aggregating findings on the use of specific modalities tends to obscure rather than clarify understanding of CAM utilization in the United States today. Considering CAM modalities such as chiropractic manipulation or herbal medicine separately produces very different results regarding the demographic characteristics of users than using a single CAM category. One aspect of the controversy on CAM utilization arises from definition of CAM itself. CAM encompasses myriad approaches to health and health care drawn from multiple cultures, traditions, and eras. Defining alternative medicine as everything *not* taught in US medical schools may be convenient but it is not highly amenable to productive research.

Despite improved sampling and data collection methods at the national level, especially those used to record ethnic and minority responses, there is both ethnocentric and medicocentric bias in the survey instruments. As a result, prevalence of CAM use among groups other than the non-Hispanic whites is probably underestimated. The 2002 NHIS questions about herbal medicine sought information on 35 specifically named drugs but failed to ask about herbs more commonly used by ethnic minorities. Herbs named in the NHIS survey questions tended to be those widely used by middle-class non-Hispanic whites and marketed as manufactured products. Hispanics and non-Hispanic blacks tend to use non-processed and home-grown herbs. In the folk medicine category, NHIS asked about only *curanderismo* and Native American healing, undifferentiated by tribe, without touching on many other types of healers. These limitations suggest that multi- and interdisciplinary collaboration is essential to designing culturally appropriate survey instruments that avoid ethnocentric bias in categorization and definitions. The successful delivery of health services to minorities must include increased awareness and appreciation for the cultural context of CAM use.

Evaluation of alternative treatments will require a more comprehensive approach to outcomes until appropriate end points can be identified and measured. Minority health-care use in the traditional sense will necessarily require modification to affect outcomes because poverty, lack of insurance, and primary care availability have been shown to affect health-care quality.[27] Current local and national research attempts to accurately measure use of CAM in minority groups. Survey instruments may produce more accurate results if administered at the point of care (ie, minority clinics, physician and dentist offices, churches, and schools) rather than by phone. Language-sensitive survey tools and examiners could help reduce response bias caused by language barriers, especially in the Hispanic and Asian communities. Research funding of alternative medicine use in minority communities will have to address issues of poor outcomes in cardiovascular diseases, diabetes, and cancer. That is, research funding will require answers to questions such as: "What is the relationship between alternative health-care use and health disparity?" and, "If use contributes to disparity, to what extent?"

▶ HERBAL MEDICINE

Despite differences among national studies that examine and report use of specific therapies, one finding stands out. Herbal medicine is always one of the most frequently reported alternate therapies. In 2002, Mackenzie observed an overall 19% usage rate with high prevalence among Native (29%) and Asian Americans (26%).[24] Graham reported an 18.6% utilization rate based on 2002 data.[26]

More Americans have used herbal remedies since congressional approval of the Dietary Supplement Health and Education Act in 1994. This act allows distribution of herbs and supplements without Food and Drug Administration (FDA) regulation. Labeling restrictions prevent manufacturers from making claims regarding specific disease efficacy and require documentation of content, but without standardization. As a result, there are currently many different formulations and concentrations of herbal medicines on the market, including some with potentially toxic adulterants. Vague definitions of what constitutes an herb or a supplement and what distinguishes these substances from drugs further complicate the regulatory picture.

In contrast, Germany has regulated herbs and supplements since 1978. Herbal medications are standardized to increase the likelihood that consumers will obtain the same dose and active ingredient over time. Through Commission E, a scientific review panel, 300 herbs were evaluated and 190 recognized as suitable for medical use. Although Commission E disbanded in 1994, the Federal Health Agency in Germany developed a series of monographs on the herbs tested, which are internationally accepted as definitive works on the subject.[28]

Herbs are seed-producing annuals, biennials, or perennials that do not develop woody tissue, die at the end of the growing season, and have medicinal, savory, or aromatic qualities.[29] Chinese and East Indian cultures have used herbs for thousands of years. It is estimated that one third of the US population had tried herbs by 1990 and that approximately 60 million used herbs regularly by 1997. Predictably, herb–drug interactions increased during this period and are a constant threat.[30–33]

Unlike many alternative therapies, some herbal preparations have been studied under randomized controlled conditions.[34] Although some herb trials have shown a trend toward benefit, outcomes in many cases fail to reach statistical significance. As a result, claims of efficacy are mostly anecdotal.

Studies that have examined patient disclosure of herbal medicine usage find overwhelmingly that disclosure to primary healthcare providers is the exception rather than the rule. Eisenberg found that 72% of patients failed to discuss herbal medicine use with their physicians.[2] Liu et al[35] noted more than 50% of patients undergoing pre- or postoperative cardiothoracic surgical evaluation did not mention herbal medicine use to their physicians, a situation that could have serious safety implications. Kaye et al[36] observed a 70% nondisclosure rate, and Graham estimated greater than 60% nondisclosure using 2002 NHIS data.[26] Graham also found significant differences in disclosure rates by ethnicity. Hispanics, identified as the most frequent users of herbal medicine in the 2002 NHIS survey, had the lowest disclosure rate at 31.5%. Black respondents indicated a 35% disclosure rate and whites, 42%.[26]

The risks of nondisclosure are particularly serious with respect to herbal products, which are a focus of this chapter. Approximately 15 million adults in the United States are potentially at risk for potential adverse reactions from prescription medications, herbs, vitamin supplements, or all three.[28] The chronically ill, the elderly, persons with existing renal or liver disease, and those with diabetes should all be monitored carefully for risks associated with interaction effects between herbal therapies and prescribed pharmaceuticals. Patients scheduled for surgery should be evaluated preoperatively for potential adverse herb–drug interactions and, if doubts exist, the herbal agent should be discontinued 1 to 2 weeks prior to anesthesia and surgery. Vulnerable populations such as children and pregnant women, whose response to herbal therapies have not been studied, should be counseled not to use these agents. Persons receiving anticoagulants, hypoglycemics, antidepressants, or sedatives should also be carefully monitored for herbal therapy use, because the potential for interaction effects is high.[28]

There are many reasons why patients do not disclose herbal product use to their primary physicians. Physicians sometimes avoid asking about use of herbal agents because of time constraints or in the belief that asking will be considered an endorsement or will legitimize herbal therapies in the eyes of patients. Patients may be reluctant to volunteer information because they believe physicians may consider herbal medicine a rejection of mainstream medicine, incorrectly perceive it as a value judgment on the physician's services, or because they do not realize the information is relevant. Whereas pharmaceutical agents are often perceived as costly, high risk, and designed for the treatment of disease, herbal products are perceived as natural, safe, and designed for the promotion of health. However, "natural" does not necessarily mean safe, and "safe" does not necessarily mean effective.[28]

Given the risks of herbal products, healthcare providers cannot afford a "don't ask, don't tell" approach to herbal product usage and cannot wait for patients to volunteer this information. Regardless of the patient's ethnicity or race, the physician must initiate the discussion of herbal product use. In one study, having the physician ask was the single most significant predictor of patient disclosure of herbal product use.[37]

Physicians should elicit information on patients' use of alternative medicine as part of a comprehensive medical history.[38] It is important to convey a nonjudgmental attitude in assessing herbal use[28] and to record herbal usage patterns as part of the patient's documented history and treatment plan.[39] Patients should know the risks and benefits of their choices and that herbs have good and desirable effects as well as negative and undesirable ones.[28] Finally clinicians must be aware of trends in herbal therapy and share this information with patients.[28]

There are currently hundreds of herbs available for use. The following description of common products includes common name, scientific name, method of administration, active ingredient, known or purported action, side effects, and herb–drug interactions. Some popular nutritional supplements and home remedies are also included because they fall under the control of the 1994 Dietary Supplement Health and Education Act. The majority of these preparations are not recommended for use in pregnancy.[40,41]

Black Cohosh

Black cohosh (*Cimicifuga racemosa*), also called black snakeroot and bugbane, has been used for the treatment of rheumatic disorders, sedation, as an antitussive, and for menstrual pain. More recently it has been used to treat perimenopausal and postmenopausal symptoms. The dried root is used; it can also be given as a liquid extract or a tincture (in 60% ethanol). Active constituents include tannic acid, acetic acid, triterpene glycosides, and flavonoids, which are believed to exert hormonal, antiinflammatory, and circulatory effects.

Animal studies have shown that black cohosh blocks luteinizing hormone estrogen receptors and decreases inflammation by blocking neutrophil activity. Clinical trials in menopausal women have shown relief of vasomotor symptoms and "vaginal estrogenic effects" when compared with low-dose estrogen.

Headaches, dizziness, visual disturbance, and mild gastrointestinal upset have been reported with long-term use. Black cohosh is contraindicated in pregnancy and should be used with caution for extended periods and in patients with a history of breast cancer.

Chamomile

Chamomile comes from two plants (*Matricaria recutita,* German chamomile; and *M Anthemis nobilis,* Roman chamomile) that are members of the family Asteraceae. It is used for sedation, motion sickness, as an antispasmodic, and as an antidiarrheal. The flower heads contain warfarin and flavonoids, which have benzodiazepine-like, antihistaminic, and smooth muscle–relaxing effects. The dried flower heads are used, or a tincture (in 45% alcohol). Clinical studies of German chamomile have demonstrated sleep induction in patients undergoing cardiac catheterization.

Allergic reactions, including anaphylaxis and rashes, have been reported. Chamomile use is contraindicated in those with known hypersensitivity to ragweed or celery, and the herb should be avoided by asthmatic persons. Chamomile blocks coumadin and should be avoided by patients receiving anticoagulant therapy. Its use is not recommended in teething infants.

Echinacea

Echinacea (*Echinacea angustifolia, E pallida, E purpurea*), sometimes referred to as black Sampson and coneflower, has been used as an antiseptic, antiviral, and immunostimulant. The roots can be used dried, as a liquid extract, or a tincture (in alcohol).

Animal studies have shown a documented effect on inflammatory markers (ie, tumor necrosis factor), prompting its use in upper respiratory illnesses.[42] Recent clinical trials have not shown echinacea to be of benefit in viral upper respiratory infections.

Side effects include salivation and mouth burning. Allergic reactions and cross-reactions (eg, comfrey) have occurred. Because of its actions, echinacea may interfere with immunosuppressive therapy, particularly steroids.

Ephedra (Ma-Huang) and Mistletoe

These two herbs are included in this discussion because of their danger. Deaths have been reported with both.

Ephedra, known as *ma-huang* in Chinese herbal medicine, has been used as a stimulant, aphrodisiac, and weight-loss preparation, and as a treatment for cough, congestion, and asthma. Ephedra contained in weight-loss preparations has been linked to deaths in patients with coronary disease.

Mistletoe (*Viscum album*) traditionally has been used as a treatment for high blood pressure and hysteria and may have immunostimulant and antineoplastic properties. It interacts with many blood pressure and cardiac medications. The berries are highly poisonous; hepatotoxicity, shock, and death have been reported.

Feverfew

Feverfew (*Chrysanthemum parthenium, Pyrethrum parthenium,* and *Tanacetum parthenium*) has been used to treat migraine, fever, menstrual disorders, stomachache, toothache, and insect bites. The leaves can be ingested fresh or dried, with food; leaves and stems may also be used in teas and fluid extracts. Terpenes, flavonoids, and tannins in feverfew block inflammatory platelet aggregation and prostaglandins. Modern use is limited to migraine prevention.

Clinical trials have found feverfew to be superior to placebo in migraine relief. Side effects include mouth sores, abdominal pain, indigestion, diarrhea, flatulence, skin rash, and so-called postfeverfew syndrome (nervousness, headaches, insomnia, joint pain, and tiredness on stopping use of the herb).

Feverfew is contraindicated in persons with known hypersensitivity to members of the Asteraceae family (eg, chamomile, ragweed, and yarrow) and the Umbellefereae family (eg, celery, parsnips, carrots, dill, and parsley). Self-medication is not recommended; however, the herb may be used under physician supervision when conventional migraine therapy has failed. Its use is contraindicated in patients who develop a rash on contact.

Garlic

The bulb (clove) of garlic (*Allium sativum*) has been used for its reputed antihypertensive, antibacterial, antithrombotic, and lipid-lowering properties. It is widely used as a food flavoring. As a medicinal it is available as a dried bulb, tincture (in 45% alcohol), oil, juice, or decoction.

Some studies have shown garlic has a mild effect on lowering cholesterol, triglycerides, and blood pressure. However, because of the relatively mild effect, routine use of garlic alone in these conditions cannot be recommended. Other, animal studies suggest cellular protection against chemotherapeutic injury in the heart, colon, and liver. Cellular protective properties are related to the sulfur-containing constituents.

Toxicity of garlic produces mild symptoms such as burning of the mouth. Side effects include vomiting and diarrhea. Allergy (to sulfur-containing constituents) has been reported, and the odor has been shown to appear in breast milk. Theoretically, garlic could potentiate anticoagulants, antiinflammatory drugs, and agents used to treat hypertension, diabetes, and hyperlipidemia. It may also interfere with therapy for acquired immunodeficiency syndrome (AIDS).

Ginkgo Biloba

Ginkgo (*Ginkgo biloba*) has a history of medicinal use dating back to 2800 BC. The most important active ingredients in ginkgo extract are ginkgo flavonoids and terpenes lactones. In traditional Chinese medicine, the seeds were used for therapy as an antitussive, expectorant, and asthma treatment. Today the leaves are concentrated into extract (available in capsules) and used to treat memory loss, intermittent claudication, and cerebrovascular-induced tinnitus and vertigo.

Several studies have investigated the cognitive effect of ginkgo, and much has been written in the literature. Animal models have demonstrated an improvement in behavior and memory along with circulatory improvement. Other studies claim a cardioprotective effect against cardiotoxic chemotherapy. Human tissue culture studies suggest antioxidant properties may be the mechanism for neuroprotective effects. However, overall, the efficacy in the treatment of the listed conditions has not been seen in human trials of patients with Alzheimer dementia or healthy volunteers. Double-blind, randomized control trials are ongoing.

There have been some reports of allergic reactions to ginkgo; however, most of these reports involve fruit pulp and seeds, which should not be ingested. Side effects include headache, palpitations, gastrointestinal upset, and skin rashes. Excessive bleeding has occurred in some patients taking anticoagulants or antiplatelet agents.

Ginseng

Ginseng (*Panax ginseng, P notogingseng, P quinquefolius, P trifolus,* and *Eleutherococcus senticosus*) is an herb that comprises several species cultivated in different parts of the world. American varieties include *P quinquefolius* and *P trifolus;* other varieties are the Chinese *P ginseng* and *P notogingseng;* Russian (Siberian) *Eleutherococcus,* and Korean *P ginseng.*

The genus name *Panax* derives from the Greek word meaning "all-healing." The root of this herb, which resembles a human figure, has been used for over 2000 years to strengthen the body and improve vitality. It has been used to treat many conditions including asthenia, atherosclerosis, and colitis. Its main use has been as an antistress agent to stimu-

late the body and improve cognitive and physical performance. The main ingredient in the root, a chemical glycan, has hypoglycemic and cholesterol-lowering effects.

Ginseng can be consumed as a tea and is available in tablet and extract form. Side effects include anxiety, diarrhea, hypertension, bleeding, and changes in glucose and cholesterol metabolism. Ginseng can interact with anticoagulants, stimulants, and monoamine oxidase inhibitor (MAOI) antidepressants, as well as antidiabetic and cholesterol-lowering agents.

Kava-kava

Kava-kava (*Piper methysticum*) is a large shrub cultivated in Fiji and other islands of the South Pacific. The dried roots are used as a sedative and sleep aid, and for treatment of anxiety. There are more than 60 varieties, but the black and white types are most popularly used as a drink, consumed at room temperature. Kava drink has been compared with the Western cocktail for its relaxation properties. Kava ingredients produce analgesia and euphoria not blocked by naloxone (nonopiate pathway).

Toxic doses may cause muscle weakness and vertigo. Chronic ingestion (so-called kavism), characterized by a puffy face, scaly rash, dry discolored skin, and red eyes; it may be related to impaired cholesterol metabolism. Alcohol markedly increases the risk of toxicity.

Milk Thistle

Milk thistle (*Silybum marianus*) seeds and fruit have been used for disorders such as jaundice and colic and for diseases of the liver, gallbladder, and spleen. Current interest focuses on its hepatoprotectant properties. Silymarin, the main ingredient, is a combination of many compounds that have antioxidant properties.

Animal studies have shown hepatic cellular protection from many toxic compounds. Clinical trials in patients with alcoholic liver disease have shown improvement in liver enzymes. There have been many case reports in Europe of improvement in liver function when milk thistle is given early after death-cap mushroom (*A phalloides*) poisoning.

There are no known serious side effects. Mild laxative effects have been reported. Because long-term safety data are lacking, excessive use should be avoided. Milk thistle is contraindicated in persons with known hypersensitivity to the family Asteraceae, which includes ragweed, chamomile, and yarrow.

Saw Palmetto

Saw palmetto (*Serenoa repens*) has been used as a diuretic, and to increase breast size. More recently it has shown benefit in treating benign prostatic hypertrophy (BPH). The dried fruit of the herb, which may be used as a decoction (boiled solution), is composed of carbohydrates (sugars), fixed fatty acid oils, steroids, and flavonoid (antioxidants). It is also available as a standardized tablet.

It is believed sterol hexane compounds in the fruit block $5\{\alpha\}$-reductase conversion of testosterone to dihydrotestosterone (DHT) in several tissues, including the prostate. DHT, a more potent compound than testosterone, is known to be the major player in the development of BPH. In clinical trials, saw palmetto has been compared favorably with prazosin and finasteride.

Mild gastrointestinal side effects have occurred, as well as mild headache. The herb should not be used in patients with known prostate cancer. It may interfere with hormonal therapy, including birth control pills.

St John's Wort

St John's wort (*Hypericum perforatum*) is somewhat unique among herbal products in that it has been widely studied in randomized trials and found to be effective in the treatment of mild depression. Although the mechanism of action is not definitely known, it is thought to affect metabolism and uptake of both serotonin and dopamine. The dried, powdered, aboveground portion of the plant may be taken as a tea, tincture, tablet, or capsule.

More than 20 trials have shown St John's wort to be as effective as tricyclic antidepressants. The active ingredient, hypericin, is extracted from the stem of the plant and is available as tablets, capsules, and extracts. There are some relatively mild side effects, but more significantly, interactions with pharmaceuticals, especially HIV/AIDS drugs, digitalis, warfarin, and oral contraceptive pills.

Valerian

Valerian (*Valeriana officinalis*) is an herb native to temperate areas of the Americas, Europe, and Asia. The herbal product is produced from the dried, powdered root of the plant. Valerian is used as a sedative, particularly in the treatment of insomnia, and virtually all herbal sleep aids contain valerian. This herb contains many compounds that act synergistically, but sesquiterpenes are the primary source of its pharmacologic effects.

Valerian produces dose-dependent sedation and hypnosis. These effects appear to be mediated through modulation of $\{\gamma\}$-aminobutyric acid (GABA) neurotransmission and receptor function. In experimental animals, valerian increases barbiturate-induced sleep time. In one case study, valerian withdrawal mimicked acute benzodiazepine withdrawal syndrome after the patient presented with delirium and cardiac complications following surgery. Symptoms were attenuated by benzodiazepine administration. Based on these findings, valerian should be expected to potentiate the sedative effect of anesthetics and adjuvants, such as midazolam, that act at the GABA receptor.

Pharmacokinetics of valerian constituents have not been studied, although their effects are thought to be short lived. Avoid abrupt discontinuation of use in patients who may be physically dependent. With such patients, it may be prudent to taper the does of valerian over several weeks before surgery under close medical supervision.[39]

▶ NUTRITIONAL SUPPLEMENTS

DHEA (Dehydroepiandrosterone)

DHEA is a prohormone (a compound that is converted into a hormone in the body). It is produced primarily in the adrenal gland but also found in testes, ovaries, and brain tissue. DHEA is found midway in the synthetic pathway of cholesterol to testosterone in the adrenal gland. It is also converted to many other hormones in various tissues when needed. Ultimately testosterone increases body muscle mass, energy, and libido. DHEA supplements are marketed to improve bodybuilding, energy performance (vitality), and improve immunity. The compound is synthesized from wild yams in the laboratory.

Humans do not possess the enzyme necessary to extract DHEA from wild yams. Supplementation increases the body's supply of so-called downstream hormones. There appears to be no feedback control mechanism for DHEA; hence, supplementation is not believed to lower natural levels. However, effects on the feedback mechanism for downstream hormones and long-term, high-dose effects are not known. Reported side effects include increased facial hair, acne, menstrual irregularity, increased perspiration, and adverse effects on the prostate gland.

Glucosamine Sulfate and Chondroitin Sulfate

Both substances are building blocks of cartilage. Glucosamine (chitin) is found in yeast, fungi, arthropods, and various marine invertebrates, whereas chondroitin comes from sources such as shark and sheep cartilage or pig intestines. These compounds are often used together to treat osteoarthritis.

There is considerable controversy over oral absorption of chondroitin because of its large molecular size. The absorption of chondroitin is 0% to 13%, whereas the absorption of glucosamine is 90% to 98%. Chondroitin has been used as a drug delivery system for some of the older nonsteroidal antiinflammatory drugs (NSAIDs; eg, diclofenac and flurbiprofen). Clinical trials of glucosamine plus chondroitin compare favorably to ibuprofen, although effects may be attributable to glucosamine more than chondroitin. When compared with placebo in clinical x-ray studies of knee osteoarthritis, glucosamine use suggested cartilage regeneration. Comparative studies using magnetic resonance imaging of the knee are pending.

Mild gastrointestinal upset appears to be the predominant side effect. Maintenance use may cause increased bleeding or interaction with aspirin and NSAIDs.

Melatonin

Melatonin (*N*-acetyl-5-methoxytryptamine) is a hormone of the pineal gland whose release is stimulated by darkness. Secretion starts at 9 PM and peaks at 2 to 4 AM. Although not approved by the FDA as a drug, melatonin has been classified as an orphan drug for treatment of circadian rhythm sleep disorders in blind people since 1993. It is commercially available as a nutritional supplement either as a synthetic product or derived from animal pineal tissue. The FDA warns: "users are taking it without any assurance that it is safe or that it will have any beneficial effect." Further, use of the animal product is discouraged because of an increased risk of contamination or viral transmission.

Studies in the past decade have investigated melatonin use for treatment of jet lag, insomnia, pregnancy prevention, boosting the immune system, preventing cancer, protecting cells from free radical damage, and even extending life. Side effects include headache, depression, menstrual irregularity in women, and residual somnolence.

Soy (Tofu)

Soybeans (*Glycine max leguminosae*) are used as a dietary source of fiber, protein, and minerals, particularly in Eastern cultures. Products derived from soybeans include soy milk (used by those allergic to cow's milk), flour, curd, tofu (a cheeselike cake high in protein and calcium), sauce, oils, and drinks, among others. Asian cultures consume on average 2 to 3 ounces per day compared with Western diets, which include one tenth that amount.

Isoflavones in soy may have anticancer effects, alleviate menopausal symptoms, and combat cardiovascular disease. The so-called phytoestrogens in soy are believed to be responsible for longer menstrual cycles and reduced breast cancer rates in Asian women, as well as for lower incidence of prostate cancer in Asian men. Clinical studies of menopausal hot flushes showed up to 45% reduction in women taking 45 g soy flour daily. Modest lowering of cholesterol has been shown with increased fiber in soy and oat bran.

Side effects include bloating and flatulence. Soy dust inhalation has caused allergic asthma.

▶ HOME REMEDIES

So-called home or folk remedies have been a mainstay of treatment for a wide range of common ailments by people of many cultures. A few of the more common remedies are described here; for more information, the reader is referred to references 40 and 41, listed at the end of this chapter.

Aloe Vera

Aloe has been used in ointments and creams to assist in healing of wounds, burns, eczema, and psoriasis. Anti-inflammatory effects have been seen in intradermal animal studies. Aloe has been associated with hypoglycemia when ingested.

Castor Oil

Castor oil (*Ricinus communis*) is used medicinally as a laxative and for other conditions in the African American community (eg, colds, external skin eruptions, and various other conditions).

Cranberry

Several species of cranberry are native to North America, including the large, or bog cranberry (*Vaccinium macrocarpon*) and other variants (*V edule, V erythrocarpum, V oxycoccos,* and *V vitis*). Cranberry juice has antiseptic properties and has been used for prevention of urinary tract infections. It is known to prevent attachment of *Escherichia coli* to the bladder wall. The dose used in clinical trials for the prevention of urinary tract infections is 300 mL cranberry juice cocktail (containing 30% cranberry concentrate) daily for 6 months. Caloric content should be borne in mind for those who require caloric reduction. Diabetic patients should be encouraged to use sugar-free preparations. There are no known serious side effects, although some patients have developed diarrhea.

Green Tea

Green tea is produced from leaves of the tea plant (*Camellia sinensis*), which is native to India and China. Different processing of the leaves produces black tea. Compounds in green tea leaves are believed to reduce cancer risk, lower lipids, and reduce dental caries through antioxidant effects. Caffeine, tannins, and flavonoids, which are also present in the leaves, are believed to be responsible for side effects, which include nervousness, insomnia, and tachycardia.

In one human study, 9 cups per day of green tea were required to lower lipid levels. Recently, green tea has replaced ephedra in herbal diet preparations. Animal and culture studies have demonstrated the ability of compounds in tea to inhibit microbial growth and cellular transformation (mutagenesis).

Vinegar

Vinegar contains acetic acid, which has no known medicinal purposes and may cause esophageal or gastric erosion if swallowed full strength. It has been used by hypertensive African American patients for blood pressure control, and by diabetic patients for glucose control. It has no known therapeutic effect in either condition.

Witch Hazel

Witch hazel (*Hamamelis virginiana*), which grows as a small shrub or tree in North America, was used by Native Americans to treat swellings and injuries. An extract of the bark has astringent properties and is used as an antiseptic. Stomach irritation occurs when ingested, and internal use is not recommended.

▶ FAITH-BASED MEDICINE

Faith and religious treatment methods are integral parts of the health-care systems of many cultures (Native American, African American, and many others). Special prayers for the sick and shut-ins are part of most African American church services. Some sources of research have confirmed statistically better health outcomes in "religious" versus "nonreligious" patients.[43,44] Use of charms, amulets, and other external articles to promote healing has deep roots in Native American and African cultures. Native American sweat lodges, which were the site for ritual healings replete with aromatics and prayers, are another example of faith-based healing. The effect of belief as a tool in healing continues to be studied.

Intercessory Prayer

This form of prayer seeks to affect health outcomes by invoking spiritual support on behalf of the patient (knowingly or unknowingly). Reports of benefit in religious patients with conditions such as depression, alcoholism, smoking, colon cancer, breast cancer, and coronary heart disease have been described in medical journals. Theoretical mechanisms for these outcomes include changes in electromagnetic energy fields, changes in DNA conformation, and immune system enhancement. The ancient Eastern art of meditation is believed to exert positive effects through some of these mechanisms, and similar concepts are believed to underlie several of the other modalities described in Appendix 31-A, whose effect is thought to be a result of influences on consciousness.

Hoodoo and Voodoo

Hoodoo and voodoo are faith-based practices that have the potential to influence health care. These terms are often used inaccurately and interchangeably, usually by peoples of European origin. Although both practices are distinctly African American, with very prominent African origins, they are quite noticeably different.

Hoodoo is believed to have originated in East and Central Africa.[45] Since the days of slavery, African Americans on the East Coast of the United States have practiced hoodoo (also called *root medicine* because of the strong herbal influence). This practice was particularly popular on the barrier islands of South Carolina and Georgia. Practitioners concoct potions, balms, and powders, and wear charms, usually to obtain positive outcomes.

Voodoo, also called *vodun,* is one of the world's oldest religions, which originated among the Yoruba tribe in Africa. Slaves brought the religion to the Americas by way of Haiti. Voodoo is also practiced by African peoples in South American countries such as Brazil, where it is called *candomblé.* The basis of the religion can be found in the translation of *vodun,* which means "spirit." Practitioners of voodoo believe that "every spirit is connected to every other spirit," and that these spirits can be controlled through incantation and will.[46] In this way, good health and bad health, for instance, can be controlled

► ESTABLISHING EFFICACY

The selective integration of CAM with conventional medicine must be approached with caution. CAM, like conventional medicine, has pros and cons, promotes good ideas and bad ones, and has both risks and benefits.[47] Without critical assessment of what should be integrated and what should not, the United States risks developing a health-care system that costs more, is less safe, fails to address management of chronic disease in a publicly responsible manner, and may contribute to disparities in health status.

In the United States, there is little incentive to test alternative therapies via randomized controlled trials.[48] Before corporate inventors of new therapies embark on the stringent process of FDA approval and regulation, there must be some potential for economic gain. Alternative medicine products are openly available as well as nonproprietary ones, which eliminates the research incentive for many corporations. Acting in the public interest, the US government promotes CAM research through the National Center for Complementary and Alternative Medicine, and it has played a key role in development of therapies for rare diseases that have limited markets for related inventions.[48]

The first step toward establishing a CAM evidence base was taken in 1996 when the Cochrane Collaboration created a complementary medicine field within its database. The Cochrane Collaboration produces, maintains, and disseminates systematic reviews on all topics in health care through its database and the Cochrane Controlled Trials Registry. Both are updated quarterly. Systematic reviews provide a cogent method for synthesizing and summarizing evidence on a given topic.[34]

► SUMMARY AND RECOMMENDATIONS

National surveys document the fact that significant numbers of Americans, including ethnic and racial minorities, use alternative therapies, either alone or in conjunction with conventional medicine. Some CAM therapies are deeply rooted in centuries of cultural tradition. But it is also clear that lack of medical insurance and the resulting lack of access to allopathic health services accounts for some use of CAM by ethnic and racial minorities, particularly Hispanics.

The 21st century has begun with dramatic advances in medical technology. Treatments that are standard today, such as lasers and photodynamic therapy, gamma knife surgery, and gene splicing, would have been considered alternative several decades ago. As science better understands and controls the energies of the atomic and subatomic world, refines its computational abilities, and decodes genetic mysteries, its ability to evaluate alternative healing measures in existence for thousands of years will greatly improve.

Selection of the "right" treatment for the "right" patient with the "right" disease at the "right" time will become much easier. Herbal remedies, for instance, may prove to be the most appropriate treatment for select patients with mild hyperlipidemia or osteoarthritis. Exposure to concentrated electromagnetic, nuclear, or proton energy fields might be used to treat patients with varied conditions such as depression, autoimmune disease, or asthma. Science may have to redefine its methods of measuring benefit until it develops the technologic capacity to measure elusive end points.

Ignoring or treating CAM as something outside the normal processes of medicine and science is no longer an option. Research in alternative medicine will help establish what is safe and effective and what is not.[47] Given the broad use of alternative medicine, as well as the possibility some therapies will prove beneficial, clinicians must endorse legitimate efforts to evaluate conventional and alternative treatments. Armed with these data, harmful or useless practices can be abandoned and physicians better positioned to help their patients make informed decisions that allow them to reach health-related goals.[38] As public use of healing practices outside conventional medicine accelerates, ignorance about these practices by physicians and scientists risks broadening the communication gap between the public and the health professions that serve them.[47]

▶ REFERENCES

1. Snyder M, Lindquist R. *Complementary/Alternative Therapies in Nursing,* 4th ed. New York, NY: Springer; 2002:xiii.

2. Eisenberg DM, Kessler RC, Foster C, et al. Unconventional medicine in the United States: Prevalence, costs, and patterns of use. *N Engl J Med* 1993;328(4):246–252.

3. Wetzel MS, Eisenberg DM, Kaptchuk TJ. Courses involving complementary and alternative medicine at US medical schools. *JAMA* 1998;280(9):784–787.

4. Barrett B. Complementary and alternative medicine: What's it all about? *WMJ* 2001; 100(7):20–26.

5. Struthers R, Nichols LA. Utilization of complementary and alternative medicine among racial and ethnic minority populations: Implications for reducing health disparities. *Ann Rev Nurs Res* 2004;22:285–313.

6. Ernst E. Complementary medicine: A definition. *Br J Gen Pract* 1995;45:506.

7. Ni H, Simile C, Hardy AM. Utilization of complementary and alternative medicine by United States adults: Results from the 1999 National Health Interview Survey. *Med Care* 2002;40(4):353–358.

8. Eisenberg DM, Davis RB, Ettner SL, et al. Trends in alternative medicine use in the United States, 1990–1997: Results of a follow-up national survey. *JAMA* 1998;208(18):1569–1575.

9. Astin JA. Why patients use alternative medicine. *JAMA* 1998;279(19):1548–1553.

10. Barnes PM, Powell-Griner E, McFann K, et al. Complementary and alternative medicine use among adults: United States, 2002. Advance data from vital and health statistics; No. 343. Hyattsville, Md: National Center for Health Statistics; 2004.

11. Bausell RB, Lee WL, Berman BM. Demographic and health-related correlates to visits to complementary and alternative medical providers. *Med Care* 2001;39(2):190–196.

12. Oldenick R, Coker AL, Wieland D, et al. Population-based survey of complementary and alternative medicine usage, patient satisfaction, and physician involvement. *South Med J* 2002; 93(4):375–381.

13. Rafferty AP, McGee HB, Miller CE, et al. Prevalence of complementary and alternative medicine use: State-specific estimates from the 2001 Behavioral Risk Factor Surveillance System. *Am J Pub Health* 2002;92(10):1598–1600.

14. Georges CA. President Clinton's new racial and ethnic disparities initiative. *Ethn Dis* 1998;8(2):257–258.

15. Anderson NB. Behavioral and sociocultural perspectives on ethnicity and health: Introduction to the special issue. *Health Psychol* 1995;14(7):589–591, 1995.

16. Elo IT, Preston SH. Racial and ethnic differences in mortality at older ages. In: Martin LG, Soldo DJ, eds. *Racial and Ethnic Differences in the Health of Older Americans.* Washington, DC: National Academy Press; 1997.

17. Bernard MA, Lampley-Dallas V, Smith L. Common health problems among minority elders. *J Am Diet Assoc* 1997;97(7):771–776.

18. *Report of the Working Group on Research in Coronary Heart Disease in Blacks.* Washington, DC: National Heart, Lung, Blood Institute; 1994:1–94.

19. Manuel RC. The physical, psychological, and social health of black older Americans. In: Livingston IL, ed *Handbook of Black American Health.* Westport, Conn: Greenwood Press; 1994:300–314.

20. Levine RS, Foster JE. Black–white inequalities in mortality and life expectancy 1993–1999: Implications for Healthy People 2010. *Public Health Rep* 2001;116(5):1–9.

21. US Dept of Health and Human Services. *Healthy People 2010,* conference ed. Washington, DC: DHHS; 2000.
22. US Dept of Health and Human Services, Task Force on Black and Minority Health. *Report of the Secretary's Task Force on Black and Minority Health.* Washington, DC: DHHS; 1985.
23. Smedley BD, Stith AY, Nelson AR. Unequal treatment: Confronting racial and ethnic disparities in health care. Washington, DC: National Academy Press; 2003.
24. Mackenzie ER, Taylor L, Bloom BS, et al. Ethnic minority use of complementary and alternative medicine (CAM): A national probability survey of CAM utilizers. *Altern Med* 2003;9(4):50–56.
25. Keith VM, Kronenfeld JJ, Rivers PA, et al. Assessing the effects of race and ethnicity on use of complementary and alternative therapies in the USA. *Ethn Health* 2005;10(1):19–32.
26. Graham RE, Ahn AC, Davis RB, et al. Use of complementary and alternative medical therapies among racial and ethnic minority adults: Results from the 2002 National Health Interview Survey. *J Nat Med Assoc* 2005;97(4):535–545.
27. Rust G, Fryer G, et al. Modifiable determinants of healthcare utilization within the African-American population. *J Nat Med Assoc* 2004;96(9):1169–1177.
28. O'Malley P, Trimble N, Browning M. Are herbal therapies worth the risks? *Nurs Pract* 2004;29(10):71–75.
29. Bauer BA. Herbal therapy: What a clinician needs to know to counsel patients effectively. *Mayo Clin Proc* 2000;75(8):835–841.
30. Harnack LJ, Rydell SA, Stang J. Prevalence of use of herbal products by adults in the Minneapolis/St. Paul, Minn, metropolitan area. *Mayo Clin Proc* 2001;76(7):688–694.
31. Rogers EA, Gough JE, Brewer KL. Are emergency department patients at risk for herb-drug interactions? *Acad Emerg Med* 2001;8(9):932–934.
32. Izzo AA, Ernst E. Interaction between herbal medicines and prescribed drugs. A systemic review. *Drugs* 2001;61(15):2163–2175.
33. Ebbesen J, Buajordet I, Erikssen J, et al. Drug-related deaths in a department of internal medicine. *Arch Intern Med* 2001;161(19):2317–2323.
34. Ezzo J, Berman BM, Vickers AJ, et al. Complementary medicine and the Cochrane Collaboration. *JAMA* 1998;280(18):1628–1630.
35. Liu EH, Turner LM, Lin SX, et al. Use of alternative medicine by patients undergoing cardiac surgery. *J Thorac Cardiovasc Surg* 2000;120:335–341.
36. Kaye AD, Clarke RC, Sabar R, et al. Herbal medicines: Current trends in anesthesiology practice—a hospital survey. *J Clin Anesth* 2000;12(6):468–471.
37. Busse JW, Heaton G, Wu P, et al. Disclosure of natural product use to primary care physicians: A cross-sectional survey of naturopathic clinic attendees. *Mayo Clin Proc* 2005;80(5):616–623.
38. Sugarman J, Burk L. Physicians' ethical obligations regarding alternative medicine. *JAMA* 1998;280(18):1623–1625.
39. Ang-Lee MK, Moss J, Yuan CS. Herbal medicines and perioperative care. *JAMA* 2001;286(2):208–216.
40. Barnes J, Anderson L, Phillipson JD. *Herbal Medicine 2002.* London, England: Pharmaceutical Press; 2002.
41. *A Guide to Popular Natural Products.* Philadelphia, Pa: Facts and Comparisons/Kluwer; 1999.
42. Turner RB, Bauer R, Woelkart K, et al. An evaluation of *Echinacea angustifolia* in experimental rhinovirus infections. *N Engl J Med* 2005;353(4):341–348.
43. Byrd RC. Positive therapeutic effects of intercessory prayer in a coronary care unit population. *South Med J* 1988;81:826–829.
44. Joyce CRB, Weldon RMC. The objective efficacy of prayer: A double-blind clinical trial. *J Chronic Dis* 1965;18:367–377.
45. Yronwode C. *Hoodoo in Theory & Practice, Introduction to African-American Rootwork.* 1995–2003. http://www.luckymojo.com/hoodoo.html
46. West African Dahomean Vodoun: Historical Background. Available at: http://www.mamiwata.com/history.html
47. Jonas WB. Alternative medicine–learning from the past, examining the present, advancing to the future. *JAMA* 1998;280(18):1616–1617.
48. Eskinazi DP. Factors that shape alternative medicine. *JAMA* 1998;280(18):1621–1623.

APPENDIX 31-A

Complementary and Alternative Therapies Listed in the NHIS Survey

The following table provides descriptions of the 10 provider-based and 8 self-administered therapies listed in the Alternative Health/ Complementary and Alternative Medicine sup- plemental questionnaire of the 2002 National Health Interview Survey (NHIS). For more de- tailed information, the reader is referred to the many other resources available on these topics.

Provider-Based Therapies

Acupuncture

Acupuncture is an ancient Eastern discipline that dates to 1500 BC and derives in part from the principles of Taoism.[1] A basic premise is that health is a balance of *Qi* (pronounced chee), the energy flow of the body. Disease results from an imbalance of *yin* and *yang,* the dark and bright sides of health (for further explanation of this concept, see the discussion of qi gong, below). Organ function and dysfunction are classified as yin or yang, and organs are further classified according to their relationship to the five elements (natural resources): wood, fire, earth, metal, and water. Disease or dysfunction is viewed as the result of disproportion in the elements, causing an imbalance of yin and yang and obstruction of the natural flow of Qi. Acupuncture treatments are believed to restore the natural flow through modalities described below. Traditional Chinese medicine (TCM) incorporates acupuncture and herbal medicine to achieve balance.

Modification of the body's energy flow (Qi) in acupuncture is accomplished by focusing on longitudinal lines, called *meridians,* that run in and around the body. Twelve major meridians exist, along with a number of divergent meridians, producing a total of 361 acupuncture points. Each meridian is connected to a specific yin or yang organ. Each acupuncture point is related to an anatomic structure and has a name and serial number. Practitioners use small-gauge, stainless-steel needles at so-called acupoints to adjust Qi (the FDA has mandated disposable needles in the United States). The technique of needle insertion and manipulation may take several forms, including "cupping," twisting, heating (moxibustion), pressure (acupressure), and electrical stimulation.

Many of the meridians and acupoints are associated with underlying nerve structures, and acupuncture has been shown to be ineffective below the level of neurologic injury in quadriplegics and paraplegics. Investigators have found electrical properties associated with acupoint manipulation, and human and animal studies have shown release of neurotransmitters associated with acupuncture treatments.[2-5] Moreover, the effect of acupuncture can be abolished by pretreatment with procaine and blocked by naloxone (an opiate antagonist), effects not seen with placebo. Alcohol and steroids inhibit the effect of acupuncture, and patients are advised to avoid their use before therapy.

Continued

The use of acupuncture has grown remarkably in the United States over the past two decades and today totals 10 to 12 million patient visits per year. Expenses are usually out of pocket. Patients are more likely to be white or Asian than African American or Hispanic. The typical consumer is a 25- to 49-year-old white woman with a college degree.

Acupuncture has been used in the treatment of many conditions, including osteoarthritis and other pain syndromes, hypertension, anxiety, substance abuse, chemotherapy-induced and postoperative nausea, and preoperative anesthesia. Studies of acupuncture treatments in many disease states are ongoing by the National Institutes of Health. Side effects include warmth, relaxation, increased energy, local irritation, and, rarely, vasovagal episodes at initial needle insertion. Very rare cases of hepatitis B, pneumothorax, and pericardial tamponade have been reported.

Ayurvedic Medicine

Ayurveda (pronounced aa-yoor-VAY-da) is an East Indian system of holistic medical practice that attempts to treat diseases and maintain health through several methods, including herbs, aroma, massage, purgatives, and meditation. The central principle of Ayurveda is the belief that beings and their organs are related to elements (space, air, fire, water, and earth), which are in balance with essences or *doshas* (*Vata, Pitta,* and *Kapha*). The combination of elements and essences make up the character of the organ and the individual. Disease and dysfunction are the result of imbalance. Multiple therapies are required to restore balance and health.

Biofeedback

Biofeedback consists of therapeutic procedures that use electronic or electromechanical instruments to measure, process, and feed information about neuromuscular and autonomic functions back to patients and their therapists. Feedback is delivered in the form of analog or binary auditory or visual signals. The objectives of this therapy are to help the patient develop greater awareness of his or her physiologic processes and increase voluntary control over them by controlling the external signal and using cognitions, sensations, and other cues to stop or reduce the associated somatic expression.[6]

Chelation

Chelation therapy has been approved in the United States for treatment of heavy metal poisonings (ie, lead and mercury, arsenic poisoning, or iron overload). Several different compounds are able to bind to metals in blood, causing subsequent removal from the body through urine. EDTA (ethylenediaminetetraacetic acid) is recommended for acute lead and mercury poisoning. Other chelating substances include dimercaprol, BAL (British anti-Lewisite), d-penicillamine, and deferoxamine. Naturally occurring human chelating substances include vitamin B_{12}, heme molecules in hemoglobin, and porphyrins. A common component of all chelating molecules is a metallic center, which helps the molecule attach to other metals. Intravenous administration is required for chelating substances used in poisonings.[7]

Recent claims of the success of chelation in reducing atherosclerotic plaques have not been supported by clinical studies (calcium binding, an adjunctive effect of chelation, is the basis for these claims). Oral and rectal forms of EDTA are marketed for use, but it is doubtful they enter the bloodstream or tissues because of their water solubility. Other conditions for which benefit has been claimed include peripheral vascular disease, Alzheimer disease, and aging.[8,9] Renal damage is the main side effect of chelation therapy.

Continued

Continued

Chiropractic

Chiropractic is a nonpharmacologic discipline and one of the manipulation and touch therapies that focuses on spine and joint alignment and manipulation to effect treatment of several painful and nonpainful conditions. According to chiropractic theory, subluxation (forward movement of the bony spine) compresses nerve roots, producing pain, disease, and dysfunction. Realignment yields pain relief as well as correcting disease states. There are over 50,000 chiropractic doctors in the United States. By 2010, this number is expected to double to more than 100,000. Chiropractic services are utilized by 11% to 20% of the US population.

Energy Healing (Reiki)

Reiki (pronounced RAY-key) is a Japanese form of energy healing that focuses on restoring order in a person whose vital energy has become unbalanced. Practitioners use specific techniques in an attempt to restore and balance energy within the patient's body and enhance the body's natural ability to heal itself.

The concept of *chakra* is foundational to several disciplines of alternative medicine and TCM and is used in reiki, as well as meditation, yoga, and therapeutic touch. Practitioners of these disciplines view *chakras* (from the Sanskrit word for "wheel") as electromagnetic energy centers that are a manifestation of consciousness and the physical body. According to this view, the body has seven major chakras and several minor ones. Disease represents abnormal flow, and treatment and cure represent establishment of natural flow, in effect, a healing of consciousness that heals the body.

Most reiki treatments do not involve actual touching. Rather, the practitioner holds his or her hands over the patient's body and seeks to manipulate the energy field from there. Reiki practitioners may also incorporate other alternative healing practices, such as meditation and aromatherapy.[10]

Folk Medicine

Refer to the discussion of "Home Remedies" in Chapter 31.

Hypnosis

Hypnosis is an altered state of consciousness characterized by a state of intensified attention, receptiveness, and an increased responsiveness to suggestions or sets of ideas. Individuals in a hypnotic state show heightened suggestibility, narrowed awareness, selective wakefulness, and focused attentiveness. The goal of hypnotic therapy is to produce desirable changes in habits, motivations, self-image, and lifestyle.[11]

Massage[12]

Massage therapies can be classified into three groups: (1) manipulative techniques, (2) energy methods, and (3) hybrid therapies that include both. In addition to producing a pleasurable feeling, massage therapy theoretically relaxes muscle tension and allows more oxygen and nutrients to reach body cells and tissues. Massage therapy is accompanied by the release of natural painkillers (eg, serotonin) and enhanced immune function.

The most common form of massage in the United States is Swedish massage, which is usually given on a massage table or special massage chair, often using aromatic oils as a lubricant. The oil is stroked and kneaded on all parts of the body using smooth stroking (*effleurage*) and kneading (*petrissage*) movements up and down the back and across the shoulder and neck muscles and the backs of the legs, feet, arms, and hands. Stroking on the front is done across the stomach, front of the legs and arms, face, and forehead.

The Trager method, named after its developer, involves gentle holding and rocking of body parts. The arms and legs are held individually in different positions suspended to the side or above the body, then gently rocked back and forth. This is a gentle form of massage, and the Trager method is preferred for people with generalized pain because no pressure is applied to sore tissues.

Reflexology procedures are centered on particular points of the hands, feet, and ears. Reflexology is considered an energy method, although it also could be called a massage therapy because it involves kneading, stroking, rubbing, and other massage procedures. Reflexologists believe energy from the point that is touched is transmitted across a network of nerves to other parts of the body, such as the back or stomach. The feet and hands are considered to be connected to the rest of the body (the heel to the lower back; the middle of the foot to the stomach area; the ball of the foot to the heart and lungs; and the toes to the head, eyes, and mouth). Thus, when one of these points is touched, its connecting structure is affected. Little is known about the origins of this therapy, and no empiric data are available on the use of this method.

Naturopathy

Naturopathy is an eclectic form of health care that incorporates many different complementary modalities in the treatment and prevention of disease. It is not limited to a single modality of healing and cannot be identified with any one therapeutic approach. Treatment protocols are integrative in nature, combining the most suitable therapies to address the individual patient's needs.[13]

Self-Administered Therapies

Herbal Medicine

Also called *botanical medicine;* refer to the discussion of "Herbal Medicine" in Chapter 31.

Homeopathy

The German physician Samuel Hahnemann developed the practice of homeopathy in the late 1700s. His theory of treatment was based on a "law of similars," which claimed that the administration of small dilutions of offending substances would produce a cure in patients. This assertion is the exact opposite of the dose–response principle demonstrated by the pharmaceutical industry. Current estimates indicate Americans spend $200 million annually on homeopathic care.[14] There is no scientific evidence to support the efficacy of homeopathic treatments.

Megavitamin Therapy

Megavitamin therapy, also known as *orthomolecular therapy,* is generally defined as ingestion of one or more vitamins in amounts 10 or more times the recommended daily allowance (RDA) established by the Committee on Dietary Allowances of the Food and Nutrition Board, US National Research Council. The popular literature on megadoses of vitamins often claims efficacy and makes recommendations for usage based on theories portrayed as fact, preliminary findings, or extrapolation of vitamin effects observed in deficiency syndromes. There is a paucity of well-designed randomized controlled trials establishing these claims, and consumers are rarely aware of toxicities associated with some vitamins when ingested in megadoses.[15]

Qi Gong[16]

Before discussing qi gong (pronounced chee-gung), it is helpful to explore the concept of Qi in Chinese culture. *Qi,* which may be translated as "air," "puff," or "power," refers to the universal life force that exists in all living things. No comparable word exists in English. In Japanese, it is called *Ki* (as in rei*ki*), and in Sanskrit, *Prana.*

Qi can be compared with the electrical charge in a battery. A new battery has a full electrical charge, which can be used to operate a radio, boom box, or electric toy. When the battery is old, exhausted of all electrical charge, it no longer can be used for any battery-powered item. When a person is full of Qi, he or she can work or be active without fatigue. When the body is low in Qi, it becomes tired easily. A person with chronic fatigue syndrome can be said to be chronically low in Qi. When a person's body is exhausted of Qi, the person is dead. Qi gong (which roughly translated means "cultivating energy") and tai chi (discussed later) are techniques that use special exercises designed to increase Qi in the body.

Continued

Continued

A verbal tradition of practices resembling qi gong may go back 10,000 years in China.[16] The inventors of these practices imitated animals and nature to invent different sets of exercises to enhance Qi and prolong life. It is estimated that there are 7000 to 8000 different sets of qi gong exercises. The exercises integrate physical postures, breathing techniques, and focused intention. Some qi gong exercises are specific for certain illnesses or diseases, such as breast cancer and Parkinson disease. Qi gong and tai chi exercises differ from traditional physical exercises in the following ways: (1) they are performed slowly (the slower one performs these exercises, the more effective they are); (2) they require full focus and concentration; (3) they involve attention to breathing, which is used to direct the flow of Qi within the body; and (4) they require relaxation (because even the slightest tension can impede the flow of Qi).

Relaxation Techniques

Meditation, guided imagery, progressive relaxation, and deep-breathing exercises are techniques that are often recommended to patients as ways to reduce anxiety, stress, and chronic pain. These techniques help to reduce tension and produce a state of relaxation. The physiologic effects may be similar to those produced by massage, described earlier.

Meditation is a self-directed practice for relaxing the body and calming the mind. Most meditative techniques used in the West are derived from the religious practices of India, China, and Japan, but related concepts are found in many cultures worldwide. In recent decades, meditation has been studied as a way to reduce blood cortisol levels (an indicator of stress), high blood pressure, chronic pain, and anxiety.[17]

Guided imagery uses the mental process of imagining to induce a state of relaxation and alleviate stress. It has been used as an adjunctive therapy to reduce symptoms in cancer patients and to control pain in a variety of settings.[17]

Special Diets

The 2002 NHIS asked respondents about their use of six special diets:

1. **Vegetarian diet.** In its broadest definition, being "vegetarian" means avoiding foods from animal sources. Instead, plant sources of food—grains, legumes, nuts, vegetables, and fruits—form the basis of the diet. Variations of vegetarian diets include the following[18]:
   a. **Lacto-ovo-vegetarian.** A person who chooses an eating approach with eggs and dairy products but no meat, poultry, and fish. The prefix "lacto-" refers to milk; "ovo" refers to eggs. Most vegetarians in the United States fit within this category.
   b. **Lacto-vegetarian.** A person who avoids meat, poultry, fish, and eggs (including egg derivatives such as albumin or egg whites) but eats dairy products.
   c. **Strict vegetarian.** Also termed *vegan* (VEE-gahn or VEHJ-ahn), a person who follows an eating plan with no animal products; that is, no meat, poultry, fish, eggs, milk, cheese, or other dairy products.
   d. **Semivegetarian.** A person who usually follows a vegetarian eating pattern but occasionally eats meat, poultry, or fish.
2. **Macrobiotic diet.** A macrobiotic diet is an extremely restrictive diet that includes some grains and a few vegetables. It gradually eliminates food categories and restricts fluids. Macrobiotic diets do not follow basic principles of healthful eating and are deficient in many essential nutrients.[18]
3. **Atkins diet.** The Atkins diet is a low-carbohydrate diet plan that focuses on consumption of nutrient-rich unprocessed foods and nutrient supplementation. Carbohydrate consumption is limited to 20 g/day, primarily from leafy greens and nonstarchy vegetables. The Atkins diet strictly controls consumption of processed and refined carbohydrates such as high-sugar foods, bread, pasta, cereal, and starchy vegetables.[19]

Continued

4. **Pritikin diet.** The Pritikin diet, developed by Nathan Pritikin, is a low-fat, high-carbohydrate diet plan. It stresses calorie reduction for weight loss, but instead of calculating calories per food item, dieters plan the calorie content of a meal. The focus is on unprocessed foods such as fruit and vegetables. The diet incorporates a healthy range of foods and generous portions, which are filling but low in calories.[20]

5. **Ornish diet.** The Ornish diet is a low-fat, mainly vegetarian diet plan that is part of a lifestyle modification program developed by Dean Ornish in the 1980s with the goal of reversing the effects of cardiovascular disease. Meat, poultry, and fish are not recommended and only a few low-fat dairy products are allowed.[21,22]

6. **Zone diet.** The Zone diet, created by Barry Sears, is designed to produce a physiologic state in which hormones governed by dietary intake (insulin and eicosanoids) are maintained within zones that are neither too high nor too low. The goals for daily intake are 40% carbohydrates, 30% fat, and 30% protein, but diets are personally calculated for each individual and are not generalizable to others. The diet rigidly prescribes amounts of foods that can be eaten, with the goal of achieving consistent insulin control, and requires supplementation of high-dose fish oil to modulate synthesis of arachidonic acid. The Zone diet involves a significant calorie reduction for most users.[23]

Tai Chi [16]

Tai chi has been practiced by the Chinese for thousands of years. The word *Tai* means "big, extreme," and *Chi* means "utmost, excellence." Approximately 1700 years ago, the Chinese physician Huo To emphasized physical and mental exercises as a means of improving health. He believed that humans should exercise and imitate the movements of animals—such as birds, tigers, snakes, and bears—to recover original life abilities that had been lost. He organized these exercises into a folkloric fighting art called *Five Animals Games*. This was the first Systematized martial art in China.

Over the centuries, various martial arts were developed in China. These can be divided into the so-called external and internal marital arts. The external martial arts (kung fu, tae kwon do, karate, and others) emphasize training techniques and building up the body. These martial arts rely on a person's physical brute strength (*Li*) to defend against and overcome opponents. Internal martial arts (such as tai chi) emphasize, first, the development and building up of Qi in the body, and later, the application of Qi to the physical techniques of self-defense.

There are many different types of tai chi, but all derive from an original set of 13 movements imitating the natural movements of animals. The most popular type in the United States is called yang-style tai chi. Its slow-motion movements—which involve a combination of balance, movement, strength development, and body awareness—are often recommended as a means of improving mobility in older people, because they help to stretch and strengthen muscles, improve balance, and increase circulation to the extremities.

Yoga[24,25]

Yoga developed in India as a school of Hindu philosophy that advocates and prescribes a course of physical and mental disciplines for attaining liberation from the material world and union of the self with the Supreme Being or ultimate principle. For its devotees, yoga is a way of life that comprises ethical precepts, diet, and physical exercise. In the United States, the physical techniques are practiced by many people who do not subscribe to the full philosophical approach. These physical exercises include a series of postures and breathing exercises practiced to gain control of the body and mind and achieve tranquility. Researchers have investigated the therapeutic potential of yoga to control physiologic parameters such as blood pressure, heart rate, respiratory function, metabolic rate, and body temperature.

Continued

Continued

[1] Dorfer L, Moser M, Spindler K, et al. 5200-year-old acupuncture in central Europe? *Science* 1998;282:242–243.

[2] Knardahl S, Elam M, Olausson B, et al. Sympathetic nerve activity after acupuncture in humans. *Pain* 1998;75:19–25.

[3] Sjolund B, Terenius L, Erickson M. Increased cerebrospinal fluid levels of endorphins after electro-acupuncture. *Acta Physiol Scand* 1977;100(3):382–384.

[4] Chen HX, Han SJ. All three types of opioid receptors in the spinal cord are important for 2/15, Hz electroacupuncture analgesia. *Eur J Pharmacol* 1992;211:203–210.

[5] Dawidson I, Angmar-Mansson B, Blom M, et al. The influence of sensory stimulation (acupuncture) on the release of neuropeptides in the saliva of healthy subjects. *Life Sci* 1998;63(8):659–674.

[6] Schwartz FA, Andrasik F. *Biofeedback: A Practitioner's Guide.* New York, NY: Guilford; 2003:35.

[7] Gilman AG. *The Pharmacologic Basis of Medical Practice.* New York, NY: Macmillan; 1990.

[8] Pentel P, Jorgensen C, Somerville J. Chelation therapy for the treatment of atherosclerosis. *Minn Med* 1984;67(2):101–103.

[9] Guldager B. EDTA treatment of intermittent claudication: A double-blind, placebo-controlled study. *J Intern Med* 1992;231:261–267.

[10] Reiki. Available at: http://www.holistic.com/Reiki.

[11] Crasilneck HB, Hall JA. *Clinical Hypnosis: Principles and Applications,* 2nd ed. Orlando, Fla: Grune and Stratton; 1985:1,18.

[12] Field T. Massage therapy. *Med Clin North Am* 2002;86(1):163–171.

[13] Smith MJ, Logan AC. Naturopathy. *Med Clin North Am* 2002;86(1):173–184.

[14] National Center for Homeopathy. Available at: http://www.homeopathic.org/.

[15] Woolliscroft JO. Megavitamins: Fact and fancy. *Dis Month* 1983;29(5)1–56.

[16] Chu DA. Tai chi, qi gong and reiki. *Phys Med Rehabil Clin North Am* 2004;15(4):773–781.

[17] Mind/Body Control. Available at: http:// www.holisticonline.com/hol_mindcontrol.htm.

[18] Duyff RL. *American Dietetic Association Complete Food and Nutrition Guide,* 2nd ed. Hoboken, NJ: Wiley; 2002.

[19] Available at: http://www.atkins.com.

[20] Available at: http://www.diet-i.com/diets.htm.

[21] Available at: http://www.diet-i.com/ diets.htm.

[22] Ornish D. *Dr. Dean Ornish's Program for Reversing Heart Disease.* New York, NY: Random House; 1990.

[23] Available at: http://www.diet-i. com/diets.htm.

[24] *The Random House Dictionary of the English Language,* 2nd ed, unabridged. New York, NY: Random House; 1987.

[25] Mind/Body Control. Available at: http://www.holisticonline.com/hol_mindcontrol.htm.

CHAPTER 32

Bioterrorism Preparedness: The Challenge of Disparate Populations

ADAM M. KINGSTON, BA
MARSHA MORIEN, MSBA, FACHE
STEVEN H. HINRICHS, MD

▶ INTRODUCTION

In the wake of recent acts of terrorism and the ongoing war in Iraq, Americans have become aware of the debate regarding the adequacy of the nation's bioterrorism preparedness efforts. Although many Americans have been continually exposed to the potential threats of bioterrorism through television, newspapers, and other public health information efforts, a significant portion of the population remains unprepared. This chapter describes the challenge represented by terrorism, the preparations necessary to reach all components of US society, and the special efforts that are needed to reduce the risk of terrorism within specific populations.

Although much progress has been made, a disparity exists in the ability of federal and state health agencies to effectively communicate the risk of terrorism to specific populations. The problem of disparities in communicating concerns of terrorism to at-risk populations is an especially pressing one. The overall level of concern has been heightened due to the amount of time and effort required to address the shortcomings of the preparedness effort. Immediate efforts must be implemented to educate at-risk populations in order to prevent a potential catastrophe.

▶ POPULATIONS AT RISK

A variety of health concerns in the era of terrorism focus on disparities in the US health information delivery system. The challenge of terrorism highlights and extends the populations that are at risk. According to the National Institutes of Health, health disparities include "differences in the incidence, prevalence, mortality, and burden of diseases and other adverse health conditions that exist among population groups in the United States."[1] The Office of Minority Health (OMH) has identified

African Americans, Hispanic Americans, Asian Americans, Pacific Islanders, and American Indians and Alaska Natives as minority populations subject to health disparities.[2] With regard to bioterrorism, this definition must be modified to include groups of people who are ill-prepared to understand or cope with an act or acts of terrorism. David Satcher has suggested two factors that contribute to the development of health concerns among these populations. First, poverty inherently creates environmental health challenges; cleanliness, diet, and basic living are all adversely affected by poverty and accentuate these problems. Second, the health system itself is heavily impacted by economic factors and services; information may be accessible based on financial standing or ability to pay.[3]

The at-risk population for adverse impact of terrorism includes many more groups than those listed above and is determined by factors beyond economic standing. Populations at risk from the impact of terrorism include the mentally disabled, children, the elderly, and non-English speakers. These groups are largely at risk due to difficulties in comprehension and accessibility, but the mentally challenged may experience a wide range of unique difficulties.

- Of the 14.3 million people older than 15 years of age with a mental disability in 1997, 1.9 million have Alzheimer disease, senility, or dementia; and 3.5 million have a learning disability.[4] These conditions may limit a full understanding of the risk of terrorism, resulting in knowledge disparities that reduce the effectiveness of mitigation strategies. A special effort is needed to address the needs of individuals with these conditions, as well as those of children and the elderly.
- The tragedy in Columbine, Colorado, showed that children are not only exposed to the psychological impact of terrorism but may be victims of the physical violence as well. Effective communication and alerting measures must be in place to reduce the overall impact of terrorism and prevent sim-

ilar events at other schools. If another terrorist act occurs in the United States, preparedness efforts may limit the potential life-long negative impact on children.
- The loss of mental acuity that often accompanies the aging process may prevent the elderly from obtaining or processing vital information concerning preparedness and response.
- Populations that speak English as a second language, or not at all, may find that bilingual publications are not available for their use.

An estimate of the total number of people that may be affected by the difficulty of communicating the risk of bioterrorism can be inferred from the population groups identified in the 2000 census of 281,241,906 US citizens, summarized in Table 32–1. Because many of these groups overlap, it is difficult to determine the total number of people that may not be adequately prepared. However, it is apparent these at-risk populations account for a significant portion of the US populace.

Beyond considerations of age, mental status, and language, several less-conspicuous factors may be involved in creating disparities in bioterrorism preparedness. Discrepancies in access to media in certain communities have been cited as additional factors that contribute to creating at-risk populations, including the known disparity in number of radio stations, television access, community population concentration, and educational level.[6]

► CHALLENGES TO PREPAREDNESS

The specific challenges generated by the problem of terrorism can be categorized into four different areas: language, cultural, medical, and age related. The effective communication of vital health information to at-risk populations is a complicated and delicate process. Beyond the obvious concerns of bodily harm due to terrorist

▶ **TABLE 32-1.** Populations at Risk From the Impact of Terrorism

Group	Population (No.)[a]	Percentage of US Population
African American	34,658,190	12.3
Hispanic	35,505,818	12.5
Asian American	10,242,998	3.6
Pacific Islander	398,835	0.1
American Indian or Alaska Native	2,475,956	0.9
Mentally disabled	14,300,000[4]	5.1
Children[b]	48,068,827[7]	17.1
Elderly[c]	34,992,000[8]	12.4
Non-English speaking[d]	10,986,851[9]	3.9

[a]Statistics are from reference 5 unless otherwise noted.

[b]Determined using 2000 figure for children aged 11 years and younger.

[c]Determined using 2000 figure for people aged 65 years and older.

[d]Determined using 2000 figure for people who describe themselves as speaking English "not well" or "not at all."

acts, public health officials must be conscious of the potential for fear, anxiety, loss of control, and depression that may occur solely in response to the potential for a terrorist event to occur in a community. Even the most competent health-care professional with the proper language skills will encounter great difficulty in conveying routine health information to these select populations. Communication of information about unknown or poorly defined risks raises even greater challenges. Health-care professionals, first responders, mental health specialists, and educators will encounter inconsistencies in health literacy, language skills, and levels of trust.

Language Barriers

The most obvious impediment to effective communication is the potential barrier generated by language or dialect. Although English is the primary language of the US health-care system, it is not the primary language for many constituents of the at-risk population. Among those who use English as a second language, the complexity of medical jargon can easily limit full comprehension. In addition, patients may find

it difficult to appropriately describe their condition, further impeding the process of diagnosis and treatment. An additional complication lies in the numerous dialects and idioms that may emerge from a given language. If an emergency response operator or first responder receives a phone call requesting aid by a caller utilizing popular American idioms or slang, a clear problem may result. An emergency operator who does not recognize these common misuses may misinterpret the information and respond incorrectly. The same problem can be encountered when delivering information to the public: "Simply translating information in a 'technical manner' does not account for differences in beliefs and attitudes. If no 'cultural' translation is done, the information is not tailored to the patient."[10]

Cultural Differences

Cultural differences also factor greatly into the issue of disparity. A lack of cultural sensitivity may be the greatest barrier to administering medical assistance as well as communicating medical concerns. Chachkes and Christ note that "Culturally determined views influence which symptoms are identified, whether they are to be treated and in what way . . . the medicinal preparations and environmental conditions that are deemed necessary for treatment, and they identify the persons who are able to treat and cure."[11] Thus, it may be necessary, in some instances, to modify treatment to satisfy cultural beliefs and customs. Chachkes and Christ describe the case of a 12-year-old Hispanic boy experiencing an acute onset of auditory hallucinations; the physician wished to medicate, but the boy's legal guardian, his grandmother, believed he was possessed and insisted on an exorcism. An acceptable outcome resulted from an agreement whereby the grandmother could perform the exorcism, following which she would sign the consent and bless the medication.[11] In this example, a positive outcome was reached by altering standard medical procedure to satisfy cultural beliefs. The appropriate question relevant to terrorism preparedness is how to incorporate cultural adaptations when confronting the challenge of communicating an unknown risk.

Medical Challenges

Other important medical challenges exist beyond the problem of communication. Although extensive knowledge exists regarding agents of bioterrorism, including their mechanism of causing disease and the proper methods for treatment, a lack of trust in the medical delivery system may reduce its effectiveness. In many respects, health-care agencies have done a poor job of relaying vital information to the general public. For example, certain populations remain more concerned or fearful about bioterrorism than others.[12] Impoverished individuals who must constantly deal with questions of what is available to eat and where to sleep have limited time to focus on terrorism preparedness. These hard-to-reach populations are entitled to understand preparations that must be made and how these pertain to their safety and that of their country.[12] Some observers believe population disparity is a complex problem of

imprecise knowledge and risk assessment. Allan Brandt of Harvard University notes that:

> There has been a lot of imprecision in communicating with the public, in general, about bioterrorism. Erratic or imprecise communications are amplified by disparities in literacy. As a result, the way people understand, perceive, and act on information can be highly variable. It is also a problem of dealing with the unknown. Given the current limits in knowledge of bioterrorism, it is very difficult to make rational risk assessments.[13]

Age-Appropriate Messages

The last challenge presented by terrorism is how to tailor the message appropriately to the age of the audience. A common maxim of modern mass communication is that the language employed should not exceed the eighth-grade level. The National Adult Literacy Survey, conducted in 1992, demonstrated that literacy is directly correlated with level of education. In addition, it showed that blacks and Hispanics, on the average, have lower literacy proficiencies than whites.[14] Thus, tailoring the educational materials to a moderate literacy level, as aforementioned, is essential to maximize the amount of information that can be delivered to the most people. With regard to bioterrorism education, this requires a high degree of preparation and discretion on the part of health agencies. For example, although it may be obvious that an educator cannot deliver the same message to a group of war veterans as to a kindergarten class, it is less clear how to alter the message for high school students. These young Americans need to be educated in preparedness, but extreme caution must be taken to effectively convey the message without creating undue stress. The possibilities for confusion and development of psychological unrest and damage are too great.[13] Without taking age into account through proper censoring and modification, it is possible to create unnecessary fear and anxiety.

Lessons can be derived from an example based on an HIV education program for children. Health educators have the responsibility to assert the dangers of human immunodeficiency virus (HIV) infection and the ways in which it is transmitted. However, overstating the risk and leading children to think that bleeding from a paper cut is a biohazard does not prepare them well, but rather creates pathologies. The same can be said about bioterrorism; minor phobias do not prevent bioterrorism, but they do produce phobic populations.[13]

▶ SOLUTIONS

Much attention has focused on the progressive decline in public health activities over the past decade and the positive impact of new money resulting from bioterrorism preparedness efforts. One of the most important questions facing the United States today is whether the September 11 attacks and anthrax-related deaths have brought public health onto the national agenda in a lasting way. One clear observation from the tragedy of 9/11 is that the attacks exposed an obvious shortcoming in the US public health network—an inability to effectively communicate public health concerns to at-risk populations.

David Satcher states that a strong public health infrastructure is essential to cope with bioterrorism and notes: "That infrastructure has three major components: the public health agencies at the federal, state, and local levels; health care providers, including physicians, pharmacists, and nurses; and the public."[3] Indeed, a strong public health infrastructure is needed to effectively mitigate the current public health dilemma. However, this infrastructure must place greater focus on those populations that are most at risk in terms of preparedness. These at-risk populations fall too easily between the cracks and are left unprepared.

The challenges of communicating public health concerns to the general public have been grossly oversimplified. According to Allan Brandt, "The right message for one community is not necessarily the most effective for another community. It is not just studying the information; it is also studying the populations to whom you are communicating it."[13]

As defined by OMH, "Cultural and linguistic competence is the ability of health care providers and health care organizations to understand and respond effectively to the cultural and linguistic needs brought by patients to the health care encounter."[15] In pursuit of this aim, OMH published the *National Standards for Culturally and Linguistically Appropriate Services (CLAS)* in December 2000. This publication took a monumental step forward in recognizing some limitations of the public health system. Although all the recommendations focus on important issues, items 11 and 12 of the publication are especially relevant to the communication of bioterrorism preparedness efforts to at-risk populations:

> 11. Health care organizations should maintain a current demographic, cultural, and epidemiological profile of the community as well as a needs assessment to accurately plan for and implement services that respond to the cultural and linguistic characteristics of the service area.
>
> 12. Health care organizations should develop participatory, collaborative partnerships with communities and utilize a variety of formal and informal mechanisms to facilitate community and patient/consumer involvement in designing and implementing CLAS-related activities.[15]

These two items address some of the most important problems plaguing bioterrorism preparedness efforts in the United States. Of the 14 recommendations, only 4 were mandated by grant guidelines for all recipients of federal funds; items 11 and 12 were not included but only recommended for adoption.

In 1998, the Office for Domestic Preparedness initiated a grant program for all 50 states, the District of Columbia, the Commonwealth of Puerto Rico, American Samoa, the Commonwealth of Northern Mariana Islands, Guam, and the US Virgin Islands to "enhance the capacity of state and local jurisdictions to prevent, respond to, and recover from incidents of terrorism involving chemical, biological, radiological, nuclear, or explosive (CBRNE) weapons and cyber attacks."[16] Mandatory implementation of items 11 and 12 of CLAS within the grant guidelines would have a significant impact on meeting the threat of bioterrorism.

The level of concern is heightened due to the immediacy of the threat and the time needed to adequately prepare. The process of resolving this dilemma must begin at the highest levels of government. Policy must be written that requires a behavioral change on the part of public health; the problem is that too few agencies are engaged in investigating the causes for our limited ability to connect with specific at-risk populations and developing effective measures to resolve the issues.[16] At the same time that funds are being procured to produce multi-million dollar biocontainment facilities, it is imperative to allocate funds to educate the public about why these facilities exist. It is vital that the opinions of the community be assessed, their leaders consulted, and their customs respected. Consider the current plan to build a biosafety Level-4 laboratory in Roxbury, Massachusetts, where, according to the local media, "some of the most dangerous pathogens on earth will be studied."[17] The proposed laboratory would be built in a crowded neighborhood of nearly 55,000 residents. Residents are currently aligning themselves against the plan, stating there is no way to guarantee their safety despite government claims that the facility will be secure.[17] Ultimately, it appears the laboratory will be built, but the question remains whether the residents will ever again feel safe and provide their critical support to the academic community. Had the need for the laboratory and a risk assessment been appropriately communicated to the community prior to the announcement of the intention to build, the current anxiety might have been minimized or prevented.

Currently, the OMH maintains minority health consultants in each of the 10 regional offices of the Department of Health and Human Services.[2] It is the task of these consultants to establish relationships with state agencies and assist in the establishment of community-oriented minority organizations. This is a good start in addressing the problem; however, the capacity of these individuals and organizations must be dramatically expanded. Ultimately, it is necessary to establish organizations that are capable of reaching everyone in a given community.

This recommendation goes well beyond typical minority groups. One of the biggest challenges will be investigating and implementing the proper method of educating communities. A primary recommendation of this work is that liaisons from the community be incorporated to gather information about the community and establish themselves as the sources of vital health information. In short, people who are trusted within their communities must be identified, and their time compensated for their vital contributions to the health communications network. Marilyn McGary, president of the Urban League of Nebraska, Inc., believes that through existing social agencies, community representatives can be found to work with the community on a day-to-day basis. Because of their standing in the community, a level of trust has already been established to facilitate the sharing of vital information.[12] Using this approach, federal money allocated to bioterrorism preparedness might serve a dual purpose: In addition to bioterrorism preparedness and response, a communications pathway and network would be put in place for all other emergency and hazardous situations. This added benefit could contribute to the future success of all public health activities.

The establishment of a public health communications network is essential to developing the appropriate message for individual communities. Only after surveying the racial, ethnic, and linguistic makeup of a population can this be accomplished. An adequate public health communications network will allow educators to assess the population in order to accurately tailor the message. However, more than the communications network is needed to make the system work; namely, health educators proficient in cross-cultural communication. These persons must know when and how to present the material in a way that respects cultural values, but also how to modify the information when necessary.[18] The message itself must be written in such a way that it does not create a secondary pathology within the target population. Allan Brandt likens this process to considering the side effects of drugs:

> Any educational or communication program without considering the side effects would be like giving someone a serious new medication without thinking about the consequences. Are there unanticipated side effects that we should be monitoring and developing feedback information to assure that even if we have an unanticipated side effect, we can at least address it when it arrives?[13]

In support of the communication pathway, it is necessary to have an inventory of all the resources available to a particular community or population in order to maximize effectiveness and efficiency. The first step is to create state or local databases of epidemiologists, mental health providers, physicians, and other health-care professionals, listing their relevant skills and ethnic backgrounds. Such databases would allow each community to access the proper information and assistance in the most efficient manner possible.

Action plans must be developed for each community based on the premise that an emergency of some type will occur. To effectively prepare each community to face the types of threats that may arise, the action plans must not be ad hoc measures. A drilling process should be implemented, whereby communities can practice the appropriate responses for particular situations. For example, in the Midwest, grade school students are routinely drilled on the proper action to take in the event of a tornado. The same drilling procedure can be modified to apply to other emergencies. This type of practice can reduce the amount of panic and indecision that often accompanies stressful situations. These drills should be routinely evaluated by the appropriate health-care and emergency officials and improved and updated when necessary.

▶ **SUMMARY**

Currently, large inconsistencies exist in the ability of the United States to communicate to its citizens the risks and mitigation strategies concerning bioterrorism. Multiple sources for this problem exist, including the inability of local health-care and social agencies to adequately survey and accommodate the needs of the community. The ongoing threat of bioterrorism has brought this shortcoming to national attention and illustrated these problems. It has been shown that these problems go well beyond typical minority populations to include the mentally disabled, children, the elderly, and persons who speak English as a second language or not at all.

The age of bioterrorism has also created an opportunity for increased visibility and growth in emergency management. In response, the federal government has allocated funds for state use in upgrading public health systems. This re-energizing of the public health infrastructure will ultimately serve a dual purpose because the system will also function in times of hazard and emergency.

A community action plan must be developed and shared with the general populations, allowing adequate consideration and time for community comment. Times of stress and anxiety serve to bring communities together. This bond can ensure the safety of the community when it comes to preparedness for emergencies of all types, including natural disasters. If information is made available and communicated appropriately to the population, then communities will embrace the efforts and prepare themselves appropriately.

▶ REFERENCES

1. National Institutes of Health. *What Are Health Disparities?* Available at: http://healthdisparities.nih.gov/whatare.html.
2. Office of Minority Health. *Protecting the Health of Minority Communities.* Available at: http://www.omhrc.gov/rah/indexnew.htm.
3. Satcher D. David Satcher takes stock [interview by Fitzhugh Mullan]. *Health Aff (Millwood)* 2002; 21(6):154–161.
4. US Census Bureau. *Americans with Disabilities: 1997.* Available at: http://www.census.gov/Press-Release/www/2001/cb01-46.html.
5. US Census Bureau. *Overview of Race and Hispanic Origin: 2000.* Available at: http://www.census.gov/prod/2001pubs/c2kbr01-1.pdf.
6. Boyd Ford V, personal interview, August 23, 2004.
7. US Census Bureau. *Children and the Households They Live In: 2000.* Available at: http://www.census.gov/prod/2004pubs/censr-14.pdf.
8. US Census Bureau. *The United States in International Context: 2000.* Available at: http://www.census.gov/prod/2002pubs/c2kbr01-11.pdf.
9. US Census Bureau. *Language Use and English Speaking Ability: 2000.* Available at: http://www.census.gov/prod/2003pubs/c2kbr-29.pdf.
10. Schaafsma ES, Raynor TD, de Jong-van den Berg LT. Accessing medication information by ethnic minorities: Barriers and possible solutions. *Pharm World Sci* 2003;25(5):185–190.
11. Chachkes E, Christ G. Cross cultural issues in patient education. *Patient Educ Counseling* 1996; 27(1):13–21.
12. McGary M, personal interview, August 30, 2004.
13. Brandt AM, Harvard University History of Science Department, telephone interview, August 24, 2004.
14. National Center for Education Statistics. *Adult Literacy and Education in America.* Available at: http://nces.ed.gov/pubs2001/2001534.pdf.
15. Office of Minority Health. *Assuring Cultural Competence in Health Care: Recommendations for National Standards and an Outcomes-Focused Research Agenda.* Available at: http://www.omhrc.gov/clas/finalpo.htm.
16. US Dept of Homeland Security, Office for Domestic Preparedness. Available at: http://www.ojp.usdoj.gov/odp/grants_goals.htm.
17. Badkhen A. Fear follows plan to build more deadly-disease labs. *San Francisco Chronicle.* August 22, 2004.
18. Kavangh K, Kennedy P. *Promoting Cultural Diversity.* Newbury Park, Calif: Sage; 1992.

CHAPTER 33

The Benefits of Affirmative Action in Higher Education

JORDAN J. COHEN, MD

▶ **INTRODUCTION**

As evident from the latest figures from the US Census Bureau, the United States is undergoing a period of profound demographic change. Despite its historic distinction as a country of significant racial and ethnic diversity, our nation has never before witnessed the astonishing growth in its minority populations that is currently underway. In fact, population trends have reached an unprecedented tipping point, with minority populations increasing in size at a much faster rate than the majority white population. Between 1980 and 2000, the African American population increased by about 28%; the Native American population, by 55%; the Hispanic population, by 122%; and the Asian population, by more than 190%. In comparison, over the same period the country's white population grew by merely 9%. As a result of these trends, demographers anticipate that by 2050, more than half of all US citizens will be members of what are currently minority groups.[1]

These trends pose significant challenges to members of the health professions. In light of changing US demographics, stagnation or reduction in minority representation within the physician workforce will, as detailed below, have several unwelcome consequences for the health of the nation. Despite demographic shifts that are turning the United States into a true mosaic of ethnicities, races, and cultures, the composition of its health-care workforce remains distinctly unrepresentative of the general population. Moreover, the diversity gap between the general population and the health professions seems destined to widen still further in the near future; students from underrepresented minority backgrounds make up barely 11% of current medical school matriculants.[2] (Similarly, minority students comprise comparably small percentages of matriculants in most other health professions schools.)

Clearly, the only way to increase the number of minority physicians is to increase the enrollment of minority students in medical schools. The major obstacle to achieving that goal is the relatively small number of academically prepared students in the pool of medical school applicants. It is for that reason, coupled with the compelling arguments favoring more diversity in the medical profession, that I make the case for the near-term use of affirmative action in medical school admissions.

The compelling arguments favoring more diversity fall into four categories: (1) advancing the cultural competency of all physicians, (2) increasing access to health care for the underserved and addressing health disparities, (3) broadening the research agenda, and (4) ensuring that medical administrators and policy makers are adequately informed about the special needs and expectations of minority populations.

▶ ADVANCING CULTURAL COMPETENCY

Arguably the most compelling reason for increasing the number of minorities among students of the health professions is the need for all health-care providers in our increasingly diverse society to be culturally competent. In light of current demographic trends, failure to educate culturally competent providers will threaten the quality of health care for everyone.

The term *cultural competence* is meant to encompass the knowledge, skills, attitudes, and behaviors required of practitioners to provide optimal health-care services to persons from a wide range of cultural and ethnic backgrounds. Cultural competence—or cultural sensitivity, as it is sometimes called—is an essential component of effective health care; competent providers must have the ability to empathize with patients and accurately elicit and analyze their verbal health accounts. Although the scientific and technical dimensions of medical care are of crucial importance, we know that disease and well-being are influenced by myriad cultural, social, and psychological factors that are beyond the reach of technology.

Health-care professionals armed with the skills of cultural competence are prepared to gauge how and why different belief systems, cultural biases, ethnic origins, family structures, and a host of other culturally determined factors may influence the manner in which individual patients experience illness, adhere to medical advice, and respond to treatment. Moreover, health-care professionals who are mindful of the potential impact of language barriers, religious taboos, unconventional explanatory models of disease, or traditional "alternative" remedies are much more likely to satisfy their patients and to provide superior care.

Preparing health professions students to be culturally competent requires much more than theoretical knowledge. Textbooks and lectures are not enough. Sociologic research shows that true understanding of the "other" can only be acquired through actual exposure to members of different racial, ethnic, and cultural backgrounds. As cited in the Supreme Court case of *Grutter v Bollinger*, studies "confirm that racial diversity and student involvement in activities related to diversity [have] a direct and strong effect on learning and the way students conduct themselves later in life, including disrupting prevailing patterns of racial separation."[3]

Exposure to members of different ethnic, racial, cultural, and socioeconomic groups contributes to the dissolution of stereotypes, which in turn gives future health-care providers the ability to look at patients from an unbiased and culturally savvy perspective. Both minority and nonminority health-care providers must acquire the ability to transcend their own views and backgrounds and develop a sensitivity to and respect for the needs of patients from dissimilar ethnic and racial backgrounds. To acquire these essential clinical skills, health professions students of any background must be immersed in learning environments featuring a critical mass of both minority students and faculty.

One might argue that racial and ethnic concordance between physician and patient provides the best assurance of culturally competent care. And indeed, studies indicate that such concordance often results in greater patient satisfaction and better health outcomes. However, reliance on racial and ethnic concordance to achieve culturally competent care is not only impractical, it is abhorrent in an egalitarian society. All members of a responsible and responsive medical profession should be prepared to meet the needs personally or through proper referral of all those seeking their care.

▶ INCREASING ACCESS FOR THE UNDERSERVED AND ADDRESSING HEALTH DISPARITIES

Another compelling reason for having more diversity among students in the health professions is to improve access to high-quality care for the underserved. Many of the areas in the United States that have a shortage of health-care providers are populated predominantly by ethnic and racial minorities, and abundant data now exist documenting that African American, Hispanic, and Native American physicians are much more likely than white physicians to choose practice sites within these underserved communities.[4] In addition, African American and Hispanic physicians are more likely to provide care to the poor and to those receiving Medicaid.[5] Thus, achieving greater diversity among physicians and health-care professionals generally would help address one of the most refractory problems currently plaguing the US health-care system: unequal access to even basic health care services.

In addition, even among those who do have access to the system, abundant studies document the existence of racial and ethnic disparities in health and health-care services. The eradication of health disparities is one of the prime targets of *Healthy People 2010,* the US Surgeon General's call to arms for tackling the nation's top health priorities.[6]

Increasing the diversity of the health professions workforce is key to solving many of the problems responsible for health disparities in our country. The Institute of Medicine's landmark report, *Unequal Treatment: Confronting Racial and Ethnic Disparities in Health Care,* cited a host of contributing factors residing both within the knowledge, skills, and attitudes of individual health-care providers, and within

the structure and processes of the health-care system.[7] Virtually none of the factors cited can be dealt with effectively until the health professions workforce is adequately populated with individuals from minority backgrounds who can bring their own experiences and values to bear on the policies of health-care institutions and on the norms of behavior characterizing the provider–patient relationship.

▶ BROADENING THE RESEARCH AGENDA

Many of the common diseases and disabilities that continue to plague the United States occur with disproportionate frequency among minority populations. This variance may be particularly striking for problems rooted, as so many are, in social, cultural, and behavioral determinants of health. More research targeted at these problems offers the only real hope of finding solutions. Although funding agencies have a strong influence on the country's research agenda, there is little doubt that the interests of individual investigators also constitute a powerful determinant of the problems that attract attention and the questions posed in grant applications. Similarly, there is little doubt that individual investigators tend to undertake research into problems that they "see" and that interest them. And what normally excites people's interest and curiosity depends to a greater or lesser extent on their personal, cultural, and ethnic backgrounds. It is reasonable to conclude, therefore, that finding timely solutions to health problems that disproportionately affect minorities, even being able to conceptualize what the real problems might actually be, will require a research workforce that is much more racially and ethnically diverse than is currently available. Creating that workforce begins with ensuring a diverse student body and faculty, particularly in MD, PhD, and MPH programs.

The extent to which the needed research will require reasonable participation by patients from minority groups constitutes yet another argument for a more racially and ethnically diverse cadre of investigators. A study in the *Archives of Internal Medicine* found that 8 in 10 African Americans feared they would be used as guinea pigs for medical research. The same study found that African Americans were less likely than whites to trust their physicians to explain fully the risks of participation in research.[8] Yet another study of the attitudes of African Americans toward participation in cancer-related clinical trials found considerable distrust of government-backed medical research, with African American men citing the infamous Tuskegee syphilis experiment as their main source of concern. In agreement with other research, this study's participants also expressed a preference for health-care providers and researchers who "looked like them," an attitude that was found to be an important factor in their willingness to participate in clinical trials.[9]

On two counts, then, (the need to broaden the research agenda and the need to encourage more participation by patients from key population subgroups) the paucity of investigators from underrepresented minority backgrounds constitutes an important barrier to advancing the nation's health.

▶ DIVERSITY IN RELATED WORKFORCES

A fourth reason for seeking more diversity in health professions education is to augment the pool of medically trained executives and policy makers available to assume key management and governmental roles in the health-care system. Providing optimum health-care services to an increasingly more diverse population is bound to pose a difficult management challenge for provider organizations, health-care funders, public and private program managers, as well as local, state, and national governments.

Leaders in many sectors of the US economy are coming to realize that it makes good business sense to have a managerial staff that reflects the racial and ethnic makeup of their respective clientele. As the "clients" of health-care organizations become increasingly more diverse, the availability of a diverse physician workforce from which to recruit leaders and managers who can anticipate the needs and deal effectively with a variety of individuals will be a critical factor in success.

Likewise, policy makers who are trained in one of the health professions and who more accurately reflect the diversity of the US public can have a substantial influence on the future of health-care policy for all Americans. The dearth of such professionals in the current health-care workforce and influential policy-making posts is yet another barrier to the achievement of high-quality health care for all Americans.

▶ THE USE OF AFFIRMATIVE ACTION IN MEDICAL SCHOOL ADMISSIONS

Acknowledging that greater racial and ethnic diversity among medical students is in the public interest, how is it to be achieved? Given the differential influence of race and ethnicity on students' preprofessional educational opportunities and resultant levels of academic achievement, the inescapable reality of contemporary American life is that affirmative action remains an essential tool to achieve that public interest. The simple fact is that relatively few medical school applicants from underrepresented minority backgrounds currently present academic credentials (ie, college grade point averages [GPAs] and scores on the Medical College Admission Test [MCAT]) that are equivalent to those typical of most successful applicants. That being so, to achieve even modest degrees of diversity, admission standards need not be lowered but greater weight must be placed on other equally important indicators of merit when evaluating many underrepresented minority applicants.

Medical school admission committees have proven to be extraordinarily adept at identifying such applicants who, despite their less-impressive numerical academic credentials, evidence the strength of mind and character to succeed in medical school, earn their MD degree, and become productive physicians and scientists. The graduation rate for minority medical students is only slightly lower than that of other students.[10]

Suppose affirmative action did not exist, and medical school admissions committees were obligated to make their admissions decisions without knowledge of their applicants' race and ethnicity. In this hypothetical scenario, admissions committees would, of course, use all other relevant information, that is, GPAs, MCAT scores, and the host of other "nonquantitative" sources used to assess a student's motivation, maturity, dedication, compassion, and the like. Suppose, further, that underrepresented minority applicants, as a group, exhibited these other nonquantitative factors to no greater degree than did majority applicants. Under these circumstances, one could calculate, from the spectrum of GPAs and MCAT scores of the successful nonminority applicants in a given year, the number of underrepresented minority applicants who would have been admitted in the absence of affirmative action and compare that number to what actually transpired. Making this calculation for the cohort of medical schools applicants and matriculants for the class entering medical school in the fall of 2001 revealed that, in the absence of affirmative action, the number of underrepresented minority students admitted that year would have been reduced from 1697 to 513, a level reminiscent of the era in which frankly discriminatory practices severely limited minority access to the medical profession.[11] Few, if any, would now view such a result as just.

▶ THE SUPREME COURT SPEAKS: DIVERSITY IS A COMPELLING INTEREST

Persuaded that diversity in higher education is a compelling public interest, the Supreme Court, in *Grutter v Bollinger,* upheld the use of nar-rowly tailored affirmative action programs in admissions to postsecondary institutions. Thus, except where prohibited by state law, the Court affirmed its 1978 decision in *Bakke,* which gave medical schools a green light to take race and ethnicity into account in their holistic evaluation of applicants.[12]

Fundamental to the Court's reasoning was a willingness to defer to a school's judgment that adequate diversity in higher education was essential because of the benefits that flow to the education of all students. But as welcome as the Court's deference to educators' judgment was, the written opinion in *Grutter* is laced with cautionary statements that schools must heed to minimize the likelihood of legal challenge to their admissions processes. For example, schools are admonished to clarify why diversity is important to their institutions, to consider whether alternatives to affirmative action exist that might suffice to achieve the desired diversity, and to conduct periodic assessments to confirm the continued need for race- and ethnicity-conscious admissions procedures.[13] Nevertheless, the Court's ruling in *Grutter* has removed the cloud of uncertainty about the legality of affirmative action in higher education admissions and should result in a significant and welcome increase in the participation of underrepresented minorities in all of the health professions.

▶ SUMMARY AND RECOMMENDATIONS

The inexorable transformation of the United States into a truly multicultural, multiracial society—a society without an identifiable majority—has huge implications for the health professions, and particularly for the medical profession. Abundant evidence exists that the paucity of underrepresented minorities among physicians precludes attainment of appropriate cultural competence within the profession, limits access to quality health-care services, weakens efforts to eliminate health disparities, stifles needed research to address pressing health problems, and denies health administrators and policy makers the expertise needed to improve the performance of individual institutions and the system as a whole.

The only short-term means for increasing racial and ethnic diversity in medicine is the continued use of affirmative action in medical school admissions. Fortunately, the Supreme Court, in *Grutter v Bollinger,* has upheld the legitimacy of narrowly tailored affirmative action programs to achieve the public's compelling interest in the educational benefits that flow from a diverse student body.

Justice O'Connor, writing for the majority in *Grutter,* expressed her hope that in 25 years affirmative action in higher education will no longer be needed. Although devoutly to be desired, that hopeful vision will become a reality only if national priorities begin to reflect the enormous amount of work required to achieve it. Affirmative action will no longer be needed when the academic credentials of applicants to competitive higher education institutions no longer differ along racial and ethnic lines. For that to happen, America's primary and secondary education systems must be in a position to provide students from all racial and ethnic backgrounds with equivalent educational opportunities and encouragement.

Only then can race-blind higher education admissions be relied on to achieve the classroom diversity now clearly established as a compelling public interest. And only then will medicine and the other health professions be able to rely on the full participation of individuals from all sectors of society to fulfill its moral obligation: delivering quality health care to everyone.

▶ REFERENCES

1. US Census, *Statistical Abstract of the United States: 2001.* Washington, DC: US Census Bureau; 2001:17, Table 15.

2. Association of American Medical Colleges Data Warehouse. Applicant Matriculant File; 2004.

3. Regents of the University of Michigan: Expert Report of Patricia Gurin for *Gratz et al v Bollinger et al,* No. 97-75321, and *Grutter et al v Bollinger et al,* No. 97-75928, 2004. Available at: http://www.umich.edu/~urel/admissions/legal/expert/gurintoc.html.

4. Kington R, Tisnado D, Carlisle D. Increasing racial and ethnic diversity among physicians: An intervention to address health disparities. In: Smedley BD, Stith AY, Colburn L, et al, eds. *The Right Thing to Do; The Smart Thing to Do: Increasing Diversity in the Health Professions.* Washington, DC: Institute of Medicine, National Academies Press; 2001:64–68.

5. Cantor JC, Miles EL, Baker LC, et al. Physician service to the underserved: Implications for affirmative action in medical education. *Inquiry* 1996; 33(2):167–180.

6. US Dept of Health and Human Services. *Healthy People 2010: Understanding and Improving Health,* 2nd ed. Washington, DC: US Government Printing Office; November 2000.

7. Smedley B, Stith A, Nelson A, eds. *Unequal Treatment: Confronting Racial and Ethnic Disparities in Health Care.* Washington, DC: Committee on Understanding and Eliminating Racial and Ethnic Disparities in Health Care, Board on Health Sciences Policy, Institute of Medicine, National Academy Press; 2002.

8. Corbie-Smith G, Thomas SB, St George DM. Distrust, race, and research. *Arch Intern Med* 2002; 162(21):2458–2463.

9. Stark N, Paskett E, Bell R, et al. Increasing participation of minorities in cancer clinical trials: Summary of the "Moving Beyond the Barriers" Conference in North Carolina. *J Natl Med Assoc* 2002;94(1):31–39.

10. *Minority Students in Medical Education: Facts and Figures,* Vols VII–XII. Washington, DC: Association of American Medical Colleges; 1993–2002.

11. Wightman LF. The threat to diversity in legal education: An empirical analysis of the consequences of abandoning race as a factor in law school admissions decisions. *N Y Univ Law Rev* 1997:1–3.

12. *Regents of the University of California v Bakke,* 429 US 953 (1978).

13. *Grutter v. Bollinger.* See Chap. 23, Ref. 59 on p. 426 of this text.

CHAPTER 34

The Role of Government in Minority Health: A Surgeon General's Perspective

DAVID SATCHER, MD, PhD

▶ INTRODUCTION

From the founding of the United States to the present day, the right to good health and well-being has been a basic tenet the nation holds dear. The US Constitution, with its affirmation of the right to "life, liberty, and the pursuit of happiness," implies the right to the pursuit of good health. The best example in modern history of this nation's commitment to the right to good health is the role the government plays at the federal, state, and local levels as it seeks to provide increased protection of citizens from the spread of infectious diseases. I was privileged to spend nearly 9 years serving the American people in leadership in the Public Health Service—5 years as director of the Centers for Disease Control and Prevention (CDC) and 4 years as Surgeon General of the United States, 3 of which I concurrently served as Assistant Secretary for Health. Today I am more convinced than ever of the need for government to remain vigilant in protecting the health of its citizens.

Attitudes toward governmental services vary widely from person to person. I often illustrate

this by relating what some consider to be the two biggest lies in history. The first one is, "The check is in the mail." The second one is, "We are from the government and we're here to help." However, I agree with those who believe that government is perhaps the only institution that can be representative of and responsible to all the people. Implied in this statement is the belief that, regardless of race, creed, color, gender, religion, social standing, or sexual preference, the US government has a responsibility to protect the health of all of its citizens. Throughout my tenure in government, whether it was as director of the CDC, Surgeon General of the United States, or Assistant Secretary for Health, this was a responsibility I took very seriously.

When I began as director of the CDC in 1993, one area we focused on closely was immunization rates, believing that government had the responsibility to ensure that all of its citizens were immunized. That year, just over 50% of US children were being immunized by 2 years of age, and the rates for African American, Hispanic, and American Indian children were much lower than those for their majority

547

counterparts. There were also striking variations in immunization rates in certain regions of the country. For example, immunization rates for children up to age 2 in the state of Vermont, which has a population that is over 95% white, approached 70%; but in the city of Detroit, which is predominately African American, the immunization rate for children in the same age group was less than 30%. Disparities also existed in adult immunization rates, despite the fact that Medicare covered immunizations. Concern over these and the many other examples of health disparities, coupled with the government's responsibility to promote the health of all of its citizens, led me to adopt a new approach for eliminating disparities. In the year 2000, we made the task of eliminating health disparities among different racial and ethnic groups one of the two goals of *Healthy People 2010,* the nation's health plan for the decade leading up to 2010.[1]

In this chapter, I explore the critical role government plays in social programs aimed at improving health and health outcomes for minority groups and the underserved. One thing is clear: the US government continues to play a significant role in protecting and enhancing the health of citizens at the local, state, and federal levels. In fact, over 50% of the current expenditures for health care in the United States are made by the government or the public sector.[2] This level of expenditure by the government provides significant leverage in the nature of health services delivered. Beyond that, the interaction between public and private sectors increasingly is shaping the nature of health expenditures and services.

▶ A BRIEF HISTORY OF THE GOVERNMENT'S ROLE IN PUBLIC HEALTH AND HEALTH CARE

There is a long history of governmental involvement in the nation's health. In 1798, President John Adams signed the Act of Congress that gave rise to the Marine Hospital Service. This service grew out of a concern for the health of merchant seamen, who often became ill or disabled during their voyages at sea. In many cases, the diseases they contracted were contagious and could spread throughout the communities to which they returned. One of the better-known examples occurred with the yellow fever epidemic of 1793 in Philadelphia. It is also one of the best-documented events in public health history. It was so notable that, in 1998, the Public Health Service, which grew out of the Marine Hospital Service, revisited the Philadelphia sites hardest hit by the epidemic as part of its bicentennial commemoration.[3]

In its early years, the Marine Hospital Service consisted of several hospitals located near ports where merchant seamen embarked and disembarked. In 1871, out of concern for controlling the spread of major infectious diseases, including yellow fever, tuberculosis, and smallpox, Dr John Maynard Woodworth was appointed as the nation's first Supervising Surgeon. In 1873 his title became Surgeon General. His responsibility was to coordinate a national response to this threat and provide leadership for the Marine Hospital Service. He began by appointing a corps of physicians to assist him, which he assigned to the various marine hospitals. In 1889, this corps of physicians officially became known as the Commissioned Corps, which consists today of 6000 health professionals of various training. As responsibilities for the Marine Hospital Service grew in scope and complexity, its name was changed in 1912 to the Public Health Service and its oversight assigned to the Surgeon General.[3]

In 1953, the Department of Health, Education and Welfare (DHEW) was established under President Dwight D. Eisenhower and a Secretary appointed to oversee it. The Public Health Service became a part of DHEW and reported to the Secretary directly or to the Assistant Secretary for Health, although for many years the Surgeon General retained all of his authority. In 1979, the Department of Education Organization Act was signed into law, which provided for a separate Department of Education. This resulted in a name change from the Department of Health, Education and Welfare to the Department of Health and Human Services (DHHS). In 1995, the Social Security Administration was split off to became a separate agency. This time the department's name did not change because it continued to be responsible for services to the elderly and to children.[3]

The government's role in health and health care, in part, is defined by the various DHHS agencies. Figure 34–1 shows how the department is organized and defines its role in areas such as research, prevention, quality oversight,

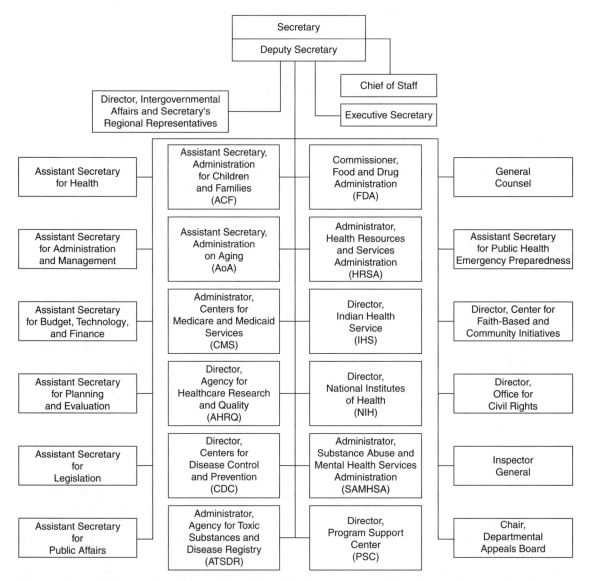

Figure 34–1. Organizational structure of the US Department of Health and Human Services.

regulation, and health care for the poor and elderly.

▶ MAJOR GOVERNMENTAL AGENCIES INVOLVED IN MINORITY HEALTH

The major governmental programs dealing with the health and health care of the American people are centralized within DHHS. By far, the Centers for Medicare and Medicaid Services (CMS) (formerly the Healthcare Financing Administration or HCFA) incurs the largest governmental expenditures to support health care for the elderly through Medicare and health care for the poor through Medicaid. Although Medicare is a federal program funded by a trust established though payroll taxes, Medicaid is jointly funded by federal and state governments based on a formula involving proportional contributions that vary from state to state. Participation among African Americans and other minorities in Medicare is fairly proportionate to their representation in the overall population, but the same is not true for Medicaid. Minorities are generally over represented in Medicaid programs, due to their higher rate of poverty when compared with the majority population. Recent Medicare reform legislation expanded Medicare to include prescription drug coverage for the elderly through a complex formula that is beyond the scope of this discussion. This is the first time since the establishment of Medicare in 1965 that such a major reform has taken place. Dually eligible persons covered under both Medicare and Medicaid because of their age and low-income status will receive prescription drug coverage through the Medicare Prescription Drug Benefit instead of Medicaid. It is not yet clear how this will affect the ability of these individuals to access drugs compared with the present coverage through Medicaid.[4]

Other DHHS programs influencing the care of minorities are funded through the Health Resources and Services Administration (HRSA). One of HRSA's most significant roles is the funding of community health centers, which provide health care in underserved communities. HRSA also funds the National Health Service Corps in an effort to increase the representation of physicians and other health professionals in underserved communities, and it supports the funding of medical education for minority groups. In addition, HRSA funds loan forgiveness programs and other strategies aimed at increasing the representation of minorities in the health professions, tying it to a commitment to underserved communities.[5]

The Indian Health Service (IHS) provides health care to Native Americans on reservations through contractual arrangements with tribal governments. A major challenge confronting this arrangement is delivery of health-care services. Today more than half the Native American population lives outside of the reservations in primarily urban communities, making them ineligible for IHS coverage. The IHS has in recent years received funding from the CDC and the National Institutes of Health (NIH) to implement programs for the prevention, early detection, and treatment of diabetes, a disease that disproportionately affects the Native American population. These programs are developing innovative strategies aimed at preventing the onset of type 2 diabetes, as well as detecting the disease early in its course to prevent complications such as end-stage renal disease.[6]

As the nation's prevention agency, the CDC targets many of its programs to minority communities, where health problems have a disproportionate impact. For example, in 1993 when I began as director of the CDC, we set a goal of increasing childhood immunization rates from just over 50% to 75% by 1996. Because low-income minority communities tended to have the lowest immunization rates for children 2 years of age and under, we focused a great deal of energy on them. Among other things we partnered with such organizations as the Congress of National Black Churches, the Women, Infants and Children Program (WIC), and other established programs that were well positioned to reach low-income communities. Perhaps one of the best examples of CDC programs targeted to minority communities is the Racial and Ethnic Approaches to Community Health (REACH) program, which was conceived in 1998 as part of the federal initiative to eliminate disparities in health. To date more than 40 communities have been funded through this program to develop innovative approaches for reducing and ultimately eliminating disparities in health.[7]

Within the US government is the largest research institution in the world: the National Institutes of Health (NIH). This is the agency through which the government funds most biomedical research. During a 5-year period from 1997 through 2002, Congress doubled the NIH budget from $13 billion to $27 billion, further strengthening its ability to influence research. There has been concern that not enough NIH-funded research has targeted disparities in health that affect minority communities. In January 1999, the Institute of Medicine (IOM) released a report[8] that looked at disparities in research relative to cancer. This report demonstrated that the level of NIH research funding that would influence cancer rates in minorities was, in fact, inadequate.[8] As a result, in 2000 Congress passed legislation establishing the National Center on Minority Health and Health Disparities (NCMHD) at NIH. This center not only makes grants for research geared toward the reduction and ultimately the elimination of disparities but also works with the other NIH institutes to support the targeting of research funding to problems that disproportionately affect minorities. For a 1-year period, from 2002 through 2003, all NIH institutes underwent a strategic planning process to define how they would work to better target their resources toward the elimination of health disparities. This plan represents a major step forward in NIH's efforts to focus on the elimination of disparities in health.[9]

Using funding from Congress and through DHHS, the IOM completed and released a report in 2002 entitled, *Unequal Treatment: Confronting Racial and Ethnic Disparities in Healthcare*.[10] This report documented dispari-

ties in the quality of health care received by minorities in the United States. These disparities persisted even when studies controlled for differences in socioeconomic status, insurance coverage, and the nature of the complaints with which patients presented.[10] The major DHHS agency concerned with the quality of health care is the Agency for Healthcare Research and Quality (AHRQ). AHRQ has now funded several Centers of Excellence in health-care quality research or disparities. As part of the national effort to eliminate disparities, in 1999 the agency was also mandated by Congress to submit an annual report tracking health disparities, entitled the *National Healthcare Disparities Report*.[11] The 2004 report on the quality of care and disparities was met with much concern by members of Congress as well as by persons in the private sector. Representative Henry Waxman (D-CA), members of the Congressional Black Caucus, and others expressed concern that the report lacked a sense of urgency when it came to the elimination of disparities and significantly downplayed the magnitude of the problem and the nature of the concern. A major concern centered on the danger of losing momentum and a sense of urgency and importance regarding the nation's efforts to confront and eliminate disparities.

▶ THE NATION'S HEALTH PLAN: HEALTHY PEOPLE 2010

In 1979, Surgeon General Julius Richmond, while also serving as Assistant Secretary for Health, issued a report on health promotion and disease prevention in the United States.[12] His report led to the beginning of the strategy of planning for the health of the American people by issuing goals and objectives for each decade and monitoring progress toward them. The nation is now in its third decade of the Healthy People initiative, as it works toward the goals of Healthy People 2010. In my role as Assistant Secretary for Health and Surgeon General, I oversaw the development of the 2010 plan, which hinges on two goals: (1) increasing the quality and years of healthy life, and (2) eliminating disparities in health among different racial and ethnic groups.

Supporting Healthy People 2010's two goals are 467 objectives. The majority are measurable and can therefore be used to monitor the nation's progress throughout the decade. Several objectives are not measurable and are labeled "developmental" because they lack the baseline information necessary to track and monitor progress.

Perhaps no Healthy People goal has received as much attention and targeted support as the goal of eliminating disparities in health. This goal has sparked a spirit of rejuvenation in public health, as both the public and private sectors have become engaged in achieving it. As stated earlier, Congress acted to create the NCMHD at NIH, and it has begun to fund Centers of Excellence for the elimination of disparities. The NCMHD is also working with other institutes at NIH on the development of their strategic plans and targeting their resources to elimination of health disparities. NIH obviously must be a major player if the nation is to be successful with this goal of Healthy People 2010. In addition to funding communities through its REACH program to develop models for the elimination of disparities in health, CDC also plays a major role in health promotion and disease prevention, especially in dealing with the nation's epidemic of overweight and obesity. This epidemic disproportionately affects African American and Hispanic women and children.

When Healthy People 2010 was launched in 2000, it was also the first time any Healthy People plan included leading health indicators (LHIs). With assistance from the IOM, 10 LHIs were defined, which are geared toward helping communities target their efforts as they become involved in working to reach the goals of Healthy People 2010. One or two measurable objectives are associated with each LHI. The indicators can be grouped into three categories: (1) health system, (2) environment and environmental quality, and (3) lifestyle. Included in the health system category are access to quality health care, access to mental health care, and access to immunizations. Two indicators are included under the category of environment and environmental quality: injury and violence prevention, and the enhancement of environmental quality as it affects individuals physically, socially, and spiritually. Included under the lifestyle indicators are physical activity, overweight and obesity, tobacco use, substance abuse, and responsible sexual behavior.

These LHIs, in and of themselves, represent an opportunity for better communicating to the American people the goals of Healthy People 2010 and the strategies that must be implemented to reach the goal of eliminating disparities in health. For example, although the lifestyle indicators focus attention on individual responsibility for being physically active and eating right, it is also clear there are major community responsibilities for providing access to healthy lifestyles. If, for example, communities do not provide safe places for people to walk or engage in physical activities or if there are no parks in the neighborhoods, the community is not living up to its responsibility for promoting healthy lifestyles. Likewise, if schools do not require physical education for all students from kindergarten through grade 12, then they are not living up to their responsibility to promote healthy lifestyles. It is clear from both examples that minorities will be disproportionately affected, because they are more likely to live in urban areas where there are fewer parks, trails, and safe areas to be physically active, and children in minority groups are most likely to reside in communities that lack the resources to support physical activities in their schools.

Another major barrier to eliminating disparities in health is the US health-care system itself—a system that excludes over 43 million uninsured people, including 36% of Hispanics and over 25% of African Americans.[13] Likewise, inadequate emphasis on health promotion and disease prevention also has a major impact on the health of minorities. At present, less than 3% of the national health budget is spent on population-based prevention, and those who suffer most from this neglect are clearly minorities. Another major concern with the health system is the underrepresentation of minorities in the health professions, which leads to other problems, including distrust and the inability of the system to relate to different cultures. Whereas underrepresented minorities make up 25%–30% of the US population, they constitute only 10% of health-care professionals.[14] Unfortunately, the future does not look bright, given that government programs to correct this underrepresentation have been losing support as challenges to affirmative action continue to mount. The importance of increasing the number of minorities in the health professions cannot be overstated because of the added benefits they bring to the system overall. It is clear that minority health professionals are more likely to care for other minorities, more likely to practice in underserved communities, and more likely to accept patients on Medicaid. These advances do not just benefit people in minority groups, they benefit the nation's health system as a whole.

Finally, the role of government in programs to improve minority health can be viewed from the perspective of the functions of public health. In a landmark report released in 1988, the IOM defined the following three functions of public health: assessment, assurance, and policy development. In carrying out these functions, the IOM declared that public health was in disarray.[15] But it also noted it was not too late for government to get it right. Nowhere is that challenge and opportunity more clear than in the Healthy People 2010 goal of eliminating disparities in health among different racial and ethnic groups.

In the area of *assessment,* we look to governmental programs—especially the CDC's National Center for Health Statistics (NCHS)—to define the health status of minorities as a baseline for setting measurable objectives and to monitor progress in the reduction and ultimate elimination of disparities in health. For example, in 1999, the infant mortality rate for white infants was 5.8 per 1000; for black infants, it

was 14 per 1000 births, a mortality rate that is 2.4 times higher.[16]

As we implement programs in communities throughout the country to reduce disparities in health, we look to data from NCHS to measure the ultimate impact on this national figure. This function of assessment also applies to areas such as cardiovascular disease, cancer, diabetes, human immunodeficiency virus (HIV) infection, and acquired immunodeficiency syndrome (AIDS).

The role of government does not end with assessment. The second role of public health as defined by the IOM was that of *assurance.* The assurance of access to basic health services such as immunizations, prenatal care, and emergency medical care has often defined public health for many people. For the millions of Americans who are uninsured and underinsured, public hospitals, community health centers, and Medicaid have been critical elements of public health assurance.

Although African Americans and Hispanics in the United States comprise about 25% of the population, they account for over 50% of the uninsured. When asked if they have a personal physician or health-care provider, over one third of African Americans and almost half of Hispanics say they do not.[17]

Too often public health programs, such as public hospitals and Medicaid, are the first to be cut when there are budgeting problems at the state level. Yet it is clear that without reasonable access to care, minorities will always lag behind in health status. Disparities in health cannot be eliminated without governmental assurance of access to care.

In great part, the role of *assurance* includes the assurance of a diverse health professional workforce. If health professionals do not speak the language of patients or understand their culture, then access is not a reality for those patients. Studies also show that minority health professionals are more likely to care for minorities, more likely to practice in underserved communities, and more likely to accept Medicaid for payment. Thus, the continued underrepresentation of minorities in the health professions is also a failure of assurance on the part of the government. HRSA programs, such as the National Health Service Corp, which tie scholarships or loan repayment for medical or dental education to a period of service in underserved communities, enhance access to care and represent the public health function of assurance.[5]

Central to all functions of government or public health is policy development. Public health generally conducts or supports research needed to aid policy development. It also communicates information in such a way as to improve the understanding of policy makers and their constituents about the need for policy, the effectiveness of existing policy, and the indications for new policies. This can be illustrated by considering the points of attack for the elimination of disparities in health. These points of attack include access to quality health care, environmental quality, lifestyle enhancement, and research to identify cases and interventions that might be effective.

At present, the United States stands alone among industrialized countries in not providing universal access to health care. As previously discussed, this lack of access disproportionately affects minorities. In 2000, the annual report of the World Health Organization (WHO)[18] ranked the US health system below 36 other member nations, despite the fact that the United States spends more money overall, more per capita, and a greater percentage of its gross national product on health care than virtually any other country in the world. The WHO report pointed to two major weaknesses in the US health system: the lack of universal access, as indicated by the fact that so many people are excluded from the health system, and the lack of balance in the system, as reflected in the fact that over 90% of US health-care expenditures are for treating diseases and their complications, many of which are preventable. At the same time, the United States spent just 2% of its health budget on population-based prevention.[18]

The policy changes necessary to assure universal access to care and a more balanced health system are critical to achieve the goal of eliminating disparities in health among the different racial and ethnic groups that comprise the population of the United States and to ensure that the protections of the US Constitution extend equally to all of its citizens.

▶ REFERENCES

1. US Dept of Health and Human Services. *Healthy People 2010: Understanding and Improving Health,* 2nd ed. Washington, DC: US Government Printing Office; November 2000.
2. Fox DM, Fronstin P. Public spending for health care approaches 60 percent. *Health Aff (Millwood)* 2000;19(2):271–274.
3. Mullan F. *Plagues and Politics: The Story of the United States Public Health Service.* New York, NY: Basic Books; 1989.
4. Altman DE. The new Medicare prescription-drug legislation. *N Engl J Med* 2004;350(1):9–10.
5. US Dept of Health and Human Services. *Health Resources and Services Administration Annual Report FY 2002.* Washington, DC: USDHHS; 2002. Available at: http://www.hrsa.gov/annualreport/part6.htm#t4
6. National Diabetes Information Clearinghouse. *Diabetes in American Indians and Alaska Natives.* NIH Publication No. 02-4567. Bethesda, Md: National Institute of Diabetes and Digestive and Kidney Disease (NIDDK); May 2002. Available at: http://diabetes.niddk.nih.gov/dm/pubs/americanindian.
7. Centers for Disease Control and Prevention. *Racial and Ethnic Approaches to Community Health (REACH 2010); Program in Brief.* Atlanta, Ga: CDC; January 2004. Available at: http://www.cdc.gov/programs.health06.htm
8. *The Unequal Burden of Cancer: An Assessment of NIH Research and Programs for Ethnic Minorities and the Medically Undeserved.* Washington, DC: National Academy Press; 1999.
9. US Public Law 106-525. Minority Health and Health Disparities Research and Education Act. Washington, DC; November 2000.

10. Institute of Medicine, Board on Health Sciences Policy. *Unequal Treatment: Confronting Racial and Ethnic Disparities in Healthcare.* Washington, DC: National Academy Press; 2003: 764 p.

11. US Dept of Health and Human Services, Agency for Healthcare Research and Quality. *National Healthcare Disparities Report Fact Sheet.* Washington, DC: USDHHS. Available at http://www.ahrq.gov/news/nhdrfact.htm.

12. US Dept of Health and Human Services. *Healthy People: The Surgeon General's Report on Health Promotion and Disease Prevention.* Washington, DC: USDHHS; 1979.

13. Institute of Medicine, Board of Health Care Services, Committee on the Consequences of Uninsurance. *Insuring America's Health: Principles and Recommendations.* Washington, DC: National Academy Press; 2004.

14. AAMC Washington Highlights. Available at: http://www.aamc.org/advocacy/library/washhigh/2001/01oct05/_6.html.

15. Institute of Medicine, Committee for the Study of the Future of Public Health. *The Future of Public Health.* Washington, DC: National Academy Press; 1988:1.

16. National Center for Health Statistics. Infant Mortality Rates Vary by Race and Ethnicity. *National Center for Health Statistics Fact Sheets 1999.* Atlanta, Ga: Centers for Disease Control and Prevention; 1999. Available at: http://www.cdc.gov/nchs/pressroom/99facts/infmort.htm.

17. Collins SR, Doty M, Davis K, et al. *The Affordability Crisis in U.S. Healthcare: Findings from the Commonwealth Fund Biennial Health Survey.* Commonwealth Fund Report; 2004:9.

18. World Health Organization. *The World Health Report 2000 Health Systems: Improving Performance.* Geneva, Switzerland: WHO; 2000:155, tables 5–10.

Appendix

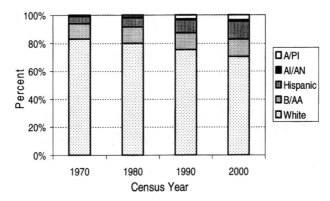

Figure A–1. US population by race or Ethnicity, 1970–2000. (A/PI, Asian or Pacific Islander; AI/AN, American Indian or Alaska Native; B/AA, black or African American.) (*Source: US Census Bureau, 2002.*)

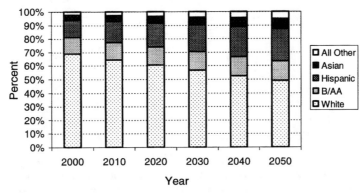

Figure A–2. Projected US population by race or ethnicity, 2000–2050. (B/AA, black or African American.) (*Source: US Census Bureau, 2002.*)

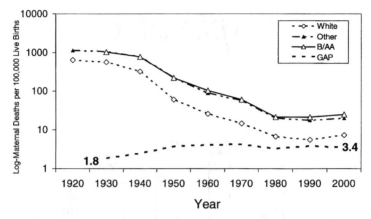

Figure A–3. Maternal mortality rates per 100,000 live births (logarithmic scale) by race, and the gap in maternal mortality rates between blacks or African Americans and whites, United States, 1920–2000. (B/AA, black or African American.) (*Source: National Center for Health Statistics, 2003.*)

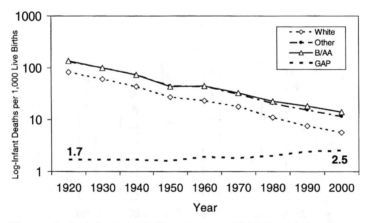

Figure A–4. Infant mortality rates per 1000 live births (logarithmic scale) by race, and the gap in infant mortality rates between blacks or African Americans and whites, United States, 1920–2000. (B/AA, black or African American.) (*Source: National Center for Health Statistics, 2003.*)

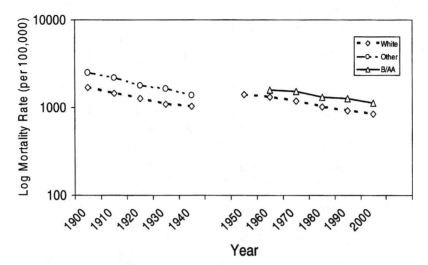

Figure A–5. Mortality rates by race, United States, 1900–1940 (not age-adjusted, whites and others) and 1950–2000 (age-adjusted, whites and blacks or African Americans). (B/AA, black or African American.) (*Source: National Center for Health Statistics, 2003.*)

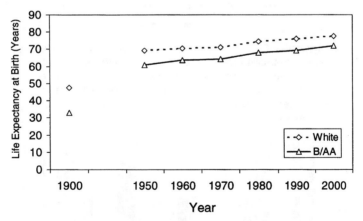

Figure A–6. Life expectancy at birth by race, United States 1900 and 1950–2000. (B/AA, black or African American.) (*Source: US Census Bureau, 2002.*)

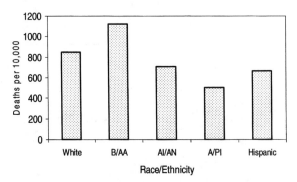

Figure A–7. Age-adjusted mortality rates per 10,000 people by race or ethnicity, United States, 2000 (A/PI, Asian or Pacific Islander; AI/AN, American Indian or Alaska Native; B/AA, black or African American.) (*Source: National Center for Health Statistics, 2003.*)

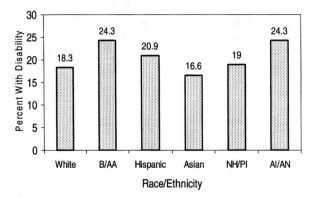

Figure A–8. Percent of people 5 years and older with a disability by race or ethnicity, United States, 2000. (AI/AN, American Indian or Alaska Native; B/AA, black or African American; NH/PI, Native Hawaiian or other Pacific Islander.) (*Source: US Census Bureau, 2003.*)

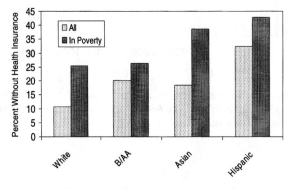

Figure A–9. Percent of people without health insurance by race or ethnicity and poverty status, United States 2002. (B/AA, black or African American.) (*Source: US Census Bureau, 2003.*)

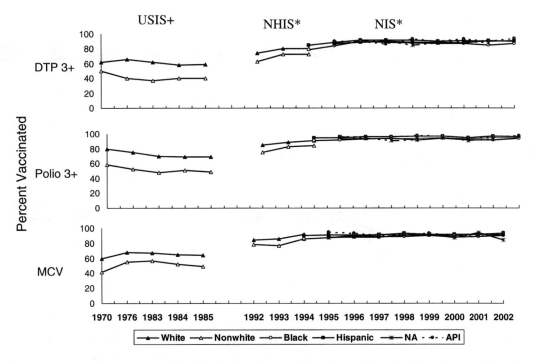

Figure A–10. Vaccination percentages.

USIS+ – United States Immunization Survey, 1-4 years of age. **NHIS*** – National Health Interview Survey, 19-35 months of age. **NIS*** -- National Immunization Survey, 19-35 months of age **MCV** -- a measles containing vaccine. **DTP3+** – 3 or more doses of ditphtheria and tetanus toxiods and pertussis vaccine. **Polio 3+** – 3 or more doses of polio vaccine. **NA**- Native American. **API** – Asian/Pacific Islander.

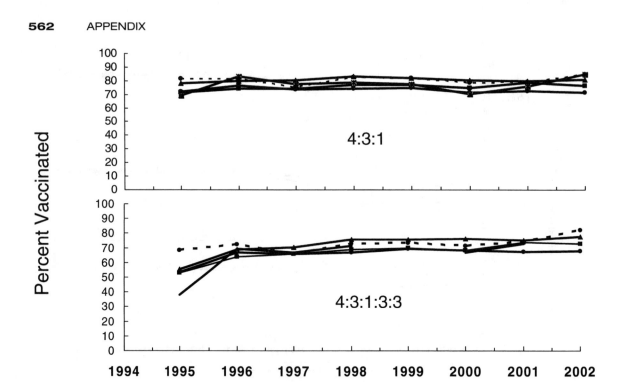

4:3:1 -- 4+ doses of DTP, 3+ doses polio vaccine, and 1 measles containing vaccine.
4:3:1:3:3 – 4+ doses of DTP, 3+ doses polio vaccine, 1 measles containing vaccine, 3 doses of Hib vaccine, and 3 doses of Hepatitis B vaccine.
NA. American Indian/Alaska Native. API – Asian /Pacific Islander.

Figure A–11. Vaccination doses.

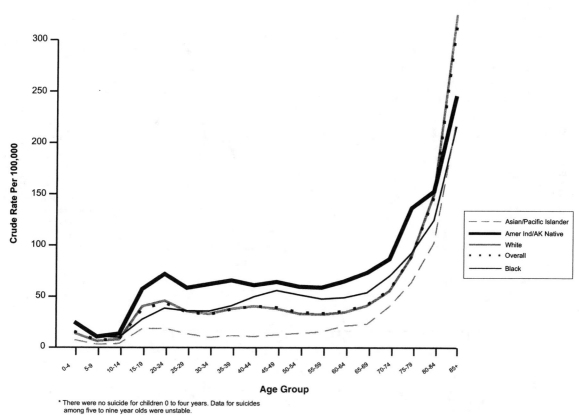

* There were no suicide for children 0 to four years. Data for suicides
  among five to nine year olds were unstable.

Figure A–12. All unintentional injury-related deaths, United States, 1990–1998. (Amer Ind/AK Native = American Indian or Alaska Native.)

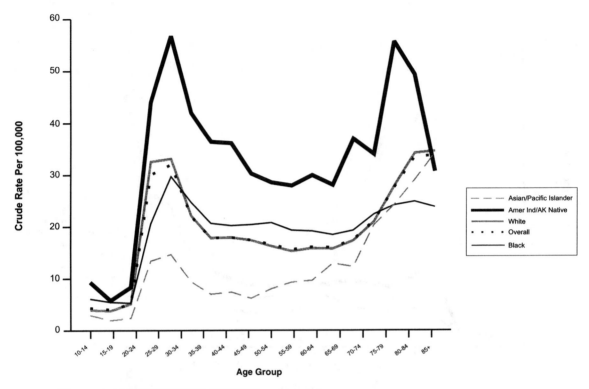

Figure A–13. All motor vehicle injury-related deaths, United States, 1990–1998. (Amer Ind/AK Native = American Indian or Alaska Native.)

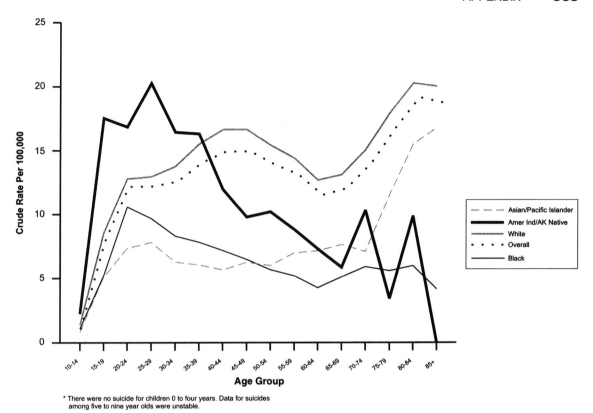

* There were no suicide for children 0 to four years. Data for suicides
among five to nine year olds were unstable.

Figure A–14. All suicide deaths, United States, 1990–1998. (Amer Ind/AK Native = American Indian
or Alaska Native.)

Index

Page numbers followed by italic *f* or *t* denote figures or tables, respectively.